Electric Fields of the Brain

Electric Fields of the Brain

The Neurophysics of EEG

Second Edition

Paul L. Nunez
Emeritus Professor of Biomedical Engineering
Tulane University

Ramesh Srinivasan
Associate Professor of Cognitive Science
University of California at Irvine

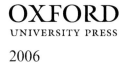

OXFORD

UNIVERSITY PRESS

2006

OXFORD

UNIVERSITY PRESS

Oxford University Press, Inc., publishes works that further
Oxford University's objective of excellence
in research, scholarship, and education.

Oxford New York
Auckland Cape Town Dar es Salaam Hong Kong Karachi
Kuala Lumpur Madrid Melbourne Mexico City Nairobi
New Delhi Shanghai Taipei Toronto

With offices in
Argentina Austria Brazil Chile Czech Republic France Greece
Guatemala Hungary Italy Japan Poland Portugal Singapore
South Korea Switzerland Thailand Turkey Ukraine Vietnam

Published by Oxford University Press, Inc.
198 Madison Avenue, New York, New York, 10016

www.oup.com

Oxford is a registered trademark of Oxford University Press

Library of Congress Cataloging-in-Publication Data
Nunez, Paul L.
Electric fields of the brain: the neurophysics of EEG/
Paul L. Nunez, Ramesh Srinivasan—2nd ed.
    p. cm.
Includes bibliographical references and index.
ISBN-13: 978-0-19-505038-7

1. Electroencephalography. 2. Brain—Electric properties. 3. Electric fields.
I. Srinivasan, Ramesh. II. Title.

QP376.5.N8'6 2006
616.8'047547 dc22   2005040874

Printed in the United States of America
on acid-free paper

Preface to Second Edition

This is a story about how brains produce dynamic patterns of electric potential on the scalp, called the electroencephalogram or EEG. Our presentation has several subplots: small- versus large-scale generators, passive volume conduction, recording strategies, spectral analysis, phase synchronization, source localization, projection of scalp potentials to dura surface, correlations between measured dynamics and brain state, and networks immersed in global synaptic fields. EEG has long been recognized as genuine "window on the mind," albeit one with inadequate literature supporting its theoretical foundation. This book provides the theoretical framework required for more sophisticated studies by neurologists and cognitive scientists, as well as engineers, physicists, computer scientists, and mathematicians interested in brain science.

The positive response of the EEG community to the first edition of *Electric Fields of the Brain: The Neurophysics of EEG* (1981) has encouraged this second edition. Our central goals remain unchanged: to explain how fundamental physical principles apply to EEG and to bridge communication gaps between complementary scientific fields. In the second edition, we follow the sage advice of EEG colleagues—do everything possible to explain things more clearly, but do so without "dumbing down" the material. To accomplish this in an EEG community with disparate backgrounds, a conversational style with generous use of metaphor is adopted. Critical equations are included, but equation development is left to the references and 12 appendices. This second edition expands the original treatment of volume conduction by more than 50% by eliminating several chapters associated with brain dynamics, a topic treated in P.L. Nunez, *Neocortical Dynamics and Human EEG Rhythms* (Oxford University Press, 1995).

This book is directed to EEG scientists and clinicians, but may also serve as a text for advanced undergraduate or graduate courses in quantitative neuroscience, applied physics, biomathematics, or biomedical engineering if supplemented with appropriate reference materials. Researchers using EEG in qualitative neuroscience, medicine, and cognitive science should find this to be a useful handbook describing the physical and physiological bases for EEG. All readers should first cover the material in chapters 1 and 2 and peruse the introductory sections of selective chapters. Beyond that, different backgrounds suggest different study strategies. The experienced EEG scientist may be interested in the high-resolution methods in chapter 8, time series analysis in chapter 9, or cognitive experiments in chapter 10, saving other material for later. The novice EEG practitioner may first choose to become familiar with recording methods and reference issues in chapter 7. Readers at the BS or MS level of physics, engineering, or mathematics may wish to read straight through, although a few difficult spots may be encountered. Wordy explanations and appendices serve to overcome these barriers. The physical science Ph.D. should have no trouble with the physical ideas; however, scientists lacking neurophysiology background may choose a reference book to consult as parallel reading. A good place to begin is M.F. Bear, B.W. Connors, and M.A. Paradiso, *Neuroscience: Exploring the Brain* (1996). Readers wanting more technical information about electric fields at cellular levels, biomagnetic fields, or EKG may consult J. Malmivuo and R. Plonsey, *Bioelectromagnetism* (Oxford University Press, 1995). Comprehensive treatment of clinical applications and related technical issues may be found in E. Niedermeyer and F.H. Lopes da Silva (Eds.), *Electroencephalography. Basic Principals, Clinical Applications, and Related Fields* (Fifth Edition, 2005).

Some scientists do not like equations; for example, presenting equations at medical conferences has been compared to showing X-rated movies in church. With this in mind, we have kept equation density much lower than that found in intermediate physics texts. This is accomplished by limiting mathematical derivations to the appendices, in a manner analogous to providing security for a loan—the appendices force us to spend our words cautiously. We could have omitted *all* equations, providing a more demo-cratic presentation in the sense that fewer readers would understand the most subtle points. That is, the presence of equations cannot reduce verbal information content, and equations have been generously supplemented with verbiage and metaphor to the best of our abilities. Another potential criticism is that the presentation level varies considerably from place to place. To this we plead guilty. Clinicians, scientists, and students have a broad range of educational experiences. One might imagine a number of books tailored to individual backgrounds; however, even if multiple books of this kind were possible, they might defeat our avowed purpose of straddling gaps between disparate scientific fields.

Chapter 1 discusses alternative philosophical approaches to science in an EEG context. Prominent issues are introduced, including interpretation of reference electrode data, source localization, and high-resolution methods. A conceptual framework is outlined in which the cell assemblies (or neural networks) believed to underlie behavior and cognition are embedded within synaptic action fields, analogous to social networks embedded within a culture. This framework provides a convenient entry point to later chapters.

Chapter 2 outlines common fallacies in EEG; supporting evidence appears throughout the book. Fallacies often originate with poor cross-field communication, but communication problems in EEG arise more frequently than the usual fuzzy interactions between biological and physical scientists. Physiologists, cognitive scientists, and clinical neurologists all record electric potentials, but have different goals and methods. Engineers and physicists develop theoretical models and apply time series analysis. Some of these methods are useful in EEG; many are not. A section on the brain's magnetic field is included to deal with EEG versus MEG controversies. Mathematical support is provided in appendix C.

Chapter 3 is an overview of electromagnetic fields with emphasis on phenomena of interest in EEG. No mathematical background beyond college calculus is assumed in this treatment. Vector fields are introduced gently and treated in more depth in appendices A, B, and C. Important conceptual distinctions are emphasized—near and far fields, microscopic and macroscopic fields, and charge sources versus current sources. Several physical systems are suggested as useful metaphors for brain dynamic phenomena: transmission lines, resonance induced by lightening strikes, and microwave ovens. Appendix B derives the quasi-static approximations appropriate for EEG.

Chapter 4 lays a theoretical foundation for macroscopic currents and fields in living tissue. Parts of this material encompass standard biophysics: Ohm's law, capacitive effects, boundary conditions, membrane diffusion, and impressed currents. Other sections are not easily found elsewhere: connections between synaptic microsources, intermediate-scale mesosources (the so-called "dipoles" of EEG), and macroscopic scalp potentials. A low-pass filtering effect caused by reduction of mesosource strength in roughly the 50–100 Hz range is suggested by a simple membrane theory. Supplementary mathematical methods are developed in appendices D, E, and K.

Chapter 5 shows behaviors of potentials and currents in a homogeneous and isotropic medium. In these examples, the spatial fall-off of potentials is determined exclusively by the geometry of the current sources and sinks. Biological examples include branched dendrites, the superior olivary nucleus, action potentials in myelinated fibers, and cortical dipole layers.

Chapter 6 is concerned with potentials in layered conductive media with emphasis on the "4-sphere" head model, an inner sphere representing brain surrounded by three spherical shells representing CSF, scalp, and skull. While the 4-sphere model is an imperfect model of volume conduction in human heads, it provides several basic properties needed to interpret EEG in terms of the underlying sources. A limited study of the effects of an inhomogeneous skull region on scalp potential is also included. Appendices F, G, and H derive supporting solutions.

Chapter 7 emphasizes several aspects of recording strategies that often receive sparse coverage in the EEG literature. The reference issue is examined in depth, including physically and digitally linked ears (or mastoids), the common average reference, bipolar recordings, and a "genuine reference" test. The reference issue is also approached using the reciprocity theorem. It is shown that all EEG recordings are essentially bipolar—the sharp distinction between recording and reference electrode is exposed as a myth that has long obscured many EEG studies. Finally, the underlying theory and limitations of temporally smoothed dipole localization methods is outlined.

Chapter 8 explains the theoretical basis for high-resolution EEG estimates obtained from the spline-Laplacian. This Laplacian estimate is shown to provide spatial band pass representations of dura surface potential. The Laplacian estimate is compared with dura imaging, an independent algorithm based on an inward continuation solution. Both the strengths and limitations of high-resolution EEG are outlined. Surface Laplacian and dura image estimates are shown to complement but not replace raw scalp potentials. Appendices I and J provide mathematical bases including (MATLAB) spline-Laplacian code for adoption in other laboratories.

Chapter 9 outlines time series analyses, especially power spectra and coherence as a means to estimate phase synchronization. The important effects of spatial filters on coherence estimates are studied with theory, simulations, and genuine EEG data. The low-pass filter forced by volume conduction and the band-pass filter provided by application of the Laplacian algorithm to this raw data are explained. Laplacian coherence is shown to remove erroneous high coherence caused by volume conduction in addition to (possible) genuine source coherence, thereby providing "conservative" coherence estimates. Other topics include comparison of ordinary with partial coherence, amplitude/coherence relationships, temporal filtering caused by spatial filtering, steady-state visually evoked potentials (SSVEPs), PCA (principal components analysis or empirical orthogonal functions), spatial-temporal spectral density functions, and estimates of EEG propagation velocity over the scalp.

Chapter 10 applies the methods of chapter 9 to several cognitive studies. Coherence changes in the theta and alpha bands during mental calculations are described. Certain pairs of electrode sites consistently exhibit enhanced phase synchronization in the theta and upper alpha bands, while synchronization at lower alpha frequencies may be reduced in the same data sets. Estimates of phase and group velocity of alpha rhythm and SSVEP are shown to be consistent with known corticocortical propagation speeds. SSVEP coherence and partial coherence are also estimated in a binocular rivalry experiment. Coherence and partial coherence increase consistently during dominance periods; that is, when the subject perceives only one flickering stimulus. These experiments are consistent with the formation of large-scale networks associated with mental tasks and conscious perception.

Chapter 11 pursues the Holy Grail of connecting psychology with physiology in the context of a global dynamic theory of synaptic action fields, first introduced to EEG by the senior author in 1972. The preface to the first edition made the following prediction: "Since this (theory) has a wide variety of experimental implications, it seems possible that it will either be established or discredited in the near future." After 25 years, neither outcome has come to pass, and the physiological bases for EEG dynamic behavior remain controversial. Nevertheless, much progress toward understanding dynamic behavior and cognition has occurred. More experimental links have been discovered, and several new dynamic theories of EEG developed; some are competitive and some are complementary to the basic global theory. Qualitative and semiquantitative connections to several EEG experiments are outlined here, and relationships of the basic global theory to other local and global theories are summarized. Appendix L outlines mathematical details and lists several efforts by other scientists to extend the basic global theory.

The appendices have several functions. Appendix A provides a simple introduction to vector fields. The quasi-static approximations in appendix B are available elsewhere, but here we emphasize that the neglect of capacitive and inductive effects in tissue are separate issues. Appendix C derives radial and tangential magnetic field components due to a dipole source at an arbitrary location. These derivations require only mid-level mathematics, but we have not found them in the literature. Appendices D, E, F, G, H, J, K, and L involve mathematics beyond the standard first-year graduate course in engineering math; this material is not easily found elsewhere.

P.L.N. was introduced to EEG by Professor Reginald Bickford in 1970 at one of the infamous California parties of the time and enjoyed a productive decade in his laboratory at the University of California at San Diego. The first edition of this book resulted from this tenure. We have attempted to remain faithful to Reg's scientific spirit, illustrated by his quote from the Foreword to the first edition, "...the authors have fallen so naturally into the lingo of the specialty while feeling free to slaughter many sacred cows that clutter the field." Reg, who died in 1998, was a clinical electroencephalographer with a keen interest in many scientific fields as well as an exceptional human being.

Ron Katznelson, author of two chapters in the first edition, made several original contributions to EEG as part of his Ph.D. research that still appear quite innovative after 25 years. He joined the communications industry upon leaving UC San Diego in 1982, acquired more than a dozen patents in a short time, founded his own successful company, and continues his career as chief technical officer.

The New Orleans spline-Laplacian algorithm used to estimate dura potential from discrete scalp samples is based on the original publication by the French group (see chapter 8). P.L.N. wrote a two-dimensional Fortran version at Tulane University in 1988, and Sam Law and Ranjith Wijesinghe later developed and tested the three-dimensional version with more than a thousand simulations. R.S. wrote the (latest) MATLAB version, which appears in appendix J for convenient implementation in other laboratories. Output tables are also supplied for two example Laplacian estimates to facilitate algorithm verification. Laplacian and spectral analysis codes may be downloaded from www.electricfieldsofthebrain.com. This site will also include updated technical information as well as feedback from the EEG community on book topics.

The experimental demonstrations in chapters 6–9 and SSVEP studies in chapter 10 were accomplished in R.S.'s laboratory at the University of California at Irvine. Much of the other experimental work in chapter 10 was carried out by Brett Wingeier as part of his Ph.D. program at Tulane University while he and the senior author enjoyed a delightful two-year sabbatical at the Brain Sciences Institute of Swinburne University of Technology in Melbourne, Australia (1998–2000). Our host and BSI founder, Richard Silberstein, is a leading practitioner of SSVEP applications to cognitive studies. He provided many hours of valuable insight. The Melbourne dura imaging algorithm used in chapter 10 was developed and first applied to SSVEP by Peter Cadusch and Richard Silberstein.

Several colleagues made helpful comments on early drafts. Many thanks to John Ebersole, Armin Fuchs, Lester Ingber, Eugene Izhikevich, Don Jewett, Viktor Jirsa, David Liley, Ken Pilgreen, Peter Robinson, Christopher Renee, David Simpson, and Cedric Walker. The van der Pol oscillator simulations of chapter 9 form a preliminary section of Bill Winter's MS thesis at Tulane University. A comprehensive review of this manuscript was provided by physicist-turned-neuroscientist Tom Ferree. We have implemented many of Tom's suggestions and thank him for his herculean effort.

Research support for the first edition was limited to several small National Science Foundation grants. By contrast, research for the second edition has enjoyed generous support over the past 20 years from the National Institute of Mental Health, National Institute of Neurological Diseases and Stroke, National Science Foundation, Australian Research Council, Swinburne University, and The Neurosciences Institute. Without this support, this expanded edition would have been impossible.

P.L.N. would like to thank his wife Kirsty for her (mostly) cheerful acceptance of book widow status. His wife and children—Cindy, Shari, Michelle, Michael, and Lisa—have helped to make the efforts worthwhile.

R.S. would like to thank his wife Surekha and son Vikram for their patience and support, and his parents for their inspiration.

Paul L. Nunez
New Orleans, Louisiana, 2005
Ramesh Srinivasan
Irvine, California, 2005

Contents

Appendices

Index

Electric Fields of the Brain

1

The Physics–EEG Interface

1 A Window on the Mind

The *electroencephalogram* (EEG) is a record of the oscillations of brain electric potential recorded from electrodes on the human scalp. Consider the following experiment. Place a pair of electrodes on someone's scalp and feed the unprocessed EEG signal to a computer display in an isolated location. Independently monitor the subject's state of consciousness and provide both this information and the EEG signal to an external observer. Even a naive observer, unfamiliar with EEG, will recognize that the voltage record during *deep sleep* has larger amplitudes and contains much more low-frequency content. In addition, the (eyes closed waking) *alpha state* will be revealed as a widespread, near-sinusoidal oscillation repeating about 10 times per second (10 Hz). More sophisticated monitoring allows for accurate identification of distinct *sleep stages, depth of anesthesia, seizures*, and other *neurological disorders*. Other methods reveal robust EEG correlations with cognitive processes associated with *mental calculations, working memory*, and *selective attention*.

Scientists are now so accustomed to these EEG correlations with brain state that they may forget just how remarkable they are. The scalp EEG provides very large-scale and robust measures of neocortical dynamic function. A single electrode provides estimates of synaptic action averaged over tissue masses containing between roughly 100 million and 1 billion neurons. The space averaging of brain potentials resulting from extracranial recording is a fortuitous data reduction process forced by current spreading in the head volume conductor. Much more detailed local information may be obtained from intracranial recordings in animals and epileptic patients. However, intracranial electrodes implanted in living brains provide only very sparse spatial coverage, thereby failing to record the "big picture" of brain function. Furthermore, the dynamic behavior of intracranial recordings depends fundamentally on measurement scale, determined mostly by electrode size. Different electrode sizes and locations can result in substantial differences in recorded dynamic behavior, including frequency content and coherence. Thus, in practice, *intracranial data provide different information, not more information, than is obtained from the scalp.*

The critical importance of spatial scale in electrophysiology can be emphasized by reference to a sociological metaphor. Experimental data obtained from large metropolitan areas will generally differ from data collected at the city, neighborhood, family, and person scales. Similarly, we expect brain electrical dynamics to vary substantially across spatial scales. Although cognitive scientists and clinicians have reason to be partly satisfied with the very low spatial resolution obtained from scalp EEG data, explorations of new EEG methods to provide somewhat higher spatial resolution continue. A reasonable goal is to record averages over "only" 10 million neurons at the 1 cm scale in order to extract more details of the spatial patterns correlated with cognition and behavior. This resolution is close to the theoretical limit of spatial resolution caused by the physical separation of sensor and brain current sources.

Scalp data are largely independent of electrode size because scalp potentials are severely space-averaged by volume conduction between brain and scalp. Intracranial recordings provide much smaller scale measures of neocortical dynamics, with scale depending on the electrode size, which may vary over four orders of magnitude in various practices of electrophysiology. A mixture of coherent and incoherent sources generates the small- and intermediate-scale intracranial data. Generally, the smaller the scale of intracranial potentials, the lower the expected contribution from coherent sources and the larger the expected differences from scalp EEG. That is, scalp data are due mostly to sources coherent at the scale of at least several centimeters with special geometries that encourage the superposition of potentials generated by many local sources.

In practice, intracranial EEG may be uncorrelated or only weakly correlated with cognition and behavior. The information content in such recordings is limited by sparse spatial sampling and scale-dependent dynamics. Furthermore, most intracranial EEG data are recorded in lower mammals; extrapolation to humans involves additional issues. Thus, higher brain function in humans is more easily observed at large scales. Scientists interested in higher brain function are fortunate in this respect. The technical and ethical limitations of human intracranial recording force us to emphasize scalp recordings. These extracranial recordings provide estimates of synaptic action at the large scales closely related to cognition and behavior. Thus, EEG provides a window on the mind, albeit one that is often clouded by technical and other limitations. This book strives for improved methods to clean up this window, allowing for more transparent imaging of the majesty of brain dynamics.

2 Brain Structures and Scalp Potentials

The three primary divisions of the human brain are *brainstem, cerebellum* and *cerebrum*, as shown in fig. 1-1. The brainstem (the brain's stalk) is the structure through which nerve fibers relay signals (*action potentials*) in both directions between spinal cord and higher brain centers. The *thalamus,* composed of two egg-shaped structures at the top and to the side of the brainstem, is a relay station and important integrating center for all sensory input to the cortex except smell. The *cerebellum,* which sits on top and to the back of the brainstem, has long been associated with the fine control

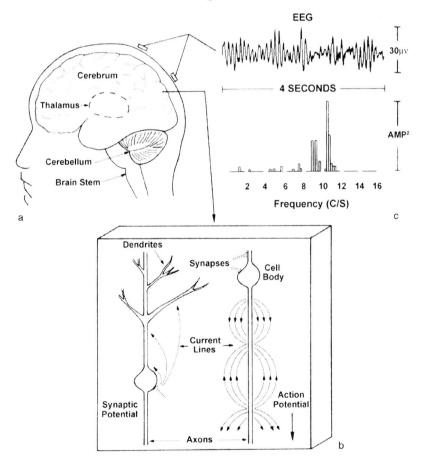

Figure 1-1 (a) The human brain. (b) Section of cerebral cortex showing microcurrent sources due to synaptic and action potentials. Neurons are actually much more closely packed than shown, about 10^5 neurons per mm^2 of surface. (c) Each scalp EEG electrode records space averages over many square centimeters of cortical sources. A four-second epoch of alpha rhythm and its corresponding power spectrum are shown.

of muscle movements. More recently, the cerebellum has been shown to play additional roles in cognition.

The large part of the brain that remains when the brainstem and cerebellum are excluded is the *cerebrum*, which is divided almost equally into two halves. The outer portion of the cerebrum, the *cerebral cortex* (or *neocortex* in mammals), is a folded structure varying in thickness from about 2 to 5 mm, having a total surface area of roughly 1600 to 4000 cm^2 and containing about 10^{10} *neurons* (nerve cells). Cortical neurons are strongly interconnected. For example, the surface of a large cortical neuron may be covered with as many as 10^4 to 10^5 *synapses* that transmit inputs from other neurons. The synaptic inputs to a neuron are of two types: those that produce *excitatory postsynaptic potentials* (EPSPs) across the membrane of the target neuron, thereby making it easier for the target neuron to fire an *action potential* and the *inhibitory postsynaptic potentials* (IPSPs), which act in the opposite manner on the output neuron. EPSPs produce local membrane *current sinks* with corresponding distributed passive sources to preserve current conservation. IPSPs produce local membrane *current sources* with more distant distributed passive sinks. In addition, several other interaction mechanisms, not involving action potentials, have been discovered by neurophysiologists. Much of our conscious experience must involve, in some largely unknown manner, the interaction of cortical neurons. The cortex is also believed to be the structure that generates most of the electric potential measured on the scalp.

The cortex is composed of *gray matter*, so called because it contains a predominance of cell bodies that turn gray when stained by anatomists, but gray matter is actually pink when alive. Just below the gray matter is a second major region, the *white matter*, composed of nerve fibers (*axons*). In humans, white matter volume is somewhat larger than that of the neocortex. White matter interconnections between cortical regions (*association fibers or corticocortical fibers*) are quite numerous. Each square centimeter of human neocortex may contain 10^7 input and output fibers, mostly corticocortical axons interconnecting different regions of the cortex, as shown in fig. 1-2. A much smaller fraction of axons that enter or leave the underside of human cortical surface radiates from (and to) the thalamus (*thalamocortical fibers*). This fraction is only a few percent in humans, but substantially larger in lower mammals. This difference partly accounts for the strong emphasis on thalamocortical interactions (versus corticocortical interactions), especially in physiology literature emphasizing animal studies. Anatomists have attached hundreds of labels to various substructures within the brain, but here we are most interested in larger structures near the surface that are more capable of generating potentials sufficiently coherent to be observed on the scalp.

Neocortical neurons within each cerebral hemisphere are connected by short intracortical fibers with axon lengths mostly less than 1 mm. In addition, human neocortex is interconnected by about 10^{10} corticocortical fibers with axon lengths in the roughly 1 to 15 cm range. Cross

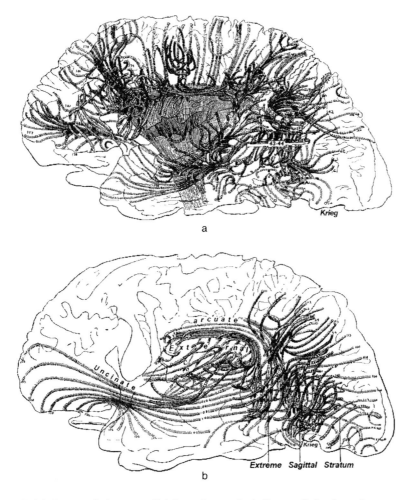

Figure 1-2 (a) Some of the superficial corticocortical fibers of the lateral aspect of the cerebrum obtained by dissection. (b) A few of the deeper corticocortical fibers of the lateral aspect of the cerebrum. The total number of corticocortical fibers is roughly 10^{10}, that is, for every fiber shown here, about 100 million are not shown. Reproduced with permission from Krieg (1963, 1973).

hemisphere interactions occur by means of about 10^8 *callosal axons* through the corpus callosum and several smaller structures connecting the two brain halves. A common view of brain operation is that of a complex circuit or *neural network*. In this view, groups of cortical cells may be imagined as analogous to electric circuit elements. The imagined circuit elements might be individual neurons or cortical columns of different sizes, perhaps containing anything between a hundred (minicolumn scale) and a hundred thousand neurons (macrocolumn scale). Intracortical axons plus cortico-cortical, callosal and thalamocortical axons might then be imagined as analogous to wires connecting the circuit elements. In this oversimplified (and probably mostly wrong) electric network picture, "circuit elements" are under external control by means of electrical and chemical input from the brainstem. More realistic views may adopt parts of this picture, but acknowledge that even a single neuron is far more complex than the most complex artificial neural network likely to be created in the near future (Scott 1995). Furthermore, neurons interact by multiple mechanisms that may not easily conform to conventional network models.

One obvious issue that arises whenever models are compared with genuine electrophysiological data is that of spatial scale. Any neural network description of brain operation must be scale-dependent so, for example, macroscopic network elements are themselves complex circuits containing smaller (*mesoscopic*) network elements. The mesoscopic elements are, in turn, composed of still smaller scale elements. Even the best imagined neural network model must break down at the membrane scale where dynamics are governed by biochemistry and ultimately Maxwell's microscopic equations and quantum mechanics. Other breakdowns of circuit analogs are evident at large scales. For example, in a simple electric circuit, signal delays take place only at circuit elements, that is, *the delays are all local*. However, neocortical interactions over large distances involve both *local* and *global delays*, the latter due to action potential propagation along axons at finite speeds. In this sense, they share some properties with electrical transmission lines like power lines or coaxial TV cables.

Transmission times for action potentials along corticocortical axons may range from roughly 10 to 30 ms between the most remote cortical regions. Local delays due to capacitive-resistive properties of single neurons are typically in the 1 to 10 ms range, but may also be longer. The brain's awareness of an external event seems to require multiple feedback between remote regions. *Consciousness takes several hundred milliseconds to develop.* The multiple mechanisms by which neurons can interact may not fit naturally into standard neural network models. Partly for these reasons, neuroscientists often prefer the term *cell assemblies*, originating with the pioneering work of Donald Hebb (1949). The label "cell assembly" denotes a diffuse cell group capable of acting briefly as a single structure. We may reasonably postulate cooperative activity within cell assemblies without explicitly specifying interaction mechanisms or relying on electric circuit metaphors.

Brain processes may involve the formation of cell assemblies at several spatial scales (Freeman 1975; Ingber 1982, 1995). We conjecture that such groups of neurons may produce a wide range of local delays and associated characteristic (or *resonant*) frequencies (Nunez 1995). Neural network models can incorporate some physiologically realistic features that are not normally present in electric circuits. However, *field descriptions* of brain dynamics may be required to model dynamic behavior and make contact with macroscopic EEG data. In this context, the word "field" refers to mathematical functions expressing, for example, the numbers of active synaptic or action potentials in macroscopic tissue volumes. Alternately, probability of neural firing in a tissue mass may be treated as a *field variable* (Ingber 1995). In the view adopted in this book, *cell assemblies are pictured* as *embedded within synaptic* and *action potential fields* (Nunez 1995, 2000a, b; Jirsa and Haken 1997; Haken 1999). Electric and magnetic fields (EEG and MEG) provide large-scale, short-time measures of the *modulations* of synaptic and action potential fields around their background levels. These synaptic fields are analogous to common physical fields, for example, sound waves, which are short-time modulations of pressure or mass density about background levels. We distinguish these short-time modulations of synaptic activity from long-timescale (seconds to minutes) modulations of brain chemistry controlled by *neuromodulators*.

Dynamic brain behaviors are conjectured by many neuroscientists to result from the interaction of neurons and assemblies of neurons that form at multiple spatial scales (Freeman 1975; Harth 1993, Scott 1995; Nunez 1995, 2000a, b). Part of the dynamic behavior at macroscopic scales may be measured by scalp EEG electrodes. This electrical activity is divided into two major categories: *spontaneous potentials* such as alpha and sleep rhythms and *evoked potentials* or *event-related potentials*. Evoked potentials are the direct response to some external stimulus like a light flash or auditory tone. Event-related potentials depend additionally on state-dependent brain processing of the stimulus (Regan 1989).

In addition to such EEG studies, electrophysiologists study potentials generated by single neurons or small cell assemblies, recorded with *microelectrodes* or *mesoelectrodes* (between micro and macro). Much work has been published on potentials recorded at smaller scales (Cole 1968; Abeles 1982; Segev et al. 1995; Destexhe and Sejnowski 2001), but this book is concerned with oscillating macroscopic potentials measured on the scalp, or in the brain, called the electroencephalogram or EEG. Meso- and microelectrode data are considered here mainly in the context of relating scalp potentials to their underlying sources.

The scalp EEG is an important clinical tool for following and treating certain illnesses (Kellaway 1979; Niedermeyer and Lopes da Silva 1999). Brain tumors, strokes, epilepsies, infectious diseases, mental retardation, severe head injury, drug overdose, sleep and metabolic disorders, and ultimately brain death are some of the medical conditions that may show up in the spontaneous EEG. EEG also provides quantitative measures of depth of anesthesia and severity of coma. Evoked and event-related potentials measured on the scalp may be used in the diagnosis and treatment of central nervous system diseases as well as illuminating cognitive processes, but often EEG abnormalities are nonspecific, perhaps only confirming diagnoses obtained with independent clinical tests.

A summary of clinical and research EEG is provided in fig. 1-3. The arrows indicate common relations between subfields. The numbered superscripts in the boxes indicate the following. (1) Physiologists record EEG from inside the skulls of animals using electrodes with diameters typically ranging from about 0.01 to 1 mm. Observed dynamic behavior generally depends on location and measurement scale, determined mostly by electrode size for intracranial recordings. By contrast, scalp-recorded

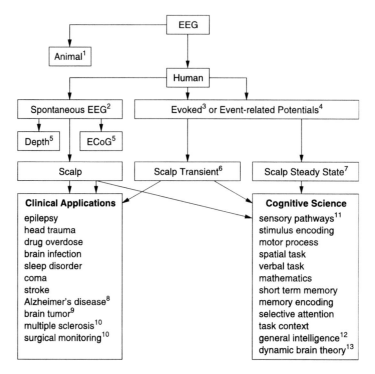

Figure 1-3 Common relationships between EEG subfields. Clinical applications are mostly related to neurological diseases. EEG research is carried out by neurologists, cognitive neuroscientists, physicists, and engineers who have a special interest in EEG. See text for a discussion of numbered superscripts. Reproduced with permission from Nunez (2002).

EEG dynamics is exclusively large scale and mostly independent of electrode size. (2) Human spontaneous EEG occurs in the absence of specific sensory stimuli, but may be easily altered by such stimuli. (3) Averaged *evoked potentials* (EPs) are associated with specific sensory stimuli like repeated light flashes, auditory tones, finger pressure, or mild electric shocks. They are typically recorded by time averaging of single-stimulus waveforms to remove the spontaneous EEG. (4) *Event-related potentials* (ERPs) are recorded in the same way as EPs, but normally occur at longer latencies from the stimuli and are more associated with *endogenous brain state*. (5) Because of ethical considerations, EEG recorded in brain depth or on the brain surface (ECoG) of humans is limited to patients, mostly candidates for epilepsy surgery. (6) With transient EPs or ERPs the stimuli consist of repeated short stimuli. The number of stimuli required to produce an averaged evoked potential may be anything between about ten and several thousand, depending on application. The scalp response to each stimulus or pulse is averaged over the individual pulses. The EP or ERP in any experiment consists of a waveform containing a series of characteristic peaks (local maxima or minima), typically occurring less than 0.5 seconds after presentation of each stimulus. The amplitude, latency from the stimulus or covariance (in the case of multiple electrode sites) of each component may be studied, in connection with a cognitive task (ERP) or with no task (EP). (7) Steady-state visually evoked potentials (SSVEP) use a continuous sinusoid modulated stimulus (a flickering light, for example), typically superimposed in front of a computer monitor providing a cognitive task. The brain response in a narrow frequency band containing the stimulus frequency is measured. Magnitude, phase, and coherence (in the case of multiple electrode sites) may be related to different parts of the cognitive task. (8) Alzheimer's disease and other dementias typically cause substantial slowing of normal alpha rhythms. Traditional EEG has been of little use in dementia because EEG changes are often only evident late in the illness when other clinical signs are obvious. New efforts to apply EEG to early detection of Alzheimer's disease are under study. (9) Cortical tumors that involve the white matter layer (just below neocortex) cause substantial low-frequency (delta) activity over the hemisphere with the tumor. Application of EEG to tumor diagnosis has been mostly replaced by *magnetic resonance imaging* (MRI), which reveals structural abnormalities in tissue. (10) Most clinical work uses spontaneous EEG; however, multiple sclerosis and surgical monitoring often involve evoked potentials. (11) Studies of sensory pathways involve early components of evoked potentials (latency from stimuli less than perhaps 10 to 50 ms) because the transmission times for signals traveling between sense organ and brain are short compared to the duration of multiple feedback processes associated with cognition. (12) The study of *general intelligence* associated with IQ tests is controversial, but a number of studies have reported significant correlations between scores on written tests and quantitative EEG measures. (13) Mathematical models of large-scale brain function are used to explain or predict observed properties of EEG in terms of basic physiology and anatomy. Although such models must represent vast oversimplifications of genuine brain function, they contribute to our conceptual framework and may guide the design of new experiments to test parts of this framework.

The clinical usefulness of quantitative EEG methods in various diseases has been assessed jointly by the *American Academy of Neurology and the American Clinical Neurophysiology Society* (Nuwer 1998). Clinical and cognitive applications of EEG have been covered extensively elsewhere, and are largely avoided here, except in some important cases where electric field concepts seem to shed new light on clinical or cognitive issues. One of our aims is to provide scientific and technical information that may lead to new EEG applications for disease states for which clinical utility has been disappointing thus far. These include mild or moderate closed head injury, learning disabilities, attention disorders, schizophrenia, depression, and Alzheimer's disease. Given the relatively crude methods of data processing currently used in most clinical settings, we simply do not now know if these brain abnormalities cause EEGs with clinically useful information. There is, however, reason to be optimistic about future clinical developments because quantitative methods to recognize spatial-temporal EEG patterns have been studied only sporadically. For example, high-resolution coherence and other measures of phase synchronization, which indicate the strength of functional connections between brain regions, are rarely used in clinical settings. High-resolution EEG generally and EEG phase synchronization are treated in chapters 8–10.

We are concerned here with the physiological bases for EEG: the nature and location of the so-called *generators* of potential and how these potentials and currents spread through brain, skull, and scalp (*volume conduction*). We also consider the possible origins of time-dependent behavior of EEG (*neocortical dynamics*), especially when this issue overlaps volume conduction considerations. These topics are directly related to the practical problems faced in recording and interpreting the EEG. Misunderstanding of electric fields and potentials often leads to fallacious and, in some cases, even absurd physiologic interpretations, as outlined in chapter 2. This book attempts to lay a more solid theoretical foundation upon which clinical and cognitive studies may rest more securely. A deeper understanding of volume conduction and dynamical issues and improved recording and computer methods should provide clinicians with more finely tuned diagnostic tools and cognitive scientists with enlightened experimental methods.

3 Human Alpha Rhythms

A central problem for the electroencephalographer or cognitive scientist is to relate potentials measured on the scalp to the underlying physiological processes. Such scalp potentials are characterized by their temporal and spatial characteristics. For example, an important human EEG category embodies several kinds of alpha rhythms, which are usually identified as near-sinusoidal oscillations at frequencies near 10 Hz. Alpha rhythm in an awake relaxed human subject is illustrated by the temporal plots and corresponding frequency spectra in fig. 1-4. The amplitude of scalp alpha oscillations is typically 20 to 50 μV, when measured between one electrode over the occipital cortex and a second electrode some 5 to 10 cm or so distant. Alpha rhythm amplitudes are typically smaller over frontal regions, depending partly on the subject's state of relaxation.

Other alpha rhythms may occur in other brain states, for example in alpha coma or with patients under halothane anesthesia. In addition to alpha rhythms, a wide variety of human EEG activity may be recorded, a proverbial zoo of dynamic signatures, each waveform dependent in its own way on time and scalp location. EEG is often labeled according to apparent frequency range: delta (1–4 Hz), theta (4–8 Hz), alpha (8–13 Hz), beta (13–20 Hz), and gamma (roughly >20 Hz). These qualitative labels are often applied based only on visual inspection or by counting zero crossings. They must be used carefully because actual EEG is composed of

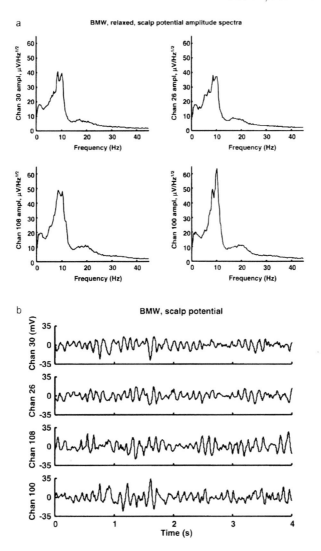

Figure 1-4 (b) Alpha rhythm recorded from a healthy 25-year-old relaxed male with eyes closed using a neck electrode as reference. Four seconds of data are shown from four scalp locations (left frontal-30; right frontal-26; left posterior-108; right posterior-100). Amplitudes are given in μV. (a) Amplitude spectra for the same alpha rhythms shown in (b) but based on the full five-minute record to obtain accurate spectral estimates. Amplitudes are given in μV per root Hz. Frequency resolution is 0.25 Hz. The double peak in the alpha band represents oscillations near 8.5 and 10.0 Hz. These lower and upper alpha band frequencies have different spatial properties and behave differently during cognitive tasks as shown in chapter 10.

mixtures of multiple frequency components as revealed more clearly by spectral analysis.

A posterior rhythm of approximately 4 Hz develops in babies in the first few months of age. Its amplitude increases with eye closure and is believed to be a precursor of mature alpha rhythms. Maturation of the alpha rhythms is characterized by increased frequency and reduced amplitude between ages of about three and ten. Normal resting alpha rhythms may be substantially reduced in amplitude by eye opening, drowsiness, and, in many subjects, by moderate to difficult mental tasks. Alpha rhythms, like most EEG phenomena, typically exhibit an inverse relationship between amplitude and frequency. For example, hyperventilation and some drugs (alcohol, for example) may cause reductions of alpha frequencies together with increased amplitudes. Other drugs (barbiturates, for example) are associated with increased amplitude of low-amplitude beta activity superimposed on scalp alpha rhythms. The physiological bases for the inverse relation between amplitude and frequency and most other properties of EEG are largely unknown, although physiologically based dynamic theories have provided several tentative explanations. For example, several salient properties of EEG are consistent with limit cycle modes as discussed in chapter 11.

Alpha rhythms provide an appropriate starting point for clinical EEG exams (Kellaway 1979; Niedermeyer and Lopes da Silva 1999). Some initial clinical questions are as follows. Does the patient show an alpha rhythm with eyes closed, especially over posterior scalp? Are its spatial-temporal characteristics appropriate for the patient's age? How does it react to eyes opening, hyperventilation, drowsiness, and so forth? For example, pathology is often associated with pronounced differences in EEG recorded over opposite hemispheres or with low alpha frequencies. A resting alpha frequency lower than about 8 Hz in adults is considered abnormal in all but the very old.

These characteristics of scalp EEG depend not only on the nature and location of the current sources, but also on the electrical and geometrical properties of brain, skull, and scalp. The connection between surface and depth events is thus intimately dependent on the physics of electric field behavior in biological tissue. Electric fields in *physical media* were understood at least 50 years before the first scalp recordings of the human EEG in the mid-1920s by the German psychiatrist Hans Berger (1928). Physical principles are directly applicable to neural tissue; we need only interpret variables and supply tissue properties to provide a good picture of head volume conduction.

There are many possible sources of electrical activity on the scalp. Eye or tongue movements, muscle contractions, and EKG can produce scalp potentials larger than EEG amplitudes. In particular, since the alpha rhythm tends to disappear with eyes open, its origin was first suspected to be a rhythmic beat of eye muscles. Convincing evidence that alpha rhythms are generated in the brain was obtained in experiments with patients having abnormal skull openings (Adrian and Mathews 1934), although this early work suggested (erroneously) that alpha rhythms originate primarily in posterior regions. Averaged over time, the largest contributions do come from occipital and parietal regions with somewhat lesser contributions from frontal regions. Modern potential maps based on long-time averages often show "hot spots" over posterior regions, thereby contributing to the (often erroneous) view of alpha as a strictly localized phenomenon. We examine this issue further later in this chapter and again in chapters 9–11 and show that *multiple alpha rhythms occur with both local and global properties.*

We now have a more accurate picture of the properties of human alpha rhythms, obtained from early cortical surface and depth recordings in epileptic patients (Jasper and Penfield 1949; Penfield and Jasper 1954; Sem-Jacobsen et al. 1953; Cooper et al. 1965; Pfurtscheller and Cooper 1975) and later with high-resolution scalp recordings (Nunez et al. 2001) reviewed in chapter 10. Some of the early findings of cortical surface recordings have recently been rediscovered. These results are consistent with the following description by EEG pioneer Grey Walter in 1964 (Basar et al. 1997).

> We have managed to check the alpha band rhythm with intra cerebral electrodes in the occipital-parietal cortex; in regions which are practically adjacent and almost congruent one finds a variety of alpha rhythms, some are blocked by opening and closing the eyes, some are not, some respond in some way to mental activity and some do not. What one can see on the scalp is a spatial average of a large number of components, and whether you see an alpha rhythm of a particular type or not depends on which component happens to be the most highly synchronized process over the largest superficial area; there are complex rhythms in everybody.

Other early EEG pioneers were electroencephalographer Herbert Jasper and neurosurgeon Wilder Penfield, famous for his studies of patient response to electrical stimulation of cortical tissue, a procedure sometimes evoking reports of past memories in patients. Numerous EEG studies of epilepsy surgery patients were also carried out by Penfield and Jasper. They recorded EEG from different regions of exposed cortex in a large number of patients. Figure 1-5 indicates that alpha rhythm was recorded (in different subjects) from almost the entire upper cortical surface. The exception was the region near the central motor strip where beta rhythms were mainly recorded.

In order to interpret these early results, note that spectral (Fourier) analysis of EEG was not in use at that time. Rather, EEG waveforms were characterized by visual inspection and number of zero crossings. This procedure tends to emphasize faster frequencies (for example, beta activity) in data containing mixed frequency content as demonstrated in chapter 9. For this reason, it is not clear how much overlap occurred between regions with dominant beta and alpha rhythms in these early cortical studies. Another issue is that widespread alpha production is mostly associated with relaxed, healthy subjects. Penfield's epilepsy patients were recorded in the operating room while awake with parts of their skulls removed, apparently not ideal conditions for relaxed subjects and robust alpha rhythm production. We have not found such detailed modern

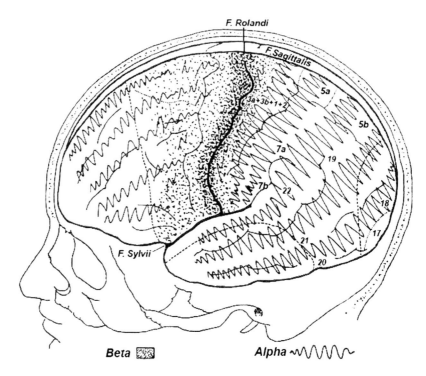

Figure 1-5 Cortical surface regions where alpha rhythms were recorded in a large population of epilepsy surgery patients are indicated by wavy lines. Dotted region near the central motor strip indicates beta activity. ECoG activity was characterized by counting zero crossings before Fourier transforms were used in EEG. Reproduced with permission from Jasper and Penfield (1949).

studies of human cortical rhythms, perhaps due partly to changing ethical standards. Another factor limiting modern data is that today's epilepsy surgery patients typically have a history of drug therapy to control seizures. Chronic drug use (whether for medical or recreational purposes) can cause long-lasting and perhaps permanent effects on normal brain rhythms. These issues complicate the extrapolation of patient data to the healthy population.

Relatively high spatial resolution EEG may now be obtained with scalp recordings using a combination of dense electrode arrays and computer algorithms to project scalp potentials to the dura surface, as discussed in chapters 2, 8, and 10. By contrast to true inverse solutions like *dipole localization, dura imaging* requires no a priori assumptions about sources. The accuracy of dura potential estimates is limited "only" by electrode density, noise, and accuracy of volume conductor model. Figure 1-6 shows eight instantaneous dura image plots; time slices are taken at successive maxima and minima of the alpha rhythm waveform in one subject. These plots are based on 131-channel scalp recordings with approximately 2.3 cm (center-to-center) electrode separation. Signal to noise ratio is quite high in these data. Furthermore, with such high spatial sampling, dura image estimates are relatively robust with respect to head model

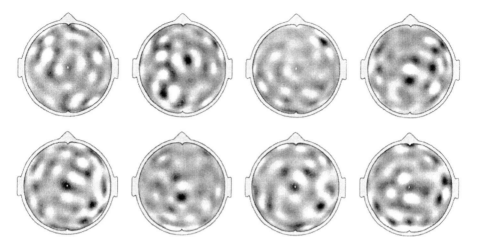

Figure 1-6 High-resolution estimates of dura potential for resting alpha rhythm at eight successive times separated by about 50 ms are shown. The plotting times correspond to alternating positive and negative peaks in the potential recorded by a posterior-midline electrode. The plots were obtained by passing 131-channel (average reference) data through the Melbourne dura imaging algorithm. The New Orleans spline-Laplacian yields similar patterns of dura potential, that is, correlation coefficients between the two high-resolution estimates are about 0.95 with the 131 spatial samples. These plots appear in color in fig. 10 of Nunez et al. (2001).

uncertainty. In fact, another high-resolution method, the New Orleans *spline-Laplacian*, which is nearly independent of head model, yields contour plots that are almost identical to those obtained by Melbourne dura imaging as discussed in chapters 8–10.

Based on these data and other evidence outlined in this book, we view alpha rhythm as a spatial-temporal dynamic modulation of cortical synaptic action, with sources widely distributed over neocortical surface. At any fixed time, patches of positive and negative potentials occur on the dura surface as suggested by fig. 1-6. These suggest alternating regions of correlated cortical source activity of opposite sign. Larger correlated regions tend to produce larger scalp potentials, which may account for observed anterior-posterior magnitude differences of alpha rhythm amplitudes. This dependence of scalp potential amplitude on characteristic correlated patch size (or effective correlation length) is demonstrated by the simulations shown in fig. 1-7. Each grid space represents a cortical macrocolumn source expressed in terms of transcortical potential, which varies between ± 200 μV (root mean square fixed at 116 μV). These transcortical potentials are consistent with intracranial recordings of spontaneous EEG in animals (Lopes da Silva and Storm van Leeuwen 1978). Filled and empty grid spaces indicate positive and negative macrocolumn sources, respectively. A head model consisting of three concentric spheres is used to estimate scalp potential contours generated by each of the source patterns.

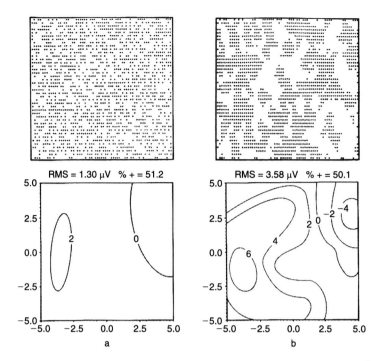

Figure 1-7 Simulated distribution of neocortical source activity over a 150 cm² square of (assumed) smooth cortical surface. Each grid space represents a cortical macrocolumn (≈ 3.5 mm²). The columnar mesosources are expressed here as local transcortical potentials to roughly match depth recordings in animals. Positive (black) or negative (white) potential differences are distributed between ±200 μV. Calculated surface potential maps (obtained with the 3-sphere head model) have progressively larger magnitudes as effective correlation lengths of the source distributions increase, that is, as source clumps become larger. The percentages of positive mesosources and corresponding RMS scalp potential magnitudes are (a) 51%, 1.3 μV; (b) 50%, 3.6 μV; (c) 55%, 7.4 μV; (d) 73%, 18.8 μV. Reproduced with permission from Nunez (1995).

The simulations shown in fig. 1-7 demonstrate that scalp potential amplitudes depend strongly on the characteristic size of the underlying correlated source patches (the amount of source synchronization). In these examples, the root mean square (rms) source strengths are held fixed at 116 μV for each simulation; only the sizes of correlated regions vary (plots a–d). When cortical source pattern is random (plot a), predicted rms scalp potential is 1.3 μV. By contrast, the large source clumps (plot d) produce a rms scalp potential of 18.8 μV. The idea that scalp potential magnitudes depend largely on source synchrony is widely recognized in clinical and research EEG environments where scalp potential amplitude reduction is often characterized as "desynchronization" (Kellaway 1979; Pfurtscheller and Lopes da Silva 1999). However, if source patterns are held fixed, scalp potential magnitudes increase in proportion to source magnitudes. These intermediate-scale (*mesoscale*) columnar sources are defined in terms of synaptic current sources in chapter 4. The

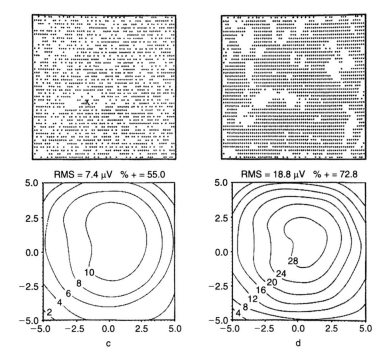

Figure 1-7 Continued.

meso-sources ($\mathbf{P}(\mathbf{r}, t)$ or dipole moments per unit volume) are simply weighted averages of membrane current sources over millimeter scale tissue masses, as given by (4.26).

Alpha rhythms can also exhibit both local and global behavior, possibly suggesting that larger amplitudes tend to occur in regions where both local and global mechanisms contribute strongly as discussed in chapters 9–11. This general picture is bolstered by volume conductor models of the head (chapters 6 and 8) that agree with observations of differences in magnitude and spectral content between cortex and scalp (Pfurtscheller and Cooper 1975) and with cortical depth recordings obtained with small electrodes to record alpha source activity in dogs (Lopes da Silva and Storm van Leeuwen 1978). Although this experimental description of sources of alpha phenomena rests on relatively solid ground, there is still no general agreement about the physiological bases for its dynamic behavior. We return to this issue in chapters 9–11.

4 A Conceptual Framework for Neocortical Dynamics and EEG

Figure 1-8 summarizes a general conceptual framework for neocortical dynamics and EEG (and *magnetoencephalograpy*, MEG). While parts of this framework are speculative, it accurately indicates, in a general sense, how volume conduction (causal connection 1-E) relates to the much

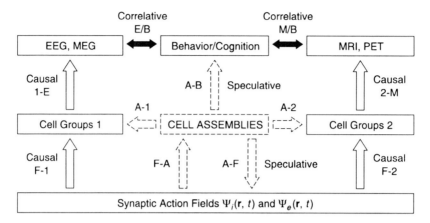

Figure 1-8 A conceptual framework for brain function. Double arrows (near top) indicate established correlative relationships between behavior/cognition and EEG, MEG, MRI, and PET. By definition, cell groups 1 generate EEG or MEG and cell groups 2 generate MRI or PET. Cell groups 1 and 2, which may or may not be part of neural networks (or cell assemblies), are embedded within the larger category (or "culture") of active synapses, the synaptic action fields $\Psi_e(\mathbf{r},t)$ and $\Psi_i(\mathbf{r},t)$. These excitatory and inhibitory synaptic action fields may be defined in terms of numbers of active synapses per unit volume or per unit of cortical surface area, independent of their functional significance. Cell assemblies and cell groups 1 and 2 may or may not overlap. Causal and correlative (may or may not be causal) interactions are indicated by hyphens and slashes, respectively. Reproduced with permission from Nunez and Silberstein (2000).

broader issues concerning EEG, brain dynamics, cell assemblies, cognition, and behavior. In any case, the fundamental principles of volume conduction rest on solid ground, independent of conjectures about other parts of the framework outlined in fig. 1-8.

The *synaptic action fields* indicated in fig. 1-8 are defined here simply as the numbers of active excitatory and inhibitory synapses per unit volume of tissue at any given time, independent of their possible participation in cell assemblies. We again caution readers about our use of the word "field" in this context. Our usage is conventional terminology in the physical sciences, but it is sometimes confusing to biological scientists. *The synaptic action fields are distinct from the electric and magnetic fields that they generate.* While controversial reports of small electric field actions on nervous tissue have been published, we do not consider the possibility of such interaction in this book. We do, however, postulate *interactions between synaptic action fields and cell assemblies.* This is simply a more efficient way of looking at established phenomena, for example, in the case of coherent synaptic activity in a large neural mass acting "top-down" on a cell assembly (or neural network). The *field description* appears useful if the field variable represents neocortical synaptic action integrated over sub-millimeter scales. The columnar structure of neocortex suggests a slightly modified definition of synaptic action fields as the numbers of active excitatory or inhibitory synapses per unit area of neocortical surface.

The idea of synaptic action fields is partly motivated by its causal connection to current sources, that is, the so-called *generators* of EEG. For example, a minicolumn of human neocortex has roughly a 0.03 mm radius, 3 mm height, and contains about 100 pyramidal cells and a million synapses (Szentagothai 1979). In mouse at least, there are perhaps six excitatory synapses for each inhibitory synapse (Braitenberg and Schuz 1991). If for the purposes of discussion we conjecture that 10% of all synapses are active at some given time, the excitatory and inhibitory synaptic action densities are about 80,000 and 14,000 per area of minicolumn, respectively. The number densities of active excitatory and inhibitory synapses, expressed as functions of time and cortical location are here assigned the symbols $\Psi_e(\mathbf{r}, t)$ and $\Psi_i(\mathbf{r}, t)$, respectively; these are *field variables*.

Each active inhibitory synapse produces a local current *source* at a membrane surface plus additional membrane *sinks* (negative sources) required by current conservation. Each active excitatory synapse produces a local negative source (sink) plus distributed membrane sources in a similar manner. The magnitude of electric potential at large distances (for example, at the local scalp) generated by a cortical column depends mainly on the distribution of synaptic and return sources over its depth and the *synchrony* of synaptic activation. For example, if excitatory and inhibitory synapses are distributed relatively uniformly through the column depth, or if synapses are randomly active in time, the strengths (*dipole moments* or *mesosources*) of column source regions will be small. Relatively large dipole moments occur if, for example, synchronous excitatory synapses act in superficial cortex (say on pyramidal cell dendrites) and inhibitory synapses act at deeper layers (say near cell bodies), a picture roughly consistent with anatomical data (Mountcastle 1979; Szentagothai 1979; Braitenberg and Schuz 1991) and electrophysiological depth recordings (Lopes da Silva and Storm van Leeuwen 1978).

A single minicolumn or even a single macrocolumn (containing about 1000 mincolumns or 100,000 pyramidal cells) is not expected to generate a dipole moment of sufficient strength to produce scalp potentials in the recordable range of a few microvolts. As a general "rule of head," about 6 cm^2 of cortical gyri tissue (containing about 600,000 minicolumns or 60,000,000 neurons forming a *dipole layer*) must be "synchronously active" to produce recordable scalp potentials without averaging (Cooper et al. 1965; Ebersole 1997). The tissue label "synchronously active" in this context is based on cortical recordings with macroscopic electrodes and must be viewed mainly as a qualitative description. In the case of dipole layers in fissures and sulci, tissue areas larger than 6 cm^2 are apparently required to produce measurable scalp potentials.

Action potential current sources contribute substantially to local extracellular potentials recorded at small scales; however, their contribution to distant scalp potentials is believed to be much smaller than that of synaptic potentials. This is expected partly because the parallel arrangement of pyramidal cell dendritic axes encourages superposition of fields from many individual synaptic sources, by forming large dipole layers. By contrast, neocortical axon orientations are more varied. The connection between current sources and extracranial magnetic field (MEG) follows similar arguments (see chapter 2). MEG is believed to be generated mainly by intracellular currents in cortical pyramidal cells rather than synaptic membrane sources. However, these currents are closely related by current conservation so no obvious advantage of this MEG feature is readily apparent.

The time dependence of EEG (or MEG) is believed to be due to modulation of synaptic action fields about background levels. To use a simple example, consider a simplified cortical model in which superficial and deep cortical layers are dominated by inhibitory $\Psi_i(\mathbf{r}, t)$ and excitatory $\Psi_e(\mathbf{r}, t)$ synaptic action, respectively, consistent with superficial current sources and deep current sinks. Short-time modulations of the synaptic action fields around background levels at cortical location $\mathbf{r}_1$ is crudely simulated in fig. 1-9. The cortical surface potential (with respect to infinity) generated by such synaptic action may be estimated at cortical location $\mathbf{r}_1$ by

$$\Phi(\mathbf{r}_1, t) \approx C_1\Psi_i(\mathbf{r}_1, t) - C_2\Psi_e(\mathbf{r}_1, t) \tag{1.1}$$

The constants C_1 and C_2 depend on the detailed distribution of sources and sinks across the cortex (including passive return current produced by each synapse) as well as volume conductive properties of the tissue. Equation (1.1) is only an approximation because genuine potentials depend on the geometric arrangement of sources (including passive return sources) across the cortex as described in chapter 4, but it serves adequately for the semiquantitative arguments of this section. Example surface potential plots calculated from (1.1) are shown in the lower row of fig. 1-9. However, an actual recorded potential in experimental work is always a potential difference between two locations. If an electrode pair is placed near locations $\mathbf{r}_1$ and $\mathbf{r}_2$, this potential difference is given by

$$V(\mathbf{r}_1, \mathbf{r}_2, t) = \Phi(\mathbf{r}_1, t) - \Phi(\mathbf{r}_2, t) \tag{1.2}$$

A second simulation for location $\mathbf{r}_2$ (perhaps an assumed reference location) with similar (but not identical) spectral content to that of fig. 1-9 plus a 1 Hz identical component (not shown), as might occur if the 1 Hz component were widespread in the cortex. The resulting potential difference is plotted in fig. 1-10. Because the 1 Hz component is common to both local potentials $\Phi(\mathbf{r}_1, t)$ and $\Phi(\mathbf{r}_2, t)$, it is absent from the simulated EEG given by $V(\mathbf{r}_1, \mathbf{r}_2, t)$. This discussion emphasizes that experimental potentials are always functions of two locations. The so-called reference location is nearly always provided in EEG publications, but often ignored

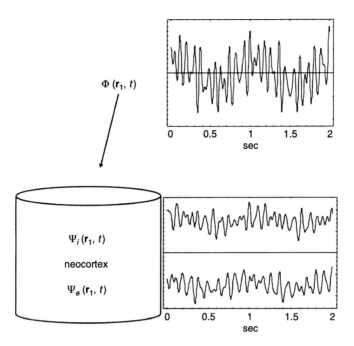

$\Phi\,(\mathbf{r}_1,\,t)$

$\Psi_i\,(\mathbf{r}_1,\,t)$

neocortex

$\Psi_e\,(\mathbf{r}_1,\,t)$

Figure 1-9 Modulations of inhibitory $\Psi_i(\mathbf{r}_1,t)$ and excitatory $\Psi_e(\mathbf{r}_1,t)$ synaptic action densities are imagined here to occur in superficial and deeper cortical layers, respectively. Each waveform shown here consists of five arbitrary frequency components in the delta, alpha, and beta ranges. The simulated cortical surface potential $\Phi(\mathbf{r}_1,t)$ is plotted as a linear combination of these synaptic field variables. A more realistic simulation might have excitatory synaptic action mainly in layers I and VI, and inhibitory synaptic action in layers II through V as indicated in fig. 11-4.

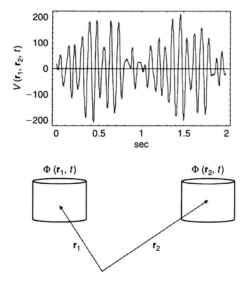

$\Phi\,(\mathbf{r}_1,\,t)$ $\qquad$ $\Phi\,(\mathbf{r}_2,\,t)$

$\mathbf{r}_1$ $\qquad$ $\mathbf{r}_2$

Figure 1-10 In genuine EEG experiments the actual recorded potential $V(\mathbf{r}_1,\mathbf{r}_2,t)$ is the potential difference between two locations $\mathbf{r}_1$ and $\mathbf{r}_2$. In this simulation the 1 Hz delta component included in the simulation shown in fig. 1-9 is common to both locations and does not appear in the recording.

23

in the interpretations of recorded data. We focus on the reference issue in chapters 2 and 7.

As implied by these simulations and shown in more detail in chapter 4, the dominant EEG frequencies below about 50 to 100 Hz are essentially the dominant modulation frequencies of synaptic action fields. Capacitive-resistive membrane properties provide low-pass filtering of these synaptic fields as a consequence of reducing mesoscopic source magnitudes, but this filtering appears to be small in the normal frequency range of EEG (below about 20 to 50 Hz).

We do not imply that EEG and synaptic field dynamic behavior are identical. Quite the contrary, we expect the neocortex to produce very complicated synaptic field dynamics that are never recorded on the scalp. This may include certain preferred frequency ranges as discussed in chapters 2, 9, and 10. Some of this "missing" dynamics may be recorded from inside the cranium. For example, relatively localized *dura* (outer brain membrane) potentials may not be sufficiently robust to appear on the scalp. But there is also a wealth of cortical dynamic behavior that cannot even be recorded on the dura. Potentials recorded inside the cranium generally depend on the size and location of the recording electrode, which determines *measurement scale*. Measurement scale is the region over which potentials are space-averaged, because of physical separation between sources and electrode, volume conduction smearing by cerebrospinal fluid (CSF) and skull (scalp potentials), or by the electrode of nonzero size (intracortical potentials).

What role is envisioned for *cell assemblies* within this conceptual framework? We view the cell assembly concept broadly here to indicate any group of neurons or neural masses (*minicolumns, corticocortical columns, macrocolumns,* and so forth) for which preferential interactions persist over time intervals of perhaps several tens of milliseconds or more. Defined this way, the existence of cell assemblies is noncontroversial, although their putative roles in behavior and cognition are poorly understood. Cell assemblies in neocortex appear more likely to form in contiguous structures as a result of dense intracortical connections, but cortical regions separated by large distances (say 10 to 20 cm) may evidently also interact preferentially. This latter idea is plausible because of the extreme interconnectedness of human brains, greatly facilitated by the numerous *corticocortical fibers* (fig. 1-2). For example, *the typical path length between any two cortical neurons is estimated to be only two or three synapses* (Braitenberg and Schuz 1991).

Given their broad definition here, cell assemblies could overlap so that, for example, one column could simultaneously be part of several cell assemblies. In this broad view of possibilities, cell assemblies could also have substantial hierarchical structures so that, for example, the 100 neurons in a minicolumn, the 100 minicolums in a corticocortical column, and (say) 10,000 *corticocortical columns* in remote cortical regions (connected by *corticocortical* or *association fibers*) could theoretically form cell assemblies at different spatial scales. However, our simple definition of synaptic action fields does not depend on such conjectures or even on the existence of cell assemblies or neural networks. *Synaptic fields cause the current sources that generate EEG and MEG irrespective of whether the active synapses are part of one or more cell assemblies.* Large scalp potentials occur because columnar dipole moments are lined up in parallel and synchronously active. There are many details to be discovered. However, the general causal connections F-1 (field-source) and 1-E (source-EEG) of fig. 1-8 appear to rest on relatively solid theoretical and experimental ground.

The synaptic synchrony requirement for large scalp potential production may favor somewhat the recording of synaptic sources that are parts of cell assemblies. However, several other source properties, apparently unrelated to cell assembly formation, are important for the relatively large scalp potentials that occur with spontaneous EEG or event related potentials. These properties include neuron geometry, synaptic distributions and source depth. The issues of overlapping and hierarchical assemblies further complicate the picture. Event related potential studies attempt to tie specific cognitive processes to averaged data. It may be argued that this averaging process tends to remove the influence of fields unrelated to the matching (time-locked) cell assembly that generates the evoked potential. Nevertheless, synaptic synchrony will still favor large evoked potentials. Furthermore, cell assembly dynamics are still expected to be influenced by synaptic fields. For these reasons, we are not generally justified in assuming that scalp EEG primarily records specific neural network activity (the A-1, 1-E path in fig. 1-8), perhaps in contrast to the hopeful views of some scientists. More generally, EEG may originate with a mixture of network and nonnetwork synaptic action. However, even if the cell assembly contribution A-1 to EEG is zero, correlations between EEG and behavior/cognition (E/B) could occur through the speculative connections A-F, F-1, 1-E in fig. 1-8. In chapter 11, we explore these ideas in more depth, including consideration of the conjecture that remote cell assemblies having no overlapping cells may become synchronized (phase locked) through resonant interactions between themselves or indirectly through global synaptic action fields.

These ideas address the so-called *binding problem* of brain science from the viewpoint of neocortical dynamics—the problem of how brains integrate disparate functions performed by different networks into coherent action and an (apparent) single consciousness. Our approach may be viewed loosely as a marriage of *Gestalt psychology* to *Hebbian neurophysiology*. However, unlike the abstract "fields" imagined by Gestalt psychologists, the synaptic action fields [$\Psi_e(\mathbf{r}, t)$ and $\Psi_i(\mathbf{r}, t)$] defined here have both a straightforward physiological interpretation and a direct connection to EEG measurements. The manner in which these synaptic fields may act on (top-down) or be acted on (bottom-up) by cell assemblies is, of course, quite speculative. Nevertheless, this approach has considerable precedent in other sciences, which further encourages our proposed conceptual framework. That is, many kinds of interactions between fields and the elements that make up the fields have been studied in sociology, economics, physics, and other disciplines. The field of *synergetics* (the science of cooperation), which deals generally with *complex systems* in this manner, is especially pertinent to brain dynamics (Haken 1983, 1987, 1999; Ingber 1995; Jirsa and Haken 1996; Uhl 1999). We return to synergetics as a relatively new way of thinking about thinking in chapter 11.

5 Currents and Potentials in Electric Circuits and Brains

A central problem for electroencephalography is to relate scalp data to brain *current sources* (*generators*). In a few applications like *focal epilepsy*, clinicians may be primarily interested in locating sources that are somewhat isolated, perhaps occupying something like 6 to 20 cm^2 of cortical surface. Or, perhaps cognitive scientists may identify specific brain regions producing large potentials associated with a particular cognitive task. However, most EEG phenomena appear to be generated by widely distributed sources, even if certain local regions (primary sensory cortex, for example) produce more consistent sources, thereby producing relatively large-magnitude waveforms in the time-averaged evoked potentials. In such cases, our goal is not localization of sources that may be anywhere and everywhere at a given time, but rather quantitative characterization of the dynamic behavior (perhaps at different scales) of multiple distributed sources. For convenience, we may view localized source activity (that generated in relatively localized cell assemblies) as a special case of generally distributed source activity. However, proper physiological interpretation of EEG data requires explicit indication of whether such localization is essentially instantaneous or refers to an average over longer times (seconds to minutes) as in the case of averaged evoked potentials.

Several concepts from electrical engineering illustrate basic source issues. Figure 1-11 shows two circuits. An *ideal voltage source* (an AC generator) is shown in (a). The circuit (b) contains an *ideal current source* (typically a separate circuit containing transistors and voltage sources). By "ideal" we mean that the magnitudes of voltage and current produced by each device are fixed properties; they are not affected by elements in the rest of the circuit (represented by the box X). Of course, this idealized representation cannot be universally valid. For example, if we open a switch in series with the current source so as to disconnect it from the rest of the circuit, its current must go to zero unless the source supplies enough power to cause electrons to jump the air gap in the switch (sparks). However, with proper source design, the ideal source assumption will be valid for any normal circuit elements in box X. The ideal voltage source

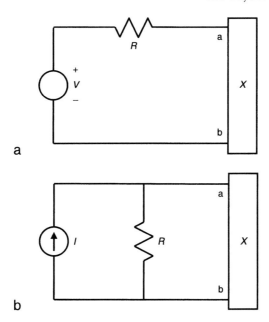

Figure 1-11 (a) A voltage source V in series with a resistor R is connected to an arbitrary electrical network represented by the box X. (b) A current source $I = V/R$ in parallel with the same resistor R is equivalent in the following sense: all the currents and voltages in the arbitrary electrical network represented by the box X (no matter how complicated) are the same when connected to either pair of ports (a, b), a result that follows from Thevenin's theorem of electrical engineering.

$(V = IR)$ in series with the resistor R is equivalent to the ideal current source I in parallel with the resistor R in the following sense. All the currents and voltages in the network represented by box X are unchanged by connecting the terminals of box X to either source circuit. This electric circuit principle (Thevenin's theorem) is valid irrespective of the complexity of the network in box X, which could contain hundreds of nonlinear circuit elements.

The equivalence of voltage and current sources also occurs in volume conductors. Small-scale electrophysiology is typically concerned with membrane potentials measured by micro- or mesoelectrodes. However, large-scale EEG data are more conveniently and intuitively related to multiple synaptic current sources produced within a macroscopic volume of tissue rather than voltage sources at complex membrane surfaces in volumes containing many cells. The current and voltage source descriptions can be regarded as equivalent in electrophysiology, just as they are in electric circuits.

An important aspect of macroscopic volume conduction of currents and potentials in brains is *linearity*. In this context, a macroscopic mass of tissue is said to be linear if *Ohm's law* is valid. For a circuit resistor of *resistance R*, Ohm's law is expressed as

$$V_1 - V_2 = RI \tag{1.3}$$

Here $V_1 - V_2$ is the potential difference across the terminals of the resistor, and I is the current through the resistor. By convention, positive current is defined as the direction of positive charge movement even though current in metal is composed of negative electron flux. By contrast, current in semiconductors is often carried by positive *holes*, that is, regions of missing electrons in a manner somewhat analogous to the flow of air bubbles in a liquid. By definition, electrons move in the direction opposite to the direction of positive current. Current moves from higher to lower potentials so positive I in (1.3) is consistent with V_1 being greater than V_2; current like water flows "downhill." We emphasize that *potential differences*, not "potentials" cause current flux, a common source of confusion in evaluating reference electrode effects by the EEG community.

In living tissue, the current carriers are positive and negative ions. The positive and negative ions move in opposite directions, and both contribute to measured current. Positive current is still defined as the direction of positive charge flow. *Impedance* is the AC equivalent of *resistance* and accounts for possible phase shifts due to capacitive and inductive properties of circuit elements. However, inductive effects are entirely negligible and capacitive effects are evidently very small in macroscopic neural tissue masses at interesting EEG frequencies (roughly 1 to 40 Hz) as indicated in appendix B. Thus, in this book we mostly use *impedance* and *resistance* interchangeably in applications of large-scale tissue volume conduction. However, even at macroscopic scales, capacitive effects may be important at electrode/tissue interfaces so the separate concept of impedance is required in such applications. Capacitive effects are, of course, critical at the microscale of individual cells.

Ohm's law in volume conductors is a more general statement than its usual form in electric circuits. It is a linear relationship between vector current density $\mathbf{J}$ (microamps per square millimeter or $\mu A/mm^2$) and the electric field $\mathbf{E}$ (microvolts per millimeter or $\mu V/mm$):

$$\mathbf{J} = \sigma\mathbf{E} \tag{1.4}$$

Here σ $(1/(\Omega \text{ mm})$ or Siemens/mm or S/mm) is the *conductivity* of the physical or biological material, typically used in mathematical models. *Resistivity* $\eta \equiv 1/\sigma$ (Ω mm) is a standard parameter mostly preferred by experimentalists. Note that when conductivity is a scalar, (1.4) is a vector equation, equivalent to three scalar equations in three directions. The simple, one dimensional version of Ohm's law (1.3) is easily obtained from (1.4) for the special case of current passing through a material of constant cross section as shown in fig. 1-12. Suppose current I is constant across the cross section (area A) of a conductor of resistivity η and length Δx, as in the case of 60 Hz current in the copper wire. In this example $\mathbf{J} = J_x\mathbf{i}$ and $\mathbf{E} = E_x\mathbf{i}$, where x indicates the direction of current and

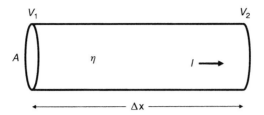

Figure 1-12 Cylindrical volume conductor of cross sectional area A composed of some conductive material with resistivity η (1/conductivity). Resistance (or impedance) to current flux I depends on both material and geometric properties of the conductor.

electric field and $\mathbf{i}$ is a unit vector in the x direction. The x component of current density is $J_x = I/A$ and electric field is $E_x \cong (V_1 - V_2)/\Delta x$. Substitution of these relations into (1.2) yields

$$V_1 - V_2 = \frac{\eta \Delta x I}{A} \qquad (1.5)$$

Comparison of (1.3) and (1.4) shows that the resistance of a wire or other cylindrical medium of resistivity η, length Δx, constant cross section A, and constant current density across the cross section is given by

$$R = \frac{\eta \Delta x}{A} \qquad (1.6)$$

Thus, *resistivity* is a basic property of the medium through which current passes and *resistance* depends on both medium and its geometric properties. By analogy, the volume of fluid that flows through a drain-pipe or blood vessel per second (*current*) depends on the pressure gradient (*voltage difference*), frictional force of fluid flowing over surface (*resistivity*), and geometry ($\Delta x/A$). Note that pressure difference not "pressure" causes fluid to flow in a manner analogous to voltage difference causing current flux.

Current flux in the head volume conductor involves several complications not normally present in simple circuits. The most obvious is that current spreads out from sources nonuniformly so that current density $\mathbf{J}(\mathbf{r}, t)$ at each location $\mathbf{r}$ is not generally constant over any cross section A. Also, head resistivity varies with type of tissue so that $\eta = \eta(\mathbf{r})$; that is, the medium is an *inhomogeneous* volume conductor. Here the scalar resistivity is expressed as a function of vector location $\mathbf{r}$; an alternative form is $\eta = \eta(x, y, z)$. Finally, tissue may be *anisotropic*, meaning that resistivity (or conductivity) is direction dependent. In white matter, for example, resistivity is evidently lower for current flux in directions parallel to axons. In anisotropic media, conductivity is a tensor (or matrix) with elements that may or may not be functions of location $\mathbf{r}$ (inhomogeneous or homogeneous).

In anisotropic conductors, Ohm's law (1.4) involves matrix multiplication. All serious volume conductor models of the head include major inhomogeneities (brain, CSF layer, skull, and scalp). However, because of the paucity of detailed experimental data and mathematical complexity of methods, today's head models nearly always assume isotropic tissue properties. Despite this approximation, head volume conductor models appear to provide good semiquantitative predictions of relations between intracranial sources and scalp potentials in most applications, as discussed throughout this book.

We should emphasize that despite the complications of conductive inhomogeneity and anisotropy, experiments indicate that living tissue is *linear* at macroscopic scales (at least for fields that are not too large). That is, Ohms law (1.4) is valid (but perhaps only in matrix form). This experimental fact is fully consistent with nonlinear conductive properties of active membranes because most externally applied current in a macroscopic mass of tissue (say 1 mm^3) flows through the extracellular fluid. Thus, we expect the addition of more cells to extracellular fluid to reduce the macroscopic conductivity of a tissue mass, but for it to remain linear. This means that *tissue resistivity can vary widely with measurement scale*. For example, a microelectrode with tip diameter of perhaps 10^{-3} to 10^{-4} cm may "see" only intracellular or extracellular fluid having substantially lower resistivity than a macroscopic tissue mass.

The fact that tissue is a linear conductor at macroscopic scales means that the principle of *superposition* is valid. That is, suppose current source I_1 at location $\mathbf{r_1}$ causes the potential V_1 at any location $\mathbf{r}$ on the head; current source I_2 at location $\mathbf{r_2}$ causes the potential V_2 at the same location $\mathbf{r}$, and so on to source I_n. Then the superposition principle says that if we "turn on" all sources $(I_1 + I_2 + \cdots + I_n)$ at the same time, the potential at location $\mathbf{r}$ will be the linear superposition or sum of individual potentials $(V_1 + V_2 + \cdots + V_n)$. Linearity of tissue also allows use of the *reciprocity theorem* as discussed in chapter 6. We emphasize that inhomogeneous and anisotropic tissue is expected to be linear; the word "linear" is not a synonym for "simple".

Ideal current sources in electric circuits can actually be composed of many circuit elements, including nonlinear elements. However, once the current source is fixed, this internal nonlinearity need not be considered in the large-scale circuit analysis. In an analogous manner, the macroscopic brain current sources discussed here are idealizations of complicated nonlinear processes at smaller scales. The number of synapses in a region roughly the size of a cortical macrocolumn (diameter ≈ 1-3 mm) is about 10^{10}. Microcurrent sources may occur near active synapses and near other parts of membranes to provide (return) current flow required to preserve current conservation. Some subset of these current sources will generally be correlated (*synchronous*) depending on the microscopic dynamical details of local cell groups. Our idealized macroscopic current sources represent space averages over such tissue volumes. We may expect macroscopic current source magnitudes to depend strongly on the degree of clustering of positive and negative microsources, as discussed in more detail in chapter 4.

6 Fluid Flow and Current Flux

In order is gain some insight into current flow in volume conductors, consider the analogy between fluid flow and electric current. The flow of fluid over an airplane wing in a wind tunnel and current in the volume conductor between the two metal plates are shown in fig. 1-13. It is customary to illustrate current flux by current lines that, in a homogeneous and isotropic conductor, have patterns identical to the electric field lines. At locations where the current density is largest, the lines of current are drawn closest together. Also, the current lines are everywhere perpendicular to the lines of constant electric potential (not shown).

When the material between the metal plates is a homogeneous and isotropic conductor, the lines of current flow are parallel and equally spaced; that is, the current density is constant everywhere between the plates, except for edge effects. If, however, an insulating body is placed between the plates as shown in fig. 1-13, the current must flow around the obstruction. One can visualize correctly that the current lines may then be squeezed together at locations close to the insulating body. It is often important to know in a quantitative way just how the current lines (and potential) are altered by the presence of the insulating body.

The lines of airflow (called *streamlines*) shown in fig. 1-13 are analogous to current lines. Every particle of air follows one of the streamlines around the wing. The volume of air crossing a unit cross-sectional area is largest

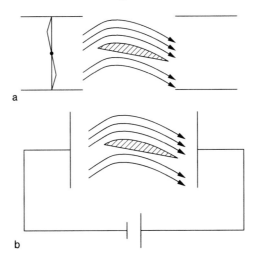

Figure 1-13 (a) Cross section of a wing placed in the test section of a wind tunnel. Arrows indicate air streamlines. (b) An insulating body placed in a conductive material between two metal plates. Arrows indicate current lines.

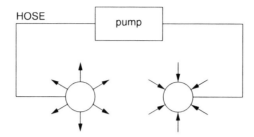

Figure 1-14 Spherical nozzles emit (source) and accept (sink) flow of some substance due to pump action. This source–sink combination is called a *dipole source*.

when the streamlines are closest together. The streamlines show the direction and magnitude of the airflow just as the current lines show the direction and magnitude of the current flow. In fact, to the extent that the air behaves as a *perfect fluid* and both the generator voltage and fan speed do not vary too rapidly with time, the pattern of streamlines around the wing is *identical* to the pattern of current lines around an insulating body of the same size and shape.

Consider now a different kind of air source, as shown in fig. 1-14. A hose is connected to an air pump. At each end of the hose are spherical nozzles with many small holes to allow air to flow in a radial direction from the nozzle surface. The pump forces air through the hose to the source on the left, through the air space between the nozzles, and into the sink (or negative source) on the right. It has proven convenient to use a single name for the source–sink geometry pictured in fig. 1-14. This source–sink combination is called *a dipole source*, an important concept in EEG applications.

Suppose now we replace the pump by an AC current source, the hose by an insulated wire and the nozzles by electrodes. If we then immerse the electrodes in a tank of conducting fluid as shown in fig. 1-15, the device consists of a *current source* $(+)$ and sink $(-)$, as indicated by the circuit on the left side of the tank. This circuit generates a potential field $\Phi(\mathbf{r}, t)$ in the salt water tank. If several conditions are met (refer to figure caption), we may record a small current $i(t)$ that is simply related to the potential difference $V_{12}(t)$ between tank locations $\mathbf{r}_1$ and $\mathbf{r}_2$.

If the stimulating electrodes are placed sufficiently close together, we speak of the combined source and sink as a *current dipole*. The current lines (solid) and lines of constant potential (dashed) for a dipole source are shown in fig. 1-16. These current lines are identical to the streamlines in a perfect fluid created by the pump of fig. 1-13. (The streamlines can, of course, be much more complicated if the fluid is not a perfect fluid.) This picture applies only to low-frequency fields. High-frequency fields cause a coupling between currents (or electric field) and an induced magnetic field. This leads to an alteration of the pattern of current flow pictured in fig. 1-16. When the field frequency is sufficiently low, magnetic induction is negligible. The currents still cause magnetic fields,

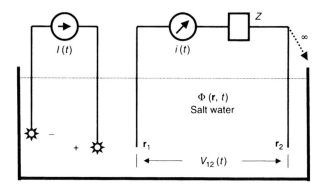

Figure 1-15 A current source $I(t)$ is used to inject AC current, thereby generating a potential field $\Phi(\mathbf{r}, t)$ in a salt water tank. A second circuit may be used to record potentials $V_{12}(t)$ at any location ($\mathbf{r}_1$) in the tank with respect to a "reference" electrode at another location ($\mathbf{r}_2$) provided that two conditions are met: (i) the series impedance Z is much larger than the impedance of the water plus electrode–water interfaces so that the small measured current $i(t)$ is simply related to $V_{12}(t)$; and (ii) the total impedance of the measuring circuit is not too large. That is, the current $i(t)$ must be large enough to meet the sensitivity requirement of the current instrument but small enough to avoid distorting the field $\Phi(\mathbf{r}, t)$. For example, if electrode $\mathbf{r}_2$ were removed from the water and attached to a perfectly insulating tank wall (dashed arrow), the measuring circuit resistance would be infinite and the current $i(t)$ zero. As a result, no potential would be recorded other than noise. The electrode ($\mathbf{r}_2$) will be a genuine reference only if placed sufficiently far from both stimulating electrodes and the recording electrode ($\mathbf{r}_1$). In this idealized case, the potential difference $V_{12}(t) = \Phi(\mathbf{r}_2, t) - \Phi(\mathbf{r}_1, t)$ will not change when $\mathbf{r}_2$ is moved to any other tank location that satisfies the same "far away" conditions. We can approximate this condition with a very large tank by placing electrodes far from the walls and water surface. However, in general, $V_{12}(t)$ depends on the location of both electrodes ($\mathbf{r}_1, \mathbf{r}_2$) and the reference electrode concept fails.

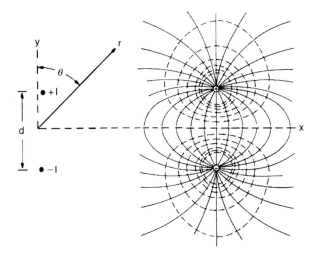

Figure 1-16 Current lines (solid) due to a current dipole source embedded in a conductive material are shown. Current density is highest when solid lines are closest together. Dashed lines are surfaces of constant potential. The current and potential patterns shown here are valid only if the medium is infinite (no boundary effects), homogeneous, and isotropic; however, the dipole concept is quite general.

33

but in the low-frequency approximation, such magnetic fields are uncoupled to the electric field and can be studied separately in MEG applications.

Finally, even when the field frequency is very high, the dipole pattern of current flow (and potential distribution) of fig. 1-16 is roughly accurate at locations close to the dipole. The electric field or potential not too far from the dipole is called the *near field*. Alternatively, the electric field pattern at very large distances from a high-frequency dipole generator is quite different from that shown in fig. 1-16. The potential at large distances is called the *far field* or *wave field*. The term *electromagnetic radiation* refers only to the *far field*. In appendix B, it is shown that all known practical problems in electrophysiology are low frequency in this context, that is, well below the megahertz range. The terms *near field* and *far field* as sometimes used in electrophysiology bear minimal resemblance to their precise definitions in the physical sciences. One never encounters a far field in electrophysiology. All potentials measured on the scalp have the same basic character (in the sense of this paragraph) regardless of whether they are generated in cortex or brainstem. Misuse of the term *far field* to describe potentials at locations "far away" from a source region is an illustration of noisy communication between physics/engineering and EEG.

7 Scalp Potentials and Electric Field Theory

How can theoretical input make a significant contribution to our understanding of the physiological basis for surface potentials? Perhaps we can obtain a tentative answers to this question in the context of locating sources of some EEG phenomenon, say the *auditory evoked potential* (AEP) and its early components known as the *brainstem auditory evoked response* (BAER). An auditory stimulus produces a potential variation with time in the midbrain that can be measured on the scalp with suitable techniques for averaging out spontaneous EEG and noise (biologic, environmental, and instrumental). A plot of the time course of scalp potential consists of at least 15 reproducible components in humans as shown in fig. 1-17. This phenomenon has clinical application since abnormality of a specific part of the BAER can be used to locate the origin of pathology. For example, abnormal delay between successive wave components may indicate reduced axon propagation speed in a specific part of the auditory nerve due to demyelination (as in *multiple sclerosis*). It is not certain to what degree the BAER reflects the passage of the compound action potential or synaptic potentials generated at the several relay stations between the auditory (VIIIth) nerve and cortex, although a stronger case for action potential origins is suggested in chapter 5.

One can imagine a number of experiments that may help to determine the origins of the BAER: for example, depth recordings from various

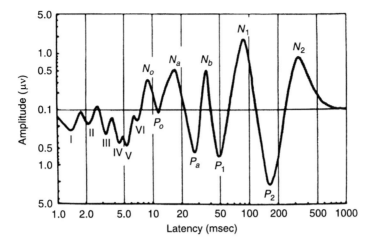

Figure 1-17 The auditory evoked potential waveform as recorded from the human scalp. A subject is presented with a series of up to several thousand tones or clicks and the time-locked EEG is averaged over the stimuli to remove the (much larger) spontaneous EEG. The first few ms of the waveform is also known as the brainstem averaged evoked response (BAER). Physiologists have assigned standard labels to each peak (N_1, P_2, and so forth). Reproduced with permission from Picton et al. (1974).

neural structures in the midbrain of an animal. From knowledge of the approximate magnitudes of these potentials, one can perhaps infer their expected magnitudes at the human scalp surface. This connection may not be so easy, however. The equations of electric field theory tell us that potentials at the surface depend on the nature of the current sources and the electrical properties of the medium. What anatomical or physiological features determine the current sources? How does the fall-off of potential with distance from a synapse differ from that of the action potential? How important is the geometrical arrangement of synapses within a nucleus in determining the magnitude of potential outside the nucleus? What about the relative sizes of different neural structures? How can we extrapolate the results of our experience with animal anatomy to that of human? What are the electrical parameters of the brain that have the most influence on the behavior of potentials? What about the effect of the skull and scalp? How can estimates of magnitudes of potential in an infinite, homogeneous medium be applied to a head surrounded by air? What can we infer from information about spatial distributions of potential over the scalp? Where should the electrodes be placed in order to maximize the information contained in the signal? What are the theoretical limits to the location of sources using surface potential information? Are the spatial properties of the BAER dependent on duration (or frequency) of the individual components?

Such questions need answers, but it is just not practical to obtain all the answers experimentally. In the absence of theory, the number of experiments required is far too large for all the physiologists and electro-encephalographers to accomplish in multiple lifetimes. A comprehensive

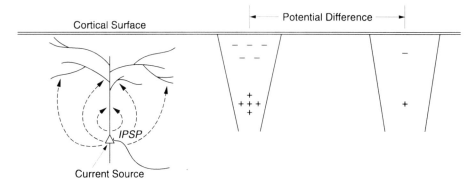

Figure 1-18 Synaptic action at membrane surfaces causes local current sources (or sinks) balanced by distributed sinks (or sources) in order to preserve current conservation. Inhibitory and excitatory synapses cause local sources and sinks, respectively. The negative surface potentials (with respect to depth or with respect to infinity) shown here may or may not be negative with respect to some other surface location.

theoretical approach is badly needed in EEG in order to construct the robust scientific framework needed for parsimonious experimental designs.

Consider how electric field theory can shed light on the basic questions surrounding the origin of scalp potentials. We know that the spatial properties of all potentials generated inside the head depend on the kind of current sources causing these potentials. The dipole source, for example, is clearly important in electrophysiology. Consider the effect of synaptic activity on a single neuron. An inhibitory synapse at the soma causes current to pass across the local membrane, through the extracellular fluid, across the dendritic and axon membranes, and back to the soma through the intercellular fluid, as shown in fig. 1-18. When viewed at the level of the single cell, this current distribution does not appear dipolar since the effective sources and sinks are distributed along the membrane surface. What then does this neuronal pattern of current flow have to do with our idealized dipoles? Here is one place where an elementary theory tells us something very important. At locations not too close to the neuron the details of the source distribution around a single neuron are not very important in determining the manner of fall-off of potential with distance. At distances larger than about three or four times the diameter of the local source region, the potential behaves as if it were produced by current flow between two poles. This is called the *dipole approximation*. It has been shown, for example, that the potential fall-off with distance from a midbrain structure (the superior olive) is approximately that of a dipole as outlined in chapter 5.

An important feature of a dipole is that it produces a potential in the surrounding medium that falls off as the inverse square of the distance (ignoring angular dependence for now). Thus, if we were to measure a potential of 25 μV at a distance of 1 cm from a dipole source, we would expect the potential due to the same dipole to be 1 μV at a distance of 5 cm. Of course, this inverse square law holds only in a homogeneous and isotropic medium; that is, in a conductor with conductivity constant in both location and current direction. We can, however, make estimates of the magnitudes of potentials based on the assumption of a homogeneous, isotropic medium and then estimate approximate corrections due to various tissue inhomogeneities.

How does the dipole concept fit known properties of cortical sources? Suppose we were to measure a potential of 100 μV at the top of the CSF. Might we imagine this potential to be generated by a single cortical dipole at a distance of 1 mm? How large should we expect the potential generated by this same dipole to be at the scalp surface? The inverse square law tells us to expect a potential of 1 μV at a distance of 1 cm. But this result appears to contradict experiment. We know that much of the EEG activity on the scalp is about 1/2 to 1/5 the magnitude of the corresponding cortical activity. It is true that we have not accounted for the effects of inhomogeneity, particularly those of the skull and finite size of the head. But these complications tend to *reduce* the estimate of scalp surface potential based on a homogeneous medium, so how can we reconcile the dipole idea with experimental EEG?

The dilemma above is resolved by realizing that we have made an incorrect choice of the *source* of the potential. Whereas the synaptic activity on a single neuron produces a dipole potential, the activity of many parallel and synchronously active neurons produces a potential due to the sum of all of them. We really have a layer (or sheet) of many dipoles. The potential fall-off with distance from a *dipole layer* is much slower than in the case of a single dipole. In fact, if the dipole layer involves many square centimeters of cortical surface, the magnitude difference between potentials at the cortical and scalp surfaces may be due *only* to the effects of tissue inhomogeneity, with no significant drop-off of potential due to increased distance from the source.

Many kinds of current sources (or source–sink geometries) exist in nature. Each one produces its own characteristic spatial behavior in the surrounding conductive medium. In order to understand the spatial behavior of potentials generated by neurons, electric field theory must be integrated with anatomical and physiological considerations. We must ask what effective sources and sinks most closely model the neural structure in question. It appears, for example, that much of the potential activity measured on the scalp can be pictured as originating from cortical dipole layers of various sizes and shapes, in and out of fissures and sulci.

Once the spatial behavior of the potential generated by a particular kind of source in a homogeneous medium is understood, we can consider the effects of inhomogeneity. Exact solutions for potentials generated in an inhomogeneous medium may require involved computations. However, there are many practical instances where approximate answers are of considerable value, particularly when partly supported by experimental data.

For example, suppose we suspect that a particular component of the human BAER is generated by the superior olivary nucleus (a deep brain auditory structure). We might first use depth recordings in cat to establish that the potential exhibits a dipolar behavior. Next, we may consider anatomical differences between the cat and human to scale our potential measurements to the human brain. Are potentials of this magnitude sufficiently large to be measured on the human scalp? It is easy to estimate the homogeneous potential at the location of the scalp; however, this estimate does not take into account the effects of various inhomogeneities.

We might guess correctly that the effect of the skull on a dipole current source is to cause a reduction in scalp potential over the homogeneous case, but by how much? Another important inhomogeneity is due to the fact that current is confined to the head; it cannot flow into the nonconducting space above the head (the electric field and potential, however, do extend into space). This current line compression near the surface actually *increases* the scalp potential over its homogeneous value. It is of interest to note that, when the source is near the midbrain, the effect of finite brain size is somewhat stronger than that of the skull. That is, the scalp surface potential due to a central dipole is roughly twice the potential that would have been generated by the same dipole in an infinite, homogeneous medium. If the dipole source is close to the surface, however, the effect of the skull on surface potential is stronger than that of finite volume conductor size. The *net* effect is a reduction to perhaps 1/4 the homogeneous potential. There are, of course, other important inhomogeneities in the head. White matter, gray matter, and CSF have different conductivities; some of their effects may be taken into account in more exact analyses.

8 Cortical Dipoles and Dipole Layers

Suppose a dipole current source is placed in an *infinite tank of salt water*. By the term "infinite" we just mean that all measurements of potential are obtained far away from tank walls and water surface as in fig. 1-15. In this case the potential $\Phi(r, \theta)$ in the tank at location (r, θ) in spherical coordinates can be expressed in terms of the current source I, separation of the electrodes d, and fluid conductivity σ, that is

$$\Phi(r, \theta) \cong \frac{Id \cos \theta}{4\pi\sigma r^2} \quad r \gg d \tag{1.7}$$

Here θ is the angle between the dipole axis and the radius vector **r**, as shown in fig. 1-19. Equation (1.7) is valid at locations **r** (measured from the center point of the two poles) that are "far" from the source region. In practice, "far" normally means $r > 3d$ or $4d$. A more accurate formula

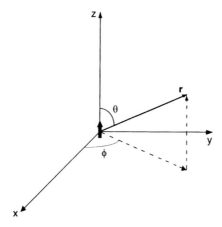

Figure 1-19 A dipole (either current or charge dipole) may be embedded in a material (either a conductor or dielectric) with the usual spherical coordinates (r, θ, ϕ) used to identify location. The potential in a conductive material generated by a current dipole is given exactly by (1.8) but is normally approximated by the more useful expression (1.7). Source symmetry about the vertical axis causes potentials to be independent of the angle ϕ in the absence of boundaries.

is based on the potentials of two monopoles located at distances r_1 and r_2 from the measuring point, that is

$$\Phi(r_1, r_2) = \frac{I}{4\pi\sigma}\left(\frac{1}{r_1} - \frac{1}{r_2}\right) \tag{1.8}$$

For example, if we approximate local current source flow from cortical layer III to layer VI in a single macrocolumn (or smaller structure), the pole separation is $d \approx 1$ mm. Suppose the current source is $I = 10$ μA and the medium is an infinite, homogeneous cortex ($\eta = \sigma^{-1} \approx 350$ Ω cm). At locations close to the source region, (1.8) for two monopolar sources is required to obtain the potential (with respect to infinity). Equations (1.7) or (1.8) may be used to predict potentials along the dipole axis ($\theta = 0$):

$$\Phi(r, 0) \cong 464 \text{ μV} \quad \text{at } r = 2.5 \text{ mm}$$

$$\Phi(r, 0) \cong 12 \text{ μV} \quad \text{at } r = 1.5 \text{ cm} \tag{1.9}$$

These estimates neglect the effects of the layers of CSF, skull, scalp, and air space above the dipole. As shown in chapter 6, the net effect of these layers of different conductivity is to reduce scalp potential due to a superficial cortical dipole to about 1/4 of the equivalent potential produced by the same sources in an infinite, homogeneous cortex. From these estimates, we can make a crude prediction of the ratio of scalp to cortical surface potential due to a dipole source in deep cortical layers. That is, for isolated cortical sources, the estimated ratio is (464)/(12/4), or roughly

$$\text{Cortical potential/scalp potential} \approx 100 \text{ to } 200 \tag{1.10}$$

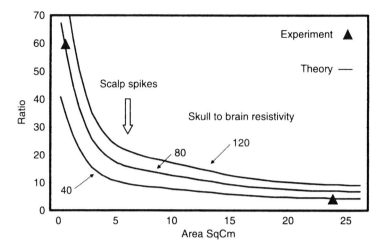

Figure 1-20 Theoretical estimates of the ratio of dura potential to scalp potential expressed as a function of "synchronous area" of active cortical sources. The three curves were generated by assuming cortical dipole layers of constant (mesoscopic) sources in the 3-sphere head model. The assumed skull to brain (or scalp) resistivity ratios are shown (40, 80, 120). The two triangles are the only available experimental points known to us (Abraham and Ajmone-Marsan 1958; Goldensohn 1979). The large arrow near the steep upturn in the curves indicates the clinical observation that epileptic spikes must be "synchronous" over at least 6 cm^2 of cortex in order be recognized on the scalp (Cooper et al. 1965; Ebersole 1997). Reproduced with permission from Nunez et al. (2001).

Many (if not most) EEG phenomena are generated by large numbers of correlated sources. In particular, if cortical sources are correlated over large distances parallel to the dura or scalp surface, scalp potential is due to the superposition of potentials due to each dipole source. We may model such cortical regions of correlated source activity as dipole layers with variable surface areas as discussed in more detail in chapters 5 and 6. Figure 1-20 shows the predicted ratio of cortical to scalp potential in a (three concentric spheres) head model as a function of area of the dipole layer on an idealized smooth cortex. The only two experimental points known to us are also plotted showing good qualitative agreement with the head model. Also shown is an arrow indicating that a dipole area of 6 cm^2 corresponds to a region of steep upward slope of the curves. This is consistent with the neurologist's rule that an epileptic spike must involve about 6 cm^2 of synchronously active "cortex" (normally meaning cortical gyri where recordings are obtained) in order to be recordable on the scalp. When the dipole area is small (less than about 1 cm^2), the cortical-to-scalp potential ratio is very large in qualitative agreement with the single-dipole estimates (1.9) and (1.10). By contrast, if a dipole layer is larger than about 10 or 20 cm^2, the ratio (1.10) is substantially reduced to

$$\text{Cortical potential/scalp} \approx 2 \text{ to } 5 \qquad (1.11)$$

Estimates (1.10) and (1.11) largely explain the following experimental observations:

(i) Root mean square amplitudes of spontaneous EEG recorded from cortex in the waking state are typically about 2 to 5 times the amplitude of simultaneously recorded scalp potentials (Penfield and Jasper 1954; Sem-Jacobsen et al. 1953; Cooper et al. 1965). These observations suggest that some focal epileptic spikes and evoked potentials from primary sensory cortex (over limited latency ranges) can apparently be crudely modeled as one or a few isolated dipoles, but, most EEG phenomena appear to originate from widely distributed sources.

(ii) At least 6 cm^2 of cortex must be synchronously active for cortical potentials (epileptic spikes for example) to be recorded on the scalp without averaging (Cooper et al. 1965; DeLucci et al. 1975; Ebersole 1997). We expect spontaneous cortical rhythms to be in the range of a few hundred microvolts based on cortical recordings in dogs (Lopes da Silva and Storm van Leeuwen 1978), cats (Abeles 1982), rabbits (Petsche et al. 1984), and humans (Cooper et al. 1965). This is consistent with fig. 1-20 since a potential range of 100 to 200 µV on the cortex implies roughly 20 to 100 µV on the scalp if the sources are widespread, but closer to 1 µV if the source is an isolated cortical dipole. Expressed another way, if a scalp alpha rhythm of 40 µV amplitude were generated by a few isolated dipoles, we would expect to record cortical potentials in the several millivolt range near the sources, based on the estimate (1.10). To the best of our knowledge, no such "super alpha" sources have been reported using macroelectrodes.

(iii) The amplitudes of alpha and sleep rhythms recorded from several centimeters deep within the brain have similar magnitudes to cortical surface potentials (Sem-Jacobsen et al. 1953). That is, no sharp increase of potential with inward movement of electrodes is evident as would be expected from deep, isolated cortical sources. In fact, potential appears to remain constant or fall off gradually with inner movement of electrodes from cortex. This is qualitatively consistent with large cortical dipole layers as the sources of such potentials.

(iv) Alpha rhythm has been recorded from a large population of epilepsy surgery patients over almost the entire upper surface of neocortex, excluding only regions near the central motor strip as indicated in fig. 1-5 (Jasper and Penfield 1949; Penfield and Jasper 1954). Widespread coverage of neocortex was not obtained in individual subjects in these studies. However, the most likely explanation for these data involves widely distributed cortical sources in each subject.

(v) In the resting alpha state, EEG frequency spectra recorded simultaneously on (subdural) cortex and scalp are similar in the range 0–15 Hz. However, much more beta activity (15–30 Hz) is recorded on the cortex (Pfurtscheller and Cooper 1975), perhaps suggesting some sort of low-pass filtering effect in tissue. However, passive temporal filtering by tissue is not consistent with published experiments or any obvious theoretical mechanism in volume conductors. Confirming this observation, these same scientists implanted dipole sources in the subject and varied current source frequency between 2 and 25 Hz. The attenuation of these signals at the scalp was independent of frequency, establishing that tissue does not act as a passive temporal filter in this frequency range.

(vi) Another explanation for the observations of paragraph (v) is clearly required. In chapter 9 we present data indicating that as temporal frequencies in the eyes-closed resting state increase from about 10 to 30 Hz in scalp data, average spatial frequencies also tend to increase. Such spatial-temporal dynamic correspondence is a near universal property of standing or traveling waves in closed systems. While the reasons for this dynamic behavior in neocortex may be controversial, ultimately they must be rooted in cortical interaction mechanisms as discussed in chapter 11. If this property of neocortical dynamics is accepted (based only on experiment with no commitment to any particular theory), we expect temporal filtering as an indirect consequence of spatial filtering by the volume conductor. That is, higher temporal frequency bands tend, on the average, to be associated with progressively smaller patches of correlated sources as temporal frequency increases. The smaller dipole layers associated with higher spatial frequencies (implying higher temporal frequencies) are more strongly attenuated as indicated in fig. 1-20, thereby accounting for observed EEG differences between cortex and scalp in the alpha state.

9 The Reference Electrode

An ongoing issue for both spontaneous and evoked potentials concerns the choice of electrode placements. Which are more suitable in a given experiment, bipolar or reference recordings? How does the reference affect physiological interpretations of EEG data? In attempting to settle such questions, much of the difficulty originates with a misunderstanding of the basic concept of electric potential. One may state that the potential at point r_1 in fig. 1-15 is (say) 10 μV, but the absolute value of this potential has no physical meaning. When we say that the potential at point r_1 is 10 μV, we often mean that the *difference* of potential between point r_1 and another point at *infinity* is 10 µV. By "infinity" we mean a location that is "far" from all sources of potential in an electrical sense. Thus, in actual measurements one might place one electrode near the sources of potential and a second electrode (the so-called "reference") at a much larger distance from all sources. For example, the electrode ($\mathbf{r}_2$) in fig. 1-15 will be a genuine reference only if placed sufficiently far from both stimulating electrodes and the recording electrode ($\mathbf{r}_1$). In this idealized case, the potential difference $V_{12}(t) = \Phi(\mathbf{r}_1, t) - \Phi(\mathbf{r}_2, t)$ and recorded potentials will not change significantly when $\mathbf{r}_2$ is moved to any other location that satisfies the same "far away" conditions. However, because all current is confined to the tank, the there may be no location in the tank that qualifies as a genuine reference. In general, $V_{12}(t)$ depends on the location of both electrodes ($\mathbf{r}_1$, $\mathbf{r}_2$) and the reference electrode concept fails.

One obvious trouble with this procedure in EEG applications is that we do not generally have prior knowledge of source locations. If the so-called *reference electrode* is placed anywhere near the head, we do not usually know in advance that it is (electrically) far enough from all sources to be considered a so-called *quiet reference* (a hopeful term long popular in EEG). If our EEG machine measured potential differences directly, a possible solution to the reference problem might be to place one electrode on the scalp and the reference electrode on, say, a distant wall of the laboratory ("infinity") as indicated in fig. 1-21. Of course, this procedure will not work. Our EEG machine would measure zero potential difference (or just

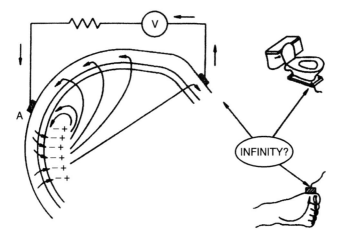

Figure 1-21 Current and potentials in the head are shown here as generated by a posterior source region. The voltage sensor V does not measure voltage directly; rather it measures the current in some measuring circuit. This measuring current (and the implied voltage) always depends on the location of both electrodes. Modern amplifiers allow accurate recording of scalp potentials when the resistance in the measuring circuit is very large. However, if one electrode (the "reference") is located off the body, the measuring circuit will have infinite resistance and no current due to brain sources will be measured. Thus, in EEG practice, one never measures potentials with respect to "infinity" and the common idea that one electrode may be characterized as "the reference" is typically misleading as illustrated in fig. 1-15.

noise) between the two locations even though the actual potential difference is far from zero. We must face the fact that our EEG machine actually measures the deflection of some recording needle, which is proportional to the current in the measuring circuit as shown in fig. 1-15. The measured current can then be related to a potential difference only when the resistance of the path for current flow between the two electrodes is sufficiently low. If the resistance of the current path between electrodes is too large, current through the measuring circuit will be too small to meet the sensitivity requirement of our instrument. This fact is, of course, well known by EEG technicians, who must often scrape a little dead skin off the scalp in order to lower the so-called *electrode resistance* (actually, the resistance of the electrode–gel–scalp interface plus the head). The resistance of this path (say 5 to 20 kΩ) must be sufficiently lower than the input impedance of the amplifiers.

Even if we could measure the potential difference between a point on the head and infinity (or the laboratory wall), we would not be interested in the result. Various noise sources from the environment cause the body potential to oscillate with time with voltages (with respect to infinity) many times larger than EEG magnitudes. This can be an important problem at power line frequencies (50 or 60 Hz, depending on country), but such external noise sources can also occur in other frequency ranges. Thus, in EEG applications, we are not really interested in scalp potential with respect to infinity. If the body is not located too close to the external electromagnetic sources, potentials induced by these environment sources will tend to be relatively constant over the body surface in the low-frequency range of EEG. This is a consequence of the fundamental property of electromagnetic fields—low temporal frequencies correspond to very low spatial frequencies.

For the above reasons, two electrodes on the head may not record environmentally generated potentials, even if the head potential with respect to infinity is quite large. Furthermore, by measuring potential differences on the head, any artifact generated by the body that produces relatively constant potentials over the head tends to be canceled. We help this measuring process by passing scalp currents through differential amplifiers that are grounded to a location close to the two recording electrodes. The grounding assists the common-mode rejection properties of the amplifier by allowing it to more accurately measure differences of potential between two recording electrodes (Cadwell and Villarreal 1999). The usual idea of a so-called EEG "reference electrode" is somewhat misleading. It is more accurate to think in terms of two recording electrodes, with the amplifier ground considered a sort of "reference." The use of shielded rooms will, of course, help to reduce the magnitude of the environment potentials but not artifact generated by the body.

In the case of isolated sources in the cortex, the usual concept of an EEG reference electrode on the head may be approximately valid. In this special case, the "recording" electrode may be located at a distance of perhaps

1 to 3 cm from a local cortical source, whereas an electrode on the opposite ear may be 10 cm or more distant. The EEG may then be sensitive to small movements of the "recording" electrode relative to sources, but fairly insensitive to movements of the "reference" electrode. It is only in this sense that we can make a distinction between recording and reference electrodes on the scalp. Clearly, such distinctions become blurred if the sources occupy large areas of cortex, are located in the midbrain or *mesial* (underside) cortex or have unknown locations.

Actually, the problem of distinguishing "reference" and "recording" electrodes is even more severe than implied by the paragraph above. There is more to the question than actual distances between source and electrodes. As shown in chapters 6 and 7, the effect of the skull is to make the current flux from a source much more widespread on the scalp than would occur in a homogeneous medium. When an electrode is (say) 1 or 2 cm from a source, but separated by high-resistivity skull tissue, it is actually much further away from the source in an electrical sense. That is, the electrical concept of a "distant" reference depends on the relative resistances of different current paths. Furthermore, we expect some tendency for current from brain sources to be focused through holes in the skull, low resistance CSF paths or both, possibly increasing local scalp potential due to distant sources. Thus, one might be careful about using the ear or nose as a reference. Another consideration is the possibility of mesial (underside) cortical sources that may contribute substantially to ear, nose, or mastoid potentials, as discussed in chapter 2.

The search for a so-called *quiet reference*, a sort of mini-holy grail of early EEG studies, has extended as far as the toe. It is argued in chapter 7 that, aside from the introduction of more EKG artifact, the toe reference is roughly equivalent to a reference on the neck. This may satisfy, in a limited sense, the requirements of a reference point. However, as a general rule, the position of *both* electrodes determines the EEG, and the concept of reference electrode for scalp recordings is of very limited value. The reference issue is discussed further in chapters 2, 7, and 8. The Laplacian estimate of dura potential (chapter 8) is reference-independent, providing additional incentive to employ this measure.

10 Philosophical Conflicts

This introductory chapter begins the task of bridging communication gaps between the distinct scientific cultures represented by clinician, cognitive scientist, physiologist, engineer, physicist, computer scientist, and mathematician whose disparate backgrounds converge on EEG work. Later, we will be concerned with the specifics of electric field behavior in the brain. Many such connections may be of practical use in EEG research. Unfortunately, the real obstacles to meaningful communication between disparate sciences cannot be overcome by simply redefining terms or by the introduction of mathematics into EEG. Problems exist at the more fundamental level of philosophical differences of approach to science. Scientists with different backgrounds often think differently, and the ultimate usefulness of the following chapters very much depends on facing up to this fact. Some of the differences are brought out by the following ratio:

$$\frac{\text{Time spent in preparation and performance of an experiment}}{\text{Time spent deciding which experiments are worth doing}}$$

This ratio seems much larger in EEG research than in physics or engineering. In the physical sciences, well-developed theories suggest experiments that are most likely to illuminate natural phenomena. In engineering, cost considerations nearly always ensure that theoretical models are developed before hardware. Engineers who fail to follow this approach tend to be eliminated by *marketplace natural selection*. In fact, many physicists and engineers believe that any *experiment that lacks a good theoretical basis is probably not worth doing*. Upon hearing of a usual experimental observation, one famous physicist is reported to have asked, "Has this data been confirmed by theory?" Of course, if this restriction on experiments were applied to EEG, its voluminous data output would be sharply curtailed. EEG theory is still in a relatively primitive state so the choice of experiments must be, of necessity, less systematic than in the physical sciences.

Although electric field theory has played a critical role in the development of physiology at the single neuron level (Cole 1968; Rall 1997; Segev et al. 1995), the relationship of theory to research on scalp EEG has been more tenuous. Certainly, physical science has had an impact: Modern machines measure and record the EEG. Data analysis is accomplished by computer. But these technological advances should not be confused with the input of fundamental ideas of electric fields and currents in inhomogeneous media. During much of the period 1930–1970 or 1980, scientists with strong physics or engineering backgrounds made minimal contribution to large-scale (scalp) EEG. Perhaps the attitude of the EEG establishment was partly responsible the slow development of a solid physical foundation for EEG research. Consider, for example, the following statement by one of the famous EEG pioneers W. Grey Walter (1961):

> When the system is homogeneous (that is, consists of identical or indistinguishable units) and when the interaction between units or systems is smoothly graded over the range of observations, a mathematical or logical description is adequate and explicit. But in biological systems, particularly in the very complex ones such as the human brain, we cannot

assume either homogeneity or linearity, and conventional mathematics is of limited value.

Although it would be inaccurate to ascribe the above opinion to all electroencephalographers, variations on this theme have often been repeated at EEG conferences (not to mention study sections making grant funding decisions). The philosophy expressed by Grey Walter's statement would seem to lie at the heart of communication barriers between electroencephalographers and physical scientists. A physicist or engineer may feel lost without equations to provide concise, unambiguous quantitative information. Equations provide a mental picture of physical phenomena that cannot be conveyed with mere words. They are the physical scientist's book of anatomical drawings, the detailed map, the tools of the trade. The equations provide the principal guidelines for choice of experiment and details of experimental design. Walter's heresy (from a physical scientist's viewpoint) must be examined closely because, if taken too seriously, the practical value of many of the following chapters of this book would be in considerable doubt.

Prospective physiologists or electroencephalographers typically take a series of elementary physics courses and later confine their studies mostly to biology. Their elementary physics courses are mostly concerned with homogeneous, linear systems. It is then perhaps not surprising that, lacking more advanced physics or engineering experience, they are left with a distorted picture. Simple systems are studied first in physics and engineering for obvious reasons. One must learn the easy material before moving on to more advanced study. There are, in fact, a large number of inhomogeneous physical systems for which our understanding is excellent. The entire field of *quantum mechanics* is concerned with probability waves in inhomogeneous media. There are experiments in the field of quantum electrodynamics which are in agreement with theory to an accuracy of one part in 10^7. Much of the industrial efforts of engineers and applied physicists are directed toward the understanding of electromagnetic radiation, plasma waves, ocean waves, seismic waves, and so forth in inhomogeneous media. Thus, the idea that the inhomogeneity of the brain itself distinguishes it from physical media is absurd.

The question of linearity is more complicated. There is no question that both linear and nonlinear processes are important in the brain. The subthreshold membrane behaves as a linear conductive medium. When its transmembrane potential approaches threshold, the neuron exhibits a conductive nonlinearity that makes possible the propagation of action potentials. However, even in this active state, the capacitive properties of the membrane seem to remain linear (Cole 1968). Furthermore, the volume conducted field of the action potential, which extends from nerve fiber to the surrounding tissue, is apparently well described by a linear equation. Over the past 30 years, the senior author has often been informed by pundits that "the brain is nonlinear." However, this statement conveys only minimal information. The question of brain linearity depends on context and the level of brain hierarchy addressed.

The question of linearity in the brain is at least partly analogous to similar questions of physical media. Consider, for example, a room full of air molecules. The interaction of two molecules is described by the linear Schrödinger equation of quantum mechanics. The interaction of a large number of molecules is described statistically by the nonlinear Boltzmann equation. If the air is not too tenuous, its movement can be described by the nonlinear Navier–Stokes equations of fluid mechanics. There are a number of applications, including the flow of air over an airplane wing (external to the inner boundary layer), for which these nonlinear fluid equations can be accurately reduced to linear equations. It is only in mathematics that a sharp distinction exists between "linear" and "nonlinear" systems. Genuine physical systems typically exhibit both kinds of behavior. Shock waves, shallow water waves, large-amplitude vibrations of structures like bridges and airplane wings, black holes, nonlinear electric circuits, and the propagation of the action potential are just some of the nonlinear phenomena that have been extensively studied, especially since the 1970s and 1980s when fast computers became more readily available. Clearly, it is invalid to associate nonlinearity only with biological systems.

It is often said that *physicists oversimplify biology*. But it must be pointed out that physicists (and engineers) also oversimplify physics. That is, they construct models of systems that contain only a small part of the real system. Once the simple system is understood, a little more is added to the model and the effects of these new complications are considered. Experience has shown that we can learn much about real physical systems from theoretical models, even though such models often neglect much that is inherent in the real systems. Thus, nonlinear systems are often studied by first obtaining a deep understanding of a similar linear system that mimics the genuine system in very special circumstances. In the following chapters, we first consider various kinds of current sources in a homogeneous and isotropic medium. Later the complication of inhomogeneity is added. In this way we can hope for a rough, semi-quantitative picture of how electric fields behave in brain, skull, and scalp.

The early chapters of this book deal with electric field theory, thereby serving as a foundation for the discussions of practical EEG problems in the later chapters. Although many practicing electroencephalographers may not wish to concern themselves with this theoretical basis, progress in EEG research is clearly dependent on *someone* having such concerns. Let us finally dispel of any notion that the *theoretical* is opposite to the *practical*. An excellent example of the critical importance of theoretical studies to practical outcomes is provided by the development of the science of fluid mechanics over the past century. We consider this story, hoping that it may provide insight into the scientific method and technological development generally, and more specifically to the importance of theory in EEG.

While sitting in an airplane, we may have looked out at the flexing wing and thought "I hope the aeronautical engineers knew what they were doing." The earliest airplane designers were not necessarily engineers or scientists. Some simply tried many new designs. Although we admire such heroic efforts, we must remember that the trial-and-error method has very serious limitations. It is one thing to build a small wood and cloth airplane that travels at low altitude and slow speeds. It is quite another to build a large plane that must fly over a wide range of speeds at both sea level and at high altitudes where the air is quite thin. It can be safely stated that without developments that took place in the science of fluid mechanics in the late 19th and early 20th centuries, there would be *no airplane travel* in the modern sense.

To illustrate the importance of the theory of fluid mechanics, let us imagine ourselves as early airplane designers with little knowledge of theory. Our imagined airplane must fulfill certain minimum requirements. In order to fly, the lift force developed by airflow over the wings must exceed the weight of the airplane. Also, the drag force must not be so large that the engine cannot bring our airplane to the desired speed. There are many other requirements, but considerations of the lift and drag will, in themselves, be quite complex. We may realize intuitively that the lift force depends on the cross-sectional shape of the wing. Air flowing over the top of the wing must move at a higher speed than the air flowing over the bottom so as to create a low-pressure region on top. The drag force is more difficult to understand. There will be resistance to the motion of the plane because of the air impinging on surfaces perpendicular to the flow. There will also be another kind of drag force due to friction between the air and the surface of the plane. Suppose that we have a particular wing in mind and wish to measure its lift and drag. We can build a physical model of the wing and put it into a wind tunnel. The wind tunnel is a circular chamber through which air is forced by a large fan. It contains a section for placing the wing model, so that forces, pressures, and air velocities at various locations along the surface can be measured, as shown in fig. 1-13.

When we try to apply the results of such measurements to our imagined airplane, substantial problems become evident. Our model wing is actually much smaller than the real wing, which would require a very large wind tunnel and be prohibitively expensive. How do we apply the values of lift and drag obtained in the laboratory experiment to the much larger airplane wing? But this is only the beginning of our troubles. Our wind tunnel contains air at sea level, but we wish to know the lift and drag when our plane is flying at various altitudes where the air has much different properties. The density, pressure, temperature, and viscosity are all quite variable with altitude. What do changes in these parameters do to lift and drag? What about the speed of our airplane? It is true that we can vary the air speed in the wind tunnel and measure the resulting effects on lift and drag, but how many measurements must be made? Can we assume that the variation of lift and drag with airflow velocity is smooth so that only a reasonable number of measurements need be made? Or must we consider the possibility of abrupt changes in lift with small speed changes? Suppose this same wing shape were to be used on a boat as a hydrofoil? Are any of our wind tunnel results applicable to water flow?

Considering all the uncertainties implicit in relating our wind tunnel results to the real airplane, we might well decide to forgo the wind tunnel experiments altogether. We might then go ahead and build our plane based on some intuitive feeling for shape, size, and strength, but even if we are lucky enough to produce a product that actually gets off the ground, our trial and error airplane will leave much to be desired. It is unlikely that we have even come close to building the most efficient machine. It will certainly require excess fuel to stay up. More importantly, we cannot predict how our plane will behave under the varying conditions of speed, attitude, and weather. Flying in our trial-and-error plane is likely to be quite dangerous.

Perhaps several accidents involving trial-and-error planes will motivate us to turn to the science of fluid mechanics. The flow of a viscous fluid over our airplane wing is described by the Navier–Stokes equations. These are a very complicated set of nonlinear differential equations, which have never been solved in the most general sense. They relate flow velocities, pressures, and frictional forces. If we were mathematicians, we might first try to obtain solutions to these equations. However, we are not mathematicians, we are airplane designers. Thus, we choose to become theoreticians for the early design stage. We are then interested in mathematics only to the extent that it can help build better airplanes. Rather than try to solve the equations, we simply take a close look at each of the individual parts of the equations and consider their physical significance. Without too much difficulty, we see that the lift and drag of a wing of a given shape depends on exactly four parameters: the size of the wing, the air velocity, the air density, and the air viscosity. This knowledge represents an enormous step forward. We have gone from knowing almost nothing about lift and drag to knowing quite a bit. We are still a long way from solving our problems of airplane design, but at least now we know some of the right questions to ask with our wind tunnel experiments.

If wings of various sizes (but fixed shape) are to operate over a wide range of velocity, air density, and air viscosity, prediction of lift and drag will depend on obtaining a large number of measurements. Let us suppose that we require 100 data points to cover the range of each parameter. We make lift and drag measurements for 100 different flow velocities in our wind tunnel. However, for each velocity, we must consider 100 different wing sizes, 100 different air densities, and 100 different viscosities. The total number of measurements required to cover the range of all four parameters is $(100)^4 = 10^8$ measurements, for each wing shape!

Even if it were possible to make a new measurement every minute for 24 hours every day, it would take us over 200 years to complete our task.

This experience has finally cured our addiction to experiments lacking genuine theoretical bases. We return to the Navier–Stokes equations, and a little manipulation shows us something rather amazing (Schlichting 1960). Although the lift and drag of a wing of a given shape depend on four parameters, the four parameters can be combined into a *single nondimensional parameter*, called the *Reynolds number*:

$$R_e = \frac{\rho v L}{\mu} \tag{1.12}$$

The Reynolds number is simply the product of the air density ρ, the air velocity v, and the wing scale L, divided by the air viscosity μ. The lift and drag depend only on this parameter. If two wings of different size but the same shape and length are operating at different air density, velocity, and viscosity, the lift and drag of the wings will be equal as long as the Reynolds number for each is equal. Thus, we can predict lift and drag for wings of various sizes operating over a wide range of conditions by making only 100 measurements instead of 10^8. We can even relate our wind tunnel results to the lift and drag of a hydrofoil. Although the density and viscosity of water is quite different from that of air, water flow also satisfies the Navier–Stokes equations. The lift and drag of our wing in airflow of a certain velocity will be equal to that produced by a hydrofoil of the same shape at a somewhat slower velocity. This slower velocity is determined by the condition that the Reynolds number for the two flows be equal. Thus, we have used the Navier–Stokes equations to transform the field of "seat of the pants" airplane design into a science, and we have done this without ever solving the equations!

We will, of course, want to do a number of experiments to make sure that we have correctly applied the Navier–Stokes equations to our airplane wing. Once this is accomplished, we are ready to go to the next step— solving the equations. Such solutions will tell us values for the lift and drag of an airplane wing of a given length, cross-sectional shape, and Reynolds number. Solving the Navier–Stokes equations thus represents our second major step forward in the field of airplane design. Intuitive feelings based on past experience will suggest that certain kinds of wings will deliver the performance desired in a particular kind of airplane. Now we can check this intuition with mathematics, perhaps discarding many potential designs as impractical. Once we have settled on several candidates, wind tunnel experiments will determine the final selection.

A deeper understanding of the fluid mechanics of airplane design depends on our ability to solve the equations; thus a summary of the historical development of practical mathematical methods in fluid mechanics is of interest (Schlichting 1960). Towards the end of the 19th century the science of fluid mechanics began to develop in two directions that had practically no points in common. On one side was theoretical hydrodynamics, which described the flow of a frictionless fluid. Elegant mathematical solutions were obtained, but unfortunately these solutions stood in glaring contradiction to experimental results. In particular, the mathematics had little relevance to the important problems of pressure losses in pipes or the drag of a body moving through fluid. For this reason, engineers, prompted by the need to solve the important problems arising from the rapid progress in technology, developed their own highly empirical field of hydraulics. The mathematicians and engineers had little contact.

At the beginning of the 20th century, these two divergent branches of fluid mechanics were unified by the famous German engineer Ludwik Prandtl. It had been long suspected that the major reason for the discrepancy between the mathematical solutions and the experiments was due to the neglect of fluid friction in the mathematics. However, owing to the great mathematical difficulties connected with the solution of these nonlinear equations (long before the development of computers), theoretical descriptions of fluid motion had not been obtained. Prandtl's genius was to show that the flow about a solid body can be artificially divided into two regions: a very thin layer close to the body (the *boundary layer*) where friction plays an essential part and the remaining region outside this layer where friction may be neglected. By this approach, Prandtl introduced a fictitious *inhomogeneity* into the mathematics in order to overcome the fundamental problem of *nonlinearity*. His solutions achieved a high degree of correlation between theory and experiment that paved the way for the remarkable success of fluid mechanics in the past century.

Considering the lack of connection between much of the current mathematics of EEG, neural networks, and other so-called "brain theory" to experimental results, one would love to mimic some of the success of 19th century fluid mechanics. In the following chapters, we pursue this goal vigorously.

11 Brain Volume Conduction versus Brain Dynamics

The physical aspects of EEG are naturally separated into two mostly disparate areas of study, *volume conduction* and *brain dynamics* (or more specifically, *neocortical dynamics*). The first area is concerned with the relationships between current sources in the brain (the so-called "EEG generators") and the scalp potentials that they produce. The fundamental laws (charge conservation and Ohm's law) that govern volume conduction are well known, although their application to EEG is nontrivial. The time variable in these laws is essentially a parameter such that the time dependence of EEG at any location is just the weighted space average of the time dependencies of all contributing brain sources. The fact that EEG waveforms can look quite different at different scalp locations and be quite different when recorded inside the cranium is due only to different weights given each brain source in the linear sum of contributions. The resulting simplification of both theory and practice in EEG is substantial. This important idea of linear superposition of source effects represents one dry island in the sea of brain ignorance. It is to be treasured in a manner similar to the Reynolds number in fluid mechanics.

The issue of brain dynamics, that is, the origins of time-dependent behavior of brain current sources producing EEG, is quite a different story. While a number of plausible physiologically based mathematical theories have been developed, we are far from a comprehensive theory. Nevertheless, even very approximate, speculative or incomplete dynamic theories can have substantial value in the formation of a conceptual framework for brain function. We have considered several such theories in earlier publications (Nunez 1995, 2000a,b) and revisit this issue in chapter 11. This book mainly considers brain dynamic behavior when this topic clearly overlaps volume conduction, medical issues, or cognitive science. Most advances in our understanding of the dynamic behavior of neural sources must be left to future generations.

References

Abeles M, 1982, *Local Cortical Circuits*, New York: Springer-Verlag.

Abraham K and Ajmone-Marsan C, 1958, Patterns of cortical discharges and their relation to routine scalp electroencephalography. *Electroencephalography and Clinical Neurophysiology* 10: 447–461.

Adrian ED and Mathews BHC, 1934, The berger rhythm: potential changes from the occipital lobe in man. *Brain* 57: 355–385.

Basar E, Schurmann M, Basar-Eroglu C, and Karakas S, 1997, Alpha oscillations in brain functioning: an integrative theory, *International Journal of Psychophysiology* 26: 5–29.

Berger H, 1929, Uber das Elektroenzephalorgamm des Menschen. *Arch. Psychiatr. Nervenk.* 87: 527–570.

Braitenberg V and Schuz A, 1991, *Anatomy of the Cortex: Statistics and Geometry*, New York: Springer-Verlag.

Cadwell MJ and Villarreal RA, 1999, Electrophysiological equipment and electrical safety. In: MJ Aminoff (Ed.), *Electrodiagnosis in Clinical Neurology*, 4th Edition, New York: Churchill Livingstone, pp. 15–33.

Cole K, 1968, *Membranes, Ions and Impulses*, Berkeley: University of California Press.

Cooper R, Winter AL, Crow HJ, and Walter WG, 1965, Comparison of subcortical, cortical, and scalp activity using chronically indwelling electrodes in man. *Electroencephalography and Clinical Neurophysiology* 18: 217–228.

Delucchi MR, Garoutte B, and Aird RB, 1975, The scalp as an electroencephalographic averager. *Electroencephalography and Clinical Neurophysiology* 38:191–196.

Destexhe A and Sejnowski TJ, 2001, *Thalamocortical Assemblies*, New York: Oxford University Press.

Ebersole JS, 1997, Defining epileptogenic foci: past, present, future. *Journal of Clinical Neurophysiology* 14: 470–483.

Freeman WJ, 1975, *Mass Action in the Nervous System*, New York: Academic Press.

Goldensohn ES, 1979, Neurophysiological substrates of EEG activity. In: DW Klass and DD Daly (Eds.), *Current Practice of Clinical Electroencephalography*, New York: Raven Press, pp. 421–439.

Haken H, 1983, *Synergetics. An Introduction*, 3rd Edition, Berlin: Springer.

Haken H, 1987, *Advanced Synergetics*, 2nd Edition, Berlin: Springer.

Haken H, 1996, *Principles of Brain Functioning: A Synergetic Approach to Brain Activity, Behavior and Cognition*, Berlin: Springer.

Haken H, 1999, What can synergetics contribute to the understanding of brain functioning? In: C Uhl (Ed.), *Analysis of Neurophysiological Brain Functioning*, Berlin: Springer, pp. 7–40.

Harth E, 1993, *The Creative Loop*, New York: Addison-Wesley.

Hebb DO, 1949, *The Organization of Behavior*, New York: Wiley.

Ingber L, 1982, Statistical mechanics of neocortical interactions: I. basic formulation. *Physica D* 5: 83–107.

Ingber L, 1995, Statistical mechanics of multiple scales of neocortical interactions. In: PL Nunez (Au.), *Neocortical Dynamics and Human EEG Rhythms*, New York: Oxford University Press, pp. 628–674.

Jasper HD and Penfield W, 1949, Electrocorticograms in man. Effects of voluntary movement upon the electrical activity of the precentral gyrus. *Archiv. Fur Psychiatrie und Zeitschrift Neurologie* 183: 163–174.

Jirsa VK and Haken H, 1997, A derivation of a macroscopic field theory of the brain from the quasi-microscopic neural dynamics. *Physica D* 99: 503–526.

Kellaway P, 1979, An orderly approach to visual analysis: the parameters of the normal EEG in adults and children. In: DW Klass and DD Daly (Eds.), *Current Practice of Clinical Electroencephalography*, New York: Raven Press, pp. 69–147.

Krieg WJS, 1963, *Connections of the Cerebral Cortex*, Evanston, IL: Brain Books.

Krieg WJS, 1973, *Architectronics of Human Cerebral Fiber System*, Evanston, IL: Brain Books.

Lopes da Silva FH and Storm van Leeuwen W, 1978, The cortical alpha rhythm in dog: the depth and surface profile of phase. In: MAB Brazier and H Petsche (Eds.), *Architectonics of the Cerebral Cortex*, New York: Raven Press, pp. 319–333.

Mountcastle VB, 1979, An organizing principle for cerebral function: the unit module and the distributed system. In: FO Schmitt and FG Worden (Eds.), *The Neurosciences 4th Study Program*, Cambridge, MA: MIT Press.

Niedermeyer E and Lopes da Silva FH (Eds.), 1999, *Electroencephalography. Basic Principals, Clinical Applications, and Related Fields*, 4th Edition, London: Williams and Wilkins.

Nunez PL, 1995, *Neocortical Dynamics and Human EEG Rhythms*, New York: Oxford University Press.

Nunez PL, 2000a, Toward a quantitative description of large scale neocortical dynamic function and EEG. *Behavioral and Brain Sciences* 23: 371–398.

Nunez PL, 2000b, Neocortical dynamic theory should be as simple as possible, but not simpler. *Behavioral and Brain Sciences* 23: 415–437.

Nunez PL, 2002, EEG. In: VS Ramachandran (Ed.), *Encyclopedia of the Human Brain*, La Jolla: Academic Press, pp. 169–179.

Nunez PL and Silberstein RB, 2000, On the relationship of synaptic activity to macroscopic measurements: does co-registration of EEG with fMRI make sense? *Brain Topography* 13: 79–96.

Nunez PL, Wingeier BM, and Silberstein RB, 2001, Spatial-temporal structures of human alpha rhythms: theory, micro-current sources, multiscale measurements, and global binding of local networks. *Human Brain Mapping* 13: 125–164.

Nuwer MR, 1998, Assessing digital and quantitative EEG in clinical settings. *Journal of Clinical Neurophysiology* 15: 458–463.

Penfield W and Jasper HD, 1954, *Epilepsy and the Functional Anatomy of the Human Brain*, London: Little Brown.

Petsche H, Pockberger H, and Rappelsberger P, 1984, On the search for sources of the electroencephalogram. *Neuroscience* 11: 1–27.

Pfurtscheller G and Cooper R, 1975, Frequency dependence of the transmission of the EEG from cortex to scalp. *Electroencephalography and Clinical Neurophysiology* 38: 93–96.

Pfurtscheller G and Lopes da Silva FH, 1999, Event related EEG/MEG synchronization and desynchronization: basic principles. *Electroencephalography and Clinical Neurophysiology* 110: 1842–1857.

Picton TW, Hillyard SA, Krausz HL, and Galambos R, 1974, Human auditory evoked potentials: I. evaluation of components. *Electroencephalography and Clinical Neurophysiology* 36: 179–190.

Rall W, 1977, Core conductor theory and cable properties of neurons. In: ET Kandel (Ed.), *Handbook of Physiology: Vol. I. The Nervous System*, Bethesda, MD: American Physiological Society, pp. 39–97.

Regan D, 1989, *Human Brain Electrophysiology: Evoked Potentials and Evoked Magnetic Fields in Science and Medicine*, New York: Elsevier.

Schlichting H, 1960, *Boundary Layer Theory*, New York: McGraw-Hill.

Scott A, 1995, *Stairway to the Mind*, New York: Springer-Verlag.

Segev I, Rinzel J, and Shepherd GM, 1995, *The Theoretical Foundation of Dendritic Function*, Cambridge, MA: MIT Press.

Sem-Jacobsen CW, Bickford RG, Petersen MC, and Dodge HW, 1953, Depth distribution of normal electroencephalographic rhythms. *Proceedings of the Staff Meetings of the Mayo Clinic* 28: 156–161.

Szentagothai J, 1979, Local neuron circuits of the neocortex. In: FO Schmitt and FG Worden (Eds.), *The Neurosciences 4th Study Program*, Cambridge, MA: MIT Press, pp. 399–415.

Uhl C (Ed.), 1999, *Analysis of Neurophysiological Brain Functioning*. Berlin: Springer.

Walter G, 1961, *The Living Brain*, London: Penguin Books, p. 15.

2

Fallacies in EEG

1 Mokita

The word *mokita*, from the Kiriwina language of New Guinea, translates roughly as, "that which we all know to be true, but agree not to discuss." Human cultures and their scientific subcultures often embrace mokita, apparently as a means of avoiding uncomfortable or self-contradictory ideas and feelings. However, there is a cost of maintaining such truths in isolation—that which we cannot discuss, we cannot change. This chapter on common EEG fallacies is presented with such human frailties in mind. Some fallacies have been repeated often, others are mainly implied. We do not suggest that EEG is necessarily more error prone than other scientific fields, but this chapter aims to be unusually proactive in the explicit acknowledgment of common fallacies, irrespective of mokita-like taboos.

When critical technical issues are properly addressed, EEG can provide robust measures of large-scale neocortical dynamic behavior that is closely correlated with brain state. It can open a revealing window on the mind, critical for new advancements in neuroscience. This feature should encourage vigorous consideration of EEG data and related theoretical tools by neuroscientists. However, EEG advances have been limited by persistent fallacies, thereby inhibiting scientific progress since the first recordings of human EEG in about 1925.

The causes of this flawed condition may be controversial, but certainly the highly interdisciplinary nature of EEG is partly to blame. Cognitive science, neurology, physiology, physics, engineering, mathematics, and computer science all have roles to play in EEG, and no one person can be expert in all these areas. In another context, the problem is not that EEG is too hard, but rather that it is too easy. As one veteran EEG expert is fond of saying, "the problem with EEG is that the entry requirements are too low." That is, EEG recording and computer processing with modern hardware and software can be accomplished with relatively small investments in time and money. Nearly anybody off the street can do it, but producing good EEG science is another matter entirely.

The fallacies outlined in this chapter are both *explicit* and *implicit*. Explicit examples involve incorrect or inappropriate experimental methods, erroneous physiological interpretations, misstatements of fact, or development of specious theories. By contrast, implicit fallacies are more analogous to crimes for which the perpetrators cannot be found guilty beyond reasonable doubt in criminal court, but are judged liable in civil proceedings. Perpetrators of implicit fallacies appear to misunderstand important principles, have failed to carry out the necessary background work or both.

Specific references to the guilty are omitted here. Gray areas separate explicit from implicit errors and from marginal fallacies; it is difficult to make such fine distinctions. Second, full citation of all errors in the EEG literature would be impossible. Thus, we avoid singling out a few unlucky targets for criticism. Our purpose is to extinguish errors not punish sinners. Finally, if the sinners were identified , fairness would require that the authors of this book cite their own errors!

This chapter's goal is to discourage both new and old EEG fallacies. Our main targets are ideas and methods that re-emerge periodically, even after they have been proven false. Our goal is facilitated by discouraging *guru science*, in which scientists or clinicians follow methods dictated by pundits without proper scrutiny. In highly interdisciplinary fields like EEG, even the so-called experts cannot be expert in all of the critical subfields. We could cite at least one publication corresponding to each of the fallacies outlined in this chapter. In most cases, multiple citations would be possible, sometimes involving citation chains where errors are propagated and even amplified. Some of our examples may seem out of date; perhaps we can be accused of beating proverbial dead horses. But old EEG horses (and the sacred cows of Reginald Bickford's Foreword to the 1981 edition) have proved remarkably robust. This time we want to ensure that they stay dead.

2 Denial of EEG as an Epiphenomenon

Some have dismissed EEG as a so-called *epiphenomenon*, apparently meaning a measure peripheral to genuine scientific interest. Yet even a naïve observer will quickly recognize that human and animal EEG generally contain different frequency and amplitude content during different brain states. More sophisticated monitoring and training allows for accurate identification of distinct sleep stages, depth of anesthesia, seizures, and other brain states. Other methods reveal robust connections of EEG to more detailed medical or cognitive events.

Smaller scale animal data recorded by physiologists and intracranial human data are available, the latter mostly from epileptic surgery patients. Such data are incorporated into our conceptual framework supporting brain function. However, let us remember that all experiments and mathematical models apply to specific temporal and spatial scales of electrophysiology and brain dynamic behavior. An important, but often difficult, task is to relate small-spatial-scale electrophysiological recordings to large-scale EEG. To date, development of such cross-scale quantitative connections has been minimal. One should be wary of hand waving arguments that trivialize efforts to bridge these gaps of scale in the neurosciences. The development of theoretical methods to relate distinct scales of measurement is responsible for the many of the successes in the physical sciences and engineering over the past century or so. The relationship between the microscopic and macroscopic versions of Maxwell's equations provides a prominent example (see chapter 3). Unfortunately, proficiency with either physiology or mathematics does not ensure that this idea is fully appreciated in neuroscience.

Modern science is rife with examples of imperfect matches between system variables that are actually measured and other variables of the corresponding model system, even in some of the most productive scientific fields. Experimental limitations often force compromises. For example, let some general experimental variable be represented by $E(\mathbf{r}_k, t_i)$, indicating data recorded at discrete times and spatial locations. The relationship of such data to supposedly similar, but continuous variables $T(\mathbf{r}, t)$ predicted by theory is often obscure. Such ambiguity does not mean that the data $E(\mathbf{r}_k, t_i)$ are "epiphenomena." Rather it means that a separate theory, new experiments, or both are needed to forge quantitative relations between the $E(\mathbf{r}_k, t_i)$ data and the theoretical $T(\mathbf{r}, t)$ variables, thereby allowing proper tests of the theory that predicted $T(\mathbf{r}, t)$ in the first place.

The mismatch between experimental and theoretical variables may be due to mismatch of spatial or temporal scale, or for other reasons. To take one example, imagine such mismatch in the electrophysiology of the action potential. The transmembrane potential of the action potential from a single axon $T(\mathbf{r}, t)$ is predicted by the nonlinear membrane theory developed by Hodgkin and Huxley. Transmembrane potential is a monophasic traveling waveform with maximum potential in the 100 mV range. Suppose the (extracellular) compound action potential of a nerve fiber containing hundreds or thousands of axons is the measured variable $E(\mathbf{r}_k, t_i)$, Do we dismiss these data as epiphenomena because they are not direct measurements of $T(\mathbf{r}, t)$? We do not. Rather, a plausible approach is to first obtain the theoretical connection between transmembrane potential $T(\mathbf{r}, t)$ and the single axon extracellular potential $\Phi(\mathbf{r}, t)$, a triphasic traveling waveform with maximum potential in the 100 μV range (a thousand times smaller than the transmembrane potential). With this connection accomplished, we are in position to compare theory with experiment. We can accomplish this by a separate theory that relates transmembrane to extracellular potential, and appropriately summing the extracellular potential from individual axons (accounting for different propagation speeds and source distributions) to predict the compound action potential. In chapters 4 and 5, quantitative relations between synaptic micropotentials and scalp EEG are derived for certain idealized source configurations. It is shown that several important qualitative and semiquantitative predictions of this procedure are robust, despite the obvious uncertainties and complications of living tissue.

Intracranial recordings provide smaller scale measures of neocortical dynamics, with scale dependent on electrode size. A mixture of coherent and incoherent sources generates the small- and intermediate-scale intracranial data. Scalp EEG is due mostly to coherent sources with the special geometries that support superposition of fields generated by many local sources. The best candidates for *EEG generators* appear to be the synaptic sources of large cortical pyramidal cells that are aligned in parallel and perpendicular to the cortical surface. Human intracranial EEG may be uncorrelated or only weakly correlated with cognition and behavior, which is typically more easily observed at large scales.

Given more than 70 years in which robust correlations between EEG and many of the most interesting aspects of higher brain function have been discovered, attempts to trivialize EEG as an "epiphenomenon" can perhaps be attributed to a *chauvinism of spatial scale*, the assumption that data and theory at one's favored scale is the most useful, or in extreme cases, an inability to recognize scientific merit outside of one's own subfield. Scale chauvinism arises in other fields as well, including economics and physics. Readers may be aware, for example, of books on particle physics aimed at the general public that adopt provocative titles like "theory of everything" or "the end of science," thereby trivializing the vast gaps between advances in particle physics and higher complex systems. The formidable problems associated with crossing hierarchies of scale in physics and neuroscience are convincingly addressed by Scott (1995). Unfortunately, some neuroscientists appear unaware of such limitations, adopting a viewpoint that one may label as *autistic reductionism.*

3 EEG Practice Divorced from Theory

As discussed in chapter 1, both theoretical and physical models are critical to advances in science and engineering. In complex or even relatively simple systems, a hierarchy of models is often evident. For example, consider the example of current sources or amplifiers containing transistors. Transistors are made of semiconductors, for example silicon (a poor conductor) doped with some added arsenic to provide donor electrons to carry small currents. At the lowest level in the scientific/engineering hierarchy are quantum mechanical models of semiconductor properties developed by solid-state physicists often having minimal interest or knowledge of circuit applications.

Up one level from these physicists are fundamentalist engineers and applied physicists, often having moderate, but not expert, knowledge of quantum mechanics. These engineers use level two models to design the current sources and amplifiers. Another group of engineers works at the third hierarchical level to design specific circuits, for example, those used in EEG systems. This higher engineering group typically takes the properties of circuit elements, provided by fundamentalist engineers at the second level, for granted in developing level three systems. Finally, the users of these circuits (EEG scientists, for example) operate at the fourth level. This outline of science and engineering hierarchy has many parallels in other fields. For example, engineers at perhaps the third or fourth level may build bridges or airplanes made of synthetic material developed by solid-state physicists, chemists, and material scientists at the first and second levels. In this book we are mainly concerned with macroscopic models, but when convenient (without drifting too far from our central focus) we forge connections to smaller scales, that is, to meso- and microelectrode data and models.

Mathematical models in EEG are of two general types: volume conductor models and models of the dynamic behavior of brain current sources. We emphasize the distinction between these two kinds of models because of the large differences in complexity, necessary assumptions, and accuracy. Brain volume conduction is far simpler than brain dynamics because we know the basic governing equation relating current sources to macroscopic currents and potentials produced in the volume conductor. The basic formulation is normally presented in terms of Poisson's equation:

$$\nabla E[\sigma(\mathbf{r})\nabla\Phi] = -s(\mathbf{r}, t) \tag{2.1}$$

Here $s(\mathbf{r}, t)$ is the volume current source function and ∇ is the vector gradient (mathematical) operator involving spatial derivatives in three spatial coordinates. Expression (2.1) involves the vector dot product, defined in appendix A. $\Phi(\mathbf{r}, t)$ is the usual scalar potential, expressed as a function of vector location $\mathbf{r}$ and time t. Tissue conductivity is given by $\sigma(\mathbf{r})$; it is a function of location $\mathbf{r}$ in *inhomogeneous tissue*. The left-hand side of (2.1) is read, "del dot sigma grad phi." The volume current source (microamperes/mm^3) on the right-hand side of (2.1) accounts for effects at some bounding surface (usually a membrane in electrophysiology) through which known source current passes, as discussed in chapter 4 and appendix K.

The neuron or neural network generating this source current $s(\mathbf{r}, t)$ is expected to involve complicated, nonlinear processes; however, (2.1) is linear in the potential $\Phi(\mathbf{r}, t)$ and may be used to determine this potential at all locations external to the source volumes. Note that if conductivity $\sigma(\mathbf{r})$ is a real function (meaning negligible capacitive effects at large scales), the time dependence of a potential is identical to the time dependence of its source. Typically, there are many EEG sources with different frequencies. The resulting tissue potential is simply the sum of all these contributions, but with unequal weights depending on volume conductor and source characteristics as given precisely by (2.1). If capacitive properties were important in macroscopic tissue volumes, conductivity would be expressed as a complex function, equal to a real plus an imaginary part, similar to capacitors in parallel with resistors in electric circuits. In this case, the imaginary part of the conductivity function describes phase shifts between source and potential. However, all tissue experiments known to us have shown negligible macroscopic capacitive properties in the 1 to 40 Hz range of interest to EEG. Thus, to a good approximation, each scalp potential is in phase with its corresponding current source. The net potential at any location is due to a linear superposition of contributions from all brain sources, generally having different frequencies and phases.

Poisson's equation (2.1) follows directly from the vector form of Ohm's law for an isotropic conductor (1.4), the law of current conservation, and the low-frequency approximation that the *curl of the electric field* (a basic vector operation described in appendix A) is zero everywhere in the volume conductor, essentially the neglect of magnetic induction in tissue (see appendix B). The latter two conditions are generalizations of Kirchhoff's laws for electric circuits. Equations (1.7) and (1.8) for dipole fields in an infinite, homogeneous conductor are special case solutions to (2.1). The anisotropic version of (2.1), applicable to tissue having different conductivities for current flux in different directions, is somewhat more complicated. However, the basic equation is still linear so that one may use superposition to calculate potentials due to multiple sources at different locations. While pundits may declare "the brain is nonlinear," volume conduction in macroscopic tissue masses is linear, at least to a first approximation. The separation of this linear theory from nonlinear source dynamics provides a critical step towards construction of a conceptual EEG framework.

An alternative formulation of volume conduction makes use of Laplace's equation, obtained by setting the current source term in (2.1) to zero and specifying the appropriate boundary conditions at the surfaces of source regions (normally cell membranes). The alternative forms of (2.1) are closely related to the equivalence of voltage and current sources (Thevenin's theorem) as indicated in fig. 1-11. The alternative formulation of Laplace's equation is often appropriate for calculation of potentials at the membrane scale. However, cell surfaces are very complicated in neural tissue masses so that macroscopic potentials are more conveniently estimated using Poisson's equation (2.1). This issue is discussed in more detail in chapter 4.

While the underlying principles of volume conduction in the head are well understood, important engineering applications of volume conduction remain. The so-called *forward problem* in electrophysiology is to solve (2.1) for potentials $\Phi(\mathbf{r}, t)$ due to known source magnitudes and locations. The forward problem always has unique solutions in the head when constrained by the boundary condition of no current flux across the outer head surface into the surrounding space. Of course, this is only an approximation (but evidently a good one) in the neck region. Obtaining accurate forward solutions (analytic or numerical) depends on knowledge of tissue conductivities and boundaries. In actual EEG practice, the scale of the microsource function $s(\mathbf{r}, t)$ is too far removed from large-scale scalp data to be used directly. Rather we employ the mesosource function (dipole moment per unit volume, $\mathbf{P}(\mathbf{r}, t)$) discussed in chapter 4. When we loosely apply the word "dipole" to a tissue mass in this book without elaboration, we mean $\mathbf{P}(\mathbf{r}, t)$, consistent with common EEG parlance.

Poisson's equation (2.1) may be used to solve forward problems, thereby using simulations to address common EEG questions. One such question concerns possible relations between local scalp potentials and the underlying synaptic action. For example, can we associate positive scalp potentials with local dendritic inhibitory postsynaptic potentials (IPSPs)? After all, IPSPs are known to produce local membrane sources and local positive intracortical potentials at the mesoscopic scale. To address this question, a simulation of surface potentials produced by 4200 (millimeter scale) dipole sources in a 3-sphere head model is shown in fig. 2-1. The source distribution includes two negative and one positive centimeter-scale source regions which remain unchanged as the background source distribution changes from random (upper left) to clumped (upper right). The lower row shows simulated scalp potential maps for each source distribution based on a right ear reference. There are no sources within about 5 cm of the right ear location, approximating a so-called "quiet reference." Comparison of the two potential maps shows that the potential over part of the positive clump changes from positive to negative and the potential over both negative clumps switches from negative to positive even though the underlying source clumps are unchanged. This simulation illustrates the general nonlocal character of scalp potentials even when no sources are located close to the reference electrode. *Generally, the potential difference between any two scalp locations depends on all sources plus the volume conductive properties of the head.*

The *inverse problem* in EEG is to find the locations and strengths of the current sources on the right-hand side of (2.1) from discrete samples of the potential V_j (with respect to some reference) on the surface of the volume conductor, as indicated in fig. 2-2. In practice, dipole searches employing sophisticated computer algorithms are based on potentials

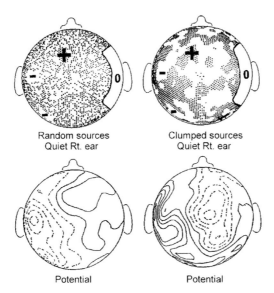

Figure 2-1 A simulation using 4200 radial dipoles (macrocolumn-scale mesosources) in a 3-sphere model of the head (brain, skull, and scalp). (*Upper row*) Filled and empty spaces indicate positive and negative source regions, respectively, with random magnitudes. The region near the right ear labeled "0" has no sources. The three clumped regions indicated by the ± signs remain unchanged as the background source pattern changes from random (upper left) to clumped (upper right). (*Lower row*) Calculated scalp potential maps predicted for a reference electrode on the right ear or mastoid. Reproduced with permission from Nunez and Westdorp (1994).

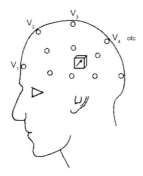

Figure 2-2 Dipole searches employing sophisticated computer algorithms are based on potentials recorded at perhaps 20 to 128 surface locations, either for fixed time slices or over some time window. If N dipoles are assumed, the algorithms attempt to calculate the $6N$ parameters that best fit the recorded data—three location coordinates, two axis angles, and one strength (dipole moment) for each dipole. Application of additional *constraints* (often assumptions) may be used to reduce the number of parameters to be found.

recorded at perhaps 20 to 128 surface locations, either for fixed time slices or over some time window. Six parameters specify each dipole: three spatial coordinates, two dipole axis angles, and the dipole moment (product of dipole current and pole separation, usually measured in microampere millimeters, µA mm). By contrast to the forward problem, the *inverse problem has no unique solution*. If one dipole provides a reasonable fit to the surface data, two or three or ten dipoles can provide an even better fit. (Although algorithms for obtaining inverse solutions for more than several dipoles often fail.) Scalp surface potentials can always be made to fit a wide range of distributed cortical sources. For example, any scalp potential map can be made to fit source distributions that are exclusively cortical, or even made to fit sources that are exclusive to cortical gyri. Of course, the constraints (physiological assumptions) required to obtain these fits may not be accurate, and *the inverse solutions (computed source locations) are generally no better than the model assumptions*.

Neocortical sources can be pictured generally as *dipole layers* (or folded "dipole sheets" in and out of cortical fissures and sulci) with source strength varying as a function of cortical location as indicated in figs. 2-1 and 2-3. Cortical sources are closer to scalp electrodes than deep sources. Furthermore, cortical neurons are strongly interconnected and aligned in parallel, facilitating the production of relatively large potentials due to superposition of many aligned and synchronous dipole sources. Cortical depth recordings have located important cortical sources of EEG rhythms. For these reasons, cortical dipole layers are believed to produce nearly all spontaneous scalp EEG of moderate to large magnitude. It should be emphasized again that the inverse problem is *very non-unique*. *Constraints* (possibly unjustified assumptions) based on separate physiological considerations must be invoked to obtain genuine inverse

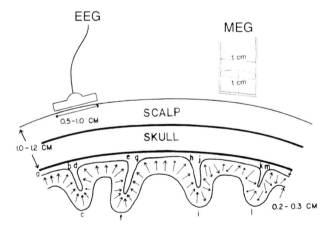

Figure 2-3 Neocortical sources can be generally pictured as *dipole layers* (or "dipole sheets," in and out of cortical fissures and sulci) with mesosource strength varying as a function of cortical location. EEG is most sensitive to correlated dipole layer in gyri (regions ab, de, gh), less sensitive to correlated dipole layer in sulcus (region hi), and insensitive to opposing dipole layer in sulci (regions bcd, efg) and random layer (region ijklm). MEG is most sensitive to correlated and minimally apposed dipole layer (hi) and much less sensitive to all other sources shown, which are opposing, random, or radial dipoles. Modified version reproduced with permission from Nunez (1995).

solutions, as discussed in section 8 of this chapter and in chapters 6 and 8. However, in many cases the most plausible constraint is that the sources are exclusively cortical. That is, if the sources are truly unknown, application of a cortical-only constraint may be a better guess than constraints based on a few isolated sources. Exceptions may occur if certain deep brain structures are implicated by other considerations, for example by known physiology (as with brainstem-evoked potential) or possibly by independent fMRI or PET imaging (Nunez and Silberstein 2000).

Given our very limited understanding of brain operation, we must view today's large-scale dynamic models very differently than volume conductor models or dynamic models of single neurons (action potential propagation, for example). Even with substantial oversimplification, dynamic models at large scales are very complex and typically contain unknown parameters, thereby making experimental connections difficult for some models and impossible for others. However, we argue that such models are critical to forming a well-posed conceptual framework in neuroscience. Such framework determines the priority of experiments to be undertaken, the specifics of experimental design, and interpretation of the resulting data. For example, our proposed framework involves *mesoscopic synaptic fields* generating EEG, as indicated in fig. 1-8. The term *field* as used here just indicates any continuous function of space and time, analogous to modulations of pressure or mass density in a fluid about background levels. Such so-called *field theories* may follow the number of active excitatory or inhibitory synapses in a tissue mass independent of their functional significance for brain operation. The field concept facilitates theoretical connections between dynamic theory and experimental EEG. That is, the inhibitory and excitatory synaptic action fields, $\Psi_i(\mathbf{r}_1, t)$ and $\Psi_e(\mathbf{r}_1, t)$, may be viewed as the origins of the macroscopic electric and magnetic fields that we record. Cell assemblies (or neural networks), believed to underlie cognition and behavior, are pictured here as immersed in these synaptic action fields. Mathematical models show how hierarchical interactions might occur with neural networks influencing macroscopic synaptic action fields (bottom-up) and these fields acting back on the networks (top-down). Brain (or specifically neocortical) dynamical issues that interface with volume conduction considerations are considered in chapters 9 through 11.

4 Misuse of Physical or Mathematical Models

Electroencephalographers are evidently more trusting of physical than mathematical models. Physical head models have been used to evaluate electrode placement strategies (including nearest-neighbor Laplacians) and accuracy of dipole localization. Other possible applications include construction of laboratory standards (*phantom heads*) with implanted current sources. One may envision EEG electrodes placed on the phantom's surface and recording potentials to be passed through the laboratory's hardware and software systems. Phantom source dynamics could also be varied to simulate different experimental subjects (producing *virtual populations*). In this manner, the laboratory's EEG hardware and software systems could be conveniently evaluated. For example, one might test software designed to improve spatial resolution, locate sources, map amplitude, covariance, or coherence, perform statistical tests on virtual subject populations, and so forth. Such a device would be welcomed in EEG laboratories. By contrast, mathematical models, even if conveniently implemented as computer software, may not be as easily accepted to test laboratory methods.

Given the (often justified) suspicion of mathematical models by medical scientists, we consider established marriages of physical and mathematical models to a variety of engineering applications where cost considerations and *market-based natural selection* have optimized methods to create profitable products. The following general approach can be expected in many branches of engineering:

(i) Physical principles are used to develop mathematical models of a proposed device, albeit models employing simplifying assumptions. However, an important caveat is appropriate here: industrial managers are well aware of the risk of being sidetracked by interesting mathematics not directly relevant to the physical system under study, an issue with some relevance to EEG.

(ii) The mathematical models are used to guide the construction of physical prototypes to be tested in the laboratory.

(iii) A multiple feedback process between steps (i) and (ii) may be required, depending on the accuracy of the original mathematical model and later modifications. A certain amount of trial and error is likely at step (ii), but step (i) is used to minimize such costly processes.

(iv) Production and sales of the new system.

Engineers do not waste time building physical models if theory predicts they will not work; however, the reverse is not true. That is, a successful mathematical model is normally a necessary, but insufficient condition to allow advance to the production step. A prototype must be shown to work first.

With this background in mind, we note that the development of anything approaching a realistic physical model of the head volume conductor must combine theory and experiment. For example, the relative conductivities of tissue layers and the electrical contact between layers, which can result in large contact impedance if one is not careful, must be fully tested. The locations and orientations of implanted sources must be known accurately. One obvious early approach is to compare potentials measured in layered spherical physical models with known mathematical solutions for concentric spherical shells. *Success at this step is required before physical models can be taken seriously.*

EEG fallacies associated with mathematical or physical models of volume conduction or brain dynamics have included:

(i) Attributing strange nonohmic electrical properties to living tissue. A lesser error involves the erroneous belief that oscillating sources produce scalp potentials that have reduced magnitude at higher frequencies; that is, passive tissue is a low-pass filter. There are, in fact, observed frequency effects on the measured ratio of cortical to scalp potential magnitude. But this is dynamic low-pass filtering, due to the nature of source dynamics, not to passive volume conduction, as discussed in chapters 1, 4, and 10.

(ii) Confusion of magnetic induction (negligible at EEG frequencies) with the ever present quasi-static magnetic field (magnetoencephalography, MEG) generated by low-frequency current sources. Magnetic induction involves the coupling of electric and magnetic fields and allows for wave propagation in the *far field*. But, inductive effects in tissue are not important below frequencies in roughly the 10^6 Hz range as shown in appendix B. There is no *electromagnetic propagation or far field associated with any measurable EEG phenomenon*. Also, action potential propagation is not "electromagnetic" in a macroscopic sense, but rather owes its origin to nonlinear membrane properties.

(iii) Confusion of charge sources that produce potentials in *dielectrics* (insulators) with current sources that produce potentials in *conductors*. These processes are mathematically identical, but quite different physically, as discussed in chapter 4.

(iv) "Correcting" volume conduction distortion of EEG using tissue boundary information obtained from CT or MRI. The problem here is that accurate corrections require both geometric and electric information. For example, knowledge of local skull thickness will not necessarily improve volume conductor models. The skull has three layers, and most of its current-passing ability is due to fluid permeating the bone, especially the inner layer (cancellous bone). If a thicker skull region occurs with thicker cancellous layer, a thick skull may pass current normal to its surface as easily as a thin skull. Furthermore, a larger inner layer may provide for more shunting of tangential current, as discussed in chapters 4 and 6. Naïve corrections of volume conductor models (based only on geometry) may actually reduce their accuracies.

(v) Placing all mathematical models in a single category. For example, head models based on a homogeneous sphere or two spherical shells have minimal use in EEG. By contrast, three or four shell models, which include the critical skull and scalp current paths, appear to provide good semiquantitative predictions of EEG observations. An essential issue is whether mathematical solutions are robust with respect to small changes in assumptions. Today's mathematical models in brain science include robust examples and others that are quite fragile.

(vi) Confusing *metaphor* with genuine *theory*. It is important to distinguish genuine mathematical theories of biological phenomena from metaphor by reserving the word "theory" for models that contain only physiological parameters. Such parameters are potentially measurable, even though they may have not yet been measured. In addition at least one predicted variable must be measurable. Thus, genuine theories make quantitative contact with existing experiments and encourage new experiments. Metaphorical models are often useful as a means to communicate theoretical ideas or as precursors to genuine theory. Metaphorical models are not able to make quantitative predictions of the outcomes of genuine physiological experiments. For example, *neural network models* often depend on a myriad of connection weights not easily connected to genuine physiology. In the absence of such relations between network parameters and genuine physiology and anatomy, neural network models must be judged as metaphor not theory. An obvious warning sign is use of words like "activity" to describe tissue state. We can measure several things in tissue: extracellular electric and magnetic fields, transmembrane potentials, different kinds of metabolic signatures, and so forth. However, the abstract entity "activity" can never be measured. Consequently, the so-called theories predicting "activity" may be predicting nothing at all.

(vii) Inappropriate crossing of *spatial scales* (*hierarchical levels*). One way to judge the issue of metaphor versus theory in electrophysiology is to determine the spatial scale of the candidate "theory." For example, one should ask the location and size of the electrode needed to record potentials appropriate for comparison with the "theoretical" potentials (if any). For many so-called "brain theories" there is no apparent answer to this question. The authors of such pseudo-theory may not even be aware that such questions are central to the creation of genuine theory. For some published material it appears that one of the following applies: (a) the mathematics is supposed to apply to all spatial and temporal scales, (b) others with stronger theoretical skills are supposed to magically find some scale that matches the derived mathematics, or (c) the author is ignorant of the importance of spatial or temporal scales in connecting genuine theory to experiment. A somewhat less serious error is the application of a successful theory at one scale to a much different scale without theoretical or experimental justification. For example, the theoretical transition from mesoscopic potentials at the membrane level to macroscopic field potentials is a nontrivial step.

(viii) Belief that spectral analysis (fast Fourier transform, FFT) is applicable only to linear systems analysis because it is accomplished by linear transformation of data. Surprisingly, this fallacy occasionally occurs even in engineering publications, apparently because of the connection to input–output relations and transfer functions in linear systems analysis. In practice, FFT methods are routinely applied to both linear and nonlinear systems (including chaotic systems) as well as stochastic systems whose origins are poorly understood. Interpretations of experimental spectra are, of course, likely to be simpler when the system is approximately linear. For the record, any mathematical function defined (or recorded) on the interval $[0, T]$ has a Fourier transform provided three conditions are met. It must be *piecewise continuous* (any discontinuities must be finite and finite in number), its *mean square integral* over $[0, T]$ must exist, and it must have a *finite number of maxima and minima* on $[0, T]$. These restrictions are so lax that nearly any function representing a genuine physical or biological process must satisfy them—it is difficult to cite even a single exception. A fourth condition is sometimes included stating that the function must be *periodic*; however, we are free to force any function defined only on $[0, T]$ to be periodic with period T. The latter condition does have practical implications for data analysis as discussed in chapter 9.

5 The Quiet Reference Myth

Searches for a so-called *quiet reference* location on the body have long occupied many EEG scientists and clinicians. Their motivation is to record scalp potentials that are essentially monopolar in nature. In extreme versions of this fantasy, recorded potentials are imagined as generated exclusively by sources directly under or at least very close to the so-called *monopolar electrode*. In order to address this issue, consider the electric circuit in fig. 2-4, which illustrates in a crude manner some of the issues of head volume conduction and reference. The circuit contains a single current source $I_1 = 50$ μA and several resistors mimicking brain, cerebrospinal fluid (CSF), skull, and scalp tissue. Of course, this is not a genuine equivalent circuit for the head volume conductor in which current spreads out nonuniformly in three dimensions rather than being confined to wires and resistors. Concentric spherical shells or more complicated volume conductor models are considered for this purpose in chapters 6 and 7. However, the resistors in fig. 2-4 are chosen in roughly

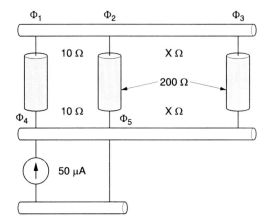

Figure 2-4 The electric circuit illustrates in a crude manner some head volume conduction and reference electrode issues. The circuit contains a current source $I_1 = 50$ μA and several resistors crudely mimicking brain/CSF (lower cylinders with horizontal axes), skull (shaded cylinders), and scalp tissue (upper cylinder with horizontal axis). The resistance path between location 2 and the reference location 3 is X Ω as shown. All the Φ indicate potentials with respect to infinity, but these cannot be measured. Rather we can measure only potential differences like $V_{13} = \Phi_1 - \Phi_3$.

the right range to match head volume conduction qualitatively. For example, a 208 Ω skull resistance occurs if uniform current is passed through a cylindrical skull plug of thickness 0.5 cm, cross section 12 cm^2, and resistivity 5 kΩ cm (see fig. 1-12).

Scalp and brain are represented by resistance per until length so that longer current paths have larger resistance. Consider two possible placements of a putative "reference" point 3, corresponding to (scalp) resistance between locations 2 and 3 of $X = 50$ Ω or 200 Ω to simulate crudely different electrical distances from the current source. The surface potential difference $\Phi_1 - \Phi_2$ (bipolar recording) is about 14 μV in either case. However, the reference potential $\Phi_1 - \Phi_3$ changes from 14 μV (when $X = 50$ Ω) to 81 μV (when $X = 200$ Ω) as the simulated reference is moved.

The general problems with the simplistic reference idea in EEG applications are as follows:

(i) We normally do not know the locations of brain sources so we do not know where to locate a reference electrode that is electrically "far" from all sources, assuming such location even exists on the body.

(ii) Sources of EEG are typically distributed throughout large regions of neocortex (and possibly the whole brain). Neocortex covers nearly all of brain surface, including the mesial surface (ventral or underside of the brain). To a first approximation, the neocortex of one hemisphere is *topologically equivalent to a spherical shell*. In fig. 2-4, the current path between source I_1 and reference has a resistance in the range of several hundred ohms. Other sources (not shown) will make even larger contributions to the reference potential Φ_3 if they are electrically closer (lower resistance paths). Because of possible complexities of brain current paths, such sources may or may not be physically closer than I_1, for example, a mesial cortical dipole layer producing a potential (with respect to infinity) at the "reference" in the range of several tens of microvolts and producing a much smaller potential at location 1. A large ear or mastoid reference potential might occur if source magnitudes are large, correlated over large regions, physically close to the reference or if current is shunted through CSF or thin skull regions. In such cases, the potential difference $\Phi_1 - \Phi_3$ may be due mostly to mesial sources affecting the reference and only minimally to the source I_1.

(iii) Even if all sources other than I_1 are electrically "far" from the reference location, a serious problem with the simplistic reference idea remains, for example if the number of (perhaps weak) sources is large and partly correlated. Suppose, for example, that our circuit contains an additional 100 sources (I_2 through I_{101}), all located electrically much further away from the reference than I_1. Let these sources be sufficiently synchronous so that each source contributes (on the average) $+0.2$ μV to the so-called "reference" potential Φ_3. In this case, the measured reference potential difference $\Phi_1 - \Phi_3$ would be decreased by about 20 μV. As in the example (ii), the source I_1 makes only a part of the contribution to the potential difference $\Phi_1 - \Phi_3$ and the simplistic reference idea fails. In chapters 7 and 8, the advantages and limitations of "reference-free" measures (the surface spline-Laplacian and average reference) are considered.

(iv) If the putative reference location actually qualifies as a genuine reference, a number of alternative reference sites should be readily available, and the EEG should not change substantially as a result of reference changes to alternative sites. However, such fundamental tests of the chosen reference are rarely (if ever) published. Unfortunately, the extra degree of freedom provided by somewhat arbitrary placement of the so-called "reference electrode" has allowed for presentation of questionable results, perhaps consistent with preconceived notions about the underlying sources. Perhaps such action is justified in certain instances. For example, a clinical neurologist may use reference EEG to confirm a diagnosis obtained by independent tests. Adopting a certain reference may also be motivated by a desire to reproduce results from other laboratories. However, in cases of unknown sources, freedom to choose *pseudo-references* can easily lead to misinterpretation of actual brain sources.

(v) The physically linked-ears and linked-mastoid references gained popularity in early cognitive studies of event-related potentials (ERPs). There are three potential problems with this approach. First, the linked-ears reference does not generally accomplish an approximation of potential at infinity as shown in chapter 7. Second, electrically linking the two hemispheres may distort natural scalp current paths, thereby distorting surface potential maps, an effect that will be more pronounced when electrode contact impedances are low in the linked path or when sources are close to the linked regions. In many cases, the resulting distortion is probably small (Miller et al. 1991); however, the physically linked ears reference violates the normal boundary conditions of zero current flux from the scalp (Katznelson 1981). It is generally difficult to estimate the distortion of scalp potentials induced by this reference choice. A third (and probably more serious) problem is that if the two contact impedances in the linked path are unequal, the effective reference is unbalanced to one side (Nunez 1991). Because normal EEG practice involves checking only that contact impedances are below some standard (say 5 to 40 kΩ) rather than matching them, *the physically linked ears reference may actually be a random reference*, as shown in chapter 7.

6 The Myth of Artifact-Free Data

EEG scientists sometimes adopt the mantra "artifact-free data" to reassure their readers. Normally this just means that the data have been examined visually and portions containing obvious artifact discarded. In studies that are insensitive to moderate artifact, this procedure may accomplish its goal nicely. However, the sensitivity of a study's main conclusions to small or moderate artifact is often difficult to determine. For example, many studies have reported small but statistically significant differences in EEG measures between populations. Such studies may be sensitive to artifact contamination, especially when population differences involve substantial contributions from delta, beta, or gamma bands. EEG power in these frequency bands is especially difficult to distinguish from small or even moderate artifact because of low signal to noise ratios. The amplitude of scalp-recorded beta and gamma activity is nearly always quite small and difficult to distinguish from muscle and other possible artifact sources. For this reason, some projects that have focused on EEG beta or gamma activity may be veiled studies of muscle artifact. The delta, beta and gamma bands are apparently quite important to brain function; however, rigorous tests are required to eliminate the possibility of artifact dominance of these frequency bands. Such tests may include the purposeful addition of known artifact and a focus on very narrow frequency bands using steady-state evoked potentials, as discussed in chapters 8 through 10.

Consider an extreme example of a naive student attempting to reduce the influence of muscle artifact. Suppose the student tinkers with the EEG system's low-pass filter settings and finds that by removing most signal power above (say) 20 Hz, the remaining signal appears to the eye to be mostly free of artifact. In this imagined study, the student then proceeds with the analysis of activity in the beta band in the "artifact-free" data. However, muscle artifact is broad band, falling off with frequency as something like $f^{-\alpha}$, where α is some small positive exponent. Thus, the beta band may still be substantially contaminated (perhaps even dominated) by muscle artifact even though the filtered data appear clean. While we are not aware of published papers in this category, it is not beyond the realm of possibilities.

Obvious artifact should, of course, be removed before submission to computer algorithms, even if artifact rejection is automated. However, more proactive measures may be required to prevent small to moderate artifact from altering major conclusions of EEG studies. Perhaps the most convincing approach involves adding separately recorded artifact (or simulated artifact) of magnitude somewhat larger than that expected in the raw data (Silberstein 1995; Nunez et al. 2001). Data analysis procedures can then be carried out with and without the added artifact. If the addition of small to moderate artifact does not cause changes in the study's central conclusions, it may be argued with more conviction that the natural artifact also did not compromise the project.

One advantage of steady-state evoked potentials, discussed in chapters 9 and 10, is the ability to follow brain responses in very narrow frequency bands (say 0.01 Hz) in which artifact contamination is small (Silberstein 1995). This is possible because artifact tends to be relatively broad band so that it may contribute minimal power in such very narrow bands.

7 Misrepresentation of Surface Laplacians or Dura Imaging

An important application of Poisson's equation (2.1) is *dura imaging* discussed in chapters 8, 9, and 10. This method projects measured scalp potentials to the dura surface. It depends on Poisson's equation (2.1), the boundary condition of no current flow out of the head, and the measured scalp potential distribution V_S. This inward continuation solution has been given several labels—*spatial deconvolution, software lens, deblurring, cortical imaging,* and *dura imaging*—the latter being the most descriptive. Such estimates of dura potential can be obtained provided that no sources are located between scalp and dura surfaces, an excellent assumption, at least if muscle and other artifact is minimal. Dura imaging will, of course, be most accurate when applied to data with relatively large signal-to-noise ratio.

The large-scale dura potential solution is unique in the sense that its accuracy depends "only" on noise, spatial sampling, and volume conductor model, independent of prior assumptions about the underlying sources. These are nontrivial limitations and studies to improve dura imaging may occupy EEG scientists well into the future. However, even today's relatively crude methods based on limited volume conductor knowledge appear to provide substantial improvements in spatial resolution over conventional EEG (Le and Gevins 1993; Gevins et al. 1994). One apparent reason is that the high-resistivity skull tends to dominate head volume conduction in EEG applications, thereby making other features of the head model relatively less important.

In chapter 8 it is shown that the *spline-Laplacian* provides an alternative method to estimate dura potential, a method largely independent of head model details. In both simulations and genuine EEG data, the Melbourne dura imaging algorithm (Cadusch et al. 1992; Silberstein 1995) and New Orleans spline-Laplacian (Law et al. 1993; Nunez et al. 1994; Srinivasan et al. 1996; Nunez et al. 2001) yield progressively more similar estimates of dura potential distribution as electrode density increases. This correspondence occurs even though the two algorithms are quite distinct. We have obtained many comparisons of the dual (Melbourne and New Orleans) estimates of dura potential from spontaneous EEG and steady-state visually evoked potentials, as well as in several thousand simulations. The correlation coefficients obtained by comparing these scalp measures to each other (electrode site by site) are in approximate ranges 0.80 (64 electrodes) to 0.95 (131 electrodes). In simulated data with zero noise, correlations between actual and estimated inner surface (dura) potential are in the same ranges (see table 8-1). Some published misunderstandings of Laplacian or dura image methods are as follows:

(i) Confusion with inverse solutions. Estimates of potential on the dura surface are just that: they are not true inverse solutions because no estimate of source location is attempted. That said, the dura potential estimate can always be matched to an equivalent set of cortical sources if this constraint is applied. Such source fits are nonunique, but are not required in many applications where good use is made of correlations of dura potential dynamics with behavior, cognition, or medical state, regardless of whether any (perhaps unnecessary) identification of dura potentials with cortical sources is obtained.

(ii) Lumping nearest-neighbor Laplacians, due originally to Hjorth (1975), spline-Laplacians, and even one-dimensional cortical depth methods into the single category *current source density* or CSD. The CSD depth methods are based on a different principle from the scalp Laplacian, which depends for its accuracy on the focusing of cortical currents by the high-resistivity skull, an issue not involved with cortical depth recordings. Nearest-neighbor scalp Laplacian estimates are often useful, but are generally much less accurate than spline-Laplacians.

(iii) Claims that coherence estimates based on spline-Laplacians are erroneously high. This idea is superficially plausible because spline fits to surface potential maps have a global character that could result in long-range spurious correlations. However, such claims have been supported only by inappropriate simulations. Later studies showed that spline-Laplacians do not inflate coherence estimates, but rather they may sometimes underestimate coherence as a consequence of the high pass nature of surface Laplacians (Nunez et al. 1997, 1999). We illustrate these ideas in chapter 8.

(iv) Belief that accurate estimates of second derivatives, as required by Laplacian algorithms, cannot be obtained in noisy data. The influence of noise on such estimates of dura potential depends on signal to noise ratio in the raw data, which varies substantially in different EEG applications. A critical issue is whether single time slices or averaged (including Fourier transformed) data are followed. When estimates are obtained from single time slices, noise may indeed be a serious limitation. However, there are also applications like estimating coherence that are based on multiple time slices. In such applications, Laplacian estimates of dura potential are minimally influenced by moderate noise levels, as shown by the purposeful addition of noise to both simulated and genuine data (see chapters 8 and 9).

(v) Belief that inward continuation solutions based on spherical surface models, which are assumed by most dura imaging and Laplacian algorithms, cannot provide useful estimates of dura potential because of inaccurate head models. There are several answers to this claim. For one thing, the goals of different EEG studies may differ substantially. For example, suppose we find that certain measures of EEG dynamic behavior are correlated with cognition at certain electrode locations, or pairs of locations in the cases of covariance or coherence estimates obtained from spline-Laplacians or dura images. Such regional cortical correlations with brain state may be important scientific findings, even if we are unable to pinpoint the specific gyri or sulci responsible due to our imperfect head model. The practical application of estimated spatial-temporal patterns on (say) a best-fit sphere in cognitive or medical studies does not require accurate localization, only robust correlations of these patterns with brain state. We emphasize that EEG's main strength lies in the quantification of spatial-temporal patterns with excellent temporal and mediocre (or worse) spatial resolution. Source localization and high spatial resolution are not natural applications of EEG or MEG, even though they have enjoyed success in certain instances.

(vi) "Proving" that some approach like the nearest-neighbor Laplacian is inaccurate using a physical model of the head with large (say 6 or 7 cm) electrode separations. Mathematical models are much more robust and convincing in making such negative evaluations; they show clearly that accurate Laplacian estimates require much smaller electrode spacing. The appropriate physical models should use small electrode separations (say 2 to 3 cm center-to-center) for which mathematical models predict moderate to good accuracy. In this manner the outer limitations of the mathematical models can be better understood.

We do not claim that that high-resolution EEG obtained with Laplacian or dura image methods approaches anything close to panacea status. However, these transformations reveal new dynamic properties of EEG by band pass spatial filtering scalp data. In general, local source effects are enhanced and global effects are suppressed by the Laplacian algorithm. In this context, the labels "local" and "global" refer to more dominant high and low spatial frequencies, respectively, somewhat analogous to the time-domain labels "fast" and "slow" oscillations. Laplacian estimates have the additional advantage of being reference free. In chapters 8–10, we demonstrate that *high-resolution EEG can substantially complement (but not replace) raw scalp potential data*.

8 Too Much Faith in Minimally Constrained Inverse Solutions in EEG or MEG

Ideally, scientists and clinicians would like to use EEG or MEG data to locate sources within the brain. All such procedures in EEG must involve inverse solutions of Poisson's equation (2.1). The nonuniqueness of unconstrained inverse solutions has been widely cited in the EEG and MEG literature. However, ubiquitous citation has not ensured full appreciation of the severity of this fundamental limitation. In particular, publications that emphasize particular algorithms used to estimate inverse solutions may appear, at first reading, to overcome nonuniqueness, *implying that fancy mathematics can somehow trump fundamental physical limitations*. In this section, we examine the uncomplicated issue of inverse solutions unconstrained by smoothing or other physiological constraints. By contrast, constrained inverse solutions are much more easily justified as discussed in chapter 6.

The potential at any location in the head volume conductor due to brain sources can be expressed as the following volume integral over the entire brain (see appendix K):

$$\Phi(\mathbf{r}, t) = \iiint_{\text{Brain}} \mathbf{G}(\mathbf{r}, \mathbf{r}') \cdot \mathbf{P}(\mathbf{r}', t) dV(\mathbf{r}') \tag{2.2}$$

Here $\mathbf{P}(\mathbf{r}, t)$ is the tissue *dipole moment per unit volume*, that is, the *mesosource strength* at location $\mathbf{r}$ and time t. This mesosource strength is defined in chapter 4 in terms of the (micro) membrane current sources. The integral in (2.2) is weighted by the Green's function $\mathbf{G}(\mathbf{r}, \mathbf{r}')$, which accounts for all geometric and conductive properties of the volume conductor. Generally, $\mathbf{G}(\mathbf{r}, \mathbf{r}')$ is large when the "electrical distance" between recording location $\mathbf{r}$ and source location $\mathbf{r}'$ is small. In an infinite, homogeneous and isotropic medium, the electrical distance equals the actual distance, but this idealization is not accurate for the head volume conductor.

In order to place the inverse problem in EEG (or MEG) in a fundamental context, we may parcel the entire brain volume into N voxels of volume ΔV, each having a mesosource strength $\mathbf{p}_n(\mathbf{r}_n, t_i) = \mathbf{P}(\mathbf{r}_n, t_i)\Delta V$ as shown in fig. 2-5. With this approximation, the scalp potential given by (2.2) may be replaced by a sum over contributions from each voxel, that is

$$\Phi_S(\mathbf{r}_k, t_i) = \sum_{n=1}^{N} \mathbf{G}_n(\mathbf{r}_k, \mathbf{r}_n) \cdot \mathbf{p}_n(\mathbf{r}_n, t_i) \tag{2.3}$$

The notation in (2.3) reflects the fact that, in EEG or MEG applications, scalp potential is sampled at discrete times t_i and discrete locations $\mathbf{r}_k$.

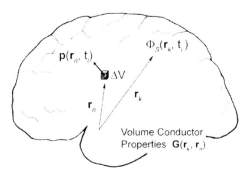

Figure 2-5 A brain volume conductor is indicated in which surface potentials $\Phi_S(\mathbf{r}_k, t_i)$ are recorded at discrete surface locations $\mathbf{r}_k$ and time t_i. The surface potentials are generated by dipole moments $\mathbf{p}(\mathbf{r}_n, t_i)$ in tissue masses (voxels) ΔV located at $\mathbf{r}_n$. All volume conductor properties are included in the Green's function $\mathbf{G}(\mathbf{r}_k, \mathbf{r}_n)$. Mesosources are defined in chapter 4 as dipole moments per unit volume $\mathbf{p}(\mathbf{r}_n, t_i)/\Delta V$.

In attempting inverse solutions using (2.3), our choice of voxel size is limited by knowledge of the head volume conductor. There is no point in seeking source resolution at subcentimeter scales if location errors due only to uncertain resistivity or tissue boundary information are likely to be in the 1 or 2 cm range or larger as appears to be the case. On this basis, it can be argued that somewhat smaller voxels are justified for MEG than for EEG applications because in the MEG inverse problem accurate head models are much closer to a homogeneous, isotropic medium. In EEG studies we might choose $\Delta V \approx 1$ cm^3 or $N = 1400$ in a typical brain volume. In this case one might naively imagine the idealized goal of assigning a source vector $\mathbf{p}_n(\mathbf{r}_n, t_i)$ to each 1 cm^3 volume of brain tissue—in a manner somewhat similar to assigning metabolic signatures to each voxel in MRI or PET studies. Of course, in EEG or MEG practice, the actual goal is much more modest—to identify a few voxels (n) located at $\mathbf{r}_n$ and their mesosources $\mathbf{p}_n(\mathbf{r}_n, t_i)$ that can account for the observed surface data.

In order to consider the fundamental nonuniqueness of the general inverse problem, here we mostly ignore algorithm, noise, and volume conductor issues. We focus only on nonuniqueness, an issue that will remain unaltered by more efficient algorithms, superfast computers, cleaner recordings, or improved head models developed in the future. Assuming a perfect head model (all $\mathbf{G}_n$'s known perfectly) and infinite signal to noise ratio (perfect knowledge of $\Phi_S(\mathbf{r}_k, t_i)$), the inverse problem boils down to solving a system of KI equations. K is the number of surface electrodes and I is the number of time samples used to determine the $3NI$ unknowns, where N is the number of voxels (number of "dipoles") and the factor of three accounts for the three components of the vector dipoles or *mesosources* $\mathbf{p}_n(\mathbf{r}_n, t_i)$.

If inverse solutions are unconstrained by smoothing in the time domain, the problem reduces to finding voxel dipole moments at each instant in time t_i. Several early dipole localization schemes proceeded as follows. Develop K equations from the forward solution (2.3) for potentials at K scalp locations generated by some assumed number Q dipoles, where Q is typically in the range 1–5. One may start by assuming a single dipole $\mathbf{p}_1(\mathbf{r}_1, t_i)$ and find the location $\mathbf{r}_1$ and dipole moment $\mathbf{p}_1$ (a total of six scalar unknowns) that best fit the experimental data. If the EEG is recorded with K electrodes (excluding reference), K equations are available to solve for the six unknown parameters that characterize a single dipole. These equations may be solved in the least-squares sense and error criteria tested to see if the single-dipole solution adequately fits the experimental data. If this one-dipole test fails, a two-dipole solution may be assumed and a new set of K equations solved to find the best two-dipole solution $(\mathbf{r}_1, \mathbf{r}_2, \mathbf{p}_1, \mathbf{p}_2)$. The error test is applied to the two-dipole solution; if this test fails a three-dipole solution is attempted and so forth.

The number of dipoles that may be recruited to fit the data in this manner is limited by the number of surface samples (electrodes) K. That is, the number of equations K must equal or exceed the number of unknowns $6Q$. Thus, if EEG is recorded with $K=64$ electrodes, it might be theoretically possible to fit the data to as many as 10 dipoles. Of course, in practice, the limitations are more severe. For one thing, separate recordings from close scalp locations may yield nearly redundant data resulting in ill-conditioned equations that produce nonsense solutions. With deep dipoles accurate inverse solutions are more difficult.

The dipole localization scheme outlined above makes good sense in applications where the underlying sources are known in advance to consist of only a few isolated sources. The best examples of this are provided by implanted sources in phantom head models or epileptic patients (Cohen et al. 1990; Leahy et al. 1998), but what about the more general case where no such prior knowledge is available? We may plausibly assume that any surface distribution of potential (or magnetic field) at fixed time t_i can, within the limits of head model and experimental error, be fully accounted for by fewer than Q_{max} dipoles. With today's head models, the number of *maximum required dipoles* in this context is probably less than 10. That is, the recruitment of dipoles in excess of Q_{max} is not expected to improve the accuracy of our data fit, even if the algorithm is able to find many more dipoles.

An essential question concerning dipole localization is then clear. How close to the actual source distribution is the solution based on Q_{max} dipoles likely to be? We can address this issue by noting that nearly every tissue mass in the brain is potentially capable of producing a dipole moment. To make our discussion more concrete, we assume a parceling of the brain into $N=1400$ voxels and recording with $K=60$ electrodes (or MEG sensors). A search for (say) 10 equivalent dipoles involves the implicit assumption that only 10 voxels produce significant dipole moments $\mathbf{p}_n(\mathbf{r}_n, t_i)$, the remaining 1390 in (2.3) are arbitrarily set to zero.

Rather than start with the assumption of a few isolated sources, we can just as reasonably (from a strictly physiological perspective) approach this problem from the opposite view of distributed sources. Ideally, we could pick any combination of $60/3=20$ voxels from the pool of 1400 voxels and solve the resulting $K=60$ equations for the 20 corresponding vectors $\mathbf{p}_n(\mathbf{r}_n, t_i)$, thereby obtaining a near perfect match to the experimental data. The number of combinations of N voxels taken $k=K/3$ at a time then yields a rough estimate of the number of inverse solutions that can be expected to fit the data perfectly. From standard probability theory

$$C_{N,k} = \frac{N!}{k!(N-k)!} = \frac{1400!}{20!1380!} \cong 3 \times 10^{44} \qquad (2.4)$$

This guess is too high because we have ignored equation sets with no solutions or ill-conditioned solutions. For example, solutions with all voxel sources located close to each other are unlikely to fit maps with large potentials over the entire scalp. Nevertheless, the number of solutions that can provide near perfect matches to scalp data appears to be greater than the number of grains of sand that could be packed into the volume of the earth ($\sim 10^{30}$). The estimate (2.4) provides some perspective on the meaning of the term "nonunique" in the context of inverse solutions. Even if we were to parcel the brain into 10 cm^3 voxels such that $N = 140$, the number of "near perfect" 20-dipole solutions is about 10^{24}. If we assume that a perfect data fit is obtained with only five dipoles and $N = 140$ voxels, there are still nearly a billion such solutions.

The arguments of this section suggest that unconstrained inverse solutions in EEG or MEG will remain forever intractable. Practical inverse solutions require substantial additional information so that plausible constraints may be incorporated into the analyses. The most common constraint is to force all but a few of the $\mathbf{p}_n(\mathbf{r}_n, t_j)$ to be zero, a procedure requiring substantial justification in each application. *The demonstration that a few dipoles provide near-perfect fits to recorded data is, of itself, a very weak argument to support the genuine presence of such isolated sources.* More information is required to support such claims. Much more plausible constraints involve smoothing in the time and spatial domains. We address the constraint question in the next section and again in chapter 6.

9 Dipole Localization: Genuine or Virtual?

Sophisticated algorithms have been developed by EEG scientists to locate implanted dipoles in mathematical and physical models and in human patients. These methods have also been applied to *interictal spikes* (between seizures) and seizure discharges in epilepsy surgery patients due to unknown sources. Both EEG and MEG localization methods have been applied. Here we summarize some of the main results:

(i) In the case of implanted dipoles in a patient (Cohen et al. 1990), dipole localization was successful using surface EEG and MEG with accuracy typically in the 1 to 2 cm range for both methods. With a single dipole planted in a physical head model (Leahy et al. 1999), both EEG and MEG methods also worked well. Typical EEG accuracy was in the 1 to 2 cm range and MEG accuracy was in the 0.5 to 1 cm range.

(ii) In simulations, several dipoles can often be successfully located accurately in concentric spheres models. The issue of how many isolated sources may be found depends partly on their locations. This number is expected to be larger if most of the sources are close to the surface. For example, the BESA algorithm (with temporal smoothing) successfully located five superficial dipoles in one blind test (Nunez et al. 1994).

(iii) In *epilepsy surgery patients* with unknown sources, the issues are much more complicated. Dipole localization algorithms are currently used in only a few clinical settings, where they are typically employed to categorize seizures much more generally than implied by the label "localization." That is, dipole algorithms are applied in combination with other clinical information to select good candidates for surgery and to choose locations for intracranial electrodes. Intracranial recordings then follow to find legitimate surgery candidates and to determine the location and volume of brain tissue to surgically remove in these patients (the *resection strategy*). Decisions to resection brain tissue based only on scalp data are made only in a carefully selected sub-set of patients.

Ebersole (1997) has discussed examples of how dipole localization algorithms are used effectively to study epilepsy surgery patients. Scalp potential distributions are expected to be more sensitive to dipole orientation than to location. Focal seizures may start in a relatively isolated deep neural structure, say in a single gyrus or sulcus of mesial cortex (underside of brain). Correctly determining the dipole axis direction may be very helpful even if the estimated location is wrong. For example, the neurologist may line up the putative dipole axis with an MRI scan of mesial cortex and assume that the equivalent dipole of the offending tissue is probably perpendicular to the local cortical surface. The area of active cortical surface is a critical issue. As a general rule, about 6 cm^2 of cortex must be synchronously active in order for the activity to be recorded on the scalp (Cooper et al. 1965; Delucchi et al. 1975; Ebersole 1997). That is, *in order for epileptic tissue dynamics to be recorded from the scalp, a seizure focus must have spread to a size that violates the dipole assumption.* Typical source regions of epileptic spikes occupy perhaps 10 to 20 cm^2 of gyral surface. In clinical practice, "dipole localization" of such activity may be interpreted as the approximate location of the center of this epileptic EEG activity, but the label "dipole" does not accurately represent such extended sources.

The examples above show how physiological interpretations of dipole localization in various circumstances can vary from *genuine dipoles* (say with known implanted sources or averaged evoked potentials from primary sensory cortex) to much less well defined ideas where the dipole solution is interpreted as a *virtual dipole* used mainly to quantify data, that is, obtain data reduction parameters. We do not argue against any method that works effectively in clinical practice. However, the following caveats apply to cases of putative locations of genuine dipoles.

Many publications of putative brain dipoles have been published without mentioning *dipole strength*. Dipole location (three parameters) and axis orientation (two parameters) may be published, but not dipole moment. Consider, for example, some EEG phenomenon with scalp potential magnitude in the 10 to 100 μV range, say one of the usual alpha or sleep rhythms or perhaps a seizure discharge. Suppose the dipole localization algorithm predicts that the measured scalp potential distribution is due to a dipole (or a few dipoles) near the center of the head. We can use (1.7) to estimate the dipole moment required to generate this measured potential, assuming the characteristic size of the source region is actually much smaller than its depth.

Consider first the case of an infinite, homogeneous conductor with resistivity $\eta \cong 300\ \Omega$ cm (brain). The maximum potential occurs along the dipole axis ($\theta = 0$). We may solve for the dipole moment Id in (1.7) for potentials at $r \cong 9$ cm (scalp) in (say) the 10 μV range. However, in chapter 6, it is shown that the combined effects of confining current to the head and adding the skull/scalp layers is to increase surface potential due to a central source to roughly twice its magnitude in an infinite homogeneous medium. From these considerations we obtain a rough estimate of the central dipole source strength in layered spherical medium:

$$Id \cong 20\ \mu A\ cm \tag{2.5}$$

Given this source strength, we can estimate the potential at (say) $r = 1$ cm above the dipole. The equation for potentials a homogeneous medium provides a reasonable estimate at such distances far from the surface. Thus (1.5) yields a rough estimate of the maximum potentials one would expect to record in depth with millimeter-scale electrodes. The predicted potential 1 cm from central dipole is then something like

$$\Phi(1,0) \cong 500\ \mu V \tag{2.6}$$

Seizures producing intracranial potentials in the 500 μV range are quite possible; however, such potentials are probably too large for normal spontaneous EEG. Actually, we have been rather conservative by making the estimate (2.6) at $r = 1$ cm. Predicted potentials closer to the dipole are higher, as might be recorded by mesoscopic electrodes, with diameters in (say) the 0.1 mm range. To make the estimates somewhat more realistic, the dipole potential (1.7) can be expressed in terms of the potential difference ΔV_S across a small radial dipole layer of area A_S as shown in chapter 5. That is, the maximum potential in (1.7) occurs directly above the dipole layer ($\theta = 0$) and may be expressed as

$$\Phi(r,0) \cong \frac{qA_S}{4\pi r^2} \Delta V_S \tag{2.7}$$

Here the equation for a radial dipole layer in an infinite, homogeneous medium has been multiplied by the correction factor q to account for the finite, inhomogeneous head. For dipole sources near the middle of the head, q is roughly equal to 2. For radial sources near the scalp surface,

q should be set to something like $1/4$ to obtain the corresponding correction for finite head size and tissue inhomogeneity. For dipole source regions in the general range of a cortical macrocolumn, A_S is roughly 0.01 cm^2. Solving (2.7) for the effective potential difference across a small dipole layer near the center of the head required to produce scalp potentials in the 10 µV range yields

$$\Delta Vs \approx 5 \times 10^6 \text{ µV} \qquad (2.8)$$

If the putative small central dipole were taken seriously, we would anticipate potentials in the roughly 5 V range to be recorded from meso-scopic electrodes (diameter in the 0.1 mm range or smaller) close to the source region. Of course, such extracellular potentials are too large by a factor of 1000 or more to be physiologically realistic. However, such considerations have not prevented reports of such magical dipoles. One wonders if this explains why source magnitudes are often not reported.

By contrast to the single dipole source, suppose the source region is a dipole layer of area (say) $A_S \approx 30 \text{ cm}^2$. Our estimate of the required source strength (2.8) from (2.7) is then reduced by a factor of 3000. Furthermore, in the case of a large *mesial source* region (on the underside of cortical surface), a good part of this region may be much closer than the assumed 9 cm to one side of the head. If, for example, the center of a 30 cm^2 mesial source region is 3 cm from the surface, our estimate (2.8) is reduced by an additional factor of $(9/3)^2 = 9$ so that (2.8) is replaced by

$$\Delta Vs \approx 100 \text{ µV} \qquad (2.9)$$

where the correction factor q was assumed to be roughly equal to one. The source strength indicated by (2.9) is quite plausible in this example of a distributed mesial source region.

By contrast to dipole localization, estimates of dura potential at large scales are unique in the sense of being limited only by sampling density, head model accuracy and noise. Model-induced errors in dura potential estimates may be smaller than the corresponding errors in deep dipole parameter estimates. This is expected because of the larger distances between scalp and locations of parameter estimation in the deep dipole case. Thus, in cases of putative isolated dipoles, *it may make sense to estimate dura potential before resorting to dipole localization algorithms.* That is, estimates of dura potential should be at least as accurate (more accurate in many cases) as estimates of dipole parameters, even when the sources are known in advance to consist of only a few isolated dipoles. One can see if the estimated dura potential distribution is too complicated to have been generated by one or two isolated sources; if so, dipole analysis could be abandoned at the outset.

In contrast, if estimated dura potential is relatively simple, it may be appropriate to use this estimated dura potential as input to dipole algorithms in place of the raw scalp data. A possible advantage of this two-step procedure (in addition to avoiding publication of absurd solutions) is that the appropriate new model for dipole localization is much closer to a homogeneous medium. That is, with potentials specified on the dura surface, one can ignore scalp and skull currents to a first approximation. Current distribution in a brain fully surrounded by a low-resistivity skull is similar to current distribution brain surrounded by empty space. If scalp potential data are the inputs to the dipole algorithm, the skull and scalp must obviously be included in the head model. By contrast, if dura potentials are the input data, the first approximation to the appropriate volume conductor is a homogeneous sphere, making the inverse EEG problem more similar to the MEG inverse problem.

10 EEG versus MEG Controversies

MEG is a relatively new and impressive technology developed to record the brain's extremely small magnetic field (Hamalainen et al. 1993). MEG has been applied mainly to evoked and event-related potentials since the early 1980s. Enthusiasm for MEG (relative to EEG) has been boosted by both genuine scientific considerations and poorly justified commercial pressures. We consider here whether MEG can add information not available in EEG or offer other advantages. A popular (but erroneous) idea, addressed below, is that MEG spatial resolution is generally superior to EEG spatial resolution.

One possible advantage (or disadvantage) of MEG versus EEG is the selective sensitivity of these measures. The external magnetic field generated by a radial dipole in a spherically symmetric volume conductor (layered or homogeneous) is zero. Thus, MEG recordings tend to filter out signals from dipole sources with axes oriented perpendicular to the scalp surface. These mesosources lay mostly along the gyral surfaces in the cortex. Gyral dipole sources tend to be more nearly perpendicular to the scalp surface than sources in fissures and sulci, although cortical surface symmetry is not fully satisfied in genuine brains. Given the irregularity of cortical surfaces, gyral sources can easily have nonnegligible dipole moments in tangential directions. For example, suppose a local gyral surface makes an angle β with local scalp. Consider a local gyral source of strength Id perpendicular to local cortex. The component of the dipole moment in the direction tangent to the scalp surface is $Id\sin\beta$. If β is (say) $20°$, the maximum extracranial magnetic field due to the gyral source is then expected to be roughly $\sin(20°)$ or 34% of the maximum extracranial magnetic field due to a dipole tangent to the local scalp with the same strength and depth. However, for the most part, MEG appears to be more sensitive to tangential dipole sources which lie principally on sulcal walls and less sensitive to sources along gyral surfaces.

By contrast, the maximum outer surface potential due to a superficial radial dipole (cortical) in a four concentric spheres model (brain, CSF, skull, and scalp) is about two to three times the maximum surface potential of a tangential dipole at the same strength and depth, as discussed in chapter 6. Thus, we expect EEG to be more sensitive to sources in cortical gyri as indicated by fig. 2-3 and less sensitive to sources in cortical sulci. *MEG and EEG are preferentially sensitive to different cortical sources.* The relative merits of MEG and EEG, either in the context of source localization or for more general analyses of spatial-temporal patterns, depend on the nature of the underlying mesosources. Unfortunately, such source information is not generally available in advance of the decision to choose between EEG and MEG systems.

Identification of special source regions may be particularly important in certain applications. Epileptic foci and primary sensory cortex located in fissures and sulci come to mind in this context. These special sources may be difficult or impossible to isolate with EEG because they are masked by larger potentials originating from other brain regions, especially cortical gyri. Thus, one can easily imagine clinical or other applications in which MEG may locate or otherwise characterize such special sources, especially in candidates for epilepsy surgery. *We emphasize that MEG's advantage in this example occurs because of its relative insensitivity to gyral sources, not because it is generally more accurate than EEG.*

MEG does indeed have an important advantage for source localization because skull and other tissues are transparent to magnetic fields. Magnetic fields generated inside the cranium are minimally distorted by tissue and form external patterns apparently close to those produced by sources in a homogeneous sphere. For this reason, there appears to be much less uncertainty in models that relate current sources in the brain to MEG, as compared to EEG, where head properties (tissue conductivities and boundaries) are only known approximately. However, in practice, EEG has an important advantage over MEG because EEG electrodes are about twice as close to cortical sources as typical MEG coils that are maintained at some distance from the scalp in a cold chamber (near absolute zero).

Some of the practical consequences of these features are demonstrated with simulations in fig. 2-6 showing a comparison of the field spreads in tangential directions due to dipole sources with axes tangent to the scalp. A 4-sphere head model predicts EEG (scalp potential), cortical potential (potential on the inner sphere) and the surface Laplacian (along the surface of the outer spherical shell). MEG (radial magnetic field) is calculated using a homogeneous sphere as head model. The plots at left and right correspond to different choices of skull conductivity and different distances between source and MEG magnetometer coils. Scalp potential and radial magnetic field (due to a tangential cortical dipole

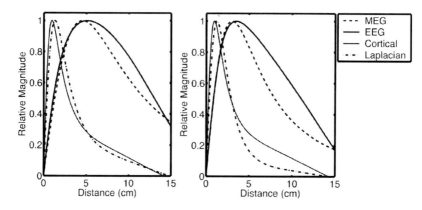

Figure 2-6 Theoretical spread of MEG and EEG measures in tangential directions from a tangential mesosource (dipole) in a spherical volume conductor. For the MEG calculation, the volume is assumed to be homogeneous with spherical symmetry. In the EEG example, the volume consists of an inner sphere and three concentric spherical shells representing brain, CSF, skull, and scalp with radii (8.0, 8.2, 8.6, 9.2 cm), our standard 4-sphere model. The brain to CSF conductivity ratio equals 0.2 and brain and scalp conductivities are assumed equal. The tangential dipole is located 0.8 cm below the surface of the inner sphere (brain). (*Left plot*) Brain to skull conductivity ratio is 40 and the MEG coil is located 2.8 cm above the scalp. The calculated fall-off with distance from the dipole source (along the outer spherical surface) of four different measures is shown. Measures plotted are: radial magnetic field (MEG) on a sphere of fixed distance above the scalp, potential on the scalp (EEG), potential on the surface of the brain (cortical), and analytic surface Laplacian of the scalp potential (Laplacian). Each measure is normalized with respect to its maximum value to emphasize relative magnitudes. (*Right plot*) Brain to skull conductivity ratio is 20 and the MEG coil located 0.8 cm above the scalp.

2.2 cm below the scalp) fall to 50% of their maxima at tangential scalp distances in the 8–14 cm range depending on head model and MEG coil location. Parameters used to construct the two plots are: brain-to-skull conductivity ratios (40 left, 20 right) and MEG coil distances from scalp (2.8 cm left, 0.8 cm right). With today's magnetometer systems, *the EEG and MEG point spread functions are in the same general range, depending critically on MEG sensor distance from the sources.* By contrast to both EEG and MEG, the surface Laplacian and other high-resolution EEG measures have theoretical point spread functions that closely follow the cortical potential with a 50% fall-off points of about 3 cm (see chapter 8). More detailed studies generally support these conclusions (Malmivuo and Plonsey 1995). Improvements in MEG spatial resolution can be obtained by using planar gradiometer coils, which are somewhat analogous to bipolar EEG recordings. The planar gradiometer configuration is less common in commercial MEG systems and can be either an advantage or disadvantage, depending on the depth of the source.

Additional insight into the differences between MEG, unprocessed EEG, and high-resolution EEG estimates obtained from the surface Laplacian is facilitated by the simulations shown in fig. 2-7. The locations of three radial dipoles are indicated by open (negative pole up) and closed

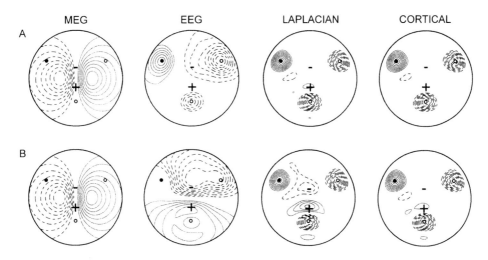

Figure 2-7 Example spatial distributions of magnetic field (simulated MEG) and potential (simulated EEG) generated by four dipole sources. Three radial dipoles are indicated by open (negative pole up) and filled (positive pole up) circles. The ± signs indicate the two poles of a single tangential dipole. Radial dipoles are located 0.2 cm below the brain surface in the spherical model. The tangential dipole is located 0.8 cm below the brain surface. The MEG field is plotted on a sphere 2.8 cm above the scalp surface. The EEG, cortical potential, and surface Laplacian were calculated using the 4-sphere model of fig. 2.6 (with brain to skull conductivity equal to 40). Each map was normalized with respect to its maximum value to emphasize relative magnitudes. Contours are plotted in steps of 10% of the maximum value. Positive field values are indicated by solid contour lines and negative fields indicated by dashed contours. (*Upper row*) All four dipoles have identical dipole moments. (*Lower row*) The strength of the tangential dipole is five times the strength of the three radial dipoles.

(positive pole up) circles. The ± signs indicate the two poles of a single tangential dipole. EEG, cortical potential (potential on the surface of the brain sphere), and scalp surface Laplacian were calculated using a four-concentric-spheres model of the head. The two rows of plots show the same four-source configuration. In row A, the four dipoles have equal dipole moments; in row B the tangential dipole has a dipole moment five times larger than the radial dipoles. In each row, the plotted spatial distribution of magnetic field is due only to the single tangential dipole, but with magnitude five times larger in case B. In case A, scalp potential is dominated by the radial dipoles. The surface Laplacian accurately locates the three radial sources and closely mimics the cortical potential. In row B, the scalp potential plot reveals the strong influence of the tangential dipole and a generally more complex potential distribution. For instance, the potential directly over the radial source in the upper left is zero, due to cancellation by the potential generated by stronger tangential dipole. In both rows, the Laplacian is effective in locating the three radial sources and closely approximates the cortical potential.

The examples in fig. 2-7 illustrate that arguments about the relative accuracies of MEG, EEG, and high-resolution EEG must depend critically on the nature of the sources. This general idea has also been confirmed experimentally in animal models using depth recordings, cortical surface recordings, and extracranial MEG and EEG (Okada et al. 1999). Row A shows that spatial distributions of potential and Laplacian indicate the positions of the three radial sources. In the examples of row A, MEG provides information that is entirely distinct from the EEG. By contrast, the examples in row B (stronger tangential dipole) show substantial similarities between EEG and MEG. Both measures provide good evidence for the stronger tangential source, while the surface Laplacian provides additional information about superficial radial dipoles that is not apparent in either the MEG or unprocessed EEG.

Several caveats are required when interpreting the plots in fig. 2-7. The MEG simulations apply only to magnetometer coils; better resolution may be obtained from gradiometer coils subject to signal-to-noise considerations. These simple simulations also fail to address issues associated with sampling density, noise, head model, and reference electrode (EEG only). Furthermore, accurate Laplacian estimates require sophisticated algorithms. For these reasons, fig. 2-6 (one point source) and fig. 2-7 (multiple point sources) cannot be used in isolation for estimating the relative accuracies of different measures. Nevertheless, we conclude that the common question of whether MEG is superior or inferior to EEG is the wrong question. The right question is whether MEG can add substantial information to that available from EEG, especially given the much higher cost of MEG. In this regard, we note that in the examples of fig. 2-7, the combination of MEG to detect deeper tangential dipoles and high-resolution EEG to detect superficial radial dipoles yields an accurate picture of the source distribution.

MEG does enjoy advantages over EEG for special applications. For example, dipole localization with MEG appears to be somewhat better than with EEG, although some controversy on this issue may remain. One reason to expect some MEG advantage in dipole localization is that the appropriate head model for MEG is much closer to a homogeneous sphere. That is, tissue conductivities and boundaries, which are known only approximately, have less influence on magnetic fields than electric fields (or potentials). Thus, accurate localization of a few isolated sources by multichannel MEG (perhaps 64 to 128 or even more coils) can be obtained using the appropriate computer algorithm and dense spatial sampling even though the point spread function for each dipole is quite broad (Leahy et al. 1998). Another reason is that the selective sensitivity of MEG to tangential dipoles reduces the number of sources to be fit. Thus, *an MEG signal is inherently more likely to be accurately explained by a small number of discrete sources* (Okada et al. 1999). This is not necessarily an MEG advantage; in most brain states we want information about all active sources.

In general, the source distributions underlying the EEG and MEG are complex and distributed over the cortex. The sources are plausibly pictured as dipole layers composed of synchronous dipoles oriented perpendicular to the local cortical surface. Each dipole, or *mesosource* $\mathbf{P}(\mathbf{r}, t)$, represents a small volume of cortical tissue as discussed in chapters 4 and 6. EEG is preferentially sensitive to large dipole layers, consisting of many gyral surfaces and the intervening sulcal folds. MEG is relatively insensitive to these types of large source distributions that appear to dominate most EEG recordings. Rather, MEG tends to detect the portions of large dipole layers that extend into sulcal walls, especially when only one side of the sulcus active, as suggested by fig. 2-3.

We have developed these arguments to identify common *MEG/EEG fallacies*. The sum of these fallacies is the idea that better laboratories are developed by replacing EEG systems with MEG systems. When judged in the context of specific scientific or clinical applications, it can be argued that an EEG laboratory will be substantially improved by an added MEG system. In other contexts, however, the MEG system may add minimally to scientific capability. In either case, it is far more difficult to justify using MEG exclusively, if only because its initial cost is perhaps 30 times the cost of EEG. In summary, common MEG/EEG fallacies include:

(i) The idea that EEG and MEG are equivalent, that is, they necessarily duplicate each other's performance in locating or otherwise characterizing brain sources. MEG and EEG are preferentially sensitive to different subsets of sources in the brain.

(ii) The idea that MEG is generally more accurate than EEG. This common belief is false since MEG is mainly insensitive to superficial radial sources and is thus likely to provide an incomplete picture of the sources relative to EEG.

(iii) The idea that MEG can generally be used to "check" the results of EEG or vise versa. While approximate correspondence between the two measures often occurs, there is good reason to view EEG and MEG as independent measures of brain function. The two methods are selectively sensitive to different sources, especially dipoles having different axis orientations. Figure 2.7 demonstrates that, depending on the number, location, and strength of the sources, MEG can be either consistent or inconsistent with EEG.

(iv) Because MEG is reference free, it has an important advantage over any EEG recording whose properties depend on choice of the reference electrode. As discussed in chapter 7, EEG potentials depend equally on the location of recording and reference electrodes. When large electrode arrays are used, the average reference often approximates reference-free recordings. Furthermore, high-resolution EEG measures such as the surface Laplacian are reference free, but require dense electrode arrays and computer processing as discussed in chapter 8.

These high-resolution EEG measures appear complementary to the MEG by emphasizing the superficial radial sources that MEG is not expected to detect. In addition, it is theoretically possible (and perhaps practical) to build capacitive-coupled sensors that measure the brain's electric field in the region approximately 1 cm above the scalp. Such electric field measures are also reference free.

11 New Data Analysis Methods in Search of Applications

Neurologists are trained to read raw (unprocessed) EEG written on vast reams of paper or, in the modern version, appearing on computer screens. For the most part, clinical data analysis has been left entirely to the clinician's well-trained brain. Similarly, cognitive scientists typically follow computer traces of evoked or event-related potentials for which simple averages over trials (stimuli) are the only automated part. Arguments against under-use of computer methods appear throughout this book. Revolutionary improvements in computer speed, cost, and convenience have occurred over the past 20 years. Thus, from one viewpoint, the general arguments for more automation of records are stronger today than when the first edition of this book was published in 1981. Despite this, substantial resistance to EEG computer analyses by some clinicians and cognitive scientists remains for both valid and invalid reasons as discussed in the context of the following *data reduction fallacies*:

(i) One old idea is that all the useful information in EEG is contained in the raw data and nothing is added by computer transformation, a view expressed to the senior author several times over the past 30 years by clinical electroencephalo-graphers. This view does, in fact, have some credibility. Highly trained EEG clinicians can be very skilled at picking out several different frequency components, including muscle or eye movement artifact, in a raw record without resorting to spectral analysis. Or, they may use a combination of bipolar EEG and EEG employing several different reference electrodes to (hopefully) locate an epileptic focus. We should not under-estimate the importance of these skills based on years of experience. *However, the essential argument here is that computer methods should complement, not replace, these human talents.*

(ii) A multichannel EEG contains spatial as well as temporal information. It is very difficult to interpret such data in three dimensions (one time and two scalp coordinates), especially if the number of channels is large. The EEG literature contains many questionable physiological interpretations of raw data. *As data become more complicated, the ability of even highly skilled brains to reduce this data fails rapidly.* Consider raw data from a radar system displayed as wavy lines similar to an EEG. Yes, all the "information" is in the raw traces, but how well could air traffic controllers use these raw traces to estimate the simultaneous locations, speeds, and directions of several airplanes? Or, suppose raw data from CT or MRI is presented as sheets of wavy lines, each representing a different brain slice. Would such traces satisfy the neurologist or neurosurgeon?

(iii) For a long time, the dominant view in EEG, often expressed to the senior author, was that adding more electrodes beyond the standard 10/20 system provides no useful information. This view may be correct if only unprocessed EEG traces are studied, but computer methods provide an excellent means to make better sense of this raw data. Given the preeminent complexity of brains, we conjecture that EEG contains many subtle dynamic properties that will be discovered only with the assistance of sophisticated data analysis tools. The studies in chapter 10 support this conjecture by establishing several global EEG properties that were unknown to earlier scientists and clinicians.

(iv) Having argued the case for more effective use of computer methods, a caveat is appropriate: *some EEG computer methods are entirely lacking in merit.* The number of ways to mathematically transform data is infinite. Transformations picked without solid theoretical reasons can be expected to obscure rather than illuminate the underlying dynamic processes. Thus, the views of the so-called old-fashioned EEG scientists cited above are partly correct. *Inappropriate computer methods are worse than no computer methods at all.* In the examples of radar signal, CT, or MRI data, physical principles are employed to transform data in ways that human brains are able to interpret in terms of genuine physical processes. A similar philosophy is required for EEG.

(v) Several tests should be considered before computer methods are applied to EEG. First, the clinical or scientific questions to be asked of the data should be clearly articulated. Does the proposed analysis work effectively in answering similar questions in other fields? If not, there is no apparent reason why it should work in EEG. Next, new methods should be tested with simulated EEG. *The best simulated sources encompass a range of dynamic properties (reflecting the uncertain dynamics of genuine data) and are located in a volume conductor model of the head.* Since the simulated source characteristics are known, the proposed methods can be evaluated for the idealized volume conductor. Of course, success at this step does not guarantee the method will work effectively with genuine brains. However, failure at this first step ensures that the proposed methods will fail when applied to EEG. The use of simulated data has the added benefit of *providing a partial check on computer codes.* Given our experience with many faulty programs, written by engineering students as well as ourselves, we are often surprised by published EEG papers where no mention is made of this critical verification step.

(vi) *No matter how sophisticated the computer method, raw data should never be ignored.* This step is especially critical for data that may contain important artifact as discussed earlier. Some glaring software errors may be discovered in this manner, for example, accidentally interchanging right and left hemisphere measures. The central issue is to remove as much as possible of the "black box" character of computer methods by matching scientific intuition with mathematics, even if this intuition is applied post hoc.

(vii) It is difficult to make blanket statements evaluating specific computer methods in EEG since any given method may be appropriate for some applications and inappropriate for others. Some methods have limited use, but are easily over-interpreted. When applied in inappropriate contexts, erroneous computer methods have included amplitude maps (especially color maps), dipole localization, correlation dimension estimates, wavelets, and even standard spectral analysis. We have been surprised, for example, at how much our subjective impressions of EEG contour maps can change with choice of *color scheme*. The color red often seems more important than other colors, as traffic engineers can attest. The issue of EEG computer processing is considered in more detail in chapters 8 and 9.

12 Treating the Entire Alpha Band as a Unitary Phenomenon

Modern studies of alpha rhythms recorded from human scalp with high-density electrode arrays and processed by dura imaging or spline-Laplacian algorithms have rediscovered several essential features observed in cortical recordings by pioneers Walter, Penfield, Jasper, Cooper, and others as discussed in chapter 1. The modern studies have also provided more detail about spectral content, spatial properties, and relationships to cognitive events (Nunez et al. 2001). The alpha band in waking humans encompasses a complex mixture of (at least partly) distinct phenomena determined by different reactivity, spatial distribution over the scalp, and frequency sub-band. For example, some tasks cause upper and lower band alpha amplitudes to change in different directions (Petsche and Etlinger 1998; Klimesch et al. 1999).

Coherence or other estimates of phase synchronization between widely separated cortical regions provide evidence of functional connections. Such measures are often sensitive to 1 or 2 Hz changes within the alpha band (Nunez 1995). For example, during moderate to difficult mental calculations in some subjects, low-alpha coherence (near 8 Hz) may be reduced over many pairs of scalp locations, whereas high-alpha coherence (near 10 or 11 Hz) and narrow band theta coherence (near 6 Hz) may mostly increase in these same data (Nunez et al. 2001). Short- (<5 cm) and long-range (>8 cm) coherence can also change in opposite directions within the same data set, consistent with changes in the spatial extents of putative cell assemblies.

These data are qualitatively consistent with cell assembly formation operating in preferred frequency bands and immersed in dynamic global environments that we characterize here as action potential and synaptic action fields, as discussed in chapters 1, 4, 9, 10, and 11. However, this (partly speculative) interpretation is not required to make the essential point that the entire alpha band (8 to 13 Hz) cannot be safely treated as a single phenomenon. Yet most of the earlier alpha studies have done so, for example, by following amplitude or coherence changes over the full bandwidth. Many such studies have reported small but statistically significant differences in such measures between populations (Often individual subject differences do not pass statistical tests.) The strategy of lumping all measures in the broad 8 to 13 Hz band into the single category "alpha" may also be confounded by the (admittedly difficult) problems associated with different subjects exhibiting different spatial and temporal dynamics associated with cognitive processes.

13 Pacemaker Icons as Means of Avoiding Brain Dynamics

The classic *EEG pacemaker* idea imagines isolated local networks, typically in the thalamus, producing signals at preferred (perhaps resonant) frequencies. This dynamical output is imagined to be forced on (input to) neocortex so that neocortical sources oscillate at the same preferred frequencies as the pacemakers. For the purposes of these general arguments concerning the standard pacemaker idea, it does not matter if the putative local pacemaker network is located in the thalamus, a region of neocortex, or some other structure.

The essential idea of a pacemaker is that its dominant frequencies are determined by local internal mechanisms, not by feedback from external tissue masses as indicated in fig. 2-8. Such pacemakers might conceivably occur at any hierarchical level between membrane and large-scale multiple networks. However, pacemakers at any spatial scale must have very restricted input in order to preserve the autonomy essential to qualify them as "pacemakers." The existence of such autonomy has been critically questioned (Lopes da Silva 1995, 1999; Basar 1997; Steriade 1999). Another problem is that the pacemaker's target system (say neocortex) can be expected to respond most strongly when the target's input frequency matches one its own resonant frequencies. However, in this case, the distinction between target system and pacemaker may be lost;

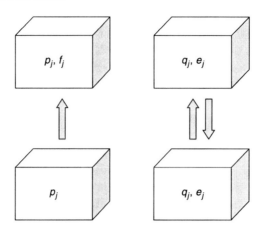

Figure 2-8 The EEG pacemaker idea is represented in the left-hand column. Oscillations in the upper system (cortex) are expected to have dominant frequencies (p_j, f_j) due to internal feedback mechanisms within each system (thalamus and cortex). By contrast, the right-hand column illustrates interactions where the "pacemaker" concept is inappropriate. In this case, oscillations in the upper system are expected to have different dominant frequencies (q_j, e_j) due to both internal and external feedback mechanisms. That is, with the addition of sufficient feedback, the two systems act as a single system.

that is, we can just as easily think of the target driving the pacemaker as the pacemaker driving its target (Nunez 1995).

To illustrate this idea, the left-hand column in fig. 2-8 indicates one-way interactions (no external feedback) between systems (or tissue masses). In this case, pacemaker frequencies p_j (resulting from internal feedback mechanisms in the lower box) are forced on the upper box. The upper box (perhaps representing a local cortical region or the entire neocortex) tends to produce oscillations with both the pacemaker frequencies p_j and the natural (or resonant) frequencies of the upper box f_j. By contrast, substantial interaction (external feedback) between the systems occurs in the right-hand column, thereby essentially creating a single system for purposes of dynamic description with natural frequencies (q_j, e_j) that depend on both internal and external interactions and can differ sub-stantially from the resonant frequencies of the isolated systems (p_j, f_j). This general kind of behavior is demonstrated in a nonlinear (van der Pol) oscillator with variable interaction strength in chapter 9.

Some physiologists have insisted on crediting each EEG frequency component to a distinct pacemaker. They apparently view brain dynamic behavior as caused by many such pacemakers, each associated with a local network, perhaps similar to multiple electric circuits with independent current sources. However, in a brain with dense thalamocortical, intra-cortical, and corticocortical connections, we may expect substantial interactions between sources, in a manner somewhat analogous to the dependent current sources in electric circuits discussed in chapter 3. In this case, the dynamic behavior of each so-called pacemaker is likely to be influenced by many other pacemakers, thereby rendering the label "pacemaker" inappropriate. The traditional pacemaker can be viewed as a special case of much more general dynamic behavior, a limiting case in which local brain sources undergo very minimal feedback from external sources. However, we suggest that substantial two-way interaction of brain sources is likely to be closer to the truth, at least in most brain states as discussed in chapters 9 through 11.

We have found minimal experimental evidence supporting EEG pacemakers, leading to suspicion that "pacemakers" are psychological crutches used to lump poorly understood physiological mechanisms into a single category, a means of dismissing scientific questions deemed inconvenient or just too hard to deal with. The pacemaker idea may work in concert with a source localization conceptual framework in which a single oscillating source underlies each EEG signal. If a genuine autonomous pacemaker of a particular brain rhythm were actually verified for an isolated tissue mass, the arguments put forward here discourage unsubstantiated extrapolation to other EEG phenomena. In essence, a *common EEG fallacy is selection of the label "pacemaker" as a catchall term, a means of avoiding difficult questions about the nature and origins of brain dynamic behavior.*

14 Summary

This chapter reviews common technical mistakes and more general errors in practice and thinking about EEG. It is presented with only minimal supporting evidence, which is distributed in other parts of the book. In contrast to much of the so-called soft sciences, the issues addressed here cannot be settled by democratic processes. Distinct schools of thought in economics, clinical psychology, and religion have their own followers. Success in these fields depends largely on finding converts with similar viewpoints. By contrast, the correct answers in brain physics are provided by nature, the ultimate dictator. We do not suggest that our interpretations are unique or that they should be immune from criticism. However, by the explicit discussions of this chapter, we invite feedback from the scientific community to facilitate scientific progress by successive approximations to the truth. Some of our views of EEG fallacies may be controversial, but as far as we can tell at this time, these views are well supported by the physical principles described in later chapters.

The major philosophical difference that distinguishes source localization from high-resolution algorithms is emphasized here. Source localization makes use of constraints based on physiological assumptions to overcome the fundamental nonuniqueness of the inverse problem. These inverse solutions depend critically on the accuracy of the chosen constraints, regardless of algorithmic sophistication or beautiful computer graphics. In other words, *fancy mathematics can never trump fundamental physics.*

High resolution EEG methods emphasized in this book do not provide non-unique inverse solutions. Rather, these methods obtain unique estimates of dura potential by inward continuation of recorded scalp potential distribution to the dura surface. The practical limitations of both source localization and high resolution methods and are discussed in more depth in chapters 6–9.

References

Basar E, Schurmann M, Basar-Eroglu C, and Karakas S, 1997, Alpha oscillations in brain functioning: an integrative theory. *International Journal of Psychophysiology* 26: 5–29.

Cadusch PJ, Breckon W, and Silberstein RB, 1992, Spherical splines and the interpolation, deblurring and transformation of topographic EEG data. *Brain Topography* 5: 59.

Cohen D, Cuffin BN, Yunokuchi K, Maniewski R, Purcell C, Cosgrove GR, Ives J, Kennedy JG, and Schomer DL, 1990, MEG versus EEG localization test using implanted sources in the human brain. *Annals of Neurology* 28: 811–817.

Cooper R, Winter AL, Crow HJ, and Walter WG, 1965, Comparison of subcortical, cortical, and scalp activity using chronically indwelling electrodes in man. *Electroencephalography and Clinical Neurophysiology* 18: 217–228.

Delucchi MR, Garoutte B, and Aird RB, 1975, The scalp as an electroencephalographic averager. *Electroencephalography and Clinical Neurophysiology* 38:191–196.

Ebersole JS, 1997, Defining epileptogenic foci: past, present, future. *Journal of Clinical Neurophysiology* 14: 470–483.

Gevins AS, Le J, Martin N, Brickett P, Desmond J, and Reutter B, 1994, High resolution EEG: 124-channel recording, spatial enhancement, and MRI integration methods. *Electroencephalography and Clinical Neurophysiology* 90: 337–358.

Hamaleinen M, Hari R, Ilmoniemi RJ, Knuutila J, and Lounasmaa OV, 1993, Magnetoencephalography: theory, instrumentation, and applications to noninvasive studies of the working human brain. *Reviews of Modern Physics* 65: 413–497.

Hjorth B, 1975, An on-line transformation of EEG scalp potentials into orthogonal source derivations. *Electroencephalography and Clinical Neurophysiology* 39: 526–530.

Katznelson RD, 1981, EEG recording, electrode placement and aspects of generator localization. In: PL Nunez (Au.), *Electric Fields of the Brain: The Neurophysics of EEG,* 1st Edition, New York: Oxford University Press, pp. 176–213.

Klimesch W, Doppelmayr M, Schwaiger J, Auinger P, and Winker TH, 1999, "Paradoxical" alpha synchronization in a memory task. *Cognitive Brain Research* 7: 493–501.

Law SK, Nunez PL, and Wijesinghe RS, 1993, High resolution EEG using spline generated surface Laplacians on spherical and ellipsoidal surfaces. *IEEE Transactions on Biomedical Engineering* 40: 145–153.

Le J and Gevins AS, 1993, Method to reduce blur distortion from EEGs using a realistic head model. *IEEE Transactions on Biomedical Engineering* 40: 517–528.

Leahy RM, Mosher JC, Spencer ME, Huang MX, and Lewine JD, 1998, A study of dipole localization accuracy for MEG and EEG using a human skull phantom. *Electroencephalography and Clinical Neurophysiology* 107: 159–173.

Lopes da Silva FH, 1995, Dynamics of electrical activity of the brain, local networks and modulating systems. In: PL Nunez (Au.), *Neocortical Dynamics and Human EEG Rhythms*, New York: Oxford University Press, pp. 249–271.

Lopes da Silva FH, 1999, Dynamics of EEGs as signals of neuronal populations: models and theoretical considerations. In: E Niedermeyer and FH Lopes da Silva (Eds.), *Electroencephalography. Basic Principals, Clinical Applications, and Related Fields*, 4th Edition, London: Williams and Wilkins, pp. 76–92.

Malmivuo J and Plonsey R, 1995, *Bioelectromagetism*, New York: Oxford University Press.

Miller GA, Lutzenberger W, and Elbert T, 1991, The linked-reference issue in EEG and ERP recording. *Journal of Psychophysiology* 5: 276–279.

Nunez PL, 1990, Physical principles and neurophysiological mechanisms underlying event-related potentials. In: JW Rohrbaugh, R Parasuraman, and R Johnson Jr. (Eds.), *Event-related Brain Potentials*, New York: Oxford University Press, pp. 19–36.

Nunez PL, 1991, Comments on the paper by Miller, Lutzenberger and Elbert. *Journal of Psycholophysiology* 5: 279–280.

Nunez PL, 1995, *Neocortical Dynamics and Human EEG Rhythms*, New York: Oxford University Press.

Nunez PL and Westdorp AF, 1994, The surface Laplacian, high resolution EEG and controversies, *Brain Topography* 3: 221–226.

Nunez PL and Silberstein RB, 2000, On the relationship of synaptic activity to macroscopic measurements: does co-registration of EEG with fMRI make sense? *Brain Topography* 13: 79–96.

Nunez PL, Silberstein RB, Cadusch PJ, Wijesinghe R, Westdorp AF, and Srinivasan R, 1994, A theoretical and experimental study of high resolution EEG based on surface Laplacians and cortical imaging. *Electroencephalography and Clinical Neurophysiology* 90: 40–57.

Nunez PL, Silberstein RB, Shi Z, Carpenter MR, Srinivasan R, Tucker DM, Doran SM, Cadusch PJ, and Wijesinghe RS, 1999, EEG coherence: II. Experimental measures of multiple coherence measures. *Electroencephalography and Clinical Neurophysiology* 110: 469–486.

Nunez PL, Srinivasan R, Westdorp AF, Wijesinghe RS, Tucker DM, Silberstein RB, and Cadusch PJ, 1997, EEG coherency: I. statistics, reference electrode, volume conduction, Laplacians, cortical imaging, and interpretation at multiple scales. *Electroencephalography and Clinical Neurophysiology* 103: 516–527.

Nunez PL, Westdorp AF, and Tucker DM, 1994, A blind test of the BESA algorithm using multiple oscillating dipoles in a head model. Unpublished data.

Nunez PL, Wingeier BM, and Silberstein RB, 2001, Spatial-temporal structures of human alpha rhythms: theory, micro-current sources, multiscale measurements, and global binding of local networks. *Human Brain Mapping* 13: 125–164.

Okada Y, Lahteenmaki A, and Xu C, 1999, Comparison of MEG and EEG on the basis of somatic evoked responses elicited by stimulation of the snout in the juvenile swine. *Clinical Neurophysiology* 110:214–229.

Petsche H and Etlinger SC, 1998, *EEG and Thinking. Power and Coherence Analysis of Cognitive Processes*, Vienna: Austrian Academy of Sciences.

Scott A, 1995, *Stairway to the Mind*, New York: Springer-Verlag.

Silberstein RB, 1995, Steady-state visually evoked potentials, brain resonances, and cognitive processes. In: PL Nunez (Au.), *Neocortical Dynamics and Human EEG Rhythms*, Oxford University Press, pp. 272–303.

Srinivasan R, Nunez PL, Tucker DM, Silberstein RB, and Cadusch PJ, 1996, Spatial sampling and filtering of EEG with spline-Laplacians to estimate cortical potentials. *Brain Topography* 8: 355–366.

Steriade M, 1999, Cellular substrates of brain rhythms. In: E Niedermeyer and FH Lopes da Silva (Eds.), *Electroencephalography. Basic Principals, Clinical Applications, and Related Fields*, 4th Edition, London: Williams and Wilkins, pp. 28–75.

3

An Overview of
Electromagnetic Fields

---

1 Introduction

This chapter consists of a "review" of electromagnetic fields in material media, although many of the ideas may be new to clinicians and cognitive scientists. The more down-to-earth EEG applications of other chapters are based on the fundamentals presented here. Readers wishing to use this book more as a handbook may skip this chapter and still make good use of the discussions of volume conduction and dynamic source behavior in later chapters. However, we do not recommend such an omission, which may deny electroencephalographers, physiologists, or cognitive scientists a richness of experience in their work that comes through a good fundamental understanding of currents and fields in living tissue as well as conceptual connections to familiar physical phenomena.

There are, of course, a number of physics and engineering books that do an excellent job of presenting electromagnetic theory at various mathematical levels. Why not replace this chapter by a list of references? There are several answers to this question. Books on circuits and electromagnetic fields are focused on issues of minimal interest in electrophysiology and, by themselves, are not very useful in EEG. Elementary electrical engineering texts are concerned with one-dimensional current in wires, rather than current flow in three spatial dimensions. Elementary physics courses emphasize fields due to charges in *dielectrics* (insulators) rather than membrane current sources in tissue generating the macroscopic electric fields recorded as EEG. Although the background provided by exercises with dielectric fields is a prerequisite for advanced physics study, the practical problems in electrophysiology require a different emphasis, one focused on current sources in conductive media.

Knowing the usual elementary relation between charges and electric fields is, by itself, of minimal use in electrophysiology. *Static membrane charge produces no electric field in tissue at the macroscopic distances of interest in EEG.* The reason is that many other charges in the conductive medium (Na, Cl, and other ions) change position so as to shield membrane charge, thereby making the electric field essentially zero at macroscopic distances from any local charge accumulation. This charge shielding issue has often been misunderstood by cognitive scientists and electrophysiologists (and even some engineers and physicists), apparently because their physics education emphasized charges as electric field sources. Another important issue in electrophysiology is the distinction between *microscopic, mesoscopic* (between micro and macro), and *macroscopic* fields in tissue. In particular, the nature of brain electric fields depends very much on the hierarchy of the brain level under study. Electric fields measured with the physiologist's microelectrode or the somewhat larger *mesoelectrode* have enjoyed comprehensive treatment elsewhere. Here emphasis is placed on electric fields measured by the scalp electrode. Relationships between electric fields (or potentials) recorded at different spatial scales are discussed in chapter 4.

A second justification for this chapter is that electrophysiological applications are nearly always concerned with fields of relatively low frequency. Later we shall be much more precise about just what is meant by "low frequency." However, it can be said with complete generality that when the field frequency is sufficiently low, electric fields are uncoupled from magnetic fields. We may calculate electric fields as if magnetic fields do not exist and calculate magnetic fields from the current source distribution in tissue, ignoring explicit interactions with the electric field. We can use pre-Maxwellian knowledge, whereby electricity and magnetism were thought to be separate phenomena. It would be difficult to overstate the enormous simplification provided by the low-frequency approximation, which makes possible this single chapter emphasizing *quasi-static electric fields* as compared to large volumes covering *electromagnetic fields.*

A third motivation for this chapter is to propose several physical analogs of possible neocortical dynamic behavior. Several physical systems are considered here in which electromagnetic fields are confined in (or near) some wave propagation medium. We are able to describe the dynamic characteristics of these electromagnetic waves in detail, with emphasis on those general properties that may be similar to certain dynamic properties of EEG, even though the underlying mechanisms, while poorly understood, are known to be quite distinct from classic electromagnetism.

The fourth reason for this chapter is perhaps both the most obvious and most important. The behavior of electric currents and fields depends very much on the medium that contains them. Fields in a plasma (ionized gas) may do quite different things from fields in a metal, liquid, or neutral gas, although, in each case, the fields are governed by Maxwell's equations. The study of fields and currents in living tissue also presents some unique problems unfamiliar to physicists lacking biological knowledge. However, biological fields are also governed by Maxwell's equations, although in nonlinear tissue like the active membrane, the connection is obscure. In the context of electric field theory, we may describe living tissue as the "fifth state of matter" (plasma being the fourth), with an apology if this seems like an overzealous characterization.

Electromagnetic theory developed largely as a result of experiments carried out over a period of roughly 80 years. Coulomb's observations of the forces between charged bodies were made around 1785. By 1864, Maxwell had published his famous paper, which contains a complete quantitative description of electromagnetism. Modern science and technology have become so dependent on knowledge of currents and fields—indeed, all our lives are so intimately involved with machines that depend on Maxwell's laws—that it is difficult to argue with the following statement by the eminently quotable physicist Richard Feynman (1962):

> From the long view of the history of mankind—seen from, say, ten thousand years from now—there can be little doubt that the most significant event of the 19th century will be judged as Maxwell's discovery of the laws of electrodynamics. The American Civil War will pale into provincial insignificance in comparison with this important scientific event of the same decade.

2 Electric Charge

There are two kinds of substance in the universe that we call positive and negative charge. We distinguish these two substances based on experimental observation of the forces between them. Charges with the same sign produce a strong repelling force and unlike charges have a similar attracting force. All matter contains a mixture of positive protons and negative electrons that are attracting and repelling with great force. The force (in newtons) between two charges q_1 and q_2 (in coulombs) is given by Coulomb's law:

$$\mathbf{F}(\mathbf{r}) = \frac{q_1 q_2 \mathbf{a}}{4\pi\varepsilon_0 R^2} \qquad (3.1)$$

Here ε_0 is a constant called the permittivity of empty space and R is the charge separation in meters. The constant $1/(4\pi\varepsilon_0)$ equals $9.0 \times 10^9 \, \mathrm{N\,m^2\,C^{-2}}$ and one newton equals about 2.2 pounds. Thus, two charges of ± 1 coulomb separated by 1 meter are attracted by a force of 20 billion pounds. Obviously, a coulomb is an enormous charge. The force vector is directed along a line between the two charges. Equation (3.1) illustrates the classic inverse square law that applies also to the gravitational force.

If we double the distance between charges, the force is reduced to $1/4$ of its original value. If we triple the distance, the force is down to $1/9$, and so on.

3 Electric Fields

The electric field at vector location $\mathbf{r}$ is defined as the force acting on a test charge of strength equal to one unit (1 coulomb, for example). From this definition and (3.1), it follows that the electric field at location $\mathbf{r}$ due to point charge at location $\mathbf{r}_1$ is given by

$$\mathbf{E}(\mathbf{r}) = \frac{q\mathbf{a}}{4\pi\varepsilon_0 R^2} \qquad (3.2)$$

as shown in fig. 3-1. Electric fields in physical media are typically measured in volts per meter (V/m). Here $\mathbf{a}$ is a unit vector pointing in the direction of a line between the charge and the field point $\mathbf{r}$. R is the magnitude of the vector $\mathbf{r} - \mathbf{r}_1$, that is, the scalar distance between charge and field point. Of course, if only one point charge is involved, it may be placed at the origin of a coordinate system so that $\mathbf{r}_1 = 0$ and $R = |\mathbf{r}|$ or just r in less cumbersome notation. The more general expression (3.2) is required since most applications involve many charges. In such cases the electric field at location $\mathbf{r}$ is due to the linear superposition of contributions from charges at locations $\mathbf{r}_n$ at different distances from the field point, given by $R_n = |\mathbf{r} - \mathbf{r}_n|$, that is

$$\mathbf{E}(\mathbf{r}) = \frac{1}{4\pi\varepsilon_0} \sum_{n-1}^{N} \frac{q_n \mathbf{a}_n}{R_n^2} \qquad (3.3)$$

Here the sum sign (sigma) simply means that we are to add up the contribution of each (nth) charge to the field until we have included all N

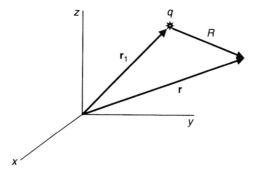

Figure 3-1 A positive charge q located at position $\mathbf{r}_1$ produces an electric field at position $\mathbf{r}$. The scalar distance between $\mathbf{r}_1$ and $\mathbf{r}$ is $R = |\mathbf{r} - \mathbf{r}_1|$. The direction of the electric field is along the line between end points of the vectors given by $\mathbf{r}_1$ and $\mathbf{r}$.

of them. The principle of superposition of electric fields embodied in (3.3) has been verified in many experiments. For macroscopic fields, typical accuracies in such experiments are one part in a thousand. At microscopic scales, accuracies of better than one part in a million have been achieved (Jackson 1975).

Note that the expression $\mathbf{E}(\mathbf{r})$ is a vector function of a vector, as indicated by the boldface symbols. That is, $\mathbf{E}$ has both magnitude and direction and it depends on the vector location $\mathbf{r}$. If there are multiple charges, (3.3) is a vector sum involving the unit vectors $\mathbf{a}_n$ pointing away from each charge q_n to the field point. One can also have a scalar function of a vector, say temperature $T(\mathbf{r})$ or electric potential $\Phi(\mathbf{r})$ as a function of location $\mathbf{r}$. An example of a vector function of a scalar is electric field as a function of time $\mathbf{E}(t)$, equivalent to three scalar functions of time, $E_x(t)$, $E_y(t)$, and $E_z(t)$, the three Cartesian components of the vector $\mathbf{E}$. Other common coordinate systems include cylindrical and spherical coordinates (radial coordinate, longitude, latitude) plus more than 10 other specialized coordinate systems useful for particular geometries. One example is prolate spheroidal coordinates to describe locations on the scalp or to account for nonspherical geometry in head models of volume conduction (Law et al. 1993). There are several motivations for the use of vector notation in science. It is shorter and less cumbersome than the equivalent scalar form. Equation derivation and other theoretical analyses are often much quicker and easier using vectors. Most importantly, the laws of physics are written in vector form to indicate their independence from human choices of coordinate system.

4 Electric Potential

All of electromagnetics, including electric circuits and electrophysiology, could be carried out without ever using the concept of *electric potential*. Electric potential was first introduced to make calculations simpler and has become part of universal practice in circuit analysis. In particular, when the oscillation frequency of fields is sufficiently low, magnetic induction is negligible and it is possible to express the *electric field vector* in terms of the scalar potential $\Phi(\mathbf{r})$ by the relation

$$\mathbf{E}(\mathbf{r}) = -\nabla\Phi(\mathbf{r}) = -\left(\frac{\partial\Phi}{\partial x}\mathbf{i} + \frac{\partial\Phi}{\partial y}\mathbf{j} + \frac{\partial\Phi}{\partial z}\mathbf{k}\right) \qquad (3.4)$$

The vector ∇ is the gradient mathematical operator, often called "del" or "grad". ∇ is defined for Cartesian (rectangular) coordinates by the terms on the far right-hand side of (3.4). The gradient of potential (electric field) is a vector whose magnitude indicates the maximum spatial rate of change of potential and whose direction is the direction of this maximum change. One may picture a mountain whose height $\Phi(x, y)$ at any location (x, y) is analogous to potential. With this analogy, the electric field at (x, y) points in the direction of the steepest ground slope, and the magnitude of the electric field is analogous to the slope in this direction. More generally, electric potential is a function of all three coordinates, that is, $\Phi = (x, y, z)$. This is more difficult to visualize since we can no longer think of the dependent variable Φ plotted in the z direction to indicate (say) height above sea level, but the principle is the same.

The gradient expression for the electric field at any location requires three variables, the three components of the electric field. By contrast, electric potential is a single variable. This is a substantial simplification. It allows, for example, specification of an instantaneous potential at each node of an electric circuit. Undergraduate engineering students can then become proficient with circuit analysis and design without any immediate need to study vector field theory. But when the field frequency is large, it is no longer possible to define electric potential in the simple manner of (3.4), to the chagrin of these same students on taking their first course in electromagnetic wave propagation. In electrophysiology, we are safe from this particular complication. Equation (3.4) may be used safely in electrophysiology because magnetic induction in tissue is negligible at field frequencies below about 10^5 or 10^6 Hz. This is just as well: we have other complications to deal with that are unique to living tissue.

The electric potential due to N charges follows from (3.3) and (3.4), that is

$$\Phi(\mathbf{r}) = \frac{1}{4\pi\varepsilon_0} \sum_{n=1}^{N} \frac{q_n}{R_n} \tag{3.5}$$

In standard engineering units (called mks for meter, kilogram, second), potentials are expressed in volts and electric fields are measured in volts per meter (V/m). In electrophysiology, potentials are normally expressed in microvolts (or millivolts) and electric fields in perhaps microvolts per centimeter (μV/cm) or microvolts per millimeter (μV/mm). The human alpha rhythm recorded on the scalp with respect to an ear reference is typically in the 40 μV range. If a 20 μV potential difference is recorded between two scalp electrodes placed 2 cm apart, the magnitude of the instantaneous electric field halfway between the electrodes is roughly 10 μV/cm. This estimate applies only to the electric field component tangent to the scalp surface, along a line between the electrodes. Estimate of a second tangential component requires a second bipolar electrode pair. Estimate of the third component of the electric field (perpendicular to the scalp) would require a different sensor, one based on capacitive effects. Such sensors of the component of the electric field normal to the scalp are currently under development.

Although electric potential is very useful, it introduces an ambiguity that has caused electroencephalographers substantial grief associated with reference electrode questions in EEG. When mathematicians or physicists speak of the "potential" at a point, they normally mean the potential difference between that point and some other point at *infinity*. Just where is this place "infinity"? In practice, it means any location where the sources of interest (charges, current sources, or voltage sources) produce negligible potentials. Thus, we use the word "infinity" to indicate not one location, but an infinite number of locations, all of which are a long way away (in the electrical sense) from all sources of interest. Inherent in the idea of a reference at infinity is the implied independence of any experimental data or theoretical calculation on the location of the reference, as long as it remains sufficiently far away. While this is a very useful concept in many physical applications, it generally fails in scalp recorded EEG because reference electrodes on the body are seldom "far away" from brain sources in the electrical sense, as discussed in chapters 2 and 7.

Do the force and electric field due to a point charge fall off *exactly* as $1/R^2$, or is this just a good approximation? The extent of human knowledge of this important exponent is perhaps surprising. Experiments have shown that Coulomb's exponent differs from two by less than one part in 10^{16}! This accuracy is possible because it turns out that the inverse square law implies that the electric field inside a conducting shell due to external static charges is always zero. This electrical shielding of the inner space occurs because charges in the shell arrange themselves in response to the external field so as to fully cancel its effects. This is also essentially the reason why static membrane charge produces zero field in the tissue. Any deviation from the inverse square law would produce a field inside the conducting shell, but no field has been measured in such experiments. The inverse law is exact as far as we can tell, at least for distances larger than about 10^{-13} cm and less than about 10^9 cm (Jackson 1975).

5 Electric Circuits and Tissue Volume Conduction

A typical electric circuit consists of various circuit elements where all voltage changes occur. We normally assume that the connecting wires are made of material with zero resistivity so that no voltage drop occurs between circuit elements. Wire current consists mainly of free electrons moving through the metal. At relatively low frequencies (say the US standard 60 Hz power frequency), current is distributed nearly uniformly across wire cross sections. By contrast, at very high frequencies, current flows mainly in a thin layer close to the wire surface called the *skin depth*. The circuit behavior is fully determined by the circuit elements and the pattern of wire connections between elements. Wire lengths and the actual positions of circuit elements in three-dimensional space have no influence on circuit behavior in this approximation. The term "lumped-parameter system" is often used to signify that the spatial dimensions of the system do not enter the circuit model. An important exception to this usual circuit behavior is the transmission line (for example, a coaxial TV cable) where system size definitely counts. In tissue, subthreshold membrane potentials are modeled by cable equations, similar to transmission line models, but without the inductive effects of transmission lines (Cole 1968; Rall 1977).

These features of normal circuits differ from tissue volume conduction in several important ways. The resistance of current pathways in tissue is proportional to the product of path length and tissue resistivity, essentially the frictional drag of the conductive medium on the movement of current carriers. Tissue current consists of positive and negative ions that move in opposite directions under the influence of electric fields. Current distribution is nonuniform in the head, depending on the locations of tissue boundaries, resistivities of different tissue, and locations of the biological current sources. The current sources themselves are products of brain dynamic behavior generated at the membrane-synapse level.

6 Current Sources and Voltage Sources

An ideal independent voltage source is a circuit element providing a specified voltage across its terminals, regardless of the current in the device and independent of the circuit in which it is placed. The circuit characteristics determine the current passing through the device. Similarly, an ideal independent current source provides a specified current, regardless of the voltage across its terminals and independent of the circuit in which it is placed. The voltage across the current source (as well as the power provided) depends on circuit characteristics. Obviously, these are idealizations that cannot always be valid. For example, an open circuit is defined as a path where no current flows, as in the example of an open switch. Suppose we place a current source in series with a switch. The idealizations of current source and open circuit are inconsistent when we open the switch. Either current must jump the switch gap (sparks!) or the current source must fail. One way or another the actual physical system no longer conforms to the model system.

Current sources and voltage sources are interchangeable in the following sense. The left-hand side of fig. 1-11a shows a resistor R in series with the AC or DC voltage source $V(t)$. Suppose we connect these two elements to some other network (represented by the rectangular box) at terminals a and b. The network in the box may be large or small. It may or may not contain nonlinear circuit elements. It may or may not contain additional current or voltage sources; it is fully arbitrary. As a result

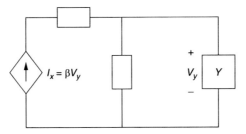

Figure 3-2 A controlled (or dependent) current source is indicated by diamond symbols in electric circuit analysis. In this example, the current through the dependent current source is $I_x = \beta V_y$ (based on interactions hidden from our view) where V_y is the voltage across the element (or network) Y. Network Y and the other two networks (empty boxes) are arbitrary.

of the connections at a and b, some pattern of currents and voltages will occur in the boxed network. Suppose now we replace the voltage source with a current source $I(t) = V(t)/R$ in parallel with the same resistor R and reconnect these elements to the boxed network at a and b, as shown on the right-hand side of fig. 1-11b. We know from circuit theory that all the currents and voltages in the boxed network will be exactly the same when connected to the current source as they were when connected to the voltage source. We make use of a very similar idea when we model EEG in terms of current sources, rather than transmembrane potentials.

Thus far, we have discussed only independent current and voltage sources, but dependent (or controlled) sources are also important in both circuits and electrophysiology. An ideal dependent voltage source provides terminal voltage determined by either a voltage or current existing at some other location in the circuit. An ideal dependent current source is similarly defined. Dependent current and voltage sources are represented by diamonds; an example dependent current source is shown in fig. 3-2. An immediate question is how do the dependent sources "know" to change their output based on changes in some other (perhaps distant) part of the circuit? The answer is that some method of interaction between the two elements (a separate circuit) must occur, but such interaction is not shown in the circuit diagram. All we are shown is the net result of this interaction, for example that the current I_x in the dependent source on the left-hand side of fig. 3-2 is proportional to the voltage across some element Y. That is, modeling of the physical system has been separated into two parts. The relationship $I_x = \beta V_y$ is obtained in the first part (based on interactions hidden from our view); and analysis of the circuit in fig. 3-2 is the second part.

A similar multistep approach to modeling is often appropriate in electrophysiology. For example, we might first assume several independent current sources and determine scalp potentials using a volume conductor model. Alternately, we might calculate dependent current sources based on some dynamic model. Such dynamic model may occur at the level of membrane, neural net, macroscopic field, or some combination. However, once the current source distribution is obtained, these same sources can be used to predict scalp potential distribution using volume conductor theory, the so-called *forward problem* in EEG.

7 Dipole and Multipole Fields

Dipoles are important actors in both physical and biological theater. We start here with the usual charge dipole studied in elementary physics, even though it is the *current dipole* not the *charge dipole* that matters in electrophysiology. In fact, the two concepts are often confused, partly because the mathematical formulations are formally identical. Consider two charges $\pm q$ of equal magnitude and opposite sign placed a distance d apart, as shown in fig. 3-3. The potential at any vector location $\mathbf{r}$ is given by the sum of individual contributions from each charge:

$$\Phi(\mathbf{r}) = \frac{q}{4\pi\varepsilon_0}\left(\frac{1}{R_1} - \frac{1}{R_2}\right) \tag{3.6}$$

In order for this expression to be more useful, the two distances R_1 and R_2 should be expressed in some convenient coordinate system, thereby making (3.6) more complicated. A more useful expression for dipole potential, valid at moderate to large distances, is

$$\Phi(\mathbf{r}) \cong \frac{qd\cos\theta}{4\pi\varepsilon_0 r^2} \tag{3.7}$$

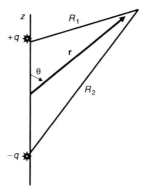

Figure 3-3 Two fixed charges of equal magnitude but opposite sign $\pm q$ form a charge dipole. Here the charges are located on the z-axis with separation distance d. The charges cause an electric (and potential) field in the surrounding dielectric (insulating) medium. The dipole field at any location in spherical coordinates $\Phi(r, \theta, \phi)$ is the "net" field due to both charges. Because of symmetry about the z-axis, this field is independent angle ϕ (longitude) measured from the (x, z) plane (normal to plane of page).

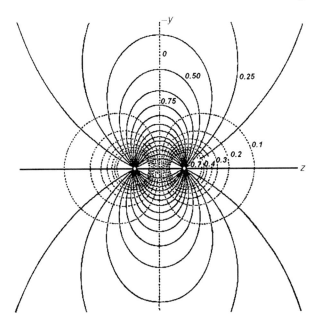

Figure 3-4 The dipole field. Solid lines are electric field lines, which point in the direction of the local electric field. Dashed lines are equipotentials. The field patterns are drawn for a charge dipole in a homogeneous, isotropic dielectric medium (no current). The axes of fig. 3-3 have been rotated 90° clockwise. These field lines are identical for a current dipole placed in a homogeneous, isotropic conductor, in which case, the electric field lines are identical to current lines. Reproduced with permission from Smythe (1950).

Here r and θ are spherical coordinates and d is the distance between charges. In summary, we started with two charges, each producing a potential that falls off like $1/R$. When we combine two such charges of opposite sign, there is a substantial cancellation effect and the two charges combine to produce a potential that falls off much faster, as $1/r^2$. (At large distances, the R and r values are approximately equal.) Equation (3.7) becomes a pretty good approximation when $r \cong 3d$ or $4d$. Electric field lines and lines of constant potential for the dipole are shown in fig. 3-4.

Most charge configurations of interest in physics and current source distributions in electrophysiology are far more complicated than the simple example of two equal sources of opposite sign. A number of other examples are shown in chapter 5; it turns out that the potential due to *all* charge (or current source) configurations can be expressed as the following series of terms called a *multipole expansion*:

$$V(r) = (\text{monopole contribution, } 1/r) + (\text{dipole contribution, } 1/r^2)$$

$$+ (\text{quadrupole contribution, } 1/r^3)$$

$$+ (\text{octupole contribution, } 1/r^4)$$

$$+ (\text{infinite number of other contributions})$$

We have shown the appropriate radial dependence (but not the angular dependence) in each parenthesis. In special cases, most of the terms in the series will be zero. For example, in the case of a single point source, all terms except the monopole term are zero, as indicated by (3.5). For the dipole sources $(r \gg d)$, all other terms are much smaller than the dipole term so that the approximate dipole expression (3.7) becomes accurate. When we are far enough away from a source containing an equal number of positive and negative charges (or current sources in the case of electrophysiology), the monopole term is zero (local charge or current conservation) and the potential typically falls off like a dipole, regardless of the detailed nature of the source distribution. Exceptions are very special cases, like that of the *quadrupole* source configuration where both the monopole and dipole terms are zero and the potential consists of quadrupole, octupole, and higher terms.

For the dipole approximation to be valid, the field point must lie at a moderate to large distance compared to the maximum dimension of the source region. It is for this reason that the dipole concept is so important to several branches of science. Note that the term "tripole" is not useful in this context. Two positive and one negative sources of equal strength along a line would produce a monopole plus dipole field. Electric field lines and lines of constant potential produced by a charge dipole in a homogeneous, isotropic dielectric medium are shown in fig. 3-4. Note that the current is zero everywhere in the dielectric. The electric field lines and potential produced by a current dipole in a homogeneous, isotropic conductor are identical to the pattern in fig. 3-4, and current lines in the conductor are identical to the electric field lines.

The field pattern due to two equal charges of the *same sign* in a homogeneous, isotropic dielectric medium is shown in fig. 3-5. At large distances, the field is that of a *monopole* since there is no cancellation effect due to the sources of opposite sign, as in the case of the dipole. A third example of charge configuration is shown in fig. 3-6. At large distances the field is that of a dipole because the total local charge sums to zero. The electric field lines and potential produced by similar current source and sink locations in a homogeneous, isotropic conductor are identical to the patterns in fig. 3-4 through 3-6, and current lines in the conductor are identical to the electric field lines.

It should be emphasized that the term "dipole field" typically refers to the approximation associated with keeping only the dipole term in the multipole expansion. Electrophysiologists have sometimes confused this concept with the simple physical dipole consisting of two point sources. Such simple source geometry is clearly not applicable to membrane biophysics where sources and sinks are distributed in complicated patterns, but this view of two point sources misses the essential issues concerning "dipoles". Even very complicated source geometry will yield dipole fields at distances that are large compared to the characteristic diameter of the source region.

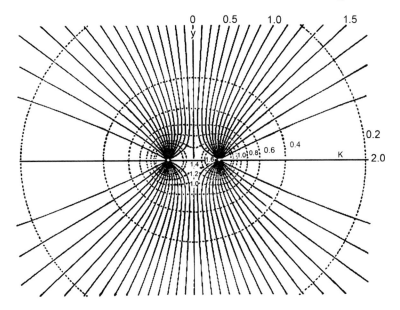

Figure 3-5 Similar to fig. 3-4, except the two charges (or current sources) are both positive. At large distances, the field is that of a monopole because total local charge (or current) does not add to zero. In the case of currents in a conductor, the current must flow to distant sinks (not shown). Reproduced with permission from Smythe (1950).

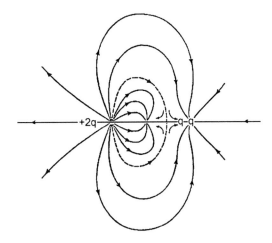

Figure 3.6 Similar to fig. 3-4, except there are three charges (or current sources) +2q, −q, and +q on a straight line. At large distances, the field is that of a dipole. Reproduced with permission from Smythe (1950).

8 What are *Fields*?

We have defined the electric field in terms of forces, but what is a force? We may think of force as the direct action of one piece of matter upon another. However, one piece of matter does not really come up against another. They are slightly separated and the effects we see are due to electrical fields acting on a small scale. Thus, it appears we have made a circular argument. We defined a field in terms of a force, but the force turns out to be due to the field!

The narrow-minded macroscopic view of forces encourages a mechanical view of nature, which dominated the thinking of physicists of the 19th century. Of course, we now call it narrow minded with the advantage of hindsight! Gradually physics was forced to move away from the mechanical viewpoint, to de-emphasize the idea of force, and to elevate the status of abstract fields (Einstein and Infield 1961). Nearly any measurable quantity that takes on values that depend on location in space and time can be considered to be a *field*, as depicted in figs. 3-4 through 3-6. For example, when an oven is turned on, the kitchen air is heated. If the air temperature at a large number of locations near the hot oven is measured, this spatial and temporal variation can be expressed with some sort of contour map or by a mathematical function $T(\mathbf{r}, t)$ or $T(x, y, z, t)$. This symbolism for temperature T simply means that the temperature depends on the location $\mathbf{r}$ of our thermometer and the time of measurement. Three scalar numbers are always required to locate a point in space. If we have chosen a rectangular coordinate system, the three numbers are the x, y, and z coordinates of the point. In spherical coordinates the field would be expressed as $T(r, \theta, \phi, t)$, for example, the worldwide atmospheric temperature, pressure, or density in terms of altitude, latitude, longitude, and time.

There are, of course, an unlimited number of quantities that can be considered as fields. For example, the altitude of the surface of the earth above sea level is a scalar function of two earth surface coordinates (latitude and longitude serve well). We could express altitude as h(latitude, longitude) or $h(x, y)$ or $h(\mathbf{r})$. The geological survey map gives us a good picture of the functional dependence of h on location. In most applications, surface height may be considered independent of time; however, inclusion of the time variable might be required for studies at geological time scales.

Temperature, mass density, pressure, and electric potential are all examples of scalar fields because they have no direction. In contrast, the gradients of these scalar fields are vector fields that point in the directions of maximum spatial rate of change. Another vector field is fluid velocity. Consider the air flow near a fan. As in the example of a temperature field, we can measure the velocity of air at various locations near the fan. However, at each location, we must know three numbers, the three components of velocity, in order to know the vector field $\mathbf{v}(\mathbf{r}, t)$. We can express the vector field as $v_x(\mathbf{r}, t)$, $v_y(\mathbf{r}, t)$, or $v_z(\mathbf{r}, t)$ for the three velocity components, which are each functions of location $\mathbf{r}$. We could express the same idea with the expression $\mathbf{v}(x, y, z, t)$ or use $v_x(x, y, z, t)$, $v_y(x, y, z, t)$, $v_z(x, y, z, t)$. All mean the same thing, but in most cases the shortest notation $\mathbf{v}(\mathbf{r}, t)$ is best because it is independent of the coordinate system. An example two-dimensional vector field plot $\mathbf{v}(x, y)$ is shown in fig. 3-7.

In neuroscience, we may define excitatory $\Psi_e(\mathbf{r}, t)$ and inhibitory $\Psi_i(\mathbf{r}, t)$ *synaptic action fields*. Short-time modulations $\delta\Psi_e(\mathbf{r}, t)$ and $\delta\Psi_i(\mathbf{r}, t)$ of active excitatory or inhibitory synapses per unit volume (or cortical surface area)

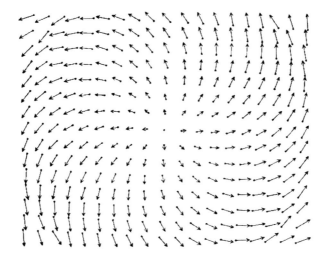

Figure 3.7 A vector field is represented by arrows with direction and length indicating local field direction and magnitude, respectively. This plot might represent a circulating fluid or an electric field, for example.

about constant background levels are shown in the example simulation of fig. 1-9. These synaptic action fields are analogous to physical fields like pressure or density fields, which are typically expressed relative to background levels. The synaptic fields are purposely defined independently of brain function because this connection is poorly understood. By contrast, the connection of synaptic fields to EEG and MEG is relatively well understood, that is, electric and magnetic fields are generated by the membrane current sources associated with synaptic action fields. We conjecture that the *cell assemblies* (*neural networks*), believed to underlie behavior and cognition, are immersed within and interact with the synaptic action fields.

Other than mathematical convenience and elegance, most field concepts are not unusually profound. For example, an excitatory synaptic action field at some cortical location (at say the millimeter scale) is just determined by mentally adding up the active excitatory synapses in (say) the local macrocolumn. Scale-dependent smoothing in time and space is implied by this definition, and the coordinate **r** associated with this scale of description locates the center of the macrocolumn. Alternatively, we may define synaptic action fields at smaller (say mincolumn) or larger scales.

Such biological fields as well as most physical fields have a known underlying structure. Temperature is due to the random motion of air molecules; velocity is their directed motion. We can also associate energy with these fields. The temperature field energy in a given volume of air is simply the total kinetic energy of the air molecules contained therein. Given this background, physicists of the 19th century tried to find an underlying structure for electric and magnetic fields for many years.

So strong was the bias toward the mechanical view of nature that all kinds of attempts were made to find the *ether,* the putative structure required to support electromagnetic fields. The ether was obliged to have somewhat strange properties in order not to disagree with known facts (Feynman 1963). For instance, the ether had to have zero mass, but also have elastic properties in order to sustain the vibrations that are inherent in the idea of wave motion. Despite such difficulties, the ether concept seemed, at the time, to be much more attractive than the alternative, which was to assume that electromagnetic disturbances could propagate without a supporting medium. After all, sound waves, water waves, and seismic waves involve physical structures in motion. However, a number of experiments failed to reveal any evidence of the ether. The most famous of these was the Michelson–Morley experiment of 1887 to measure the velocity of the earth relative to the ether. No such relative motion was found, and an alternative possibility of ether attached to the earth was in conflict with astronomical observations. These experiments, together with Einstein's special theory of relativity (1905), eventually forced the abandonment of the idea that electric and magnetic fields require a physical medium in which to propagate.

We now regard the *electromagnetic field* as something much more profound than did the early physicists. In the modern view, electric and magnetic fields retain an abstract quality (Einstein and Infield 1961). The fields are defined only in terms of the effects that they produce on charges and currents. Such measurable effects are entirely predictable by Maxwell's equations. We have mentioned that temperature and velocity fields have energy, which is simply the kinetic energy of the underlying structure. Electric and magnetic fields also have energy, an *energy contained in the field itself.* The energy density of an electric field is proportional to E^2. The energy density of a magnetic field is proportional to B^2. In mks units, the energy density is expressed in joules per cubic meter (1 joule $= 2.78 \times 10^{-7}$ kilowatt-hour). The fact that electric and magnetic fields can carry energy, without requiring an underlying mechanical structure, makes possible the transmission of the sun's energy over millions of miles of empty space, making life on earth possible.

9 Charges in Physical Dielectrics and Tissue

If the location of a number of charges is known, the potential at any location may be calculated rather easily using (3.5). Such calculations are fine exercises in elementary physics and provide useful solutions to practical problems involving dielectrics (insulators). However, in most practical problems in physical media and in *all* biological tissue, specification of the problem in terms of individual charges is impossible. A macroscopic sample of matter may contain 10^{20} or more charges, all in motion because of thermal agitation. Even if we were somehow able to know the instantaneous position of all charges in a piece of matter, the resulting microscopic potential given by (3.5) would fluctuate wildly as our probe at the observation point **r** is moved by very small distances (of the order of atomic dimensions).

Fortunately, the microscopic field is *not* the field of interest to either electrophysiologists or to many engineers and physicists working at macroscopic scales. They are interested in fields measured by electrodes that have dimensions much larger than the average distance between electrons and protons. For example, the neurophysiologist's *microelectrode*, which may have a tip diameter as small as 10^{-4} cm, is still much larger than atomic dimensions. Typically, it measures field strengths averaged over regions larger than $(10^{-4})^3 = 10^{-12}$ cm^3. Since atomic volumes are of the order of 10^{-24} cm^3, there are perhaps 10^{12} atoms in the volumes displaced by the electrode tip. It is the potential averaged over this and much larger volumes (in the case of the scalp electrode) for which we wish to present a theoretical basis in this and the next chapter. Of course, there are more than just two levels in the brain's hierarchy of fields, as depicted in table 3-1, and we will need to keep our electrode size in mind when interpreting measurements or making calculations of electrophysiological fields. We will often employ the term *mesoscopic* to indicate a spatial scale intermediate between microscopic and macroscopic, but in cortical tissue the number of distinct scales associated with tissue structure is actually more than three. Electrophysiology spans about five orders of magnitude of spatial scale, due partly to choice of electrode size. When we speak of "field" or "potential" we always mean the *space average* of these quantities over some volume of tissue, and we must be clear about just what size volume this is. Furthermore, related experimental parameters like tissue conductivity must be specified at the appropriate scale.

The distinction between microscopic and macroscopic fields is an old story in the physical sciences. Much effort has been directed by solid state, liquid, gas, and plasma physicists toward understanding the relationship between fields measured by macroelectrodes and the microfields that are more amenable to accurate theoretical description. There are, in fact, two

Table 3-1 Typical probe sizes for mapping electric fields at disparate spatial scales

Electric field location	Probe size (mm)
Inside DNA molecule	10^{-7}
Inside cell membrane	10^{-6}
Inside cell body	10^{-4}
Over minicolumn radius	10^{-3}
Over macrocolumn radius	10^{-1}
Over neocortical Brodmann area	1
Scalp EEG	10

versions of electromagnetic theory. The microscopic Maxwell's equations are entirely self-contained. Together with the Lorentz force on a charge equation, they provide a complete, unique description of the relationship between charges, currents, and the electric and magnetic fields that they generate. In contrast, the macroscopic version of Maxwell's equations, which is expressed in terms of space-averaged fields, contains more unknowns than equations even when the charges and currents are fully specified. Maxwell's macroscopic equations must be supplemented by purely experimental relations required to fill the knowledge gap between the micro- and macroscales. The three principal experimental relations needed to form a complete description of macroscopic media involve the *dielectric constant* for insulators, the *conductivity* (or *resistivity*) for conductors, and the *permeability* for magnetic materials.

We consider here the physical basis for these new parameters since their applicability to brain fields should be examined carefully. A dielectric (insulator) is a material in which charges are free to move only over atomic distances. Charge is stored by the material at microscopic scales. By contrast, some charges in a conductor flow freely under the influence of electric fields. In practice, this distinction between dielectrics and conductors is not so clear-cut. Many materials, especially biological tissue, exhibit properties of both dielectrics and conductors. This is not surprising because all materials contain different kinds of charges that may be distinguished by their different mobility.

Dielectric (or capacitive) effects in all materials are due to electronic, molecular, or other *polarization* of internal charge separation. First, consider electronic polarization. An atom has a positive charge on the nucleus, which is surrounded by a cloud of negative electrons. When an external field is applied, the nucleus will be attracted in one direction and the electrons in the other. The electron cloud will be distorted, and the "center of gravity" of the negative charge will no longer coincide with the positive nuclear charge. To a first approximation, the distorted atom is a tiny charge dipole, which produces a very small electric field pointed in a direction opposite the applied (or external) field. This *induced field*, due to polarization, reduces the *net field* inside the dielectric. As shown by our earlier discussion of dipoles, the induced field is proportional to the distance of charge separation. Furthermore, if the external field is not too large, this charge separation will itself be proportional to the local field. This latter condition defines *linearity in a dielectric*, and it has been verified in a wide variety of materials over a wide range of field strengths and field frequencies.

Next we consider molecular polarization in polar molecules. For example, in the *water molecule*, the location of the hydrogen and oxygen atoms results in a separation of charge. Each molecule has a permanent charge separation that produces a microscopic electric field. When there is no external field acting on a macroscopic volume of water, the individual molecules point in random directions, and the net electric field due to all molecules is zero. However, when an external field is applied, there is a tendency for the individual molecules to rotate so that the dipole axis lines up with the external field. At physiological temperatures, collisions between molecules in thermal motion keep them from lining up very much. However, there is some net alignment, and so some induced field. This induced electric field is called molecular polarization. Molecular polarization in water is a much larger effect than electronic polarization. It also acts in a direction opposite the external field. Molecular polarization shows up at the macroscopic level through the dielectric constant, which is large in substances like water that have relatively large internal charge separations. The relative dielectric constant of pure water is about 80.

The charge polarization effects described above can be expected with varying importance in all materials. Suppose an electric field **E** inside a conductor encounters a small dielectric body as shown in fig. 3-8. Bound charges in the dielectric will be distorted producing an electric field called the polarization $\mathbf{P}_C$ inside the dielectric. The net effect of many such small dielectric bodies is accounted for in electromagnetic theory by introduction of a new kind of electric field called the displacement vector **D** given by

$$\mathbf{D} = \varepsilon_0 \mathbf{E} + \mathbf{P}_C \tag{3.8}$$

That is, the displacement field **D** (due only to free charges) depends on the total field **E** (due to all charges) plus the polarization $\mathbf{P}_C$ (due to bound charges). In the mks system of units, **D** and $\mathbf{P}_C$ have different units from **E**, but this is only due to choice of units. Equation (3.8) is quite general. However, in a *linear* dielectric, the polarization itself is proportional to the net field, that is

$$\mathbf{P}_C = (const)\,\mathbf{E} \tag{3.9}$$

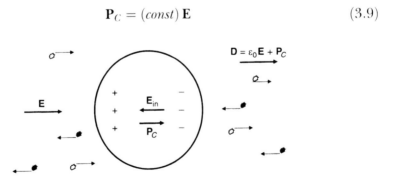

Figure 3-8 An electric field **E** inside a conductor encounters dielectric bodies (perhaps molecules or living cells). The bound charges in the dielectric bodies are slightly distorted by this field, producing an opposing electric field and polarization vector $\mathbf{P}_C$ in the same direction. The displacement vector **D** is essentially an electric field, but it is associated only with the free positive charges shown moving from left to right. The total current includes negative charges (negative ions in tissue) moving right to left. For more detail, see Jackson (1975).

Relation (3.9) is not always valid. It must be verified by experiment for any particular material. However, experience with a wide range of physical materials has shown that it is often an excellent approximation, provided that the applied field is not extremely large. By combining (3.8) and (3.9), we obtain the usual description of a *linear* dielectric medium:

$$\mathbf{D} = \varepsilon\mathbf{E} \tag{3.10}$$

Here the proportionality constant ε is called the *permittivity* of the medium. As suggested by fig. 3-8, a macroscopic mass of living tissue has both conductive and dielectric properties due to extracellular fluid and membrane charge storage, respectively. Dielectric effects are often expressed in terms of the *relative dielectric constant* of the material, defined by $\kappa = \varepsilon/\varepsilon_0$, where ε_0 is the permittivity of empty space. Equation (3.10) implies that, to a good approximation, all our ignorance about the repositioning of perhaps 10^{20} bound charges due to an applied electric field can be lumped into a single parameter ε (or κ). It is perhaps surprising that this linear description works so well in a very wide variety of materials and over a broad range of field strengths. In a nonlinear dielectric material, one can use the idea of permittivity or dielectric constant in an approximate sense only if the field is not too strong.

Linear ideas must be applied to living tissue with care; however, it appears that both the intracellular and extracellular fluids are probably well described by linear dielectric constants similar to water, that is, with $\kappa \approx 80$. The membrane may also be a linear dielectric in most instances. A number of experiments have found a membrane capacitance of about 1 microfarad/cm^2, a value that appears to be independent of both field frequency and excitation (Cole 1968). This fact implies linearity of the membrane in the dielectric sense since capacitance is, by definition, directly proportional to dielectric constant. For example, the capacitance (charge capacity) of a parallel plate capacitor is (in mks units)

$$C = \frac{\varepsilon A}{d} \tag{3.11}$$

Here A is the area of the plate and d is the plate separation. Note that the dimensions of capacitance in mks units are farads (F). If $C/A = 1\ \mu F/cm^2$, and the membrane has a thickness $d = 100\ \text{A} = 10^{-8}$ m, (3.11) implies that the relative dielectric constant of membrane material is $\kappa = \varepsilon/\varepsilon_0 \approx 11$ (Plonsey 1969). Note that capacitance depends on the geometry, whereas dielectric constant (or permittivity) is only a property of the material itself.

10 Macroscopic Polarization in Living Tissue

The electronic and molecular polarization effects discussed thus far occur on a microscopic level. There is, however, a third source of polarization, which originates at mesoscopic levels and is a critical property of living tissue. We have shown that polarization effects occur in materials when there is some internal mechanism to effect (bound) charge separations, thereby producing local dipole fields at relatively small scales. Quantum mechanical effects keep electrons at distances of roughly 10^{-13} cm from nuclei and keep hydrogen and oxygen atoms separated by distances of the order of 10^{-8} cm. In living tissue, the semipermeable membrane provides for charge separations of 10^{-6} cm. We often wish to consider electric fields in a mass of tissue large enough to contain many cells. This mass of tissue may then be treated as if it were a homogeneous medium with a certain average electrical polarization. The detailed mechanisms of tissue polarization are not as well understood as the analogous phenomena in physical media. However, we expect applied fields to cause membrane charge rearrangement that produces an internal field to oppose the applied field as in fig. 3-8. Experiments have indicated that a macroscopic mass of living tissue can have a relative dielectric constant of $\kappa \approx 10^{6}$ or 10^{7} at field frequencies below about 10 Hz (Polk and Postow 1986). At higher field frequencies, the dielectric constant is considerably reduced. In chapter 4, we consider experiments that compare dielectric and conductive effects in tissue.

11 Charges in Conductors

A dielectric can be thought of as a material in which positive and negative charges are tied together by elastic strings. When acted on by an external field, the charges are allowed to move slightly further apart and to align themselves with the field, but they cannot move beyond atomic distances. In a conductor, the strings between some charges are cut. Free charges move large distances under the influence of external fields, although charge motion is impeded by collisions with other charges as measured by *medium resistivity*. In biological tissue, the charges are carried by positive and negative ion flux through the extracellular fluid and to a much lesser extent through cell membranes having large resistivity. Because tissue contains both bound and free charges, it exhibits some of the properties of both dielectric and conductor, although it is the conductive behavior that is of most interest in applications involving the low frequencies of interest in EEG.

Consider the following thought experiment involving the introduction of a single new charge (a *test charge*) in any conductor, including biologic tissue. When we place a positive test charge inside the conductor, two separate effects occur. A polarization effect due only to bound charges (dielectric properties) will occur. In addition, free charges will produce a second (conductive) effect. In either laboratory electrolyte solutions or tissue, charged ions are free to rearrange themselves. The positive test charge will be very quickly surrounded by a "cloud" of negative charge,

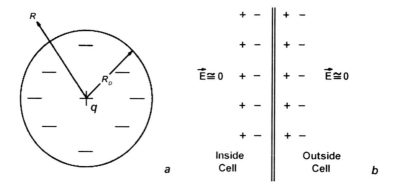

Figure 3-9 (a) Debye shielding of a test charge q by other charges in a conductive medium. The resulting electric field is due to all charges. (b) Similarly, the field due to a double layer of membrane charge is zero at all macroscopic distances because of the same shielding behavior.

which then shields most of the electric field, as shown in fig. 3-9. In other words, the effect of the (induced) cloud of negative charges almost but not quite cancels the effect of the positive test charge.

The potential due to a test charge in an electrolyte solution was developed using statistical arguments in the mid-20th century and is given by

$$\Phi(r) = \frac{q}{4\pi\varepsilon_0\kappa R}e^{-R/R_D} \tag{3.12}$$

Here R_D is called the *Debye shielding distance*. Equation (3.12) is an extension of (3.5) with $N = 1$ charge in a vacuum, but here polarization effects of the medium are included with division by κ, and medium conductive shielding causes multiplication by the exponential function. When $N = 1$, $\kappa = 1$, and $R \ll R_D$, (3.12) is essentially identical to (3.5). However, R_D is on the order of several angstroms in biological tissue. Thus, modification of the vacuum formula for potential (3.5) by the exponential function (due to conductive shielding) is a drastic one. For example with a typical $R_D = 3 \times 10^{-7}$ mm, the exponential part of (3.12) is roughly $10^{-4,000,000}$ at a field point $R = 3$ mm. This gives us an idea of the size of the error created by ignoring charge shielding in a conductor. Equation (3.12) indicates *the potential due to a test charge in biological tissue is negligibly small at all macroscopic distances.* Debye shielding depends on the freedom of motion of the ions in solution, and thus R_D is a function of temperature and charge density. Equation (3.12) does not apply to regions *inside* membranes, where the statistical arguments used in its derivation are not valid.

Elementary physics courses emphasize the fields due to charges in dielectrics with no conductive shielding. In contrast, fields in the brain must be calculated in a different manner since the location of all contributing charges is never known in practical problems. This difference has led to much confusion in the physiology literature. For example, it is not uncommon to find statements to the effect that potentials in the brain are due to some specified *charge* distribution. The problem with this idea is that the field is due not only to the specified charge, but also to all other charges in the conductive medium. In biologic tissue, current sources at membrane surfaces rather than charges are the so-called generators of EEG.

12 Electric Current in Physical Media and Tissue

Electric current is the movement of charge, regardless of the actual carriers of the charge. In living tissue, both positive and negative ions contribute to current. This situation is somewhat different than that of current in a metal, where free electrons are the principal current carriers. Regardless of the nature of the medium, current flux in a volume conductor is more complicated than current in an elementary electric circuit. In the latter case, (low-frequency) currents are uniform over the cross-section of metal wires, and one is only concerned with how the total current and node voltages vary with time in the circuit. The concept of total current will be of limited use in problems of tissue volume conduction, so it is necessary to define the more general idea of current density $\mathbf{J}$. Current density due to several different ions may be expressed as a sum over individual contributions from ions having charge density ρ_i:

$$\mathbf{J} = \sum_i \rho_i \mathbf{v}_i \qquad (3.13)$$

By convention, the current direction is defined as the direction of movement of positive charge, even in a metal where no positive charges move and the negatively charged electrons determine the current. Thus, electrons in a metal move in the direction opposite to the current direction. In (3.13), the ρ_i are free charge densities of various positive and negative ions in a ionic conductor like tissue. Free charge is free to move over distances of many molecules (or many cells); polarization charge is not free. The charge densities are equal to the value of an electron (or ion) charge multiplied by the number of free ions in a given volume of tissue. In mks units, charge density is measured in coulombs/m^3 (C/m^3). The $\mathbf{v}_i$ are the average velocities of the ions in meters per second. The current density is the amount of current passing through a cross-section of unit area measured in units of $C/(s\,m^2)$ or amperes/m^2 (A/m^2). The current density is the amount of current passing through a cross section of unit area. Note that the term "current density" is somewhat of a misnomer, since it the word "density" often implies something per unit volume, but here it is current per unit area. In general, current density is a function of both location and time in the conductive medium, that is, we may write it as $J(r, t)$, a current density field. In the special case when the current passes through a conductor of uniform cross section A, the scalar current density J is related to total current I by the relation

$$J = \frac{I}{A} \tag{3.14}$$

In a wire, the current flux is only in one direction, along the wire, so there is no need for the boldface vector sign for J.

13 Electroneutrality of Tissue

The previous discussion of Debye shielding of ions in an electrolyte solution is closely related to the condition of *electroneutrality*. This condition requires that the positive ionic charge per unit volume does not deviate appreciably from the negative ionic charge density in a macroscopic volume of electrolyte. If this were not the case, very strong electrostatic forces would be created to restore the neutrality implied by the Debye shielding effect. The membrane provides a mechanism for charge separation at mesoscopic levels; however, for the calculation of EEG fields, the volumes of interest contain many cells so that the numbers of positive and negative charges are essentially equal. When an electric field is applied to an electrolytic solution (or living tissue), both positive and negative ions contribute to the resulting current.

To illustrate the process of current flux, imagine a rude crowd, considered here to be crudely analogous to ions in solution. An announcement is made requesting that all men walk north and all women walk south. The crowd moves as directed with much pushing and shoving. We might further suppose that each person tries not to bump into someone of the same sex (charge), but does have a tendency to bump persons of the opposite sex. This crowd will have a strong tendency to preserve "sex neutrality" so that in any region of the crowd, which is large enough to contain many persons, the number of men roughly equals the number of women. If lines were drawn at the north and south ends of the crowd, we might count the number of men crossing the north line plus women crossing the south lines, thereby measuring a "current of men" or a "current of women." Since the average speed of the men and women may differ, the *total* current may have *unequal* contributions from the men and women, even though their numbers in any mesoscopic volume are nearly equal. This same analogy can be used to illustrate electrical resistance, since the average person velocity is clearly limited by the frequency and strength of all the pushing and shoving. We might further imagine other physical obstacles to the movement that most people go around, but a few energetic ones manage to climb over. Such physical obstacles are analogous to membranes that have large resistance to current flow.

14 Ohm's Law for Linear Conductors

Thus far in this chapter our discussions of current flow have been general; they apply to both linear and nonlinear conductors. We have avoided an important question. What will be the average velocity of ions in an electrolyte or the velocity of electrons in a metal? The current density is proportional to this velocity, which is limited by collisions with other ions. The details of this process can be quite difficult to work out. Statistical mechanics and either Newton's law (in fluids) or quantum mechanics (in solids) may be used to calculate how many collisions per second are experienced by a charge and how its velocity is changed by each collision. Despite all the complications, it often turns out that the drag force on a charge moving in a conductor is proportional to its velocity. This result is consistent with Ohm's law, a relation between current density and applied electric field that defines the medium as *linear in the conductive sense*, that is

$$\mathbf{J} = \sigma\mathbf{E} \tag{3.15}$$

Current density is proportional to electric field with the proportionality constant σ called the *electrical conductivity* of the medium. In mks units, conductivity has units of 1/(ohm m) (same as Siemens/m or S/m) but in biologic tissue it is often more convenient to use the units 1/(ohm cm) or 1/(ohm mm) or (S/mm). *Resistivity* is the inverse of conductivity and may be measured in ohm cm or ohm mm. The experimental resistivities of several physical and biological tissues are listed in table 4-1. For example, macroscopic resistivity of neocortex is about a million times larger than copper resistivity. Whereas (3.15) can be derived from microscopic theories (making use of plausible assumptions), it is its widespread experimental verification that makes it so important to macroscopic field theory.

Biological membranes selectively pass some ions more readily than others, thus membranes provide a mechanism to maintain different concentrations of each ion across the membrane, that is, between the inside and outside of living cells. The concentration gradients produce *diffusion currents* that occur in addition to *ohmic currents* caused by electric fields. The total current density across the membrane due to both electric fields and diffusion is given by the Nernst–Planck equation:

$$\mathbf{J} = \sigma\mathbf{E} + \sum_i D_i \nabla \rho_i \tag{3.16}$$

Equation (3.16) is only valid for membranes operating well below the threshold transmembrane potential at which action potentials are initiated. *Action potentials* are remarkable nonlinear phenomena "designed" by natural selection so that the conductivities of individual ions become separate functions of transmembrane potential (or electric field), that is $\sigma \to \sigma_i(\mathbf{E})$ in (3.16). The D_i are ion diffusion coefficients and the ρ_i are charge densities of the individual ions. The gradient operator ∇ indicates that diffusion current is proportional to concentration gradient for each ion. Electrochemical equilibrium occurs when the total current density is zero, that is, when ohmic current just balances diffusion current. In genuine biological membranes, an important additional process is the *active transport* of specific ions across the membrane, for example, the *sodium and potassium pumps*. If such processes occur, more terms must be added to the right-hand side of (3.16).

Equation (3.15) is the usual form of Ohm's law for a linear volume conductor; (3.16) is the linear modification to account for membrane diffusion. Low-frequency currents in circuits are uniformly distributed across wire cross sections and (3.15) relates total current I to current density J. Furthermore, the voltage difference between two points (1 and 2) separated by a small distance d follows directly from the definition of electric potential (3.4):

$$V_1 - V_2 \approx Ed \tag{3.17}$$

By combining (3.14), (3.15), and (3.17), the elementary form of Ohm's law for current in an electric circuit is obtained as

$$V_1 - V_2 = IR \tag{3.18}$$

Note that the sign of the current I is consistent with current moving from a region of higher to lower potential, analogous to water flowing down hill in a pipe. The *resistance* R of a length of wire d is related to the wire conductivity σ and geometry by

$$R = \frac{d}{\sigma A} \tag{3.19}$$

The resistance R is expressed in ohms. Resistance (like capacitance) depends on the geometry of the conductor, whereas resistivity or conductivity (like dielectric constant) depends only on the property of the material. For example, it makes no sense to speak of the resistance of copper or tissue. Rather, we speak of the resistivity of materials. The resistance of a long wire (or long tissue path) of small cross section is larger than the resistance of a short wire (or short tissue path) of large cross section, if the materials are the same.

As shown in chapter 4, a volume conductor having important capacitive effects (charge storage) in addition to conduction can be described by a complex conductivity $\sigma = \sigma_R + j\sigma_I$. In this case, a mass of tissue acts like a resistor in parallel with a capacitor, and the resistance R in (3.19) may be interpreted as impedance. While capacitive effects are critical at membrane scales, their effects in macroscopic tissue appear negligible at EEG frequencies.

One must be somewhat careful about interpretations of "constant conductivity." Conductivity is independent of electric field strength (or potential) in linear media. In fact, this condition defines a *linear conductive medium*. However, both conductivity and dielectric constants of linear media generally vary with field frequency. For example, the conductivity of a macroscopic mass of cortical tissue has been reported to increase by about 25% as frequency is increased from 5 to 1000 Hz (Polk and Postow 1986). Small conductivity changes with frequency do not appear important in EEG applications where only a narrow frequency range is of interest and much larger conductivity differences are, in any case, associated with different tissues.

The conductivity of head tissue is considered in chapter 4. In summary, cortex, blood, cerebrospinal fluid, white matter and scalp have conductivities that may vary by perhaps a factor of five or so. Bulk skull conductivity is apparently between 1/80 and 1/20 of cortical conductivity. In addition to the effects of tissue inhomogeneity, head volume conduction is influenced to an unknown degree by tissue anisotropy. White matter appears to be anisotropic because current evidently flows more easily parallel to axon fibers. Skull is composed of three layers; the inner layer has the largest conductivity because it contains the largest spaces containing fluid. This implies that bulk skull (treated as a single tissue layer) must be *anisotropic* because, for a fixed path length, current evidently passes more easily inside the middle layer. Note that tissue homogeneity (no variation with location) and isotropy (no variation with direction) are separate issues, an occasional source of confusion in electrophysiology.

The tissue properties discussed above complicate our picture of electric fields in the brain and make practical calculations and algorithm development more difficult. Nevertheless, we emphasize that tissue inhomogeneity, anisotropy, dielectric (capacitive) effects, and their variations with field frequency are usually all *linear effects*. In a general sense, these complications are not unique to living tissue; however some important details evidently are unique. As much as possible, we build on known phenomena involving electric fields in physical media. In some cases new analyses are required. In other cases, we need only provide the proper physiological interpretation of existing physical theory.

15 Nonlinear Conductors

For the most part, violations of Ohm's law in physical media occur only under conditions incompatible with life. The electric field may be very large or the material very hot or very cold. Superconductivity, in which current may flow with essentially no impressed electric field, is a phenomenon that occurs in special materials at very low temperatures. By contrast, nonlinear effects in brain tissue are caused by the peculiar properties of cell membranes. The cell membrane also provides a good example of a medium that simultaneously exhibits both dielectric and conductive properties. To a first approximation, membranes well below threshold for action potential generation have linear conductive properties, and linear dielectric properties even during active action potentials. The core conductor model of the neuron, which is based on an idealized linear network of resistors and capacitors, has been quite successful in explaining important aspects of subthreshold membrane behavior.

The active membrane presents quite a different story. When transmembrane potential (or electric field inside the membrane) is changed from its equilibrium value of roughly -65 mV (inside negative with respect to outside) closer to its threshold of perhaps -40 mV, the membrane becomes a nonlinear conductor. At threshold, the membrane exhibits a remarkable nonlinear conductive behavior, the propagation of the action potential. As a result, (naturally selective) violations of Ohm's law within the membrane allow signals to be transmitted over large distances within the body with no appreciable spatial attenuation. This process is quite distinct from volume conduction in which potentials are strongly attenuated with distance from a small source region, but spread out nearly instantaneously. By contrast, action potentials propagate with velocities in the approximate range 0.1 to 100 m/s, depending on axon diameter and myelination. Typical action potential speeds in myelinated cortico-cortical axons (forming most of the subcortical white matter in humans) are 5 to 10 m/s. The fastest speeds occur in sensory and motor axons that carry signals between the brain and remote body regions.

Linear phenomena are often conveniently characterized as either wave or diffusion processes, although many important phenomena involve both, as in electromagnetic wave propagation through a conductive medium. The action potential can be described as a *nonlinear diffusion process* from the perspective of the basic theory of *Hodgkin–Huxley*, but in several important ways it behaves as a *propagating wave*, analogous to wave propagation along transmission lines. The fact that axons allow for propagation at relatively low speeds in a closed medium, suggests the possible existence of traveling and standing waves of synaptic action at macroscopic scales. Supporting experimental evidence for such waves is discussed in chapters 9 and 10; a theoretical basis is proposed in chapter 11.

The fundamentals of electric field theory underlying electrophysiology have been presented in the first part of this chapter. The remaining material in this chapter is not generally required in electrophysiological applications. Thus, some readers may wish to go directly to chapter 4. The remainder of this chapter is concerned with magnetic fields in physical media and in brains, the relationship of electrostatics to electromagnetic fields, near and far fields, and electromagnetic resonant phenomena. The latter subject provides a metaphor for ideas about the nature of neocortical dynamics and the so-called *brain binding problem*, discussed in chapter 11.

16 The Brain's Magnetic Field

At the low frequencies of brain dynamics, electric and magnetic fields are uncoupled. Thus, magnetic fields are due only to currents and may be calculated from the Biot–Savart law, a special case of Maxwell's equation (3.24):

$$\mathbf{H} = \frac{\mathbf{p} \times \mathbf{r}}{4\pi r^3} \tag{3.20}$$

Here $\mathbf{H}$ is the magnetic field, $\mathbf{p} = I\mathbf{d}$ is the vector current dipole moment, and $\mathbf{r}$ is the vector from the dipole to the field point. It is assumed in (3.20) that r is much larger than the spatial extent d of the dipole. Consider a straight current element of length 1 mm, for example, inside a pyramidal cell or bundle of cells oriented tangent to the local scalp surface. If the total current magnitude is 4π µA, the magnitude of magnetic field at a distance of $r = 1$ cm is

$$H = \frac{4\pi \times 1\,\text{mm} \times 10\,\text{mm}}{4\pi \times 10^3\,\text{mm}^3} = 0.01\ \text{µA/mm}$$

The direction of $\mathbf{H}$ is circular, wrapped around the dipole axis so that magnetic field lines exit and reenter the scalp with field intensity that first increases and then decreases at progressively larger distances from the scalp location directly above the dipole axis, as indicated by the tangential dipole in fig. 2-6. Currents form closed paths. Ideally, we may imagine the magnetic dipole current to be exclusively intercellular and its return current to be distributed in a symmetric manner about a cylindrical cell in the extracellular fluid. In this idealized picture, the net contribution to $\mathbf{H}$ from all the external return loops will be zero due to perfect cancellation. The magnetic field at the scalp will then be due only to intercellular current (Hamaleinen et al. 1993). While this picture is quite plausible, it is not known how closely it matches genuine brain sources. Advances in superconductors have made it possible to record the extremely small magnetic fields of the brain, called magnetoencephalography or MEG. In chapter 2, we consider the selective sensitivity of MEG and EEG to different kinds of sources and compare their relative accuracies.

17 Maxwell's Equations

There are two versions of Maxwell's equations, the microscopic and macroscopic formulations. These equations, representing one of the supreme intellectual achievements in human history, are listed in table 3-2 (Jackson 1975). We have numbered the equations for easy reference; there is no standard order. The microscopic version of Maxwell's equations together with the Lorentz equation (force on a moving charge) and Newton's laws provide a complete classical description of the dynamic interaction of charged particles and electromagnetic fields. In fact, by adding one more equation, the gravitational force between two bodies, *all of classical physics* (everything known before Einstein's special relativity in 1905) would be expressed by these few equations (Feynman 1963)! If we think of the enormous variety of physical phenomena that result from these simple-looking equations, "the unreasonable success of mathematics in science" (Wigner 1960) is suggested. The rather smug attitude of many 19th century physicists is perhaps also understandable. A common idea at the time was that all physical laws had been discovered and that physicists of the future would be mainly concerned with the dull task of finding the next decimal point in preexisting calculations.

Table 3-2 Microscopic and macroscopic versions of Maxwell's equations

Microscopic fields	Macroscopic fields	Approximate description	
$\nabla \cdot \mathbf{E} = \rho_t/\varepsilon_0$	$\nabla \cdot \mathbf{D} = \rho$	The first kind of spatial rate of change (*divergence*) of electric field ($\mathbf{E}$ or $\mathbf{D}$) is proportional to charge density (ρ_t or ρ)	(3.21)
$\nabla \times \mathbf{E} = -\dfrac{\partial \mathbf{B}}{\partial t}$	$\nabla \times \mathbf{E} = -\dfrac{\partial \mathbf{B}}{\partial t}$	The second kind of spatial rate of change (*curl*) of electric field $\mathbf{E}$ is proportional to time rate of change of magnetic field $\mathbf{B}$	(3.22)
$\nabla \cdot \mathbf{B} = 0$	$\nabla \cdot \mathbf{B} = 0$	The first kind of spatial rate of change of magnetic field $\mathbf{B}$ is zero	(3.23)
$\nabla \times \mathbf{B} = \dfrac{\mathbf{J}_t}{\varepsilon_0 c^2} + \dfrac{1}{c^2}\dfrac{\partial \mathbf{E}}{\partial t}$	$\nabla \times \mathbf{H} = \mathbf{J} + \dfrac{\partial \mathbf{D}}{\partial t}$	The second kind of spatial rate of change of magnetic field ($\mathbf{B}$ or $\mathbf{H}$) is proportional to the current density $\mathbf{J}$ plus the time rate of change of electric field ($\mathbf{E}$ or $\mathbf{D}$)	(3.24)

The microscopic equations relate electric and magnetic fields to each other and to sources of total charge density and current. If we know all the charges and currents (that is, all charges and their velocities) in some region, we can unambiguously determine the resulting electric **E** and magnetic **B** fields. By "total charge" we mean both free and polarization charge. We must also know the currents of all bound atomic electrons in addition to free electron current. The microscopic equations work very well for a few charges and currents isolated in a near vacuum. However, in a macroscopic medium like tissue, they are of no use except to shed light on the macroscopic version.

Since we cannot possibly know the positions of all charges in biological tissue, only the macroscopic version of Maxwell's equation in the second column of table 3-2 is useful in electrophysiology. The displacement vector **D** was introduced by (3.8) to include the cumulative effects of internal charge polarization of any medium with capacitive properties. In order to account for molecular currents, the macroscopic magnetic field **H** (due only to macroscopic currents) is defined in terms of the magnetic induction **B** (due to all currents) and the material magnetization **M**:

$$\mu_0 \mathbf{H} = \mathbf{B} - \mathbf{M} \tag{3.25}$$

The relationship of magnetic field **H** to the magnetic induction **B** is analogous to the relationship of the displacement field **D** to the electric field **E**. The field **B** is often called the magnetic induction to distinguish it from the magnetic field **H**. The lack of perfect similarity between (3.8) and (3.25) results from their early relations to experiments rather than any theoretical issue. Here μ_0 is a constant called the *permeability* of free space. In linear magnetic materials, the fields are simply related by

$$\mathbf{H} = \frac{\mathbf{B}}{\mu} \tag{3.26}$$

where μ is the *permeability* of the magnetic material. Linear relation (3.26) is analogous to linear relation (3.10). In nonlinear magnetic materials, especially ferromagnetic substances, (3.26) must be replaced by a nonlinear relationship. While the distinction between the **B** and **H** fields is very important in magnetic materials, its only consequence in MEG applications is that the two fields have different units. This follows because normal tissue is nonmagnetic. In tissue as in empty space, (3.26) connects the two fields with μ replaced by μ_0.

Having defined the new fields **D** and **H** for macroscopic volumes of material, we turn our attention to the differences between the microscopic and macroscopic versions of Maxwell's equations in table 3-2. Suppose that, in each case, the currents and charges are known and we wish to calculate the fields. The microscopic version consists of 8 scalar equations

(2 vector plus 2 scalar) and 6 scalar unknowns (2 vector fields). This tells us right away that Maxwell's microscopic equations contain redundancy. The macroscopic version also consists of 8 scalar equations, but it contains 12 scalar unknowns (4 vector fields). Thus, the macroscopic version cannot be solved without additional information. Here is where the experimental relations for a linear conductor (3.15), a linear dielectric (3.10), and a linear magnetic material (3.26) come to the rescue. If all three experimental vector relations are valid, 9 more scalar equations are obtained for a total of 17 scalar equations and 12 unknowns, again a redundant system. Of course, a linear dielectric need not be a linear conductor or linear magnetic material so the count can be somewhat different in different applications. However, often the macroscopic equations plus experimental (*constitutive*) relations provide a redundant system.

In formal electromagnetic theory, the inherent redundancy of Maxwell's equations is typically removed by expressing the electric and magnetic fields in terms of one scalar and one vector potential (4 scalar variables) in 4 scalar equations. From a purely mathematical viewpoint, this is far more satisfactory; however, the untransformed Maxwell's equations are normally viewed as the fundamental equations perhaps partly for historical reasons, but especially because of their close connection to the experiments that led to their original formulation.

Nearly all materials can have capacitive (polarization), conductive, and magnetic properties. If a material is linear in all three senses, three parameters (σ, ε, μ) characterize the material. If any of the three properties is nonlinear, more parameters are required. Perhaps we can see why some scientists appear confused by the term *linear*. A linear conductor can, at the same time, be a nonlinear dielectric or magnetic material. A nonlinear conductor can also be a linear dielectric as in the active membrane. In biological tissue especially, linearity can also depend very much on the hierarchical level considered. A macroscopic mass of tissue, containing many conductively nonlinear membranes with substantial capacitive properties, can typically be described as a linear conductor with negligible capacitive properties.

In this chapter, we have glossed over many of the subtle aspects concerning the connections between microscopic and macroscopic electric and magnetic fields, as well as the (perhaps surprising) widespread validity of the linear constitutive relations. In fact, many physicists have spent a large fraction of their professional lives working on theoretical and experimental projects that forge cross-scale connections. In this abbreviated description, we may appear to have justified the macroscopic equations based on the more concise microscopic equations, but the historical record is quite the opposite. The microscopic version of Maxwell's equations was developed largely on the basis of experiments performed at macroscopic scales. Extension of these principles to microscopic scales was far from obvious and required a mix of intuition, mathematical skills, and clever new experiments (Jackson 1975). *There is an important lesson here for scientists who would trivialize relationships between electrophysiological data recorded at different spatial scales, ranging from the "microelectrode" with tip diameter in the 10^{-4} cm range to the scalp electrode recording source activity from at least several square centimeters of cortical tissue.*

Implicit within Maxwell's equations are energy and charge conservation. In particular, the conservation of free charge follows directly from macroscopic equations (3.21) and (3.24):

$$\nabla \cdot \mathbf{J} + \frac{\partial \rho}{\partial t} = 0 \qquad (3.27)$$

where $\mathbf{J}$ is the macroscopic current density. This expresses the fundamental law that charge is neither created nor destroyed. This principle was known early on and was, in fact, used by Maxwell to obtain (3.24). Although his derivation was mostly wrong, his answer was correct! Equation (3.27) is a basic conservation equation; the same formalism describes mass and radiation energy conservation, the latter also implicit in Maxwell's equations.

18 Electromagnetic Radiation and Other Waves

This brief summary of Maxwell's equations would be absurdly inadequate without some discussion of *electromagnetic radiation*. This phenomenon requires substantial coupling between the electric and magnetic fields. It is a high-frequency phenomenon of little apparent importance in electrophysiology. Before 1864, knowledge of electricity and magnetism was essentially that which we now formalize as Maxwell's equations, with the exception of the far right-hand term in (3.24), $\partial \mathbf{D}/\partial t$. It was Maxwell's genius to realize that this critical addition was required to preserve the principle of charge conservation (3.27). Forging this connection was far more difficult at the time because vector field theory had not yet been developed. With this powerful tool we can now show that the $\partial \mathbf{D}/\partial t$ term is required in a few short steps. The addition of the new term on the right-hand side of (3.24) led to an uncountable number of changes in the world because the complete equations yield a quantitative understanding of electromagnetic radiation. The equations show that phenomena associated with static charges, magnets, microwaves, radio waves, visible light, and more are all part of the same fundamental process and allow us to manipulate this process in a myriad of new ways into the foreseeable future.

Maxwell's equations combine to form wave equations, either in terms of the electric and magnetic fields components or, in a more concise formulation, the scalar and vector potentials. The equations tell us that a local AC current distribution (in an antenna, for example), if oscillating at sufficiently high frequency, will produce an electromagnetic field that becomes "detached" at some distance from the source region and propagates through empty space with the velocity of light, given by

$$c = \frac{1}{\sqrt{\varepsilon_0 \mu_0}} \tag{3.28}$$

Electromagnetic fields consist of electric and magnetic fields that oscillate in both time and space, but remain perpendicular to each other and perpendicular to the direction of propagation; they are *transverse waves*. The field vectors may either have fixed direction or rotate about the propagation direction in various ways described as *wave polarization* Here the word "polarization" is used as in optics, a different usage than in a dielectric. For the special case of one-dimensional propagation in a wave guide, one might picture an active spatial region containing a *wave packet* (a local group of wave components) traveling in a straight line. With no wave guide, wave packets generally spread out from the source region with energy contained in an expanding spherical shell. A two-dimensional analog is a water wave packet spreading out from a surface disturbance like a raindrop.

Electromagnetic waves travel through material media with velocity given by (3.28) with the permittivity μ_0 and permeability ε_0 of empty space replaced by their equivalents μ and ε for the particular medium. As a result, electromagnetic propagation through a material medium is somewhat slower than in a vacuum. Up until the time of Maxwell's contribution, the constant c was just an "electromagnetic constant." Maxwell realized that c was, in fact, the velocity of light. Thus, one of the great unifications of science was made. *Light is just electromagnetic waves* with field frequencies in a rather narrow range, and electromagnetic waves occur over a very broad frequency range. *Wave phenomena* generally involve transmission of energy or information over long distances with minimal attenuation of signal and no permanent distortion of the wave medium. Another important characteristic of waves is that many of their properties depend on the wave medium, independent of the source of the waves. *Wave dispersion* and *propagation speed* depend only on the medium, for example. The dispersive properties of the medium determine how the wave packet distorts and spreads out as it propagates. Electromagnetic wave packets in a vacuum maintain constant form as they propagate: they are *nondispersive waves*. By contrast, electromagnetic waves propagating in a material medium, water waves, and most other waves in nature are dispersive. The *dispersion relation* for a particular kind of wave and medium follows directly from the Fourier transform of the appropriate linear wave equation. For waves propagating in one dimension, the dispersion relation takes the general form

$$\omega = \omega(k) \tag{3.29}$$

Here $\omega = 2\pi f$ is the angular frequency where f is frequency in Hz. The spatial frequency or wavenumber is $k = 2\pi/\lambda$, where λ is the spatial wavelength. In the case of nondispersive waves, the dispersion relation is

$$\omega = ck \quad \text{or} \quad f = c/\lambda \tag{3.30}$$

This is the familiar relation indicating that wave frequency is proportional to the medium's characteristic velocity and inversely proportional to the wave's spatial wavelength. It holds for electromagnetic propagation in a vacuum, simple sound waves, standing waves in a violin string, and other phenomena. In fact, many engineers take this relation for granted by referring to certain frequency ranges in terms of their corresponding spatial wavelengths λ; the label "microwaves" is an example.

Most waves in nature are dispersive; that is, they spread out and distort as they propagate. The relationship between frequency and spatial wavelength is more complicated in this general case—we cannot so easily infer temporal frequency from spatial wavelength. We emphasize that linear partial differential equations produce, by Fourier transform, nonlinear dispersion relations in all but the simplest case, but such waves are still "linear". The *single fiber action potential* behaves similarly to a linear nondispersive wave pulse in a wave guide or transmission line, even though the underlying physiological bases involve nonlinear diffusion of various ions across the membrane. The traveling transmembrane potential of the single fiber action potential satisfies (3.30) with propagation speed c dependent on axon diameter and axon myelination. The *compound action potential* of a bundle of axons (a nerve) behaves as a dispersive wave due to a mix of contributions from axons of different diameter having different action potential speeds. We have suggested that some EEG phenomena consist at least partly of standing waves of synaptic action, as discussed in chapters 9–11. Such EEG waves are predicted by physiological theory to occur at higher hierarchical levels, but owe their origins to the nonlinear membrane properties that allow for axon propagation at relatively low speeds.

Electromagnetic propagation through a material is generally much more complicated than vacuum propagation. The reason is that the electro-magnetic fields that make up the wave induce new currents in the medium, which act back on the wave to alter the wave's properties. A number of new phenomena occur, and their study in a variety of materials (in the four or more states of matter) occupied many scientists and engineers throughout the 20th century. Typically, the focus is on wave dispersion, which is closely aligned with both theory and experiment. When dispersion is very large, it may not even be possible to define a clear propagation velocity. This ambiguity can occur as a result of large wave distortion so there is no identifiable reference point in the wave packet after it has traveled some distance. Several different kinds of wave velocity are defined for radiation through a material, or for other dispersive waves, like water waves. For example, *phase velocity* refers to the velocity of a single component wave in a wave packet. *Group velocity* is normally the velocity of energy transfer for the entire wave packet; it is sort of the velocity of the "center of mass" of the wave packet. Phase and group velocities are equal for nondispersive waves.

Linear partial differential equations produce, by Fourier transform, nonlinear dispersion relations in all but the simplest case. In many applications, the complications of wave dispersion are entirely linear; however, important nonlinear effects may also occur. A propagating wave may grow steep and then break, as in ocean waves approaching the shore. Shock waves caused by supersonic jets are nonlinear sound waves.

19 Near and Far Fields

Consider what happens to Maxwell's equations when all fields are constant with the passage of time. The time derivatives in (3.22) and (3.24) are zero. (3.21) and (3.22) govern the electric field, independent of magnetic field. Also (3.23) and (3.24) govern the magnetic field behavior, independent of electric field. This limiting case provides an enormous simplification. We can calculate or measure electric fields as if magnetic fields do not exist and call this subfield *electrostatics*. We can calculate or measure magnetic fields as if there were no electric fields (provided we know all the currents) and call this study *magnetostatics*. If the fields are changing with time, but at sufficiently low frequency, the fields will be uncoupled to a first approximation and we may speak of a *quasi-static* approximation to Maxwell's equations. EEG and MEG are quasi-static phenomena, as shown in appendix B.

At high frequencies, electric and magnetic fields become closely linked and we speak properly of *electromagnetic fields*. Consider the dipole antenna of characteristic size d with current oscillating at frequency f as shown in fig. 3-10. The electromagnetic fields generated in empty space by antennas generally have complicated spatial characteristics. To simplify matters, it will prove useful to distinguish two regions occupying two spherical shells surrounding the antenna. The *near zone* is defined for intermediate distances r from the antenna such that $d \ll r \ll \lambda$. The *near fields* vary with distance and frequency according to

$$E \propto \frac{1}{r^3} \quad B \propto \frac{f}{r^2} \quad \text{(near fields)} \tag{3.31}$$

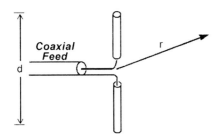

Figure 3-10 Dipole antenna used to generate an electromagnetic field (a *far field*). The electric and magnetic fields close to the antenna comprise the *near field*.

The near electric field is just the static dipole field, but oscillating in time. The near magnetic induction field vanishes as $f \to 0$. The far zone (or wave or radiation zone) is defined as $d < \lambda \ll r$. The *far fields* satisfy

$$E \propto \frac{f^2}{r} \quad B \propto \frac{f^2}{r} \quad \text{(far fields)} \tag{3.32}$$

In (3.31) and (3.32) we have shown the field dependence only on radial distance from the antenna r and field frequency f; the more complicated angular dependence is not shown. The near electric field falls off as $1/r^3$, an identical fall-off to the quasi-static dipole (potential falls off as $1/r^2$) as expected. In the far zone, both electric and magnetic fields go to zero if source frequency is zero. The far electric and magnetic fields have identical attenuations with distance r, which is not surprising since they comprise the unitary *electromagnetic field*. The terms "near field" and "far field" have been occasionally used in EEG to distinguish scalp potentials due to midbrain sources from potential due to cortical sources. Such use of these terms in EEG bears minimal relation to their standard use in electromagnetic theory.

The electromagnetic field carries energy, energy contained in the field itself. The electric and magnetic field energy densities (joules/mm³) are proportional to E^2 and B^2, respectively. Imagine that the antenna current is turned on for a fixed time τ so that the resulting wave packet is located entirely in an expanding spherical shell of thickness $c\tau$ and average radius r. The volume of this shell increases as r^2. Thus, the total energy in the electromagnetic wave packet (product of energy density with volume) remains constant as the spherical shell expands. Radiation energy is conserved in a vacuum as expected.

20 Transmission Lines

In the next two sections, we consider electromagnetic wave propagation in confined spaces, thereby causing multiple traveling waves to interfere and form standing waves. Often standing waves occur as a result of reflection from boundaries, as in the mechanical example of a violin string. However, here we consider a different kind of boundary condition, the *periodic boundary condition* that also leads to wave interference and standing waves.

These physical systems with periodic boundary conditions are chosen as metaphors to conjecture possible aspects of EEG dynamic behavior. The reason is that the *neocortex–white matter system* carries signals with finite velocity and each cortical hemisphere is approximately *topologically equivalent to a spherical shell*, thereby making periodic boundary conditions on synaptic action variables the appropriate choice.

The first analog system is the transmission line. Transmission line waves transmit electromagnetic power and information, typically using power, telephone, television, and computer lines. The fundamental processes that cause action potentials and transmission line waves are quite different. The action potential is based on selective nonlinear ion diffusion across neural membranes. Transmission line waves result from linear inductive, capacitive, and resistive properties of the lines; however, the net results of these disparate processes have important properties in common. Both processes typically involve pulses of electric potential traveling over long distances with finite speeds, minimal attenuation and dispersion of the waveform, and no permanent alteration of the underlying medium. In addition, both processes can repeatedly transmit coded information along their respective "fibers" to local "computers" or "relay stations."

When viewed from the higher hierarchical levels of EEG dynamic behavior or cognitive science, the general operational features of action potentials discussed above may be as important as the underlying membrane details. In other words, we are suggesting that a plausible conceptual framework for macroscopic dynamic EEG behavior can be formulated based partly on higher-level properties of action potentials, largely independent of their underlying physiological mechanisms. To use another analogy, the physical mechanisms underlying Ohm's law for solids differ from those for fluids. However, if Ohm's law is valid, it can be used effectively in macroscopic electromagnetic study, independent of the microscopic details supporting this law.

A transmission line typically consists of two conductors separated by a dielectric (insulating) material. The line may have any of several cross sections, the coaxial cable being a convenient choice. The line carries transverse electromagnetic waves in one dimension along the line. The equivalent circuit for an incremental section of a transmission line is shown in fig. 3-11. In the coaxial line, the inner and outer conductors are represented by a series resistance R_1 and inductance L_1 per unit length. The dielectric material between the conductors is represented by a capacitance C_2 and conductance G_2 per unit length. The conductance is acknowledged as nonzero to account for current leakage across the dielectric. If a voltage is applied between the inner and outer conductors at one end of the line, the voltage difference propagates along the line according to the standard transmission line equation. When Fourier transformed, this wave equation yields the dispersion relation (real part) given by

$$\omega^2 = \omega_0^2 + v^2 k^2 \tag{3.33}$$

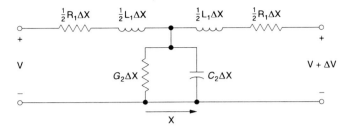

Figure 3-11 The equivalent circuit for a transmission line in terms of resistance R_1 and inductance L_1, per unit length. Dielectric conductance G_2 and capacitance per unit length C_2 are indicated. If inductance $L_1 = 0$, this is also the equivalent circuit for a subthreshold membrane with intracellular and extracellular fluids analogous to inner and outer conductors of the transmission line. The membrane is analogous to the dielectric with conductance (current leakage) per unit length G_2. Reproduced with permission from Nunez (1995).

The oscillation frequency ω has two parts, a *local part* given by

$$\omega_0^2 = \frac{R_1 G_2}{L_1 C_2} \tag{3.34}$$

and a *global part* $v^2 k^2$, where k is the wavenumber of a propagating wave component.

The labels "local" and "global" refer here to physical mechanisms underlying the field oscillations, parlance consistent with the neocortical dynamic theory outlined in chapter 11. This is a somewhat different context than our discussions of EEG data, in which case "local" and "global" refer to more dominant high and low spatial frequencies, respectively.

The transmission line dispersion relation also has an imaginary part (not shown) corresponding to resistive losses that convert wave energy into heat. Wave packets are typically composed of some mixture of wavenumbers (or spatial wavelengths) determined by the spatial details of the initial disturbance at the end of the line. The characteristic speed of the transmission line v is given by

$$v = \frac{1}{\sqrt{L_1 C_2}} = \frac{1}{\sqrt{\varepsilon \mu}} \tag{3.35}$$

Here μ and ε are the permeability of the conductive material (inner cylinder and outer cylindrical shell of the line) and permittivity of the dielectric (middle cylindrical shell), respectively. When μ and ε are replaced by their values for empty space, μ_0 and ε_0, respectively, v equals c the velocity of light in a vacuum.

Generally, a wave packet will contain some distribution of waves with different wavenumbers k. *Phase velocity* v_P and *group velocity* v_G for the packet are given by

$$v_P = \frac{\omega}{k} \quad \text{and} \quad v_G = \frac{d\omega}{dk} \tag{3.36}$$

In the transmission line this yields

$$v_P v_G = v^2$$

The velocity of the wave packet (group velocity v_G) is less than v and the velocity of a single k component (phase velocity v_P) is greater than v. Thus, transmission line waves are generally dispersive so that a wave packet spreads out and distorts as it propagates. The transmission line wave packet behaves like a compound action potential in this sense, even though the two underlying mechanisms differ substantially. The equivalent circuit for a section of transmission line (shown in fig. 3-11) is identical to that used to describe the spatial-temporal subthreshold membrane responses to synaptic input, except for the critical inclusion of electromagnetic induction in the transmission line. Without induction, potential follows a linear diffusion process. The induction parameter L_1 represents concisely the coupling of electric and magnetic fields, thereby allowing for wave propagation (with some diffusion) in the transmission line. By contrast, action potential propagation occurs as a result of selective nonlinear resistive (conductive) properties of the membrane as described by Hodgkin and Huxley.

While physical transmission lines are not normally constructed in closed loops, we consider this example as a useful metaphor for putative standing waves in neocortex. In a closed transmission line loop, waves propagate with the speeds v_P and v_G and distort according to the same dispersion relation (3.33). Waves traveling in opposite directions around a loop of length a interfere in such a manner that only the following wavenumbers are allowed:

$$k_n = \frac{2n\pi}{a} \qquad n = 1, 2, 3, \ldots \tag{3.38}$$

That is, only standing waves with an integer number of waves with wavelengths given by $\lambda = 2\pi/k_n = a/n$ can persist in the closed line. This restriction is necessary to satisfy periodic boundary conditions, essentially that any genuine potential must be a single-valued function of position in the closed line. This is similar to standing waves in a violin string or other systems where waves are reflected from boundaries, except that with periodic boundary conditions, no wave reflection occurs in the circumference direction and no half-integer waves are allowed such that derivatives of potential are also continuous. Rather, wave interference and the resulting standing waves in the closed transmission line are due to periodic boundary conditions. The resonant frequencies of the closed transmission line are then given by (3.33), but with wavenumbers restricted by (3.38), that is

$$\omega_n^2 = \omega_0^2 + v^2 k_n^2 \qquad n = 1, 2, 3, \ldots \qquad (3.39)$$

The resonant frequencies consist of the *fundamental frequency* or *mode* ($n = 1$) and the *overtones* ($n = 2, 3, 4, \ldots$). Because of the local contribution ω_0, the overtones are not *harmonics* in this system, in contrast to the resonant frequencies in a simple violin string. Our use of the terms "local" and "global" to describe the separate frequency contributions in (3.39) is hopefully now clear to our readers. The local part can be determined from analysis of a small section of the line, independent of its length a and characteristic line speed v. This is also the case if different sections of the line produce somewhat different local frequencies. Local frequencies ω_0 will then depend on location along the line. By contrast, the global frequencies are the same everywhere in the transmission line, but theoretically an infinite number may occur.

21 Schumann Resonances

The *Schumann resonances* and standing transmission line waves provide useful metaphors to facilitate our proposed conceptual framework for EEG dynamic behavior at large scales (Jackson 1975). A number of scientists have proposed local cortical or cortical–thalamic networks in which characteristic (or resonant) EEG frequencies are due to local neuronal delays, especially postsynaptic rise and decay times of transmembrane potential near cell bodies (see chapter 11). Others have proposed global resonant frequencies due to finite axonal propagation in the closed cortical–white matter system, which is topologically equivalent to a spherical shell (Nunez 1974, 1981a,b,c, 1995; Katznelson 1981). This makes the system somewhat analogous to the spherical shell formed by the earth's surface and the bottom of the ionosphere. In this region electromagnetic waves generated by multiple, near-simultaneous lighting strikes travel with velocity c and interfere to form standing waves, the so-called Schumann resonances (see fig. 3-12). In chapter 11, we suggest that characteristic EEG frequencies may have both local and global contributions, with relative contribution strength depending on brain state. The recorded scalp potentials are not generally due to action potentials. Rather scalp EEG is believed to be the summed synaptic potentials from generally large cortical regions. Nevertheless, action potentials may

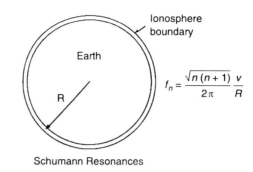

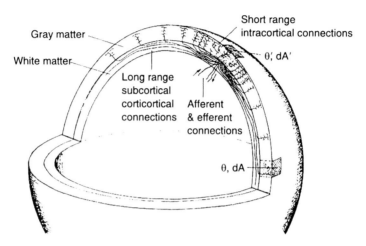

Figure 3-12 (*Top*) Spherical shell formed by the earth's surface and the inner surface of the ionosphere. Electromagnetic waves created by multiple on-going lighting strikes cause waves traveling away from each epicenter with the velocity of light $v = c$. Wave interference and periodic boundary conditions in the shell result in discrete preferred frequencies of field oscillations, the *Schumann resonances* given by the expression for f_n (3.41). (*Bottom*) A similar phenomenon is postulated for *brain waves*. The brain-like structure results from mentally inflating the folded cortical surface of one hemisphere. The characteristic velocity corresponds to the peak in the velocity distribution function for corticocortical transmission of roughly 6 to 9 m/s. Reproduced with permission from Katznelson (1981) and Nunez (1995).

provide important time delays that partly determine EEG dynamic behavior.

Maxwell's equations may be solved in a thin spherical shell of (average) radius R, that is, with periodic boundary conditions applied to waves traveling around all circumferences within the shell (Jackson 1975). These electromagnetic waves are generated by near continuously on-going lighting strikes in the atmosphere. Each lighting flash is an electric field source that produces a wave packet spreading out from the source in a manner analogous to a water wave packet on a pond surface generated by a rain drop. Multiple wave packets interfere to produce a large cancellation effect. As a result of this interference, only waves with wavelengths dictated by the shell geometry can persist. For a homogeneous medium with characteristic speed v and no local frequency contributions, the resonant frequencies in a thin spherical shell are

$$\omega_n = \frac{v\sqrt{n(n+1)}}{R} \qquad n = 1, 2, 3, \ldots \qquad (3.40)$$

As in the transmission line, the resonant frequencies consist of fundamental ($n = 1$) and overtones ($n = 2, 3, 4, \ldots$). Also in this example, the overtones are not harmonics, but here lack of harmonic overtones is due to the spherical geometry, rather than local properties in the transmission line. In neocortex, we conjecture the possibility of both local and global effects on characteristic frequencies so that EEG overtones are not expected to be harmonic.

For electromagnetic waves in the atmosphere, R is the earth's radius and v is the velocity of light. The first seven Schumann resonances from (3.40), expressed in Hz are

$$f_n = \omega_n/2\pi = 10.6, 18.3, 25.8, 33.4, 40.9, 48.4, 55.8 \qquad (3.41)$$

These frequencies were predicted by Schumann in 1952. If they are multiplied by the constant correction factor 0.78, they agree closely with the experimental frequencies ($8, 14, 20, 26, 32, 37, 43$ Hz) first recorded in the 1960s. The correction factor is required because the original theory depended on the crude approximation that the ionosphere and earth boundaries are perfectly conducting.

Suppose we naively apply (3.40) to human neocortex, using the square root of folded cortical surface area (1600 to 4000 cm^2) to determine an effective radius $R \approx 11$ to 18 cm and an estimated range for the propagation speeds in corticocortical axons of $v \approx 600$ to 900 cm/s (Nunez 1995). This exercise yields an estimated fundamental mode for putative "brain waves":

$$f_n = 7 \text{ to } 18\,\text{Hz} \qquad (3.42)$$

with overtone frequencies similar to those in (3.41). This estimate of brain wave frequencies does not, by any stretch of the imagination, constitute a theory. It is merely a preliminary calculation to see if the idea of standing waves in the brain is worth additional consideration. Equation (3.42) predicts EEG frequencies in roughly the correct range for humans. Perhaps it has sufficient physiological substance to have motivated an experimental search for human EEG frequencies in this general range had the estimate been obtained before the first human EEG recordings in the mid-1920s. In chapter 11, we consider both a general conceptual framework and a specific physiological theory of brain waves that includes both global effects analogous to Schumann resonances and local network effects. Such theory will ultimately be judged by its consistency with existing data and its ability to make predictions that are both new and correct.

22 Microwave Ovens, Spectroscopy, and Top-Down Resonance

Our proposed conceptual framework for brain operation in general and neocortical dynamics in particular, described in chapters 1 and 11, involves *cell assemblies* (or probably less accurately *neural networks*) immersed within synaptic action fields. We propose that both top-down and bottom-up interactions between the synaptic action fields and cell assemblies may be important to brain function. We here consider two electromagnetic analogs that illustrate the general concepts of top-down energy transfer and resonant interaction between oscillating systems. The first example is microwave cooking, popular because food is cooked more rapidly and uniformly than with conventional cooking. In a conventional oven, inner oven walls and air are heated. Heat energy is then transferred from the oven's internal air to the food surface and into the food interior by ordinary conduction. This process is relatively slow and inefficient and provides much faster cooking at the surface than in the interior. By contrast, microwaves do not heat the air and walls so nearly all microwave energy is absorbed by the food, mostly over a depth of 1 to 2 cm, at least when the food is placed in a nonabsorbing container. Deeper heating occurs mostly by conventional conduction heating from the outer layer.

For our purposes the critical issue is that electromagnetic fields (and other waves) interact with matter in three basic ways. Waves may be reflected (or scattered) at the walls of a microwave oven. Waves may be transmitted with minimal distortion, as in the examples of air inside an oven or microwave-safe containers used to hold food. Finally, wave energy may be absorbed, as in the example of cooking food in microwave ovens (similar to energy losses in transmission lines). The deep heating effect of microwaves is also the basis for *medical microwave diathermy*, in which beneficial heating may be delivered to injured or inflamed tissue inside the body without overheating the skin.

The question of whether electromagnetic wave energy is reflected, transmitted, or absorbed by a material depends on several factors, including the frequency of the field. Electric fields passing through electrically conductive media induce currents. If a medium is a very good conductor (for example, a metal with free electrons to carry current), penetration of fields into the medium (the *skin depth*) is very small. Most wave energy is reflected from the region near the surface. In the case of food or tissue, the current carriers are ions. Electrical conductivity of food is much lower than that of a metal (typically by a factor of a million or so) and skin depth is much larger. The ions collide to produce heat. This *Joule heating* is apparently the main mechanism by which food is cooked in a microwave oven. The second heating mechanism is due to interactions between the electric field and polar molecules that attempt to align with the applied field. The molecules tend to oscillate back and forth at the frequency of the field, but such oscillations are resisted by intermolecular forces. The work done by the electric field in overcoming these forces is converted into heat. By contrast to Joule heating, this *dielectric heating* occurs in both conductors and insulators.

Dielectric heating in materials can be a very sensitive function of field frequency because intermolecular or interatomic interactions typically involve resonant behavior. Such resonance is analogous to mass/spring systems, electric circuits designed as filters, closed transmission lines, and violin strings that respond much more easily to external forces or fields at their resonant frequencies. For example, water and oxygen cause substantial attenuation of microwave energy from extraterrestrial sources passing through our atmosphere. This effect occurs with water when microwave frequency matches the water molecule's resonant frequencies. Such resonance is also the basis of *molecular microwave spectroscopy*. Each molecule has electronic, vibrational, and rotational energy and absorbs electromagnetic energy preferentially in narrow frequency bands, the resonant frequencies of the absorption lines. In spectroscopy, the absorption lines provide signatures indicating the presence of specific molecules.

The resonant interaction of physical wave fields with matter provides a metaphor for putative global/local synaptic interactions in brain tissue. First, it should be emphasized that such physical interactions are not limited to electromagnetic fields (which have no underlying mechanical structure). Consider the dramatic demonstration of an opera singer producing a pure tone at one of the resonant frequencies of a wine glass, causing it to break. This experiment is analogous to microwave spectroscopy if we imagine a room filled with many glasses of different sizes and shapes, each with its own set of known resonant frequencies (fundamental and overtones that are not generally harmonics). These sets of frequencies provide signatures for each glass, depending on size, shape, thickness, material, and so forth. We further imagine perfectly reflecting walls of the room and very sensitive instruments to measure sound wave energy as a function of frequency. A singer or microphone produces a wide range of pure tones. The resonant absorption lines of the recorded sound can tell us which glasses are present in the room.

Chapter 11 is concerned with neocortical dynamics, that is, the dynamic behavior of the current sources of EEG. The proposed conceptual framework adopts the idea of synaptic action fields $\Psi_e(\mathbf{r}, t)$ and $\Psi_i(\mathbf{r}, t)$. These fields are defined simply as the numbers of active excitatory and inhibitory synapses per unit volume of neocortical tissue at macroscopic location $\mathbf{r}$ and time t, independently of whether or not the synapses are part of cell assemblies. Such synaptic action densities are analogous to the mass densities of (say) two kinds of molecules in some medium. Sound is produced by short-time modulation of total mass density (or pressure) about some equilibrium level. The two kinds of molecules correspond metaphorically to short-time modulations of excitatory and inhibitory action about background levels in a neural tissue mass.

The introduction of synaptic action fields should be noncontroversial. There is no doubt that such fields exist: it is merely a question of whether the idea is useful to neuroscience. Following the classic ideas of Donald Hebb (1949, 1980), we conjecture cell assemblies operating at multiple hierarchical levels as the principal structures underlying behavior and cognition. Hebb viewed cell assemblies as diffuse cell structures, acting as closed systems for short periods. However, if we accept Hebb's ideas, why do we even need a synaptic field theory? The first reason is straight-forward: EEG is generally not a direct measure of cell assembly activity. Rather, EEG is a selective large-scale measure of brain activity that depends on passive volume conduction. EEG is directly related to synaptic field oscillations, independent of their function. Thus, synaptic fields are practical constructs to help us bridge the gap between the putative cell assemblies and scalp potentials.

The second reason for introducing synaptic action fields is more speculative. We conjecture that these fields may have a more profound significance that just a convenient bridge between theory and EEG data. That is, we advance the speculative idea that preferred (resonant) inter-actions may take place between the global fields and cell assemblies having matching resonant frequencies. Such fields may be modulated at certain preferred (resonant) frequencies determined partly by global properties of the cortical/corticocortical fiber system, an idea with several kinds of experimental support.

This speculative top-down mechanism addresses the so-called *binding problem* in neuroscience. For example, it allows for selective interactions (phase locking, for example) between remote cell assemblies having no direct fiber connections. The proposed phenomenon is somewhat similar to microwave spectroscopy or the resonant sound wave experiment, with the molecules or wine glasses analogous to local cell assemblies. However, in the neocortical system, a precisely tuned external source (opera singer) is not required to act as a "pacemaker." Rather, the neocortical system is conjectured to act similarly to a resonant cavity (as in the example of Schumann resonances in the atmosphere) in that it band-passes synaptic noise input and selects only certain preferred frequency ranges for the global synaptic action fields. These macroscopic fields can then act on *local cell assemblies* (top-down) and be influenced in turn (bottom-up) by the local cell assemblies (or *neural networks*). It should be emphasized that the existence of such resonant mechanisms in the brain is based mainly on dynamic theory and apparent consistency with known phenomena. It fits nicely into a conceptual framework for brain operation and serves as a useful working hypothesis. In a very general sense, our proposed conceptual framework combines *Hebb's cell assembly* idea with that of *brain fields*, providing a loose connection between cell assemblies and the abstract "fields" imagined by *Gestalt psychologists*.

23 Summary

We have presented a brief overview of electromagnetic theory with special emphasis on topics that appear relevant to large-scale neocortical dynamics and EEG (electroencephalography). In particular, quasi-static approximations to Maxwell's equations are considered with focus on electric potentials generated by current sources in conductive media. The quasi-static approximation applies to all volume conduction properties of interest in EEG; that is, the passive spread of currents and potentials in a spatially extended but finite conductive medium. We emphasize that any local distribution of sources and sinks at membrane surfaces, no matter how complicated, generates a potential that can be expressed in terms of a multipole expansion. Retaining only the dipole term in such expansions is sufficiently accurate in many EEG applications.

Our motivation for outlining electromagnetic phenomena differs from that of quasi-statics. The outline of electromagnetics is mainly intended to suggest plausible metaphors for some neocortical dynamic behavior. The physiological mechanisms underlying neocortical dynamic behavior (the collective behavior of membrane current sources) have little to do with mechanisms responsible for the physical waves discussed in this chapter. Nevertheless, the macroscopic dynamic behavior of neocortex may exhibit several phenomena that appear similar to physical waves, including propagation of disturbances with finite speeds, interference phenomena, dispersion relations, influence of periodic boundary conditions, and linear approximations to inherently nonlinear phenomena. The apparent importance of these generic properties of spatially extended dynamic systems and their connection to genuine physiology is discussed in chapters 9–11.

References

Cole K, 1968, *Membranes, Ions and Impulses*, Berkeley: University of California Press.

Einstein A and Infield L, 1961, *The Evolution of Physics*, New York: Simon and Schuster.

Feynman RP, 1963, *Lectures on Physics*, Vol. 2, Palo Alto, CA: Addison-Wesley.

Hamaleinen M, Hari R, Ilmoniemi RJ, Knuutila J, and Lounasmaa OV, 1993, Magnetoencephalography-theory, instrumentation, and applications to noninvasive studies of the working human brain. *Reviews of Modern Physics* 65: 413–497.

Hebb DO, 1949, *The Organization of Behavior*, New York: Wiley.

Hebb DO, 1980, The structure of thought. In: PW Jusczyk and RM Klein (Eds.), *The Nature of Thought*, Hillsdale, NJ: Lawrence Erlbaum Associates, pp. 19–35.

Jackson JD, 1975. *Classical Electrodynamics*, 2nd Edition, New York: Wiley.

Katznelson RD, 1981, Normal modes of the brain: neuroanatomic basis and a physiologic theoretical model. In: PL Nunez (Au.), *Electric Fields of the Brain: The Neurophysics of EEG*, 1st Edition, New York: Oxford University Press, pp. 401–442.

Law SK, Nunez PL, and Wijesinghe RS, 1993, High-resolution EEG using spline-generated surface Laplacians on spherical and ellipsoidal surfaces. *IEEE Transactions on Biomedical Engineering* 40: 145–152.

Nunez PL, 1974, The brain wave equation: a model for the EEG. *Mathematical Biosciences* 21: 279–297.

Nunez PL, 1981a, *Electric Fields of the Brain: The Neurophysics of EEG*, 1st Edition, New York: Oxford University Press.

Nunez PL, 1981b, A study of the origins of time dependencies of scalp EEG: I. Theoretical basis. *IEEE Transactions on Biomedical Engineering* 28: 271–280.

Nunez PL, 1981c, A study of the origins of time dependencies of scalp EEG: II. Experimental support of theory. *IEEE Transactions on Biomedical Engineering* 28: 271–280.

Nunez PL, 1995, *Neocortical Dynamics and Human EEG Rhythms*, New York: Oxford University Press.

Plonsey R, 1969, *Bioelectric Phenomena*, New York: McGraw-Hill.

Polk C and Postow E, 1986, *CRC Handbook of Biological Effects of Electromagnetic Fields*, Boca Raton, FL: CRC Press.

Smythe WR, 1950, *Static and Dynamic Electricity*, New York: McGraw-Hill.

Wigner E, 1960, The unreasonable effectiveness of mathematics in the natural sciences. In: *Communications in Pure and Applied Mathematics*, Vol. 13, New York: Wiley.

4

Electric Fields and Currents in Biological Tissue

1 Basic Equations for Macroscopic Fields in Conductive Media

Electric fields and currents at the macroscopic scale in neural tissue obey a simplified version of Maxwell's macroscopic equations (table 3-2) together with the purely experimental (*constitutive*) relations that depend on tissue properties. The formulation of well-posed problems in electrophysiology, in which the number of equations equals the number of dependent variables (unknowns) requires this combination of fundamental and experimental relations. These *basic field equations of linear electrophysiology* are introduced in chapter 3 in the much broader context of general electromagnetic theory and are summarized here as follows:

$$\text{Conservation of charge: } \nabla \cdot \mathbf{J} + \frac{\partial \rho}{\partial t} = 0 \qquad (3.27)$$

$$\text{Gauss' law: } \nabla \cdot \mathbf{D} = \rho \qquad (3.21)$$

$$\text{Ohm's constitutive law for linear conductors: } \mathbf{J} = \sigma \mathbf{E} \qquad (3.15)$$

$$\text{Constitutive law for linear dielectrics: } \mathbf{D} = \varepsilon \mathbf{E} \qquad (3.10)$$

$$\text{Defines scalar potential for low-frequency}$$
$$\text{(quasi-static) fields: } \mathbf{E} = -\nabla \Phi \qquad (3.4)$$

For convenience, these symbols are redefined here with their mks (meter, kilogram, second) units in parentheses.

- $\mathbf{E}(\mathbf{r}, t)$ The *net macroscopic electric field* (volts/meter or V/m) at location $\mathbf{r}$ and time t in a tissue mass. By "net" we mean that $\mathbf{E}$ is proportional to the field due to free (*conduction*) charges $\mathbf{D}$, less the field due to dielectric (*polarization*) charges $\mathbf{P}_C$. In tissue $\mathbf{P}_C$ is due mainly to membrane charge, which is much larger than the molecular and atomic charge effects common to physical materials.
- $\mathbf{D}(\mathbf{r}, t)$ The *macroscopic electric displacement vector* (couloumbs/meter^2 or C/m^2) in a tissue mass, proportional to the electric field due only to free (conduction) charges.
- $\Phi(\mathbf{r}, t)$ The *scalar potential* (volts or V).
- $\mathbf{J}(\mathbf{r}, t)$ The *free macroscopic current density* (amperes/meter^2 or A/m^2 or μA/mm^2) in a tissue mass. The word "free" distinguishes this conduction current from polarization currents that occur at atomic, molecular, and cellular scales.
- $\rho(\mathbf{r}, t)$ The *free (conduction) charge density* (coulombs/meter^2 or C/m^2).
- $\sigma(\mathbf{r})$ The *macroscopic electrical conductivity* ($1/(\Omega\,m)$ or Siemens/meter or S/m) of a mass of tissue. In an inhomogeneous medium, σ varies with location $\mathbf{r}$, for example, across boundaries separating different tissues. In tissue, σ varies weakly with field frequency, but is normally considered constant within the EEG band.
- $\eta(\mathbf{r})$ *Resistivity* (ohm meter or $\Omega\,m$) equals inverse conductivity $1/\sigma(\mathbf{r})$.
- $\varepsilon(\mathbf{r})$ The *permittivity* (second/(meter ohm) or S s/m) of a tissue mass that measures the ability of tissue to store charge. Tissue permittivity is a sensitive function of field frequency, typically becoming very large at the low frequencies of EEG as a result of membrane charge accumulation. The permittivity of empty space in mks units is $\varepsilon_0 = 8.84 \times 10^{-12}$.
- $\kappa(\mathbf{r})$ The *relative dielectric constant* of a tissue mass equal to $\varepsilon/\varepsilon_0$ (unitless).
- ∇ The vector *gradient operator* (1/m) involving first spatial derivatives in three spatial coordinates. A mathematical operator is just a rule to be applied to the expression to its immediate right, as in the definition of potential in terms of electric field given by (3.4). Appendix A contains more discussion of mathematical operators.

In addition to the variables listed above, several additional variables are defined that are convenient for describing macroscopic currents and fields in tissue. These are:

- $s(\mathbf{r}, t)$ The *volume current source function* or membrane *microsources* (μA/mm^3).
- $\mathbf{P}(\mathbf{r}, t)$ The *mesosource function* of a tissue mass (μA/mm^2). This terminology or simply *mesosources* is shorthand for *current dipole moment per unit volume at mesoscopic scales*, for example in cortical

columns or other tissue masses with linear dimensions in the approximate range 0.1 to 1.0 mm.

- $\Psi_e(\mathbf{r}, t)$ or $\Psi_i(\mathbf{r}, t)$ The *synaptic action fields*, that is, the numbers of active excitatory or inhibitory synapses per unit volume of tissue $(1/\mathrm{mm}^3)$ at mesoscopic scales. Or, numbers of active synapses per unit area of cortical surface $(1/\mathrm{mm}^2)$.

2 Comments on the Basic Equations in the Context of Macroscopic Electrophysiology

A *microelectrode* with tip diameter $\sim 10^{-4}$ cm records potentials at a small electrophysiological scale. The tissue volume displaced by the micro-electrode tip is then on the order of 10^{-12} cm^3, containing roughly 10^{12} molecules. The macroscopic fields of Maxwell's equations (and the quasi-static versions above) are accurate as space averages over material volumes containing many molecules. Thus, even the so-called microelectrode recordings of electrophysiology qualify as "macroscopic" from the view-point of Maxwell's equations. For historical reasons, we must live with this inconsistent terminology that developed mostly independently in the physical and biological sciences.

The *basic field equations of linear electrophysiology* listed above consist of three vector plus two scalar equations, or a total of 11 scalar equations. Experimental electrophysiology spans about five orders of magnitude of spatial scale, ranging from microelectrode ($\sim 10^{-4}$ cm) to scalp recordings (~ 10 cm). The 10 cm scale is cited as the upper limit because scalp electrodes actually record neural activity space averaged over cortical surface regions much larger than scalp electrode diameter due to field spreading between electrode and sources. How do we apply our basic field equations at these disparate spatial scales? The answer depends on experimental circumstances. Charge conservation (3.27) and Gauss' law (3.12) are fundamental laws: they apply to all scales and experiments. The scalar potential equation (3.4) is valid whenever magnetic induction is negligible, essentially in all electrophysiological applications as discussed in chapter 3 and appendix B. By contrast, the (linear) experimental conductive (3.15) and dielectric (3.10) relations may or may not be valid. Even when these relations are valid, their interpretations must be con-sidered carefully.

The conductivity σ and dielectric constant κ must always refer to space averages over tissue volumes of a certain size. These parameters have different meanings that depend on measurement scale. For example, the neuron is a large structure compared to the microelectrode tip. Field measurements can be expected to fluctuate greatly when small electrodes are moved over distances of the order of cell body diameters, as pictured in fig. 4-1. Theory at this small scale is concerned with the parameters (σ, κ) defined separately for intercellular and extracellular fluid and membrane.

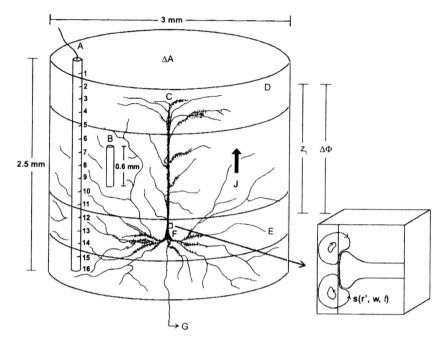

Figure 4-1 The macrocolumn scale in neocortex is defined by the spatial extent of axon branches E that remain within the cortex (*recurrent collaterals*). The large pyramidal cell (C) is one of 10^5 to 10^6 neurons in the macrocolumn. Nearly all pyramidal cells send an axon (G) into the white matter, most re-enter the cortex at some distant location (*corticocortical fibers*). Each large pyramidal cell has 10^4 to 10^5 synaptic inputs (F) causing microcurrent sources and sinks $s(\mathbf{r}', \mathbf{w}, t)$. Field measurements can be expected to fluctuate greatly when small electrode contacts (A) are moved over distances of the order of cell body diameters. Small-scale recordings measure space-averaged potential over some volume (B) depending mostly on the size of the electrode contact. An instantaneous imbalance in sources or sinks in regions D and E will cause a diffuse current density **J** and potential difference $\Delta\Phi$ across the cortex. Reproduced with permission from Nunez (1995).

The fluid and membrane electrical properties, which are lumped into just these two parameters, owe their origins to complicated processes at the much smaller molecular scales.

Macroelectrode recordings present quite a different picture. For example, the scalp electrode measures fields due to neural activity in tissue masses containing perhaps 10^8 to 10^9 neurons. In this case, conductivity and dielectric constant must refer to average properties in a similar size volume of tissue. The dielectric constant of a tissue mass depends much more on membrane charge separation than on the microscopic effects at atomic and molecular scales. The conductivity (or resistivity) of tissue can be expected to depend strongly on the packing density of the cells because membranes provide relatively high-resistance current pathways.

The membrane *microsources* currents $s(\mathbf{r}, t)$ and synaptic action fields $\Psi_e(\mathbf{r}, t)$, $\Psi_i(\mathbf{r}, t)$ are distinct but closely related physiological variables. Separate variables are defined here to describe similar physiological processes for several reasons. First, our membrane current *microsource function* $s(\mathbf{r}, t)$ must include both active sources at the synapses and passive (return) current from more distant locations on the cell, whereas the synaptic action fields $\Psi_e(\mathbf{r}, t)$, $\Psi_i(\mathbf{r}, t)$ simply indicate the number densities of active synapses in mesoscopic (millimeter scale) tissue volumes. Thus, microcurrent source distributions depend on capacitive-resistive membrane properties of cells within the volume in addition to synaptic action density. Second, nonsynaptic current sources like action potentials may in some instances contribute to recorded potentials, and we want our theoretical formalism to be expressed in the general terms of current sources, irrespective of their physiological origins.

3 Resistive Tissue Properties

The validity of Ohm's law (3.15) in tissue depends on measurement scale. At the membrane scale, membrane state is critical. That is, Ohm's law is strongly and (naturally) selectively violated inside active membranes, making action potential propagation possible. However, we are mostly concerned here with much larger spatial scales, for which the appropriate tissue mass contains many cells. Most of the current in a macroscopic cell suspension (consisting of a mixture of cells and fluid) is expected to bypass the cells. Partly for this reason, the medium is expected to be linear in the conductive sense, at least for the relatively weak electric fields of EEG. Discussions in this book refer both to *conductivity* and its inverse, *resistivity*. We need both terms because conductivity is more commonly used in equations, whereas resistivity is the more common experimental measure.

Over a century ago, Maxwell (1891) calculated the theoretical resistivity of a homogeneous suspension of uniform spheres of certain resistivity, as indicated in fig. 4-2. Rayleigh (1892) obtained a similar expression for a suspension of cylinders for the case of current direction normal to cylinder axes. For the special case where the spheres or cylinders are

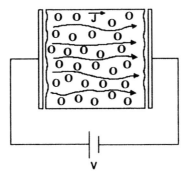

Figure 4-2   Current passing through a fluid containing nonconducting bodies in suspension. The macroscopic mass of material (or tissue) has a resistivity that is higher than the resistivity of the conducting fluid and depends on the density of the added material.

nonconductive, the Maxwell–Rayleigh formula for the ratio of suspension resistivity η to fluid resistivity η_s is

$$\frac{\eta}{\eta_s} = \frac{1 + h\alpha}{1 - \alpha} \tag{4.1}$$

Here α is the fraction of volume occupied by the insulating bodies. The parameter h is determined by their geometrical shape: h is ½ for spheres and 1 for cylinders. It has been estimated that neurons comprise perhaps 40 to 50% of cortical volume and glial cells about 35 to 56%. The extracellular space has been estimated to occupy between 2 and 20% of cortex (Van Harreveld 1966). Although the original derivation of (4.1) was based on the assumption that the fractional volume occupied by the insulating bodies was small ($\alpha \ll 1$), later experiments and theory indicate that (4.1) is valid for high concentrations, that is, $\alpha \to 1$ (Cole 1935; Cole et al. 1969). As $\alpha \to 1$, the resistivity of the cell suspension predicted by (4.1) approaches infinity since the cells are assumed in this context to be perfect insulators. In this limit, the cell suspension theoretically becomes a perfectly insulating wall blocking all current. Of course, genuine cells will pass some current, but tissue cell resistivity is at least several orders of magnitude higher than that of extracellular fluid. This theory and a number of experiments establish the conductive linearity of tissue masses containing large numbers of cells, at least for the small electric fields of EEG.

If a tissue mass is linear in both the conductive and dielectric senses, its electrical properties can be fully described by just two parameters: either the resistivity $\eta(\mathbf{r}, f)$ or conductivity $\sigma(\mathbf{r}, f)$ and the relative dielectric constant $\kappa(\mathbf{r}, f)$. The functional dependencies of these parameters on tissue location $\mathbf{r}$ and field frequency f are indicated explicitly. In EEG applications, a fixed conductivity is normally assigned to each kind of tissue so that conductivity changes occur only at the borders between distinct tissues, especially neocortex, cerebrospinal fluid (CSF), skull, and brain. The linear constitutive relations (3.10) and (3.15) provide for an enormous simplification of the most general case where fields and currents are due to the repositioning of massive numbers of charges at atomic, molecular, and cellular scales.

The brain is *inhomogeneous*; that is, conductivity $\sigma(\mathbf{r}, f)$ and dielectric constant $\kappa(\mathbf{r}, f)$ vary with location. In addition, fibrous tissue like white matter is expected to be *anisotropic* in the conductive sense. That is, conductivity is generally expected depend on whether current passes parallel to or across nerve fibers. However, in macroscopic tissue volumes, this issue may be complicated by lack of consistent fiber directions within tissue masses so that measurements of tissue anisotropy appear to be sensitive to spatial scale and tissue location. In EEG applications, skull properties are of major importance, apparently more

Table 4-1 Typical resistivity of several materials and tissues

Material	Resistivity (Ω cm)
Copper	2×10^{-6}
Seawater	20
CSF	64
Blood	150
Spinal cord (longitudinal)	180
Cortex (5 kHz)	230
Cortex (5 Hz)	350
White matter (average)	650
Spinal cord (transverse)	1200
Bone (100 Hz)	8,000–16,000
Pure water	2×10^7
Active membrane (squid axon)	2×10^7
Passive membrane (squid axon)	10^9

important than any other tissue in determining volume conduction between cortical sources and scalp.

Resistivities for a variety of biological materials are listed in table 4-1. For comparative purposes, a few physical materials are also included. For the most part, the approximate values listed have been confirmed by several investigators. The experimental methods used to measure resistivity can be found elsewhere (Schwan and Kay 1957; Ranck 1963a, b; Ranck and BeMent 1965; Geddes and Baker 1967; Plonsey 1969). In some instances, resistivity was measured *in vitro*, but the neurological data are mostly from *in vivo* studies. A few generalizations about the resistivity of biological materials are possible (Geddes and Baker 1967; Kosterich et al. 1983, 1984; Polk and Postow 1986). The resistivities of all body fluids are relatively small because they are rich in dissolved salts. Materials with the lowest resistivities are the cell-free fluids—urine, amniotic fluid, bile, CSF, and blood plasma. The addition of cells in normal concentrations to blood plasma may increase experimental resistivity by factors of two or three, consistent with the theoretical relation (4.1). Brain tissue resistivity is variable. Average white matter resistivity is higher than gray matter resistivity, and white matter resistivity is apparently anisotropic.

4 Skull Resistivity

The resistivity of skull tissue strongly influences EEG volume conduction. Because the skull resistivity question is complicated and remains unsettled, we have included this separate section to outline the issues involved. Human skull consists of a sandwich of three layers: two compact layers, the inner and outer tables (*cortical bone*), plus a spongy middle layer (*diploe* or *cancellous bone*) with more fluid spaces as indicated in fig. 4-3. Most of the skull's current-passing ability is due to fluid permeating the

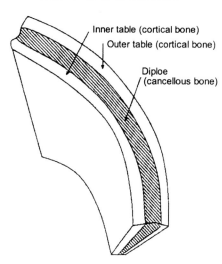

Figure 4-3 Human skull consists of three layers, the compact inner and outer tables (*cortical bone*) and a midde layer with more spaces for fluid (*diploe* or *cancellous bone*).

bone, and the inner layer contains more spaces for fluid. Thus, we expect skull taken as a whole to be both inhomogeneous and anisotropic. At the same time, the tissue within each individual skull layer may be closer to homogeneous and isotropic at large scales. If tissue is linear but anisotropic in the conductive sense, Ohm's law (3.15) remains valid, but conductivity is a *tensor* (or matrix), with at least three conductivity components (the diagonal elements of the matrix) required to indicate separate tissue properties in three perpendicular directions.

A number of scientists have proposed corrections to inverse solutions or high-resolution EEG estimates by using CT or MRI to find local variations in skull thickness. In a single-layered skull (homogeneous in directions normal to its local surface), the local resistance of a skull plug of constant resistivity η, thickness d, and cross-sectional area A is given by

$$R = \frac{\eta d}{A} \tag{1.6}$$

Since local skull current is largely determined by this resistance, the product of local resistivity with local thickness acts as a single parameter to a first approximation (Nunez 1987). Thus, if skull resistivity variations over the surface were small compared to thickness variations, corrections to volume conductor models based on more accurate skull boundaries would be expected to improve head models. Several tests of this idea were obtained by measuring resistance of hydrated skull plugs of different thicknesses drilled from multiple surface locations (Poulnot et al. 1989; Law 1993). It was found that the resistance of skull plugs was uncorrelated or perhaps even negatively correlated with skull thickness; that is, (1.6) does not apply to skulls (at least dead skulls). The apparent reason for this discrepancy is that thicker skull regions occur mainly as a result of increased thickness of the middle layer of cancellous bone, which may be largely absent in thin skull sections (Law 1993). The resistance of a three-layered skull plug is given by

$$R = \frac{\eta_1 d_1 + \eta_2 d_2 + \eta_3 d_3}{A} \tag{4.2}$$

Resistivity measurements on live human skull flaps indicate that resistivities of the inner and outer compact layers (η_1 and η_3) generally differ from each other and are perhaps three to six times larger than the resistivity of the middle layer η_2 (Akhtari et al. 2002). Given these data, it is plausible that an experimental scatter plot of R versus total skull thickness ($d_1 + d_2 + d_3$) could have a zero or even negative slope as observed experimentally. For this reason, *attempts to correct volume conduction models of the head using only total skull thickness information may actually reduce model accuracy.* While corrections based on individual thickness variations of the three layers appear to be more promising, the important issue of resistivity variations within each layer over the surface remains.

The ratios of skull resistivity to other tissue resistivities determine current flow patterns in the head and, as a result, scalp potential distribution. Over the past three decades many theoretical papers have adopted an assumed skull-to-brain resistivity ratio of 80 based on the classic study of Rush and Driscoll (1968, 1969). This 80 ratio was suggested as an overall average fit between recorded data and predictions made using a 3-sphere head model with (assumed constant) skull and scalp thicknesses of 6 mm each. The resistivity ratio estimate was based partly on experiments in a dead, hydrated skull (Rush and Driscoll 1968) and partly on estimates obtained in four living subjects using frontal scalp current injection (Driscoll 1970). Estimates of *in vivo* skull resistivity ratio ranged from 33 to 93 with an average of 58.

These large skull resistivity ratio estimates have been challenged in studies of a fresh cadaver skull and two living subjects (Oostendorp et al. 2000). The *in vivo* studies used scalp current injection and three-layered head models constructed from MRI images. Skull thickness varied over the surface with an average value of 7 mm. The average skull to brain resistivity ratio was estimated to be about 16. Interpretations of these (apparently conflicting) estimates of skull resistivity ratio or direct skull resistivity measurements should take into account the following arguments.

In the usual 3 and 4-sphere head models, the *skull-to-brain resistivity ratio* is based on the assumption that all other tissues close to the surface have equal, isotropic resistivities. This is only a rough approximation. Thus, when evaluating skull resistivity measurements, *there may be substantial differences between the resistivity of skull plugs measured in vivo and the effective resistivity that is most appropriate for the particular volume*

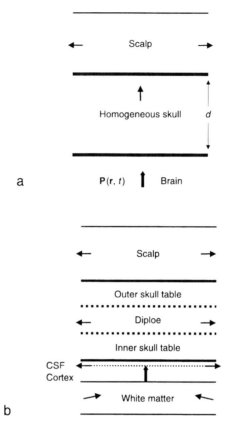

Figure 4-4 (a) A common volume conductor model of the head is the *three-sphere model*. It consists of an inner sphere (brain) and surrounded by two concentric spherical shells (skull and scalp). More complicated models may not be more accurate if tissue boundaries and (especially) tissue resistivities are not known with sufficient accuracy. (b) A more realistic geometric model consists of two additional skull layers and a layer of cerebral spinal fluid (CSF). Current shunting through the middle skull layer (diploe), CSF, and scalp is indicated by arrows. The effective skull resistivity in the *three-sphere model* (a) is larger than the actual skull resistivity in (b).

conductor model of the head. Figure 4-4 illustrates some of the issues. Imagine two skull plugs of equal resistance, one homogeneous and one three layered as indicated in fig. 4-3. The arrows depict shunting of current through the relatively low resistance pathways of the CSF and inner skull layers. Other factors to consider are possible tangential current shunting by blood vessels in the skull and by anisotropic white matter. Such current shunting may cause additional spread of the scalp potential due to a local cortical mesosource $\mathbf{P}(\mathbf{r}, t)$. Thus, the effective resistivity ratio appropriate for a 3-sphere model of the head may be substantially larger than the actual resistivity ratio. Also, the "best" resistivity ratio used with a 3-sphere model may differ substantially from the "best" ratio used with a 4-sphere model (including a CSF layer) or a model with varying skull thickness. In chapter 6, we show that a 4-sphere model with an actual brain-to-skull conductivity ratio of 30 spreads currents due to intra-cranial sources in a manner nearly identical to a 3-sphere model with a brain-to-skull conductivity ratio of roughly 40 to 60, where this ratio depends on thickness and conductivity of the CSF layer. Since the thickness of the CSF layer tends to be larger in old age, the effective skull-to-brain resistivity ratio appropriate for n-sphere models may also increase with age.

Many other volume conduction parameters can influence the effective brain-to-skull conductivity ratio for idealized head models. For example, one experimental study using scalp current injection in six living adult subjects found wide range of brain-to-skull conductivity ratios with an average ratio of 72 when a spherical model was adopted as the head model (Goncalves et al. 2003a,b). But with realistic geometry, the effective ratios were in the 20–50 range. In a study of five children (ages 8–12) using a 3-sphere model, Lai et al. (2004) found effective conductivity ratios in the 18 to 34 range.

Not surprisingly, several experiments have reported large resistivity differences between hydrated dead and living skulls as well as variations between and within subjects (Oostendorp et al. 2000; Akhtari et al. 2002; Hoekema et al. 2003). For all the reasons outlined above, estimates of skull resistivity obtained by scalp current injection in living subjects are not generally expected to match direct measurements of dead (or perhaps even living) skull plug resistance. Skull resistivity measurements are summarized in table 4-2. Taking into account all these data, our best guess for the effective brain-to-skull conductivity ratio recommended for use with the 3-sphere model is in the range 20–80, with substantial variation between individual subjects expected.

Relatively accurate cortical dipole localization can be obtained from EEG using inaccurate head models if the dipoles are widely separated. Deep dipole localization accuracy appears to be limited to something like 1 or 2 cm by the uncertainty of tissue resistivities, even if perfect knowledge of tissue boundaries is available. However, such limitations on localization do not invalidate high-resolution estimates of regional

Table 4-2 Skull resistivity reported in the literature

Skull condition	Resistivity (Ω cm)	Frequency (Hz)	Reference
Dead, dry	10^{13}		Rush and Driscoll 1969
Dead, hydrated	10,000–20,000	500	Rush and Driscoll 1969
Dead, hydrated	13,000–21,000	100	Law 1993
Dead, suitures	3,500–10,000	100	Law 1993
Dead, hydrated	13,000–86,000	20	Akhatari et al. 2000
Live, 3 layers	4,600–21,000	20	Akhatari et al. 2000
Live	7,700	10–1000	Oostendorp et al. 2000
Dead, hydrated	6,700	$10–10^5$	Oostendorp et al. 2000
Live	1,200–3,100	10	Hoekema et al. 2003

Modified from Hoekema et al. (2003).

dura potential patterns and associated measures. For example, high-resolution estimates of coherence between electrode pairs separated by more than several centimeters may reveal robust changes with changes in brain state. These data can provide important insight into relationships between large-scale brain dynamic behavior and brain function, even when accurate estimates of source locations are not obtained. We return to this issue in chapters 8–11.

5 Capacitive Effects in Tissue

A macroscopic tissue mass with relatively high conductivity and low charge storage at the field frequency of interest is labeled *purely resistive*, indicating that capacitive effects are negligible for the analysis at hand. However, different experimental or theoretical studies of the same tissue might require inclusion of capacitive (dielectric) effects. Small-scale analysis might require such inclusion, for example. Capacitive effects, that is, charge storage effects, are described by the second term on the left-hand side of the conservation of charge equation (3.27). In appendix B, it is shown that *a macroscopic mass of tissue subjected to an oscillating electric field of frequency f behaves similarly to a resistor in parallel with a capacitor.* The frequency-dependent condition by which capacitive effects may be neglected in tissue is

$$\frac{\text{Capacitive current}}{\text{Resistive current}} = \frac{2\pi f \varepsilon(f)}{\sigma(f)} \ll 1 \qquad (4.3)$$

The ratio (4.3) may expressed in terms of relative dielectric constant for specific tissue. Using a cortical conductivity of $0.3\,\text{S/m}$ (table 4-1), the ratio (4.3) is about $2 \times 10^{-9}\kappa(10)$ at $10\,\text{Hz}$. Thus, for most EEG purposes, large-scale capacitive effects are negligible in neocortex if $\kappa(10)$ is less than about 10^8. As shown in appendix B, even if large-scale capacitive effects were to reach this level, they would apparently have minimal influence on practical EEG studies. Small-scale capacitive effects are quite a separate issue as discussed below.

Relation (4.3) also holds for nonperiodic fields if $(2\pi f)^{-1}$ is interpreted as a characteristic time for substantial change in field magnitudes. Similar to the condition for the neglect of magnetic induction, (4.3) is frequency dependent, but it is quite a different condition. The neglect of magnetic induction becomes a progressively better approximation as the field frequency is reduced. As a result, magnetic induction is negligible in tissue at frequencies below about 10^5 or 10^6 Hz, as shown in appendix B. The frequencies for which capacitive effects are small are not immediately obvious from (4.3) because the permittivity $\varepsilon(f)$, or relative dielectric constant $\kappa(f)$, increases sharply at very low frequencies.

That is, membranes are able to store substantial charge for short times if local field directions change sufficiently slowly.

The dielectric constant (or permittivity) of many materials can be expected to be a sensitive function of field frequency since charges take some time to rearrange themselves when acted on by external fields. Such short-time charge storage in tissue can occur at atomic, molecular, and cellular scales. Tissue resistivity also varies with frequency, but in the EEG frequency range, resistivity changes with frequency are much smaller than the larger variations due to differences in tissue type and scale of measurement. Thus, in EEG applications we normally assume that resistivity is independent of field frequency.

The frequency dependence of both resistivity and dielectric constant of a mass of excised muscle tissue over the approximate range 10 to 10^5 Hz is shown in fig. 4-5. This plot provides a rough guess of what we might expect in cortical tissue. In one study of rabbit cortex over the frequency range 0.5 to 50,000 Hz, a maximum capacitive-to-resistive current ratio of 0.12 was obtained in the 50 to 100 Hz range (Ranck 1963). The ratio (4.3) has been reported to lie in the approximate range 0.1 to 10 for a wide range of electromagnetic field frequencies and tissue types (Polk and Postow 1986). The detailed (macroscopic) dielectric properties of neocortex at the very low frequencies of most interest in EEG (~1 to 20 Hz) have not been widely studied, but the available evidence suggests that capacitive effects at macroscopic scales have minimal influence on EEG volume conduction. In contrast, the following discussion in section 14 suggests that dielectric (capacitive) effects at membrane scales can have an important influence on the *strength* of *mesosources* of EEG, that is, on *cortical dipole moments per unit volume* $\mathbf{P}(\mathbf{r}, t)$ produced by the (smaller scale) synaptic current sources.

In tissue with negligible capacitive effects, the question of dielectric linearity is of no practical importance. If future applications occur where capacitive effects are important, we are likely to assume dielectric linearity in order to obtain solutions to volume conduction problems. The linearity assumption appears to have solid experimental support.

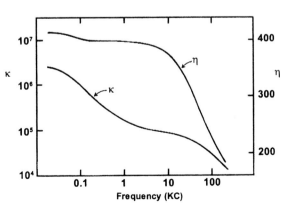

Figure 4-5 The frequency dependence of both resistivity η and dielectric constant κ of a mass of excised muscle tissue over the approximate range 10 to 10^5 Hz. Reproduced with permission from Schwan and Kay (1957).

Even the active membrane, which is a highly nonlinear conductor seems to exhibit linear dielectric properties to good approximation (Cole 1968). The Hodgkin–Huxley equations describing action potential propagation make this assumption, for example. When tissue is linear in both dielectric and conductive senses and the field oscillates with frequency f, capacitive effects are easily included in theory by introducing the *complex conductivity*:

$$\sigma_c = \sigma(f)\left[1 + j\frac{2\pi f \varepsilon(f)}{\sigma(f)}\right] \tag{4.4}$$

Complex conductivity is the volume conductor analog of *impedance* in a normal linear electric circuit containing resistors and capacitors. The real and imaginary parts of the complex conductivity correspond to conductive and dielectric properties, respectively. The main consequence of the imaginary (capacitive) part is to cause phase shifts between brain source waveforms and the corresponding potentials. The phase difference (or *phase angle*) between applied current and measured potential is simply a measure of the ratio of capacitive to resistive current. This phase angle may be measured by implanting dipole current sources in tissue and varying the source frequency. To the best of our knowledge, no human studies (for example, in epilepsy patients) have yielded measurable phase shifts between implanted sources and scalp potential at EEG frequencies.

Such putative capacitive phase shift due only to volume conduction is a phenomenon quite distinct from the ubiquitous phase differences observed between potentials at various scalp locations. The latter are due to phase differences between the many underlying current sources. *Current source phase differences between brain regions can be modeled only with dynamic brain theory*, quite separate from volume conduction and possible macroscopic capacitive effects. The dynamic problem is somewhat analogous to one involving dependent current sources in an electric circuit as discussed in chapters 2 and 3. That is, the interaction controlling the source current, which could involve a complicated nonlinear circuit, is hidden in the linear circuit diagram.

6 Boundary Conditions for Inhomogeneous Media

Different regions of the brain have different conductivities; thus, problems of practical interest involve tissue boundaries. At macroscopic scales, the most obvious boundaries involve the poorly conducting skull and air space surrounding the head. At cellular scales, membrane–fluid interfaces provide critical boundaries between tissues with different electrical properties. Generally, we are interested in volume conduction problems in layered tissue separated into distinct regions, with constant conductivity within each region. The electric potential $\Phi(\mathbf{r}, t)$ will normally have a different solution $\Phi_i(\mathbf{r}, t)$ in each of the regions i having constant conductivity σ_i. When no sources occur in the head regions i or j the *basic field equations of linear electrophysiology* reduce to a simple form in each region:

$$\nabla^2 \Phi_i = 0 \tag{4.5}$$

$$\nabla^2 \left(\sigma_j \Phi_j + \varepsilon_j \frac{\partial \Phi_j}{\partial t} \right) = 0 \tag{4.6}$$

The subscript i indicates source-free brain regions in which capacitive effects are negligible or the fields are sinusoidal and the tissue behaves as a linear capacitor. In this case, (4.5) is the governing principle; that is, potentials are solutions of Laplace's equation. Thus, (4.5) essentially applies to all of large-scale electrophysiology and (4.6) is not needed in such applications. The subscript j refers to regions in which linear capacitive effects occur, but the fields are nonsinusoidal. In electrophysiology (4.6) is applied to membranes and fields generated at small scales. Equation (4.6) depends on the validity of Ohm's law. Thus, it is not strictly valid inside membranes where the electric field and diffusion currents due to concentration gradients, indicated by the Nernst–Planck equation (3.16), as well as active ion transport (the Na–K pump and so forth) govern membrane behavior (Plonsey 1969; Malmivuo and Plonsey 1995). Nevertheless, the basic cable equation describing spread of transmembrane potential due to an applied synaptic (or electrode) stimulus across a subthreshold membrane is derived from (4.5) and (4.6) in section 8 and appendix D by treating the membrane as a simple passive j region. This is a crude (but useful) approximation based on lumping all membrane properties into two parameters—an effective composite conductivity (or resistance) for all ions that cross the membrane and an effective dielectric constant (or capacitance).

There will always be one equation for the one unknown potential [$\Phi_i(t)$ or $\Phi_j(t)$] for each region. Each of these equations has an infinite number of solutions, but 19th century mathematicians have established the required mathematical foundation by determining the necessary and sufficient conditions required to obtain unique solutions. The proper choice of these field constraints (the *boundary conditions*) is based on physical not mathematical considerations. Equations (4.5) and (4.6) are to be solved subject to the following boundary conditions at the interface between any two regions labeled m and n:

$$\sigma_m \frac{\partial \Phi_m}{\partial u} = \sigma_n \frac{\partial \Phi_n}{\partial u} \tag{4.7}$$

$$\frac{\partial \Phi_m}{\partial w} = \frac{\partial \Phi_n}{\partial w} \tag{4.8}$$

The boundary conditions are expressed in terms of coordinate u, defined as everywhere normal to the local interface between regions, and two tangential coordinates, say w_1 and w_2. Condition (4.7) expresses the physical requirement that the normal component of current density must be continuous across any interface. This follows directly from the conservation of charge (3.27); it is similar to Kirchhoff's current law in electric circuits. The only exception to (4.7) occurs when sources are located on the boundary; an example is shown in appendix H. Condition (4.8) states that the tangential component of electric field must be continuous across the interface. This follows from Maxwell's equation (3.22). In the case of our n-sphere head models, (4.8) is identical to continuity of potential across interfaces. These two *boundary conditions* are fundamental to all electric field theory, linear or not.

Consider the implications of boundary conditions (4.7) and (4.8) for scalp potential problems. Let region m be the scalp and region n the surrounding air space. Since air conductivity is near zero, (4.7) just indicates that no current flows outside the scalp surface, that is

$$\frac{\partial \Phi_m}{\partial u} = 0 \qquad (4.9)$$

As in the case of the brain's magnetic field, the potential and electric field due to brain sources extend into the surrounding air space (as implied by our book cover design), but the current is confined inside. When applying volume conductor theory, we are generally not allowed to specify potential at the outer surface in advance (called a *Dirichlet boundary condition*). Rather, we must specify zero normal derivative at the outer surface (*Neumann boundary condition*). Laplace's equation is known to have a unique solution in any volume of material if either the potential or normal derivative of potential is specified over the entire surface. Or, a unique solution exists if potential is specified over part of the surface and normal derivative is given over the remaining part, that is, *mixed boundary conditions* (Morse and Feshbach 1951). However, we cannot specify both potential and normal derivative for the same surface region and obtain a forward solution.

An interesting variation on these boundary conditions occurs in the application of *dura imaging* to EEG. EEG is recorded at (say) 64 to 131 scalp locations to obtain estimates (at each time step) of the distribution of potential on the scalp. The normal derivative of scalp potential at its outer surface is known to be zero so this procedure involves over-specification of the normal boundary value problem associated with Laplace's equation. Suppose both the potential and normal derivative were known over the entire outer surface (as in the idealized case of a detached head). With this idealization, the potential on any inner surface (say, the dura) can be uniquely calculated, provided no current sources are active between the two surfaces. That is, the tissue volume to which Laplace's equation applies is bounded by outer (scalp–air) and inner (dura–CSF) surfaces. If we over-specify the outer boundary conditions, the inner boundary condition (dura potential) may be calculated uniquely. While the idealization of complete outer surface sampling is not fully accurate in real applications, it is sufficiently close to provide a practical means of estimating dura potential from scalp potential measurements. This approach of dura imaging to *high-resolution EEG* is discussed in chapter 8.

7 Brain Current Sources

The so-called *forward problem* in EEG involves calculation of scalp potentials from known current sources, where the current across some boundary is specified (the *current source*). In EEG applications, this boundary might be an outer cell membrane for mesoscopic treatments or a large group of cells in the case of macroscopic studies. The combination of head model, current source distribution, and outer surface boundary condition (zero normal current) then uniquely determines the potential at every point in the head. In this section, we are concerned only with the physiological bases for these brain current sources.

Equations (4.5) and (4.6) are fully accurate representations for passive linear media (excluding active membrane processes), but require modification to be fully useful in electrophysiology. The unmodified versions require knowledge of potential or normal derivative of potential on bounding surfaces, but bounding surfaces in tissue are complicated membrane surfaces at cellular scales. We cannot easily specify the required boundary conditions in such complicated geometry. However, since the normal derivative of potential is proportional to current density in a conductor, we have the option of replacing boundary conditions on parts of the bounding surfaces by *current sources*. This procedure is similar to a well-known procedure in electric circuits. A voltage source in series with a resistor may be replaced by its equivalent: a current source in parallel with the same resistor as shown in fig. 1-11.

Consider first the membrane current due to a synaptic action as shown in fig. 4-6. An action potential in the presynaptic axon activates a neurotransmitter in the synaptic knob. This chemical diffuses across the synaptic cleft into the subsynaptic membrane. When the cell is in electrochemical equilibrium, the inner membrane surface potential is about $-65\,\mathrm{mV}$ with respect to the outer surface. If the synapse is *excitatory*, the net transmitter effect is to increase the membrane permeability to positive ions that move through the local membrane surface. The resulting transmembrane potential change is called the *excitatory postsynaptic potential* or *EPSP*. The EPSP reduces the magnitude of the potential difference, thereby bringing the postsynaptic neuron a little closer to the threshold for firing its own action potential, perhaps $-40\,\mathrm{mV}$ or so. The subsynaptic membrane acts as a *current sink* (or negative source) as

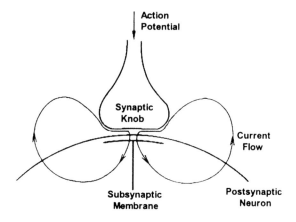

Figure 4-6 Membrane current due to local excitatory synaptic action. An action potential propagating along the presynaptic axon activates a neurotransmitter in the synaptic knob that changes local membrane conductivities to select ions, thereby producing a local current sink and more distant distributed sources to preserve current conservation.

shown in fig. 4-6 since positive ions move inward. This current flows in the intracellular fluid and exits the membrane at more distant (distributed) locations to form closed current loops. The total inward membrane current in must equal the total outward current as a result of current conservation (3.27). If the synapse is inhibitory, the trans-membrane potential change is called the *inhibitory postsynaptic potential* or *IPSP*. It acts in the opposite manner to the EPSP (with generally different magnitude) and lessens the likelihood of an action potential in the postsynaptic neuron. The IPSP then provides a local *current source* that must be matched by distributed sinks along the more distant cell surface.

The extracellular potential due to a synaptic event is determined by the full distribution of membrane sources and sinks $s(\mathbf{r}, t)$, not just the local current near the active synaptic knob. The manner in which source–sinks are distributed depends on the conductivities of intracellular and extracellular fluids and on both the conductivity and capacitive proper-ties of the membrane. Owing to the complicated three-dimensional geometry of neurons, the details of the source–sink distribution and resulting extracellular potential can be difficult to calculate. This may pose substantial problems in relating theory to experiment for electro-physiologists engaged in animal recordings with small electrodes. However, in EEG applications, we are able to bypass much of this com-plexity by traversing the spatial scales of current generation and defining an effective current dipole moment for each tissue volume. The *current dipole moment per unit volume* $\mathbf{P}(\mathbf{r}, t)$ *in cortical tissue may be considered as a cortical mesosource field that generates the macroscopic electric and magnetic fields observed on the scalp.*

To see (qualitatively) how this crossing of spatial scales occurs, consider the large cortical pyramidal cell shown in fig. 4-1. The dendritic tree provides a large surface area for perhaps 10^4 to as many as 10^5 synaptic inputs. Furthermore, there are roughly 10^5 neurons under each square millimeter of cortical surface. At any instant in time, a large number of synapses on local neurons may be active so as to produce a net current source distribution, due to both active synapses and passive (return) current. The extracellular potential measured by a small electrode within this (say) $1\,\mathrm{mm}^2$ cortical column will be very complicated, with large changes in recorded potential typically resulting from small electrode movements. At distances large compared to the characteristic size of the column, the potential due to sources and sinks confined to the column can be represented by the *dipole term* of a *multipole expansion*, as discussed in chapter 3. If many such columns are active, scalp potential will be due to the weighted sum of dipole contributions from each column. We may then describe overlapping mesoscopic source regions in terms of a continuous function $\mathbf{P}(\mathbf{r}, t)$, the *mesoscopic neocortical source strength* or *neocortical dipole moment per unit volume*, described in sections 12–16.

A major advantage of adopting this mesoscopic descriptive scale is that the results are generally independent of the detailed nature of the multiple interaction mechanisms that may occur between closely spaced neurons (Bullock 1980; Abeles 1982; Llinas 1988; Koch and Zador 1993; Stuart and Sakmann 1994). Membrane current sources may be due to synaptic or action potentials, or to active or passive transport. It does not matter if the synapses are chemical or electrical or whether action potentials occur in cell bodies, axons, or dendrites. *Reciprocal synapses* between dendrites, *fast chemical transport*, or "short-circuits" between adjacent neurons do not alter the general formalism. *Retrograde signaling* in which postsynaptic membranes release chemicals to prevent the release of inhibitory neurotransmitters in presynaptic neurons also fails to alter our picture. Of course, all these phenomena generally influence the magnitude and direction of the resulting mesosources. However, they do not change the basic idea that *some* source distribution will always occur within a local tissue mass, and that the (net) mesosource $\mathbf{P}(\mathbf{r}, t)$ essentially behaves as a dipole at distances large compared to source–sink regions. Pyramidal cell source–sink regions evidentially have characteristic separations less than cortical thickness (a few millimeters), and the closest scalp locations are about 1 to 1.5 cm distant. Thus, the dipole approximation to sources generated in cortical columns with diameters smaller than a few millimeters (macrocolumn diameter) appears to be quite acceptable in EEG studies.

The considerations above show why this book's emphasis is quite different from publications directed to *electrophysiologists working at cellular scales*. Such scientists are properly concerned with details of the very neural interaction mechanisms that we have so glibly glossed over. *EEG scientists working at macroscopic scales* have a different set of complications to worry about. In this book, we are particularly interested in scalp potentials generated by individual dipoles or more generally by *dipole layers* (or *dipole sheets*) that follow the folded cortical surface. The resulting scalp potential distributions must depend on the nature and location of the mesosources $\mathbf{P}(\mathbf{r}, t)$ forming such dipole layers and the macroscopic inhomogeneity of the head volume conductor, that is, the boundaries and resistivities of brain, CSF, skull, and scalp tissue.

8 Explicit Use of Macroscopic Current Source Regions

Unless otherwise noted, further discussion in this book considers media to be purely resistive and linear so that conductivity is real and currents obey the following simplified version of (3.27):

$$\nabla \cdot \mathbf{J} = 0 \tag{4.10}$$

It will prove useful to introduce the idea of a macroscopic current density source $\mathbf{J}_S$ such that Ohm's law (3.15) is modified to read (Geselowitz 1967; Malmivuo and Plonsey 1995)

$$\mathbf{J} = \sigma \mathbf{E} + \mathbf{J}_S \tag{4.11}$$

That is, total current in a volume conductor is often imagined to be composed of *ohmic current* $\sigma \mathbf{E}$ plus source current crossing some boundary, the so-called *impressed current* $\mathbf{J}_S$. However, this interpretation is not quite as straightforward as sometimes implied in the literature. We may also think of $\mathbf{J}_S$ simply as a convenient means of specifying boundary conditions on complicated inner surfaces as shown in appendix K. The introduction of this pseudo-current may, at first, appear artificial and mysterious, but turns out to be quite useful.

One can substitute (4.11) into (4.10) and make use of the definition of electric potential (3.4) to obtain

$$\nabla \cdot [\sigma(\mathbf{r})\nabla \Phi] = -s(\mathbf{r}, t) \tag{4.12}$$

where the volume source current is defined by

$$s(\mathbf{r},t) \equiv -\nabla \cdot \mathbf{J}_S(\mathbf{r}, t) \tag{4.13}$$

The conductivity $\sigma(\mathbf{r})$ (S/mm or S/cm) is generally spatially dependent so it appears inside the outer operator ∇. The microsource function $s(\mathbf{r}, t)$ has dimensions of current per unit volume ($\mu A/mm^3$). It can be viewed as a *volume source* of potential generated in a macroscopic medium. The reasoning supporting this idea is as follows. Any tissue volume may be subdivided such that all current source activity takes place in certain subvolumes, as indicated by the gray regions in fig. 4-7. Since the remaining tissue volumes (white) contain no sources, the potential in

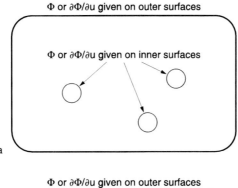

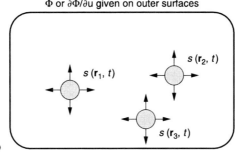

Figure 4-7 A general volume conductor is indicated by the rounded rectangle. (a) The inner regions (circles) are excluded from the volume. The potential is uniquely determined by Laplace's equation (4.5) everywhere in the volume conductor if either the potential or the normal derivative of potential is specified on outer and inner surfaces. The positive surface normal coordinate u is directed outward from the volume (into the small inner regions). (b) Rather than specify boundary conditions on the inner surfaces, we may specify volume current sources $s(\mathbf{r}, t)$ at these surfaces. In this case a unique solution for potential in the volume conductor may be obtained by solving Poisson's equation (4.12). See appendix K for a mathematical description of $s(\mathbf{r}, t)$.

these regions is determined by Laplace's equation, either (4.5) in homogeneous volumes or (4.12) in regions with variable conductivity with $s(\mathbf{r}, t)$ set to zero. However, unique solutions require that potential or its normal derivative be specified on all surfaces bounding the white regions. In the formalism of *Poisson's equation* (4.12), we have replaced standard conditions at source region boundaries by the volume current source term $s(\mathbf{r}, t)$. The negative sign in (4.12) is consistent with positive current flowing into the white (non source) regions, as discussed in appendix K. We interpret $s(\mathbf{r}, t)$ as current generated per unit volume. Boundary conditions at surfaces not involving source regions are applied in the usual manner, as in conditions (4.7) and (4.8).

Another point is that, in a purely resistive medium, the time dependence of potential $\Phi(\mathbf{r}, t)$ is identical to the time dependence of its source $s(\mathbf{r}, t)$. In a medium with important capacitive effects and a single oscillatory source $s(\mathbf{r}, t) \sim \sin(2\pi f t)$, the potential consists of an oscillation at the same frequency, but with phase shift β_{cap}; that is, $\Phi(\mathbf{r}, t) \sim \sin(2\pi f t - \beta_{\text{cap}})$. In EEG applications, the phase shift β_{cap} between source and potential may evidently be set to zero based on studies indicating negligible capacitive effects in tissue at macroscopic scales. Generally, however, there will be many source regions oscillating with different frequencies and phases. The scalp potential at any location is a linear superposition of the contributions from individual source regions, but with unequal weighting due to volume conductor properties and varying distances between sources and scalp measurement location. The manner in which such sources are weighted is considered in chapters 6 and 8.

While the mathematical transformation discussed above may seem artificial, it turns out to be quite useful in macroscopic volume conduction problems. One way to emphasize this is to compare (4.12) for the potential in a conductor (due to a current source region) to the equation for potential in a dielectric (due to a charge source region). The dielectric equation is obtained by combining (3.21), (3.10), and (3.4). This algebra also leads to *Poisson's equation for potentials in a dielectric*:

$$\nabla \cdot [\varepsilon(\mathbf{r})\nabla\Phi(\mathbf{r}, t)] = -\rho(\mathbf{r}, t) \qquad (4.14)$$

Here $\rho(\mathbf{r}, t)$ is free charge density (C/m^3 in mks units) and $\varepsilon(\mathbf{r})$ ($s/(m\,\Omega)$) is the permittivity of the dielectric. The relations (4.12) and (4.14) are both Poisson's equation, but with changed symbols; they are mathematically identical, yet their physical bases are quite different. The macroscopic free charge density $\rho(\mathbf{r}, t)$ in a conductor is essentially zero; thus (4.14) is of no direct practical use in macroscopic electrophysiology. However, many solutions of (4.14) have been published in physics texts, corresponding to various kinds of inhomogeneous properties in dielectric materials. All that is needed to apply these same solutions to conductors is to replace the medium parameter $\varepsilon(\mathbf{r}, t)$ by $\sigma(\mathbf{r}, t)$ and change the source term $\rho(\mathbf{r}, t)$ to $s(\mathbf{r}, t)$. For example, consider the special case of N "point" current sources, that is, source regions with volumes much smaller than the distances to recording electrodes. In an infinite, homogeneous, isotropic, and purely resistive volume conductor, the potential external to the source regions is analogous to the expression for potential due to point charges (3.5), that is

$$\Phi(\mathbf{r}, t) = \frac{1}{4\pi\sigma} \sum_{n=1}^{N} \frac{I_n(t)}{R_n} \qquad (4.15)$$

With a typical set of consistent units for EEG applications, the $I_n(t)$ are monopolar current sources (μA) flowing from source regions n into a volume conductor of conductivity σ ($1/(\Omega\,cm)$). The $R_n = |\mathbf{r} - \mathbf{r}_n|$ are the distances between the measuring (field) point $\mathbf{r}$ (cm) and the source locations $\mathbf{r}_n$ as indicated in fig. 3-1 with q replaced by I. For example, the potential at a distance of 1 cm generated by a current source of $(4\pi)\,\mu A$ in an idealized cortex with resistivity $\eta = 1/\sigma = 300\,\Omega\,cm$ is $300\,\mu V$. In the assumed purely resistive medium, the potential has a time dependence given by the weighted sum of all sources. In media with capacitive effects, phase shifts occur between sources and potential. For oscillatory potentials, such capacitive effects are accounted for in (4.15) by allowing the conductivity to be complex.

The mathematical equivalence of (4.12) and (4.14), or (3.5) and (4.15), has led to much confusion in electrophysiology. It would be easy to cite texts (not to mention "experts") in which this fundamental issue is misunderstood. Let us emphasize again that *the two versions of Poisson's equation represent different physical processes*. Only (4.12) or (4.15) is directly applicable to macroscopic electrophysiology. *Macroscopic potentials in tissue cannot be calculated from charge sources because we cannot know the locations of all the charges!* Any reader still confused on this point should revisit the discussion of *Debye shielding and electroneutrality* in section 11 of chapter 3.

The methods of calculating potentials using (4.15) or more generally (4.12) do not require distinctions between sources at subsynaptic membranes and sources at more distant locations required for current conservation. The latter have sometimes been referred to as "passive loads." However, as used in this book, the terms "source" and "sink" refer to current passing some boundary surface, which is defined separately in each application. Often this boundary surface will coincide with a physiological boundary like a membrane or skull surface, but (4.12) and (4.15) do not require this. The general relationship of current sources to potentials produced in macroscopic neural tissue is summarized in fig. 4-8.

9 Synaptic Current Sources and the Core Conductor Model of the Neuron

Current sources at membrane surfaces are responsible for extracellular potentials. These current sources may occur as a result of several known processes at the cellular scale, including the action potential. Here we focus on the origin of currents generated by synaptic inputs to the subthreshold neuron. Synaptic current sources in neocortex are believed to be the principal sources of scalp-recorded EEG.

The *core conductor model* describes the subthreshold electrical response of a cylindrical nerve fiber (axon or dendrite) to some stimulus (current source) as pictured in fig. 4-9.

As usually presented, the model consists of an equivalent network with resistors representing increments of intracellular and extracellular fluid and resistors in parallel with capacitors representing increments of membrane (Cole 1968; Malmivuo and Plonsey 1995). This approach is often referred to as a lumped parameter model. The circuit model is identical to that of the transmission line (fig. 3-11) except that

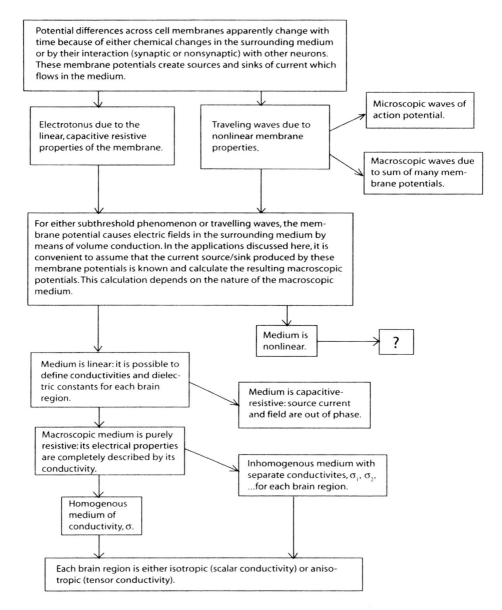

Figure 4-8 The general relationship of current sources to potentials produced in macroscopic media is summarized.

electromagnetic induction in the nerve fiber is negligible as shown in appendix B. In *comparing the nerve fiber to a coaxial cable*, the intracellular fluid, membrane, and extracellular fluid are equivalent to the inner cylindrical conductor, insulating (but leaky) dielectric surrounding the inner cylinder, and outer conductor covering the dielectric. Both linear diffusion and linear wave propagation occur in the transmission line, but the wave process must dominate if the line is to transmit signals over long distances with minimal attenuation (loss of electromagnetic energy to heat

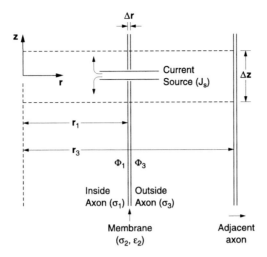

Figure 4-9 Cylindrical fiber geometry. The fiber may be either axon or dendrite subject to the assumptions listed in Section 8. A current source disturbs the equilibrium potential difference across the membrane. The *core conductor model* of the fiber describes the subthreshold electrical response of the transmembrane potential $V(z, t)$, which is governed by the membrane cable equation (4.16). Solutions (4.22) and (4.24) indicate the change in $V(z, t)$ with time t and distance z from the input location for transient (impulse response) and steady-state inputs, respectively.

energy associated with current flux). By contrast, there are no waves in the subthreshold nerve fiber, only diffusion.

The equivalent network model makes good intuitive sense; however, it must be based on (4.5) in the fluid media (where capacitive effects are negligible) and (4.6) inside the membrane (where capacitive effects are critical). That is, the essential problem involves solving three partial differential equations, one in each of the two fluid media and one in the membrane. It is instructive to use this more general approach of volume conduction. After all, we are concerned throughout this book with volume conductor problems for which equivalent circuits, if they exist at all, are unknown. A second reason for deriving the membrane equation from the fundamental principles of volume conduction is that *we are forced to make simplifying assumptions explicit*. The core conductor description of the nerve fiber is based on assumptions that are (mostly) implicit in the equivalent circuit model. We can apply the core conductor analysis to either axon or dendrite provided the following conditions are satisfied:

1. The nerve fiber is cylindrical and infinite in extent (no end conditions to worry about).
2. The adjacent cells force the extracellular current to flow mainly in the axial direction; intracellular current is also mainly axial. Current density in the extracellular space between nerve fibers is approximately constant in directions normal to the axis. This

assumption appears to be most accurate when applied to axons within a nerve (a tight bundle of axons), but is expected to be approximately valid for cylindrical dendrites surrounded by the closely packed cells of cortical tissue.

3. Membrane thickness is much smaller than the diameter of the extracellular space and the space between cells.
4. The initial stimulus is symmetric with respect to the angular location on the circular cross section of the target cell.
5. The axons are unmyelinated.
6. Inductive effects are negligible in the tissue (an excellent approximation).
7. The media are all linear (the membrane potential is well below threshold).
8. All the complications of membrane physiology (including diffusion and active transport) can be lumped into just two parameters—the effective bulk membrane conductivity (accounting for all ion transfer across the membrane) and the effective dielectric constant.

Any good electrophysiologist attempting to connect this idealized theory with intracranial electrode recordings must, of course, evaluate the accuracy of each one of these assumptions for each new scientific study. For our purposes, such details at small scales are not critical. We mainly need to understand the general character of subthreshold membrane behavior.

Let $\Phi_n(z, t)$ represent the potential at axial location z, with $n = 1$, 2, and 3 indicating the three regions: inside axon, membrane, and outside axon, as shown in fig. 4-9. We consider the potential difference across the membrane, that is, the *transmembrane potential* $V(z, t) \equiv \Phi_1(z, t) - \Phi_3(z, t)$. It is always possible to add an arbitrary constant to any electric potential. It is convenient to use such constant so as to define the equilibrium transmembrane potential as $V = 0$. Here we provide a warning to those students (and even some seasoned neuroscientists) who may carelessly use words like "potential," "dendritic potential," or similar imprecise language. Transmembrane potential is quite different from intracellular, membrane, or extracellular potential. Such distinctions are important in both intracranial electrophysiology and scalp EEG applications. Generally, our task is to solve Laplace's equation (4.5) in the two fluid regions 1 and 3 (where capacitive effects are negligible), and solve (4.6) in the membrane, region 2. The equation for region 1 requires inclusion of a source term due either to current injection with an electrode or synapse. The solutions are to be joined at interfaces (1, 2) and (2, 3) using boundary conditions (4.7) and (4.8). In complicated geometry, this is generally a difficult problem. However, the simplifying assumptions above allow for the easy solution in appendix D. That is, the subthreshold transmembrane produced by a localized current sources is shown to satisfy the following linear diffusion equation, *the basic cable equation of electrophysiology* (Cole 1968):

$$\lambda^2 \frac{\partial^2 V}{\partial z^2} - \tau \frac{\partial V}{\partial t} - V = -S(z,t) \tag{4.16}$$

The term $S(z,t)$ has dimensions of potential and is proportional to the magnitude of the current source (due to either synapse or stimulating electrode). The space and time variables are expressed in nondimensional form, that is, $z \to z/\lambda$ and $t \to t/\tau$. Here λ is the *space constant of the axon and surrounding space* given by

$$\lambda^2 = \frac{r_1 \Delta r}{2} \frac{\left(\frac{r_3^2}{r_1^2} - 1\right) \frac{\sigma_1}{\sigma_2}}{\left(\frac{r_3^2}{r_1^2} - 1 + \frac{\sigma_1}{\sigma_3}\right)} \tag{4.17}$$

The axon radius is r_1 and $(r_3 - r_1)$ is the average space between adjacent axons. Membrane thickness is Δr. By contrast to the space constant, the *time constant τ of the membrane* is independent of geometric properties; it depends only on membrane capacitive-resistive properties, that is

$$\tau = \frac{\varepsilon_2}{\sigma_2} \tag{4.18}$$

In neuroscience texts, the membrane time constant is normally written in terms of membrane capacitance and resistance. From (3.11) and (3.19), we obtain

$$\varepsilon = \frac{C \Delta r}{A} \qquad \sigma = \frac{\Delta r}{AR} \tag{4.19}$$

Here C is the capacitance and R is the resistance for current flow in any material over a distance Δr across an area of cross section A. By substituting (4.19) into (4.18), we obtain the usual expression for the membrane time constant:

$$\tau = RC \tag{4.20}$$

Actually, (4.18) is a little more illuminating than (4.20) because it shows explicitly that the *time constant is independent of axon geometry*, whereas the *space constant depends on geometry*. Thus, it is proper to refer to "membrane time constant," but not strictly correct to use "membrane space constant." Using relations (4.19), it is shown in appendix D that (4.17) yields the more familiar expression for the space constant associated with a portion of axon of length Δz, that is

$$\lambda^2 = \frac{R_2 \Delta z^2}{R_1 + R_3} \tag{4.21}$$

The membrane, internal, and external resistances are R_2, R_1, and R_3, respectively. Equation (4.21) may seem to suggest that the space constant depends on the arbitrary choice of axon segment Δz, but this is not so. Because of the cylindrical geometry, membrane resistance to radial current is inversely proportional to Δz, whereas the two fluid resistances are proportional to Δz. Thus, the right-hand side of (4.21) is independent of Δz as shown explicitly with our preferred expression for the space constant (4.17).

10 Solutions to the Cable Equation

The transmembrane potential due to a current source impulse at time $t = 0$ and location $z = 0$ is easily obtained as a solution to (4.16) by setting $S(z, t) = \delta(z)\delta(t)$. The solution corresponds approximately to a single synaptic input at (say) some part of the dendritic tree. From Rall (1977) and appendix E, the transmembrane potential at a distance z from the synapse and time t, measured from its activation is

$$V(z, t) = \sqrt{\frac{\tau}{t}} \exp\left[-\frac{(z/\lambda)^2}{4t/\tau} - \frac{t}{\tau} \right] \tag{4.22}$$

Equation (4.22) takes the indeterminate form $0/0$ when $t = 0$ as a result of the mathematical properties of the delta function input; however, it is valid in the limit $t \to 0$ and may be used for calculations with any $t > 0$. According to (4.22), transmembrane potential $V(z, t)$ at some distance z from the point source increases to a maximum at some time that we identify as the *postsynaptic potential (PSP) rise time* given by

$$\left(\frac{t}{\tau}\right)_{rt} = \frac{1}{4}\left[\sqrt{4(z/\lambda)^2 + 1} - 1 \right] \tag{4.23}$$

For example, at a distance from the source of one space constant, (4.23) predicts that the PSP rise time is about $0.3\,\tau$. At two space constants, PSP rise time is about $0.8\,\tau$ as shown in fig. 4-10. Suppose the cortical pyramidal cell membrane time constant is 8 ms (Lux and Pollen 1966) and estimate that most dendritic synapses are located within one or two space constants of the soma (Rall 1977). From (4.23) the maximum soma potential due to (simultaneously active) synapses distributed over the dendritic tree is reached in something like 3 to 7 ms from synaptic activation. We can compare these estimates with experimental work indicating the existence of at least two types of excitatory and two types of inhibitory synapses. Excitatory rise times are roughly in the 1 and 10 ms range for the two types (Segev et al. 1995).

   After the maximum transmembrane potential is obtained, $V(z, t)$ decreases more slowly to zero. The time constant τ is the characteristic

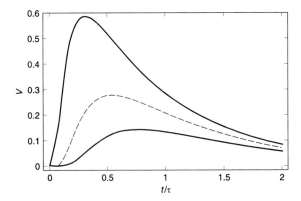

Figure 4-10 Transient solutions (4.22) to the cable equation (4.16). The transmembrane potential $V(z, t)$ is plotted at three non-dimensional distances ($z/\lambda = 1.0, 1.5, 2.0$) from the input location. The input impulse (delta function) stimulus occurs at $t = 0$. Potential is plotted in arbitrary units. Time is normalized with respect to membrane time constant τ. PSP rise time at a distance of one space constant (upper curve) is about 0.3τ.

time for the transmembrane potential inducted by an external stimulus (synapse or electrode) to spread (diffuse) along the axial direction. It is a measure of the time required for membrane charge to redistribute itself in accordance with Maxwell's microscopic equations. Such *relaxation times* are short in good conductors and long in poor conductors. Some reported experimental time constants are as follows: squid giant axon (1 ms), cortical pyramidal cell (8 ms), muscle fibers (30 ms) (Lux and Pollen 1966) and thalamic relay cells (23 ms) (Destexhe and Sejnowski 2001). The subthreshold conductivity of membrane tissue can be estimated from (4.18) and the measured time constant because membrane capacity is relatively constant over a wide variety of species (Cole 1968). Measurement of axon magnetic fields has made possible more accurate estimates of cable properties (Woosley et al. 1985).

The space constant of the axon and extracellular space is roughly the spatial extent along the membrane's axial direction that exhibits a substantial change in resting potential (at some fixed time) under the influence of a localized external stimulus, as indicated by (4.22) with t/τ fixed. When membrane conductivity σ_2 is small, transmembrane potential charges from equilibrium tend to spread out over larger distances, as in the case of myelinated axons. Alternatively, membranes with large conductivity tend to confine potential changes locally. In the limit of high conductivity, membrane charges are more free to move, and the space constant becomes somewhat analogous to the Debye shielding distance for fluid conductors (3.12). The space constant λ in (4.17) is proportional to the square root of axon radius r_1 provided r_3/r_1 is fixed. As extracellular space becomes small ($r_3 \rightarrow r_1$), λ also becomes small since the model allows for very little extracellular current.

The transient solution to the basic cable equation for a nerve fiber (4.16) is given by (4.22). The steady-state solution is also of interest in EEG.

If a localized input is a sinusoidal function of time, $S(z, t) = \delta(z)\cos(\omega t)$, the transmembrane response is derived in appendix E as

$$V(z, t) \propto \frac{\exp\left[-\sqrt{\frac{1}{2}(\sqrt{1 + \omega^2\tau^2} + 1)}\frac{z}{\lambda}\right]}{\sqrt[4]{1 + \omega^2\tau^2}}\cos(\omega t - \theta) \qquad (4.24)$$

The exponential factor in (4.24) was derived by Plonsey (1969) with the frequency-dependent denominator treated as a general constant. Here we consider all frequency-dependent terms because of our interest in cortical low-pass effects on EEG.

Transmembrane potential $V(z, t)$ decreases exponentially along the fiber from the location of source input with characteristic length λ. In the low-frequency limit $\omega\tau \ll 1$, $V(z, t)$ is independent of frequency. At higher frequencies, $\omega\tau > 1$, $V(z, t)$ decreases with frequency. In (4.24) θ is the phase difference between input and output to the membrane, given in appendix E. This phase shift θ at the cellular scale should not be confused with the putative macroscopic potential phase shift β_{cap} discussed in section 8. The *phase angle θ applies to transmembrane potential, which is roughly proportional to cellular source strength in subthreshold fibers.* By contrast, *the angle β_{cap} refers to a putative phase shift between fixed sources and macroscopic potential,* strictly a volume conduction effect. Several studies indicate that $\beta_{cap} \cong 0$ in applications associated with EEG. By contrast, transmembrane potential (and by implication dipole source strength) is predicted by (4.24) to exhibit a low pass filtering behavior. Source strength is affected because dipole moments generated by cortical columns depend on source–sink separations. Larger spreads of $V(z, t)$ over the dendrites produce larger effective pole separations leading to larger mesosources.

Any fiber input function $S(z, t)$ can be expressed as a Fourier series, that is, a sum of separate inputs with different frequencies. Thus, (4.24) provides a plausible (if substantially oversimplified) estimate of the low-pass filter properties of cortical dendrites. For example, consider a cortical pyramidal cell with time constant τ and synaptic input concentrated at nondimensional distances from the input region, expressed in effective length constants $z_S/\lambda = 1$, 2, and 3. Figure 4-11 shows the decay of transmembrane potential with frequency for these distances from the input region (any part of the dendrite) for $\tau = 8$ ms (upper) and 16 ms (lower). Each curve is normalized with respect to transmembrane potential at zero input frequency. For example at 40 Hz and $\tau = 8$ ms, transmembrane potential is predicted to fall by about 40% to 70% of its value at zero frequency depending on distance from the input region z_S/λ. Genuine neural input is distributed over dendrites with varying diameters, violating the simple cable model based on constant diameter, infinite length, and localized input. However, the discussion in the next

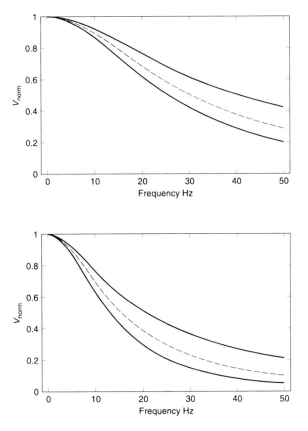

Figure 4-11 The steady-state solution (4.24) to (4.16) shows the decay of transmembrane potential magnitude with input frequency for time-dependent synaptic input at three non-dimensional distances ($z_s/\lambda = 1, 2, 3$) from the input region (any part of the fiber). Each curve is normalized with respect to transmembrane potential at zero input frequency to emphasize frequency dependence. (*Upper*) membrane time constant $\tau = 8$ ms. (*Lower*) $\tau = 16$ ms.

section indicates that a more realistic model may plausibly replace z_S/λ by an effective *electrotonic length*. For cortical pyramidal cells, this electrotonic length appears to be of order one or two; that is, in the general range assumed for z_S/λ in fig. 4-11.

Local membrane source strength for passive neurons well below threshold is approximately proportional to transmembrane potential. Thus, (4.24) provides an estimate of membrane *microsource strength* $s(\mathbf{r},f)$ as a function of frequency and distance from the synaptic input region. As indicted in section 15, the strength of mesosources produced by a cortical tissue volume is similarly reduced at higher frequencies. These arguments suggest that the low-pass characteristics of the model nerve fiber derived above are in general agreement with the observation that mammalian cortical EEG is strongly attenuated at frequencies higher than roughly 50 to 100 Hz, in contrast to much higher frequency field potentials recorded in invertebrates (Bullock 1977).

At the very large scale of scalp EEG, nearly all the signal normally occurs below about 15 or 20 Hz. This EEG frequency attenuation between cortex and scalp is believed to be caused by a mechanism quite apart from the capacitive-resistive membrane properties outlined in this section. Rather, the attenuation of higher frequencies between cortex and scalp is apparently a combined effect of *spatial filtering* by the head volume conductor and the dynamic nature of cortical sources, as discussed in chapters 2, 9, and 11. In other words, *temporal filtering between cortex and scalp is believed to be a byproduct of spatial filtering by the volume conductor and the tendency for higher temporal frequencies to occur with higher spatial frequencies above the alpha band (due to the dynamic behavior of cortical sources).*

11 Synaptic Input to Branched Dendrites

The quantitative effect of synaptic input to the branched dendrites of cortical pyramidal cells is important for our understanding of neocortical dynamics and its large-scale EEG signature. Pyramidal cell dendrites have many branches that extend horizontally in the cortex as shown in fig. 4-1. The complicated geometry makes analysis of the branched dendrite system more difficult than that of the single, cylindrical fiber. However, detailed theoretical studies have been carried out by Wilfred Rall, well known for his seminal contributions to neuron cable theory. His approach to fiber branching involves the transformation of a particular class of dendritic tree into an equivalent cylinder (Rall 1967). For a class of dendritic tree that appears to be physiologically plausible for cortical pyramidal cells and others with substantial branching, the basic cable equation for the cylindrical axon (4.16) is again appropriate, but with the space constant interpreted as an effective length constant for the entire dendritic tree. In the branched dendrite model, the nondimensional distance z/λ for the cylindrical fiber in (4.16) is replaced by a nondimensional *electrotonic distance* Z, which accounts for the variation of local length "constant" $\lambda(z)$ with dendritic diameter, that is

$$Z = \int_0^L \frac{dz}{\lambda(z)} \tag{4.25}$$

An important observation is that a typical electrotonic length, obtained by integrating (4.25) from soma to the end of a typical dendritic terminal (L) is only 1 or 2 (Rall 1977; Redman and Walmsley 1983). This implies that the *functional distance* of a cortical pyramidal cell synapse is often much less than the actual distance. By "functional distance" we mean the ability of a distant synapse to alter soma transmembrane potential, that is, to influence the firing of an action potential in its target neuron. For example, a distant synapse may easily be located 1 or 2 mm from the soma. The length constant for cortical pyramidal cells has been estimated to be about 0.2 mm (Jacobson and Pollen 1968). The branched dendrite model then suggests that the effective (functional) distance of distant synapses may be much shorter than 1 mm, perhaps only 0.2 to 0.4 mm.

Rall's theoretical studies have encouraged electrophysiologists to carry out experimental work to check his predictions. For example, one application of (4.25) to a thalamic relay cell yielded a calculated electrotonic length of 2.7 and a predicted time constant of 17 ms (Destexhe and Sejnowski 2001). However, the measured time constant was 23 ms. Evidently the discrepancy between theory and experiment occurred because this neuron had minimal branching compared to cortical pyramidal cells, thereby violating Rall's assumed branching behavior.

The issue of synaptic functional distance has important implications for neocortical dynamics (Nunez 1995). It is estimated that about 85% of cortical synapses are excitatory (Braitenberg and Schuz 1991), but excitatory synapses occur mainly on spines and dendritic branches, whereas inhibitory synapses are more concentrated near soma. That is, excitatory synapses tend to have more influence because of their higher density, but inhibitory synapses tend to compensate by acting closer to cell bodies. The branched dendrite model then suggests a relatively more important role for excitatory synapses (versus inhibitory synapses) than does the single fiber model.

A closely related issue is the relative importance of corticocortical versus thalamocortical input to cortical columns. In humans, about 98% of the input fibers are corticocortical; only a few percent are thalamocortical (Braitenberg 1977, 1978; Katznelson 1981; Nunez 1995), suggesting a dominance of corticocortical interactions in dynamic behavior. The corticocortical axons, which number about 10^{10}, are believed to be exclusively (or nearly so) excitatory and terminate mainly on the branches of dendrites of pyramidal and stellate cells with relatively few on soma (Scheibel and Scheibel 1970). The specific (primary sensory) thalamocortical axons (total number about 10^{6}) provide disproportionate inputs near cell bodies in cortical layer IV (Szentagothai 1979). The nonspecific thalamocortical axons (total number about 10^{8}) are apparently much more diffusely distributed. The branched dendrite model then suggests a more important role for corticocortical synapses (versus specific thalamocortical synapses) than does the single fiber model (Nunez 1995). We return to this issue in the context of neocortical dynamics in chapter 11.

12 Mesoscopic Source Strength as Dipole Moment per Unit Volume

Each 1 mm^3 volume of human neocortex contains, on average, about a hundred thousand neurons and a billion or so synapses. Each active synapse produces local membrane current, as well as return current from more distant membrane surfaces as required by current conservation. *Excitatory synapses* produce negative source regions (*sinks*) at local membrane surfaces and distributed positive sources at more distant membrane locations, as indicated in figs. 4-1 and 4-6. *Inhibitory synapses* produce current in opposite directions, that is, local membrane *sources* and more distant distributed sinks. The distribution of passive sources and sinks over each cell depends on capacitive-resistive properties of the cell and surrounding space. The membrane time constant and cell space constant are discussed in section 9, with subthreshold trans-membrane potentials estimated by the diffusion equation (4.16). Action potential sources may also contribute to scalp potential; however, action potential contributions appear to be much smaller than those of synaptic sources. The reason has to do with microsource geometry and synchrony rather than microsource strength, as discussed in section 13 and chapter 5.

The detailed nature of cortical potentials measured with small electrodes may be of considerable interest to electrophysiologists working at small or intermediate scales of neocortical dynamics. The intra-cranial electrode may record so-called *field potentials*, a label often used to indicate extracellular rather than transmembrane potentials in the physiologist's parlance. These extracellular potentials may be generated by anything between one and perhaps 10^5 or so neurons, depending on size and location of the intracranial electrode (Abeles 1982). Electrophysiology spans about five or six orders of magnitude of spatial scale, ranging from microelectrode with tip diameter in the 10^{-4} cm range to the 0.5 to 1 cm diameter (with contact gel included) scalp electrode. Scalp potential is an experimental measure of dynamic activity at scales larger than 1 cm due to field spreading by the volume conductor. Each scalp electrode records space-averaged potentials from tissue containing something like 100 million to 1 billion neurons, depending on scalp electrode density and on whether high-resolution methods are employed to project scalp data to the dura surface, as described in chapter 8.

How are the disparate spatial scales of electrophysiology related? In order to address this fundamental question, we here recruit the powerful theoretical tools developed by physicists in the 19th and 20th centuries. Recall from chapter 3 that there are two versions of Maxwell's equations, the microscopic and macroscopic formulations listed in table 3-2. The microscopic equations allow exact calculations of electric and magnetic fields, provided the locations and magnitudes of all charges and currents (charges and their velocities) are known in advance. The obvious trouble with Maxwell's microscopic formulation is that we cannot possibly know the details of all the atomic, molecular, and cellular charges in even a very small volume of tissue. Thus, Maxwell's microscopic theory is of no direct use in macroscopic problems: we must use the macroscopic version.

The issue of cross-scale connections in electromagnetic field theory is similar to cross-scale connections in electrophysiology. We can make good use of the mathematical identity of the two versions of Poisson's equation, that is, (4.14) for the electric potential due to charges in a dielectric and (4.12) for potential due to current sources in a conductor. This means that our comparison is not just qualitative: it is quantitative. We can make excellent use of the established formalism developed for physical dielectric materials (Jackson 1975) by changing the names of the variables and parameters. The remaining discussions in this chapter make substantial use of established physical theory.

The *current dipole moment per unit volume* $\mathbf{P}(\mathbf{r}, t)$ of a tissue mass is defined as a weighted space average of all the microsources $s(\mathbf{r}, t)$ within the volume as shown in fig. 4-12. The vector $\mathbf{r}$ locates the *center of the volume W* within the brain and the vector $\mathbf{w}$ locates the microsources inside this volume; thus, we replace the notation $s(\mathbf{r}, t)$ by $s(\mathbf{r}, \mathbf{w}, t)$ when appropriate. We are relatively free to choose the size of the tissue volume between (say) 1 and 10^{-2} mm^3 in various applications involving electrodes of different size. Thus, we refer to $\mathbf{P}(\mathbf{r}, t)$ as a *mesoscopic source function* or *dipole moment per unit volume*. It is defined by the following triple integral over the tissue volume element W:

$$\mathbf{P}(\mathbf{r}, t) = \frac{1}{W} \iiint\limits_{W} \mathbf{w}s(\mathbf{r}, \mathbf{w}, t)dW(\mathbf{w}) \qquad (4.26)$$

The weighting vector $\mathbf{w}$ locates each current source within the volume W. Equation (4.26) is useful in EEG when the volume sizes W are roughly between the minicolumn and macrocolumn scales. At these scales, neocortex may be treated as a continuum so that $\mathbf{P}(\mathbf{r}, t)$ is a continuous *field variable*. There are, however, some limitations to this approach. First, the *tissue volume should be large* enough to contain many microsources $s(\mathbf{r}, \mathbf{w}, t)$ due to local synaptic activity as well as their passive return currents, but its characteristic size should be much smaller than the closest distance to the scalp. The former condition suggests that the total strength of

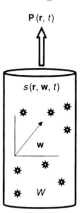

Figure 4-12   A mesoscopic tissue volume W, for example a millimeter-scale cortical column containing millions of membrane microcurrent sources $s(\mathbf{r}, t)$ is indicated by stars. The tissue mass produces a *current dipole moment per unit volume* $\mathbf{P}(\mathbf{r}, t)$, also called the local *mesosource strength*. The notation $s(\mathbf{r}, \mathbf{w}, t)$ indicates the explicit dependence of microsource strength on the column vector coordinate $\mathbf{r}$ and its vector location within the column $\mathbf{w}$. Cortical or scalp potential $\Phi(\mathbf{r}, t)$ due to brain sources is the weighted integral of $\mathbf{P}(\mathbf{r}, t)$ over the brain volume, or in the case of exclusively cortical sources, the integral over the cortical surface.

microsources will be approximately balanced by an equal strength of microsinks such that the monopole contribution of the tissue volume W is approximately zero, that is

$$\iiint\limits_{W} s(\mathbf{r}, \mathbf{w}, t) dW(\mathbf{w}) \cong 0 \qquad (4.27)$$

The second condition *that the volume W be sufficiently small* ensures that quadrupole and higher order terms will make negligible contributions to scalp potential. If both conditions on W are satisfied, the dipole term in the general multipole expansion expressing scalp potential is dominant. Refer to Jackson (1975) and chapter 3 for the analogous discussion of microscopic effects in physical dielectrics.

Equation (4.26) is identical to the definition of charge polarization in a dielectric if the current sources $s(\mathbf{r}, \mathbf{w}, t)$ are replaced by charge sources. As discussed in chapter 3, the condition of *electroneutrality* holds in any macroscopic mass of conductive tissue so that macroscopic charge polarization $\mathbf{P}_C$ is everywhere zero. However, *current polarization* or *current dipole moment per unit volume* $\mathbf{P}(\mathbf{r}, t)$ is generally not zero. The volume microsources $s(\mathbf{r}, \mathbf{w}, t)$ and *mesoscopic source strength* $\mathbf{P}(\mathbf{r}, t)$ have typical units of $\mu A/mm^3$ and $\mu A/mm^2$, respectively. Thus, $\mathbf{P}(\mathbf{r}, t)$ has units of current density. In section 13, it is shown that *for idealized source distributions, this dipole moment per unit volume is essentially the (negative) diffuse macroscopic current density across the cortex.*

The mesoscopic source strength $\mathbf{P}(\mathbf{r}, t)$ is a vector, indicating that it has separate strengths in each of three directions. However, approximately 85% of neurons in mammalian cortex are pyramidal cells oriented normal to the cortical surface (Braitenberg and Schuz 1991). For this reason, we emphasize the local cortex-normal component of $\mathbf{P}(\mathbf{r}, t)$, which is a function of time t and cortical macroscopic location $\mathbf{r}$ of the volume element W. The time dependence of $\mathbf{P}(\mathbf{r}, t)$ is determined by the time-dependent behaviors of the microsources $s(\mathbf{r}, \mathbf{w}, t)$. The distribution of such sources within W and the resulting *mesoscopic source strength (dipole moment per unit volume $\mathbf{P}(\mathbf{r}, t)$)* depend on capacitive-resistive membrane properties, as discussed in section 15.

For purposes of visualizing the relationship between *microsources* $s(\mathbf{r}, \mathbf{w}, t)$ and *mesosources* $\mathbf{P}(\mathbf{r}, t)$, it is may be convenient to think of $\mathbf{P}(\mathbf{r}, t)$ as generated by sources $s(\mathbf{r}, \mathbf{w}, t)$ in volumes W of roughly 1 mm^3. This particular choice, made largely independent of cortical morphology, is a good one for two reasons. First, the macrocolumn scale is well below the typical spatial resolution of extracranial recordings, even with the best high-resolution EEG or MEG. We cannot distinguish spatial patterns at this scale; the mixing of positive and negative mesosources within a cortical column of this size will simply tend to reduce its dipole moment. All we are able to record from the scalp is the net result from a large tissue volume. The 1 mm scale is also much less than the 1.0 to 1.5 cm distance between cortex and scalp. Thus, scalp potential due to a *1 mm scale mesosource* is, to a reasonable approximation, a characteristic *dipole potential*, such that the quadrupole and higher order terms discussed in chapters 3 and 5 may be neglected. Second, the orientation of the axes of cortical pyramidal cells, which varies greatly in cortical fissures and sulci, is approximately constant over each 1 mm^2 area of macrocolumn. Thus the concept of local normal sources at this scale appears well-justified. We are free to define $\mathbf{P}(\mathbf{r}, t)$ in (4.26) based on cubical volume elements (voxels) as long as the volume W is large enough to contain a large number of cells. This implies that $\mathbf{P}(\mathbf{r}, t)$ is a continuous function of cortical location $\mathbf{r}$. In applications involving scalp potentials, it is perhaps more convenient to think of W in terms of overlapping cortical columns with diameter in the 1 mm range and height roughly equal to cortical thickness, approximately in the 3 mm range. If each 1 mm^2 cortical column were a discrete entity any neocortical source activity would consist of a hundred thousand or so macrocolumn "dipoles" (the *mesosources*) of varying strength and direction given by $\mathbf{P}(\mathbf{r}, t)$. However, macrocolumn boundaries overlap and vary with brain activity, thus $\mathbf{P}(\mathbf{r}, t)$ is usually more accurately pictured as a continuous field variable.

The explicit relation between the microsources $s(\mathbf{r}, \mathbf{w}, t)$ and mesosource strength $\mathbf{P}(\mathbf{r}, t)$, given succinctly by (4.26), yields several useful insights even in the absence of any calculations. This fundamental equation shows that *mesosource strength at any fixed time is generally proportional to the instantaneous strength of the microsources* as expected. However, there is much more to the relation than this. *Mesosource strength increases as the typical separation between positive and negative microsources increases.* Thus, if both positive and negative microsources are nearly equally distributed through the volume W, mesosource strength will tend to be small, even with relatively large microsources. The so-called *closed field* of electro-physiology is an example of uniform mixing of positive and negative microsources. In contrast, clustering of positive sources in one part of the tissue mass W and negative sources in another part can lead to relatively large mesosources $\mathbf{P}(\mathbf{r}, t)$ even when the underlying microsource magnitudes are not large.

13 Simulations of Mesosources Generated in a Tissue Mass

The importance of microsource distribution within cortical columns is demonstrated here by several numerical simulations. For convenience, we assume discrete microsources rather than more realistic distributed microsources. This assumption has minimal influence on the central ideas presented in this section. In the first example, 2000 synchronous microsources are assumed to be randomly distributed (random locations $\mathbf{w}$) throughout a volume W as shown in fig. 4-13 (upper). This

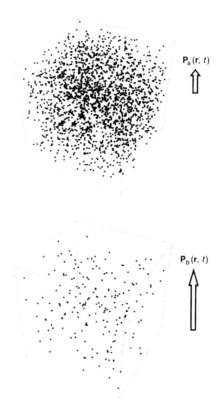

$\mathbf{P}_a(\mathbf{r}, t)$

$\mathbf{P}_b(\mathbf{r}, t)$

Figure 4-13   (*Upper*) The dots indicate 2000 synchronous microsources and sinks $s(\mathbf{r}, \mathbf{w}, t)$ mixed with random locations $\mathbf{w}$ within a tissue volume W. The *mesosource* or *dipole moment per unit volume* $\mathbf{P}_a(\mathbf{r}, t)$ is small, due only to statistical fluctuation. (*Lower*) 100 synchronous microsources $s(\mathbf{r}, \mathbf{w}, t)$ constrained to the upper half of the volume W plus another 100 microsinks constrained to the lower half of the tissue volume. $\mathbf{P}_b(\mathbf{r}, t)$ is about 4.5 times larger (on average) than $\mathbf{P}_a(\mathbf{r}, t)$ even though the synaptic action densities $\Psi_e(\mathbf{r}, t)$ and $\Psi_i(\mathbf{r}, t)$ are only 10% as large as those indicated in the upper plot. This occurs because of the relatively large average separation between sources and sinks in the lower plot.

random source simulation was repeated 50 times. We can think of the repeated simulations as representing estimates of mesosource strength $\mathbf{P}(\mathbf{r}, t_j)$ at different times t_j. The microsource magnitudes $s(\mathbf{r}, \mathbf{w}, t_j)$ are assumed to vary randomly between 0 and 100 (say in units of $\mu A/mm^3$), but for each of the 1000 positive current sources a negative source (sink) of the same magnitude is included. This procedure was chosen to satisfy the *condition of local current conservation*; that is, that the integral of $s(\mathbf{r}, \mathbf{w}, t_j)$ over the volume W is zero (4.27). Note that the integrand in (4.26) is weighted by the vector $\mathbf{w}$, so the integral in (4.26) is generally not zero.

There is essentially no difference between the average magnitudes of the x, y, and z components of $\mathbf{P}_a(\mathbf{r}, t_j)$ as expected. The magnitude of the z component of the mesosource vector $|P_{za}(\mathbf{r}, t_j)|$ is plotted for a succession ($j = 1, 50$) of random microsource distributions, indicated by the lower plot in fig. 4-14. Note that $P_{za}(\mathbf{r}, t_j)$ can be positive or negative,

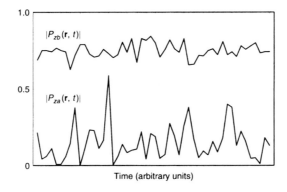

Figure 4-14 Simulated dipole moments per unit volume (z component of $\mathbf{P}$ in arbitrary units) generated by the model tissue masses (or cortical column) of fig. 4-13 are simulated for 50 discrete "times," that is, with different choices of random source magnitudes and locations. The lower trace shows the simulated P_{za} due to 1000 microsources and 1000 matching microsinks with random magnitudes and locations corresponding to the upper plot in fig. 4-13. The upper plot is the estimated P_{zb} due to 100 microsources randomly placed in the upper half of the tissue mass and 100 microsinks of matching magnitudes placed in the lower half. The same (random) magnitude range of microsources was used to generate both plots. As expected the 200 microsource–sinks with nonrandom location produce about four or five times the average magnitude of the 2000 random microsource–sinks, as predicted by the ratio $200/(2000)^{1/2} = 4.47$.

but its sign is not indicated. Mesosource strengths in this first example are due only to statistical fluctuation in the tissue volume. That is, although every microsource was balanced by another microsource of the opposite sign (sink), the average separation distances are not fully balanced. As a result, small mesosource strengths roughly in the $0.5\,\mu\text{A}/\text{mm}^2$ range were obtained (assuming a $1\,\text{mm}^3$ volume W).

The second simulation study is similar to the first. The strength distribution of the microsources is unchanged. However, the 2000 randomly located sources are replaced by a much smaller set of 100 microsources that are constrained to the lower half of the volume W plus another 100 microsinks constrained to the upper half, as partly indicated in fig. 4-13 (lower). The idea is to simulate inhibitory and excitatory synaptic action occurring at deep and superficial cortical depths, respectively, consistent with genuine cortical anatomy and physiology.

The magnitude of the z component of the tissue mesosource vector $|P_{zb}(\mathbf{r}, t_j)|$ is shown in the upper plot in fig. 4-14. This simulation demonstrates that only 200 sources with nonrandom locations generate mesosource magnitudes in the $2\,\mu\text{A}/\text{mm}^2$ range, or on average about four or five times larger than mesosources generated by the 2000 randomly placed microsources of the same average strength. This magnitude difference is easily explained as the ratio of the number of nonrandom sources to the square root of random sources or $200/(2000)^{1/2} = 4.47$. A more realistic simulation might compare two macrocolumns each containing 10^{10} sources (roughly the number of synapses). In this case, the estimated ratio of nonrandom to random mesosource magnitude is $10^{10}/(10^{10})^{1/2}$. In this example, the average magnitude of the mesosource generated by the nonrandom column is about a hundred thousand times larger than that generated by a column with random distributions of microsources.

Equation (4.26) has important implications for determining the underlying sources of scalp-recorded potentials. EEG, like other brain data, provides a selective measure of the underlying microsources. In each application, we should do our best to understand what brain activity we are most likely to be measuring with EEG and what we are almost certainly not measuring. Discussions of these issues occur in various contexts throughout this book. These mesosource simulations have implications for studies of *co-registration* of fMRI or PET with EEG. Several possible physiological causes for mismatches between metabolic and electrical measures of brain function are discussed by Nunez and Silberstein (2001). As a first guess, we might expect that the tissue mass with the largest density of microsources (fig. 4-13 upper), which in this example produces the smaller mesosource, should produce the stronger metabolic signatures. However, this issue is unclear for a number of reasons, for example, the neural mass with nonrandom sources (fig. 4-13 lower) might generate more action potentials, substantially increasing local metabolic activity.

By adopting the concept of meso-sources as the so-called *generators* of EEG, we can, to a large degree, divorce our macroscopic description from many of the detailed issues that occupy electrophysiologists working at smaller scales. The *scale-crossing* arguments may be illustrated as follows. Suppose, for purposes of argument, that future scientists somehow overturn much of today's neurophysiology. Perhaps intracortical action potentials (rather than synaptic potentials) are shown to make the dominant contribution to EEG (unlikely). Or new mechanisms of neuron–neuron interaction may be discovered. It has been suggested that the computational complexity of a neuron is greatly increased over the classic model by reciprocal synaptic interaction between dendrites (Segev et al. 1995). Or, chemical release by subsynaptic neurons can inhibit the release of GABA in the presynaptic neuron; such inhibition of inhibition is equivalent to excitation (Nicoll and Alger 2004).

Such advances in our understanding of small-scale electrophysiology may dramatically influence our views of neurophysiology and micro-source dynamics $s(\mathbf{r},\mathbf{w},t)$ and have profound scientific consequences. However, these events will not change the validity of (4.26): they only influence the details of the calculations. That is, the only factors determining mesosource strength in any tissue volume W are microsource strengths and the distribution of these microsources within the volume. In theory, many distinct physiological processes can produce the same distribution of microsources $s(\mathbf{r},\mathbf{w},t)$, and many different distributions of $s(\mathbf{r},\mathbf{w},t)$ can produce the same mesosources $\mathbf{P}(\mathbf{r},t)$. We must remember, however, that scalp potential is determined by $\mathbf{P}(\mathbf{r}, t)$, independent of the underlying details of the microsources.

All *microsources* $s(\mathbf{r}, \mathbf{w}, t)$ considered in these simulations are assumed to be *synchronous*. That is, they tend to "turn on" together for some interval and then "turn off" together. Clearly, the contribution of *asynchronous microsources* to $\mathbf{P}(\mathbf{r}, t_j)$ will be much lower. Random-in-time contributions of microsources to mesosources are expected to be similar to the random-in-space contributions of fig. 4-13; that is, proportional to the square root of the number density of active microsources. The idea of *coarse graining* in time is appropriate in this context; that is, if our volume element W contains many synapses, we expect temporal overlap of synaptic activation within each volume to facilitate microsource synchrony at the relatively low temporal frequencies of EEG.

14 Simple Interpretation of Mesosource Sources in an Idealized Tissue Mass

Figure 4-15 depicts a cortical macrocolumn, although any mesoscopic tissue mass (or voxel) will do just as well. Small electrode studies in animal cortex often record only minimal changes in extracellular potential as electrodes are moved parallel to the cortical surface over small distances (Mountcastle 1979; Eccles 1984; Abeles 1982). This electrophysiological data reflects columnar cortical morphology, that is it matches anatomical observations that changes in neocortical tissue characteristics are much larger in surface normal (depth) than in tangential directions.

In order to provide an idealized example of a mesosource, we here choose a case where inhibitory and excitatory synaptic sources are

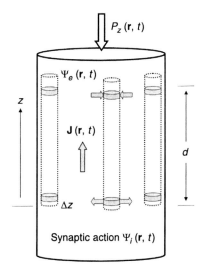

Figure 4-15 A cortical macrocolumn is suggested, although any mesoscopic tissue mass (or voxel) will do just as well. In this greatly oversimplified example, excitatory sinks (upper) and inhibitory sources (lower) are assumed to occur only within narrow depths of the column (distributed return membrane current neglected here). In this idealized case, the dipole moment per unit volume $\mathbf{P}(\mathbf{r}, t)$ equals $-\mathbf{J}(\mathbf{r}, t)$, the diffuse extracellular current density across the cortex.

confined to the deep and superficial disk regions, respectively. In this idealized picture, current sources are confined to two thin layers: a deep layer of positive sources due to inhibitory synapses and a superficial layer of negative sources (sinks) due to excitatory synapses (Szentagothai 1979, 1987). For simplicity, we assume that the passive (return) currents, mainly from regions between the two synaptic layers, cancel perfectly. The volume source density is also assumed to be constant over each thin cylindrical layer. Column cross-sectional area and volume are given by A and W, respectively. The magnitude of total extracellular current generated in each disk-shaped source region is I. The microsource current density is assumed to be independent of coordinates parallel to the surface and is given by

$$s(\mathbf{r}, z, t) = \frac{\pm I}{A\Delta z} \qquad (4.28)$$

Here the assumed positive source region is $(0 < z < \Delta z)$ and the negative source region is $(d - \Delta z < z < d)$. All other regions are assumed to lack sources. The dipole moment per unit volume (mesosource) is directed along the column axis with unit vector direction $\mathbf{a}_z$. Its magnitude follows from (4.26) and (4.28) with $\mathbf{w} = z\mathbf{a}_z$ (Nunez 1995), that is

$$\mathbf{P}(\mathbf{r}, t) = -\mathbf{J}(\mathbf{r}, t) \qquad (4.29)$$

In this idealized example the dipole moment per unit volume is simply the diffuse extracellular current density across the column, $\mathbf{J} = J_z\mathbf{a}_z$. The sign of J_z is determined by the direction of movement of positive ions from deep sources to superficial sinks. Some of this current exits the bottom of the column, passes through brain, CSF, skull, and scalp and returns to superficial sinks. Most current remains inside the cranium, but some passes through the skull into the scalp. Such skull "sources" cause the scalp potentials we record as EEG. The positive ion current flow is matched by the movement of negative ions from sink to source regions, consistent with the condition of *electroneutrality*. This example corresponds crudely to the case of clustered excitatory and inhibitory synaptic input to superficial and deep cortex, respectively. While we have failed to include several effects, including return current distributed along dendritic surfaces, such inaccuracies do not change our main point: *the mesosource strength is an approximate measure of the diffuse current density along the column axis.*

While the simple physical interpretation of the mesosource function $\mathbf{P}(\mathbf{r}, t)$ embodied in (4.29) depends on an idealistic view of cortical microsource distribution, the fundamental integral given in (4.26) is not so limited. That is, the mesosource function may be determined from (4.26) regardless of the complications of genuine cortical morphology and physiology, and this mesosource function provides a parsimonious bridge of the large gap between microsources and scalp potentials.

15 Low-Pass Filtering of the Mesosources P(r, t)

We have emphasized that volume conduction is, for most practical purposes, independent of source frequency in the range of EEG frequencies, roughly 1 to 50 or 100 Hz. Thus, if we were to implant a physical dipole in a subject's brain and vary the frequency of its (constant amplitude) AC current source, we would expect no change in scalp amplitude with frequency. In fact, this prediction was verified experimentally in at least one human experiment (Cooper et al. 1965); there is no attenuation of scalp potential due to increasing source frequency provided the rms amplitude of the implanted dipole current and pole separation (that is, dipole moment) are held fixed. This is not to say that mesosource strength of genuine physiological sources $P(r, t)$ might not be attenuated at high frequencies, as suggested by the following analysis.

In this example, we illustrate the variable contribution from passive membrane sources that depend on the temporal behavior of the synaptic input. Inhibitory synapses are again assumed to be confined to a thin deep layer in fig. 4-16; no excitatory synapses are included in this example. The inhibitory synaptic action causes local current sources at membrane surfaces and return current sinks mostly distributed over more superficial cortical layers. The distribution of sources in the cortical depths depends on the capacitive-resistive properties of cells and extracellular fluid. If most of the pyramidal cells are passive (well below threshold), the cable equation (4.16) provides a rough approximation to transmembrane potential $V_i(z, t)$ for each cell i as a function of distance along dendritic axes aligned in the z direction. The effects of dendritic branching are accounted for approximately by expressing solutions to (4.16) in terms of an effective space constant of the cells given by (4.25) rather than the space constant for a cylindrical axon (4.17).

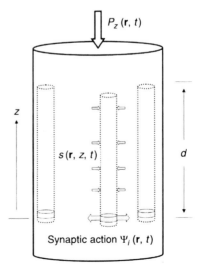

Figure 4-16 Inhibitory synapses are again assumed to be confined to a thin deep layer, but no excitatory synapses are included in this example. The inhibitory synaptic action causes local current sources $s(r, w, t)$ at membrane surfaces and return current sinks distributed over more superficial cortical layers. In this idealization, symmetry across the column (identical parallel fibers) is assumed so that microsource strength depends only on depth within the column, that is, $s(r, w, t) \rightarrow s(r, z, t)$.

In order to account for temporal filtering by membrane capacitive-resistive properties, we note that any input function due to a large number of synapses that become active at generally different times can be Fourier transformed. In this manner, synaptic input may be expressed as a function of frequency rather than time. The resulting (Fourier transformed) transmembrane potentials $V_i(z,f)$ are functions of distance z from the input region and frequency $f = \omega/2\pi$. For pyramidal cells well below threshold, the membrane current source distribution is approximately proportional to transmembrane potential. *Thus, (4.24) provides an estimate of the (return) current source density distributed across the cortex due to synaptic input that is localized to a thin cortical layer.*

Equation (4.24) may be used to define a new, nondimensional length constant $\Gamma(f)$ that includes the effects of both dendritic branching and input frequency to dendrites. The transmembrane potential amplitude may be expressed as a function of distance z from the input region as

$$|V(z,f)| \propto \frac{\exp\left[-\dfrac{z}{\Gamma(f)}\right]}{\sqrt[4]{1 + (2\pi f\tau)^2}} \tag{4.30}$$

Comparison of (4.30) with (4.24) yields our estimate of axon transmembrane potential in terms of the new nondimensional length constant $\Gamma(f)$, where

$$\Gamma(f) = \frac{\lambda}{\sqrt{0.5\left(\sqrt{1 + (2\pi f\tau)^2} + 1\right)}} \tag{4.31}$$

Here λ is the length constant associated with constant input ($f \to 0$), which may include the effects of dendritic branching effects if λ is interpreted as the effective (*electrotonic*) length constant as indicated by (4.25). This definition is based on the dominance of the exponential term in (4.30). As the frequency f becomes large compared to $1/\tau$, the effective length constant $\Gamma(f)$ falls off approximately as $f^{-1/2}$.

An example application of these ideas is provided by an estimate of the expected source strength of a model minicolumn consisting of a clump of parallel, cylindrical dendrites as indicated in fig. 4-17. If the dendrites in the minicolumn are essentially identical, mesosource strength across the cortex may be estimated from (4.26). We idealize the source region as a thin disk of area A from which membrane current I emerges in the upward direction and re-enters cells higher in the cortex. In this approximation, (4.30) provides a rough estimate of membrane microsource strength expressed as a function of frequency:

$$s(z,f) = \frac{I\delta(z)}{A} - \text{Const}|V(z,f)| \tag{4.32}$$

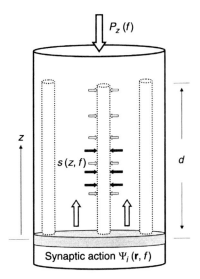

Figure 4-17 An alternative view of the process in fig. 4-16, with total source current I (due to synapses on many cells) assumed to be generated inside a thin disk of area A in the lower part of the column. In this example, we imagine the Fourier transformation of all variables to express them as functions of frequency rather than time. Synaptic action $\Psi_i(\mathbf{r}, t) \rightarrow \Psi_i(\mathbf{r}, f)$ may cause microcurrent source strengths in the deep layer that are independent of frequency, but the passive return currents that spread vertically at low frequencies (gray horizontal arrows) tend to be more confined to lower layers at high frequencies (black horizontal arrows). This is expressed in terms of the frequency-dependent space constant $\Gamma(f)$ given by (4.31). As a result of this shortening of the effective pole separations at high frequencies, mesosource strength is reduced as simulated in fig. 4-18.

Here the delta function $\delta(z)$ indicates that all synaptic input is assumed to occur in a thin layer located near $z = 0$. The constant multiplying the transmembrane potential $|V(z, f)|$ must be chosen to force the electroneutrality condition (4.27). Substitution of (4.32) into (4.26) yields the following expression for our rough estimate of the mesosource strength of the cortical column as a function of frequency:

$$P_z(f) = \frac{I}{A} \left\{ \frac{1 + \dfrac{\Gamma(f)}{d} \left\{ 1 - \exp\left[\dfrac{d}{\Gamma(f)}\right] \right\}}{1 - \exp\left[\dfrac{d}{\Gamma(f)}\right]} \right\} \tag{4.33}$$

Columns containing fibers with effective space constants equal to fiber length ($\Gamma(f) = d$) produce mesosources strengths $P_z(f) = 0.42 I/A$. The limit of very large length constants $\Gamma(f)/d \rightarrow \infty$ yields $P_z(f) = 0.5 I/A$. This mesosource strength is half the strength that would have occurred if both sources and sinks were confined to thin layers separated by distance d as in fig. 4-15. In the latter approximation, the dipole moment and volume of the column are Id and Ad, respectively, yielding a dipole moment per unit volume I/A. If the space constant is not much shorter

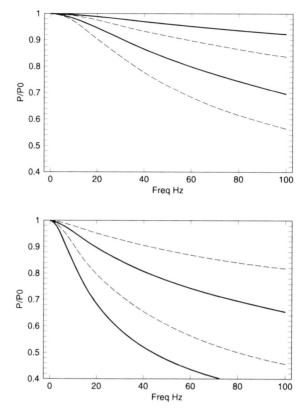

Figure 4-18 Estimates of the magnitude of the normalized mesosource function $|P_z(f)/P_z(0)|$ generated in a cortical column are plotted versus synaptic input frequency based on the simple cortical model shown in fig. 4-17 and the assumption that membrane microsource magnitude $|s(\mathbf{r},t)|$ is proportional to transmembrane potential. The four plots on each graph correspond to four ratios of the effective space constant to axon length (bottom to top) $\lambda/d = 1/4$, $1/2$, 1, and 2. (*Upper*) Bulk membrane time constant $\tau = 10\,\mathrm{ms}$. (*Lower*) $\tau - 30\,\mathrm{ms}$.

than dendrite length, the dipole moment per unit volume is not sensitive to moderate changes in length constant. In contrast, the limit $\Gamma(f)/d \to 0$ yields $P_z(f) \to 0$, that is, very short length constants result in small columnar mesosources as in the upper plot of fig. 4-13.

The estimated normalized *mesosource strength* of the column $|P_z(f)/P_z(0)|$ given by (4.33) is plotted versus synaptic input frequency for various space constants λ/d in fig. 4-18. The plots correspond to (bulk) cortical cell membrane time constants τ equal to 10 ms (upper plot group) and 30 ms (lower plot group). In each example, mesosource strength magnitude (dipole moment per unit volume) is normalized with respect to its maximum value at zero frequency, thereby emphasizing frequency effects while suppressing other influences. We have plotted curves for a wide range of time and space constants because the issue of their effective values in genuine (bulk) cortical tissue appears to be quite unsettled (Segev et al. 1995; Koch et al. 1996).

Any temporal modulation of synaptic action fields can be expressed in terms of its frequency components; high-frequency components are predicted to make smaller contributions to mesosources. While this crude calculation is based on an idealized dendritic model that neglects end effects (and many other effects), more accurate analyses are likely to agree qualitatively with the following general conclusion. *Mammalian neocortex can be expected to low pass filter its mesosources (and by implication macroscopic EEG signals) below the high-frequency range* $f > 1/\tau$, consistent with EEG recordings in a wide variety of mammalian species. That is, nearly all EEG power observed in mammal cortex lies below about 100 Hz. By contrast, invertebrate EEG spectra typically exhibit substantial relative power above 100 Hz (Bullock 1977). We emphasize that this predicted low-pass filtering is due to high-frequency reductions in mesoscopic dipole moment, not bulk tissue properties.

16 Broad Classification of the Mesosource Field $\mathbf{P}(\mathbf{r}, t)$ Based on Scalp EEG

For ease of discussion, it is convenient to define the following broad classification of dipole sources at scales between roughly 1 mm (macrocolumn) and about 1 cm, depending on application and experimental accuracy of the data being considered. Our theoretical framework has emphasized $\mathbf{P}(\mathbf{r}, t)$ at more idealized scales in the minicolumn range (≈ 0.03 mm and 100 neurons) to macrocolumn range (≈ 1.0 mm and 10^5 neurons). These structures are defined anatomically and have been proposed as basic functional units of neocortex (Mountcastle 1979; Szentagothia 1979, 1987). Perhaps they are better candidates than individual neurons because of the substantial redundancy observed within columns (see review by Nunez 1995). Scalp data are, however, limited to much larger scales. The characterizations below depend on both the temporal and spatial scales of the mesosources, as dictated by specific EEG experiments. Generally, we view the mesosource function $\mathbf{P}(\mathbf{r}, t)$ as a continuous function of time and cortical location, with localized mesosources treated as a special case.

16.1 Type I. Localized and Time Stationary

In this approximation, cortical mesosources are considered to consist of a single or perhaps a few isolated dipoles that do not change location with time. A single localized mesosource of EEG at position $\mathbf{r}_0$ may be approximated by

$$\mathbf{P}(\mathbf{r}, t) \approx g(t)\delta(\mathbf{r} - \mathbf{r}_0)\mathbf{a}_n(\mathbf{r}) \qquad (4.34)$$

Here $\mathbf{a}_n(\mathbf{r})$ is the unit vector normal to the local cortical surface, in and out of cortical folds. The mesosource magnitude varies with time according to the function $g(t)$. Evoked potential waveforms are obtained by averaging EEG over periods T in order to separate small potentials time-locked to the stimulus from spontaneous EEG. In this case t may be interpreted as the latency from the stimulus. In the example of the *somatosensory evoked potential* (SEP), 1080 electric shocks to the wrist at a typical stimulus rate of six per second requires $T = 3$ minutes. The SEP is represented here by the function $g(t)$ and appears to fit category I sources approximately for some latency range, perhaps something like 20–50 ms. The lower latency corresponds to the period before arrival of substantial synaptic input from thalamus at primary sensory cortex. The later latency corresponds to the time when substantial spread of synaptic activity to secondary cortical regions has occurred, thereby invalidating even the crude dipole approximation. Of course, the appropriate latency range depends on just how serious one takes the approximation (4.34). A mixture of time-stationary and nonstationary sources in secondary cortex can be expected at longer latencies. Because of the time-averaging procedure, only the time-stationary sources contribute substantially to the evoked potential waveform.

16.2 Type II. Localized and Nonstationary

Here each dipole (mesosource) is confined to a relatively small tissue volume for short time periods, but changes its location over time. In the case of K nonstationary dipoles:

$$\mathbf{P}(\mathbf{r}, t) = \sum_{k=1}^{K} g_k(t)\delta[\mathbf{r} - \mathbf{r_k}(t)]\mathbf{a}_k(\mathbf{r}) \qquad (4.35)$$

Epileptic spikes with multiple, moving foci at locations $\mathbf{r}_k(t)$ and with time-varying amplitudes $g_k(t)$ may fit the Type II definition approximately.

16.3 Type III. Spatially Distributed and Time Stationary

In this category, current sources are distributed over relatively large cortical regions (say from a few square centimeters to the entire cortical surface) so that neither Type I nor II approximations is valid. However, characteristic spatial patterns of amplitude are approximately constant over time when one period (perhaps a long record) T is compared to the next period. For example, the amplitude distribution of human alpha rhythm may fit this category approximately in a given subject if the averaging period T is (say) one minute and physiological state is held fixed. The time-averaged potential distribution $\langle \Phi(\mathbf{r}, t) \rangle$ is simply related to the time-average dipole moment per unit volume $\langle \mathbf{P}(\mathbf{r}, t) \rangle$. That is, from the basic relation (4.39) of section 17

$$\langle \Phi(\mathbf{r}, t) \rangle \equiv \frac{1}{T} \int_t^{t+T} \Phi(\mathbf{r}, t')dt' = \iint_S \mathbf{G}_S(\mathbf{r}, \mathbf{r}') \cdot \langle \mathbf{P}(\mathbf{r}', t) \rangle dS(\mathbf{r}') \qquad (4.36)$$

where the time-averaged mesosource function is defined by

$$\langle \mathbf{P}(\mathbf{r},t) \rangle \equiv \frac{1}{T} \int\limits_{t}^{t+T} \mathbf{P}(\mathbf{r},t')dt' \tag{4.37}$$

The condition for a crude kind of stationarity based on time averages is

$$\langle \mathbf{P}(\mathbf{r},t) \rangle \approx \langle \mathbf{P}(\mathbf{r},t+T) \rangle \tag{4.38}$$

It must be emphasized strongly that this approximate equality of time averages for large T does not imply equality for small or intermediate T. For example, the human alpha rhythm is a dynamic process for which substantial changes in spatial distribution occur on timescales in the range of several tens of milliseconds. Successive instantaneous maps (based on 500 Hz sampling) of $\Phi(\mathbf{r},t)$ are quite different when separated by about 50 ms (half a cycle for a 10 Hz rhythm), with a typical reversal of positive and negative potentials in most scalp regions, as shown in chapter 10. With 100 ms separation, potential distributions are more similar, but still vary substantially on such short timescales. This behavior is superficially similar to standing waves in a drum membrane (Nunez 1995). When time averages over $T \approx 1$ s are compared, correlation coefficients comparing successive amplitude and phase distributions tend to be small to moderate (Nunez et al. 2001). Thus, the human alpha rhythm's spatial properties are nonstationary, except perhaps in the very crude sense of similarity of successive long-time averages ($T \approx 1$ minute). This experimental observation has led some scientists to promote fixed equivalent dipoles as an "explanation" of alpha rhythm. This extreme local interpretation might be taken more seriously if alpha variability could be attributed mainly to noise; however, many alpha studies have refuted this picture. We address this issue in chapters 8–10.

16.4 Type IV. Spatially Distributed and Nonstationary in Time

In this case none of the idealizations of mesosource Types I through III is valid. While such approximations may be poor in some applications and acceptable in others, the theoretical considerations of this chapter as well as much of the available EEG data suggest that Type IV sources are the rule rather than the exception. That is, in the most general case, the *mesosource field* (or *dipole moment per unit volume*) $\mathbf{P}(\mathbf{r},t)$ changes with time and is continuously distributed over the entire neocortex (and the entire brain, excluding tissue mass that is effectively passive). More localized or stationary mesosource fields are, by the basic definition (4.26), special cases of this general picture. Given this background, a prudent approach for both experimentalists and theoreticians is to select Type IV as the preliminary classification of unknown EEG or MEG phenomena. In this manner, unbiased experimental design or theoretical development is more likely. If evidence for more localized or stationary dynamic behavior is obtained, the preliminary view can be re-evaluated. For example, data presented in chapter 10 indicate that human alpha rhythms can exhibit both local and global properties based on the same data sets. In this context, the labels "local" and "global" refer to more dominant high and low spatial frequencies, respectively, somewhat analogous to the time-domain labels "fast" and "slow" oscillations. A comprehensive view of brain dynamics must encompass a wide range of potential dynamic behaviors.

17 Macroscopic Potentials Generated by the Mesosources

The mesosource function or dipole moment per unit volume $\mathbf{P}(\mathbf{r}, t)$ is viewed as a continuous function of cortical location $\mathbf{r}$, measured in and out of cortical folds. The function $\mathbf{P}(\mathbf{r}, t)$ forms a *dipole layer* (or dipole sheet) covering the entire folded neocortical surface. *Localized mesosource activity* is then just a special case of this general picture, occurring when only a few small cortical regions produce substantial dipole moments, perhaps because the microsources $s(\mathbf{r}, t)$ are asynchronous or more randomly distributed within most columns. Or perhaps, contiguous mesosources $\mathbf{P}(\mathbf{r}, t)$ are themselves too asynchronous to generate recordable scalp potentials. For example, in the case of so-called *focal sources* occurring in some epilepsies, the corresponding $\mathbf{P}(\mathbf{r}, t)$ appears to be relatively large only in selective cortical regions at the centimeter scale. Most scalp EEG is believed to be generated in neocortex, for the reasons outlined in chapters 5 and 6. In such cases, potentials $\Phi(\mathbf{r}, t)$ at scalp locations $\mathbf{r}$ may be expressed as an integral over the cortical surface, that is

$$\Phi(\mathbf{r}, t) = \iint_S \mathbf{G}_S(\mathbf{r}, \mathbf{r}') \cdot \mathbf{P}(\mathbf{r}', t) dS(\mathbf{r}') \tag{4.39}$$

as outlined in appendix K. This integral is an important special case of the volume integral (2.2) when subcortical sources may be neglected. Some of the smaller components of evoked potentials may have significant subcortical sources, but these components are generally too small to be recorded at the scalp without time averaging. If extracortical brain regions make substantial contributions to scalp potential, (4.39) may be replaced by the volume integral over the entire brain (2.2). However, here we focus the following discussion on the most important case where EEG sources are mainly in neocortex.

As indicated in fig. 4-19, all geometric and conductive properties of the volume conductor are accounted for by the (surface) *Green's function*

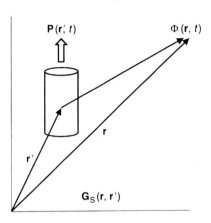

Figure 4-19 A cortical column located at **r**'
produces a mesosource (dipole moment
per unit volume) **P**(**r**', t) in cortical tissue with
Green's function G_S(**r**, **r**'). The potential Φ(**r**, t)
at any location **r** in the head is given by the
weighted integral (4.39) of **P**(**r**', t) over the cortex,
where the (surface) Green's function G_S(**r**, **r**') is
the weighting function containing all geometric
and conductive information about the
volume conductor.

G_S(**r**, **r**'), which weighs the contribution of the mesosource field **P**(**r**', t) according to source location **r**' and the location of the recording point **r** on the scalp. Contributions from different cortical regions may or may not be negligible in different brain states and applications. For example, source activity in central parts of mesial (underside) cortex and the longitudinal fissure (separating the brain hemispheres) may make negligible contributions to scalp potential in most brain states. Exceptions to this picture may occur in the case of mesial sources contributing to potentials at an ear or mastoid reference, an influence that has sometimes confounded clinical interpretations of EEG (Ebersole, 1997; Niedermeyer and Lopes da Silva 1999).

An accurate Green's function for the head volume conductor must include the geometric and conductive information and weight the integral in (4.39) accordingly. That is, G_S(**r**, **r**') will be small when the *electrical distance between scalp location **r** and mesosource location **r**' is large*. In an infinite, homogeneous medium the electrical distance equals the physical distance. However, in the head volume conductor, the two distances can differ substantially because of current paths distorted by variable tissue conductivities. Green's functions provide a standard mathematical tool used to facilitate solutions and provide physical insight for many of the partial differential equations that represent physical processes (Morse and Feshbach 1953).

In theory, a single macrocolumn could possibly produce a sufficiently large dipole moment to be scalp-recorded, but in most cases, such activity is likely to be masked by a myriad of other sources. A time-stationary macrocolumn dipole might possibly be extracted by averaging if only a single time-stationary dipole were active locally. However, this idealized case is not likely to occur in practice. In some applications source activity space averaged over (say) 10 cm^2 or more of neocortex has been characterized as a single dipole source. The use of such (often misleading) description is considered in chapter 6.

18 Summary

The theoretical bases for linear mesoscopic and macroscopic electro-physiology have been outlined. The theoretical framework supporting all applications involving spreading of currents and fields generated by current sources in volume conductors is developed from fundamental principles. *Current conservation, electroneutrality, tissue resistivity*, and *boundary conditions* are the main structural members supporting this framework. The framework will remain valid into the foreseeable future even if future advances in physiology substantially alter our views of membrane micro-sources. In order to facilitate both physiological interpretations and field calculations, we emphasize volume current sources $s(\mathbf{r}, t)$ that replace internal boundary conditions at source region boundaries as discussed in more detail in appendix K.

The subthreshold (linear) membrane diffusion equation is presented in the dual contexts of a single cylindrical cable and branched dendritic trees. The basic cable equation is derived in appendix D, and solutions obtained in appendix E. Following Rall's classic theoretical studies, an effective neuronal space constant, the *electrotonic length*, for neurons with branched dendrites is discussed. It is suggested that electrotonic lengths may be substantially shorter than expected from (constant diameter) cylindrical dendrite models. This result generally supports the idea that synaptic input to remote dendrites can have substantial influence on transmembrane potential at cell bodies, a conclusion seeming more consistent with natural selection. That is, if remote synapses do not do anything, why are they there?

The definition of effective space constant due to branching was extended to include the effects of synaptic input frequency on meso-source strength. At high synaptic input frequencies (perhaps 50 to 100 Hz), this length constant is predicted to shorten substantially due to capacitive-resistive membrane properties. This reduction in electrotonic length implies shorter average source–sink separations in neocortex at higher frequencies, thereby reducing the magnitude of the cortical mesosource function $\mathbf{P}(\mathbf{r}, t)$ and suggesting a *macroscopic low-pass filtering mechanism in cortical tissue that tends to reduce cortical potential amplitudes at higher frequencies.*

The predicted phenomenon of reduced mesosource strength at higher frequencies is quite distinct from bulk tissue capacitive effects that could theoretically cause phase shifts between oscillating sources of fixed magnitude and scalp potentials. Several experiments with living tissue, including one using an implanted dipole source in a human patient, indicate that this capacitive phase shift effect (due to mesosources of constant strength) is negligible at EEG frequencies. Furthermore, no attenuation of tissue potential occurs at higher frequencies if source strength is held fixed across frequencies.

One of the great hallmarks of human scientific progress is the ability to break down complex problems into a subset of simpler problems. Two such *breakdown simplifications* are presented here. First, the fundamental relationship between the membrane *microsources* $s(\mathbf{r}, \mathbf{w}, t)$ and tissue *mesosources* $\mathbf{P}(\mathbf{r}, t)$, given by (4.26), allows us to avoid many complications inherent in smaller-scale electrophysiology. The term "mesosource" is our shorthand for current *dipole moment per unit volume at mesoscopic scales*, for example in cortical columns or other tissue masses with linear dimensions in approximately the 0.01 to 1.0 mm range. The idealized example of section 14 shows that $\mathbf{P}(\mathbf{r}, t)$ is an approximate measure of diffuse current density across the cortex. Alternatively, mesosource strength may be expressed (approximately) in terms of mesoscopic transcortical potential V_C, cortical conductivity σ_C, and cortical thickness d_C using (4.29), that is

$$P \approx \frac{\sigma_C V_C}{d_C} \tag{4.40}$$

Using a typical value from animal experiments $V_C \approx 300\,\mu\text{V}$ and a cortical resistivity $\eta_C \approx 3000\,\Omega$ mm, (4.40) yields $P \approx 0.1\,\mu\text{A}/\text{mm}^2$, which represents the net dipole moment per unit volume after substantial cancellation effects at smaller scales (Nunez 1995).

It is also shown that *scalp potential can generally be expressed in terms of dipole moment per unit volume (or per unit area of cortex) at macrocolumn or smaller scales* as given by (4.39) or its equivalent volume integral over the entire brain (2.2). This formalism conveniently separates the effects of distributed source strength $\mathbf{P}(\mathbf{r}, t)$ from properties of the (generally subject-dependent) head volume conductor, given by the Green's function $G_S(\mathbf{r}, \mathbf{r}')$. Thus, the dynamic (time-dependent) behavior of scalp potential $\Phi(\mathbf{r}, t)$ in a linear conductive medium like the human head is just a linear weighted sum (or integral) of all the mesosource activity $\mathbf{P}(\mathbf{r}, t)$. Of course, the mesosources themselves owe their origins to both linear and non-linear neural interaction mechanisms producing the underlying *microsources* $s(\mathbf{r}, \mathbf{w}, t)$.

Evidently, this underlying dynamic behavior of microsources $s(\mathbf{r}, \mathbf{w}, t)$ may originate at multiple spatial scales ranging from single neurons to cell assemblies of different sizes to the entire neocortex and its (white matter) corticocortical and thalamocortical interconnections. The possible physiological bases for the dynamic behavior of brain sources or the closely associated synaptic actions fields $\Psi_e(\mathbf{r}, t)$ and $\Psi_i(\mathbf{r}, t)$ are considered in chapter 11.

References

Abeles M, 1982, *Local Cortical Circuits*, New York: Springer-Verlag.

Akhtari M, Bryant HC, Mamelak AN, Heller L, Shih JJ, Mandelkern M, Matlachov A, Ranken DM, Best ED, and Sutherling WW, 2000, Conductivities of three-layer human skull. *Brain Topography* 13: 29–42.

Braitenberg V, 1977, *On Texture of Brains*, New York: Springer-Verlag.

Braitenberg V, 1978, Cortical architechtonics. General and areal. In: MAB Brazier and H Petsche (Eds.), *Architectonics of the Cerebral Cortex*, New York: Raven Press, pp. 443–465.

Braitenberg V and Schuz A, 1991, *Anatomy of the Cortex. Statistics and Geometry*, New York: Springer-Verlag.

Bullock TH, 1977, *Introduction to Nervous Systems*, San Francisco: WH Freeman.

Bullock TH, 1980, Reassessment of neural connectivity and its specification. In: HM Pinsker and WD Willis (Eds.), *Information Processing in the Nervous System*, New York: Raven Press, pp. 119–220.

Cole KS, 1935, Electrical impedance of suspensions of Hipponoe eggs. *Journal of General Physiology* 18: 877–887.

Cole K, 1968, *Membranes, Ions and Impulses*, Berkeley: University of California Press.

Cole KS, Choh-luh L, and Bak AF, 1969, Electrical analogs for tissues. *Experimental Neurology* 24: 459–473.

Cooper R, Winter AL, Crow HJ, and Walter WG, 1965, Comparison of subcortical, cortical, and scalp activity using chronically indwelling electrodes in man. *Electroencephalography and Clinical Neurophysiology* 18: 217–228.

Destexhe A and Sejnowski TJ, 2001, *Thalamocortical Assemblies*, New York: Oxford University Press.

Driscoll DA, 1970, *An Investigation of a Theoretical Model of the Human Head with Application to Current Flow Calculations and EEG Interpretation*, Ph.D. Dissertation, University of Vermont.

Ebersole JS, 1997, Defining epileptogenic foci: past, present, future. *Journal of Clinical Neurophysiology* 14: 470–483.

Eccles JC, 1984, The cerebral cortex: a theory of its operation. In: EC Jones and A Peters (Eds.), *Cerebral Cortex: Vol 2. Functional Properties of Cortical Cells*, New York: Plenum.

Geddes LA and Baker LE, 1967, The specific resistance of biological material—a compendium of data for the biological engineer and physiologist. *Medical and Biological Engineering* 5: 271–293.

Geselowitz DB, 1967, On bioelectric potentials in an inhomogeneous volume conductor. *Biophysical Journal* 7: 1–11.

Goncalves S, de Munck JC, Verbunt JPA, Bijma F, Heethaar RM, and Lopes da Silva FH, 2003a, In vivo measurements of the brain and skull resistivities using an EIT-based method and realistic models for the head. *IEEE Transactions on Biomedical Engineering* 50: 754–767.

Goncalves S, de Munck JC, Verbunt JPA, Heethaar RM, and Lopes da Silva FH, 2003b, In vivo measurements of the brain and skull resistivities using an EIT-based method and the combined analysis of SEF/SEP data. *IEEE Transactions on Biomedical Engineering* 50: 1124–1128.

Hoekema R, Wieneke GH, Leijten FSS, van Veelen CWM, van Rijen PC, Huiskamp GJM, Ansems J, and van Huffelen AC, 2003, Measurement of the conductivity of skull temporarily removed during epilepsy surgery. *Brain Topography* 16: 29–38.

Jackson JD, 1976, *Classical Electrodynamics*, 2nd Edition, New York: Wiley.

Jacobson S and Pollen DA, 1968, Electronic spread of dendritic potentials in feline pyramidal cells. *Science* 161: 1351–1353.

Katznelson RD, 1981, Normal modes of the brain: neuroanatomic basis and a physiologic theoretical model. In: PL Nunez (Au.), *Electric Fields of the Brain: The Neurophysics of EEG*, New York: Oxford University Press, pp. 401–442.

Koch C, Rapp M, and Segav I, 1996, A brief history of time (constants). *Cerebral Cortex* 6: 93–101.

Koch C and Zador A, 1993, The function of dendritic spines. Devices subserving biochemical rather than electrical compartmentalization. *Journal of Neuroscience* 13: 413–422.

Kosterich JD, Foster KR, and Pollack SR, 1983, Dielectric permittivity and electrical conductivity of fluid saturated bone. *IEEE Transactions on Biomedical Engineering* 30: 81–86.

Kosterich JD, Foster KR, and Pollack SR, 1984, Dielectric properties of fluid saturated bone: effect of variation in conductivity of immersion fluid. *IEEE Transactions on Biomedical Engineering* 31: 369–374.

Lai Y, van Drongelen W, Ding L, Hecox KE, Towle VL, Frim DM, and He B, 2005, Estimation of in vivo human brain-to-skull conductivity ratio from simultaneous extra- and intra-cranial electrical potential recordings. *Clinical Neurophysiology* 116: 456–465.

Law S, 1993, Thickness and resistivity variations over the upper surface of human skull. *Brain Topography* 3: 99–109.

Llinas R, 1988, The intrinsic electrophysiological properties of mammalian neurons: insights into central nervous system function. *Science* 242: 1654–1664.

Lord Rayleigh (JW Strutt), 1892, On the influence of obstacles arranged in rectangular order upon the properties of a medium, *Phil. Mag.* 34: 481–502.

Lux HD and Pollen DA, 1966, Electrical constants of neurons in the motor cortex of the cat. *Journal of Neurophysiology* 29: 207–220.

Malmivuo J and Plonsey R, 1995, *Bioelectromagetism*, New York: Oxford University Press.

Maxwell JC, 1891, *A Treatise on Electricity and Magnetism*, 3rd Edition, New York: Dover, pp. 310–314.

Morse PM and Feshbach H, 1953, *Methods of Theoretical Physics*, Vol. 1, New York: McGraw-Hill.

Mountcastle VB, 1979, An organizing principle for cerebral function: the unit module and the distributed system. In: FO Schmitt and FG Worden (Eds.), *The Neurosciences 4th Study Program*, Cambridge, MA: MIT Press.

Nicoll RA and Alger BE, 2004, The brain's own marijuana. *Scientific American* (Dec.) 291: 68–74.

Niedermeyer E and Lopes da Silva FH (Eds.), 1999, *Electroencephalography. Basic Principals, Clinical Applications, and Related Fields*, 4th Edition, London: Williams and Wilkins.

Nunez PL, 1987, A method to estimate local skull resistance in living subjects. *IEEE Transactions on Biomedical Engineering* 34: 902–904.

Nunez PL, 1995, *Neocortical Dynamics and Human EEG Rhythms*, New York: Oxford University Press.

Nunez PL and Silberstein RB, 2001, On the relationship of synaptic activity to macroscopic measurements: does co-registration of EEG with fMRI make sense? *Brain Topography* 13: 79–96.

Nunez PL, Wingeier BM, and Silberstein RB, 2001, Spatial-temporal structure of human alpha rhythms: theory, micro-current sources, multi-scale measurements, and global binding of local networks. *Human Brain Mapping*, 13: 125–164.

Oostendorp T, Delbeke J, and Stegeman DF, 2000, The conductivity of human skull: results of in vivo and in vitro measurements. *IEEE Transactions on Biomedical Engineering* 47: 1487–1492.

Plonsey R, 1969, *Bioelectric Phenomena*, New York: McGraw-Hill.

Polk C and Postow E, 1986, *CRC Handbook of Biological Effects of Electromagnetic Fields*, Boca Raton, FL: CRC Press.

Poulnot M, Lesser G, Law SK, Westdorp AF, and Nunez PL, 1989, Unpublished study, Brain Physics Group, Tulane University, New Orleans.

Rall W, 1967, Distinguishing theoretical synaptic potentials computed for different soma-dendritic distributions of synaptic input. *Journal of Physiology* 30: 1138–1168.

Rall W, 1977, Core conductor theory and cable properties of neurons. In: ET Kandel (Ed.), *Handbook of Physiology: Vol. I. The Nervous System*, Bethesda, MD: American Physiological Society, pp. 39–97.

Ranck JB, Jr, 1963a, Specific impedance of rabbit cerebral cortex. *Experimental Neurology* 7: 144–152.

Ranck JB, Jr, 1963b, Analysis of specific impedance of rabbit cerebral cortex. *Experimental Neurology* 7: 153–174.

Ranck JB, Jr and BeMent SL, 1965, The specific impedance of the dorsal columns of cat: an anisotropic medium. *Experimental Neurology* 11: 451–463.

Redman SJ and Walmsley B, 1983, The time course of synaptic potentials evoked in cat spinal motoneurons at identified group Ia synapses. *Journal of Physiology* 343: 117–133.

Rush S and Driscoll DA, 1968, Current distribution in the brain from surface electrodes. *Anesthesia Analgesia* 47: 717–723.

Rush S and Driscoll DA, 1969, EEG electrode sensitivity: an application of reciprocity. *IEEE Transactions on Biomedical Engineering* 16: 15–22.

Scheibel ME and Scheibel AB, 1970, Elementary processes in selected thalamic and cortical subsystems: the structural substrates. In: FO Schmitt (Ed.), *The Neurosciences 2nd Study Program*, New York: Rockefeller University Press, pp. 443–457.

Schwan HP and Kay CF, 1957, Capacitive properties of body tissues. *Circulation Research* 5: 439–443.

Segev I, Rinzel J, and Shepherd GM, 1995, *The Theoretical Foundation of Dendritic Function*, Cambridge, MA: MIT Press.

Stuart GJ and Sakmann B, 1994, Active propagation of somatic action potentials into neocortical cell dendrites. *Nature* 367: 69–72.

Szentagothai J, 1978, The neural network of the cerebral cortex: a functional interpretation. *Proceedings of the Royal Society of London* B201: 219–248.

Szentagothai J, 1987, Architectectonics, modular, of neural centers. In: G Adelman (Ed.), *Encyclopedia of Neuroscience*, Vol. I, Boston: Birkhauser, pp. 74–77.

Van Harreveld A, 1966, *Brain Tissue Electrolytes*, Washington, DC: Butterworths.

Woosley JK, Roth BJ, and Wikswo JP, Jr, 1985, The magnetic field of a single axon: a volume conductor model. *Mathematical Biosciences* 76: 1–36.

5

Current Sources in a Homogeneous and Isotropic Medium

1 General Issues

The relationship of microsources at cell membranes to mesosources is discussed in chapter 4. At large scales, the brain closely approximates an electrical medium in which magnetic induction is negligible and Ohm's law is valid. These tissue properties allow for considerable simplification of the general problem of the interaction of electromagnetic fields with matter. The potentials generated in a volume conductor by known current sources then depend on just two conditions: the magnitudes and locations of the current sources and the conductivities and geometric shapes of various parts of the (generally) inhomogeneous and anisotropic medium.

In this chapter, sources in an idealized *infinite homogeneous, isotropic medium* are studied so that only the source issue applies. By "infinite" we mean that all boundaries between regions with different conductivity are far from all current sources and measuring points. All calculations in this chapter are based on current conservation at low frequencies (4.10), Ohm's law (3.15), and the low-frequency definition of potential (3.4). Medium linearity means that the potential due to any source–sink combination may be obtained by simply adding up (or integrating) the contributions from multiple point sources at different locations. Thus, the problems of this chapter are essentially problems of elementary geometry and calculus. Explicit application of Poisson's equation (4.12) is delayed until media with variable conductivity are treated in chapters 6 through 8.

The solutions presented here represent only rough approximations to genuine volume conduction in human heads. However, as we shall see in studies of inhomogeneous media in chapter 6, such approximations provide important intuitive insights into tissue volume conduction and, in any case, provide a necessary step to the more accurate descriptions required for inhomogeneous media.

2 Currents and Potentials in a Saltwater Fish Tank

This discussion of volume conductor current sources starts with a simple experiment using a fish tank full of saltwater, as pictured in fig. 5-1. An external circuit is used to generate an AC current $I(t)$ between two stimulating electrodes (star symbols at left). A second circuit containing recording electrodes measures the potential difference $V_{12}(t)$ in the water. In order to have an accurate measuring circuit, the input impedance of the amplifier must be large. It must be much larger than the impedance of electrode–fluid interfaces (plus water path) in order for the potential difference at the amplifier inputs to reflect the actual potential difference between tank locations r_1 and r_2. Amplifier impedance must also be sufficiently large so that the current $i(t)$ in the measuring circuit is much smaller than tank current to ensure that volume current is not distorted by addition of the measuring circuit. That is, one attempts to avoid the classic experimental error of inappropriate experimental methods distorting the natural processes to be measured.

To compare this simple experiment to EEG applications, note that the input impedance of modern amplifiers is typically in the 100 mega ohm (MΩ) range, whereas electrode contact impedance is typically in the 5 or 40 kilo ohm (kΩ) range (Caldwell and Villarreal 1999; Ferree et al. 2001). The impedance of a 10 cm diameter head (with electrodes placed on

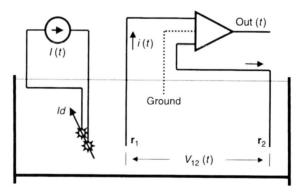

Figure 5-1 A current source $I(t)$ is used to inject AC source current into a saltwater tank. The (star) electrodes form a dipole source with arrow indicating the dipole "strength" (vector dipole moment, $\mathbf{p} = I\mathbf{d}$), where d is the pole separation. A second circuit may be used to record potential differences $V_{12}(t)$ between locations r_1 and r_2 using a differential amplifier (triangle). The amplifier is designed to produce an amplified replica of very small potential differences between its two inputs. The electrode–water interfaces produce large impedances (see fig. 5-2). A very small current through the amplifier $i(t)$ may be converted to the amplified potential difference. The ground electrode provides the amplifier with reference to (common mode) water voltages with respect to external equipment.

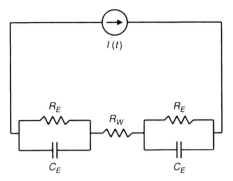

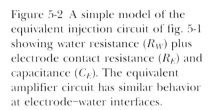

Figure 5-2 A simple model of the equivalent injection circuit of fig. 5-1 showing water resistance (R_W) plus electrode contact resistance (R_E) and capacitance (C_E). The equivalent amplifier circuit has similar behavior at electrode–water interfaces.

opposite sides) is perhaps $300\,\Omega$ (Ferree et al. 2001). Thus, in this example, head current is roughly a million times larger than amplifier current so potentials generated in the brain may be accurately measured without distorting the natural patterns of current due to internal brain sources. A possible exception involves the physically linked ears reference discussed in chapter 7.

The choice of a constant current source in the experiment of fig. 5-1, rather than a constant voltage source, allows us to largely avoid the *electrode polarization* issue. Substantial voltage changes can be expected at the interfaces between electrodes and water. That is, fish tank potentials are measured in an electrolytic medium where current consists of the movement of positive and negative ions. However, current in the metal wires consists of electron motion. Thus, chemical reactions must occur at all metal–electrolyte interfaces (Plonsey 1969; Regan 1989). Such junctions contribute their own potential changes, as indicated by an approximate equivalent circuit shown in fig. 5-2. For the purposes of this chapter, we can bypass generator circuit details, provided the current amplitude in the generator circuit is held constant.

We may also want to place the electrode shown at r_2 at the magical place called "infinity," that is, sufficiently far (*electrically far*) from the other three electrodes so that it qualifies as a *genuine reference electrode*. For location r_2 to be a genuine reference, we should be able to move it to many alternative locations (also far from the other electrodes) with minimal change in recorded potentials. For example, we might try moving the reference electrode to alternative locations close to the far right-hand wall. However, if such experiments were to yield substantial changes in recorded potential with the other three electrodes held at fixed locations, the electrode at r_2 would fail to qualify as a genuine reference. Essentially, the same arguments apply to so-called reference electrodes placed on human scalp, except that the head volume conductor typically causes more severe reference problems than suggested in fig. 5-1. This is expected because of more current and field spreading by skull and cerebrospinal fluid (CSF) tissue than occurs in the fish tank. Partly for this reason, genuine head references are more difficult to find than fish tank references. More

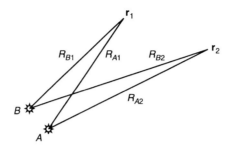

Figure 5-3 Current sources in the saltwater tank and the various distances used to calculate potentials are shown. Equation (5.1) may be used for this purpose provided all electrodes are far from tank walls and water surface.

importantly, we rarely know brain source locations in advance of our recordings (and often we still do not know locations after recording). Thus, finding a genuine reference location is not so easy.

In the idealized case where electrode 2 is a genuine reference, the potential at point $\mathbf{r}_1$ depends only on the distances R_{A1} and R_{B1} between generating electrodes A and B and the recording electrode at $\mathbf{r}_1$. In the notation appropriate for fig. 5-3

$$\Phi_1 \cong \frac{I}{4\pi\sigma} \left(\frac{1}{R_{A1}} - \frac{1}{R_{B1}} \right) \tag{5.1}$$

The approximately equal sign in (5.1) is used since this formula applies only to an infinite, homogeneous medium. The actual medium in this example consists of water of constant conductivity σ, tank walls, and surrounding air space with essentially zero conductivity. However, if the source–sink at electrodes A–B is located near the center of a large tank, an estimate of the effect of finite tank size can be obtained based on the discussion in chapter 6. The predicted effect of finite tank size is to increase the actual (or inhomogeneous) potential Φ over homogeneous potential because of compression of current paths by tank walls and water surface.

The additional error in (5.1) due to a so-called *active reference* at $\mathbf{r}_2$ can be estimated easily by treating electrode 2 as a second recording electrode, that is, in the same manner as electrode 1. The potential difference between locations $\mathbf{r}_1$ and $\mathbf{r}_2$ is then simply

$$V_{12} = \Phi_1 - \Phi_2 \tag{5.2}$$

Location $\mathbf{r}_2$ is a true reference only if $\Phi_2 \ll \Phi_1$ for many different choices of electrode locations $\mathbf{r}_2$. The EEG reference electrode issue in considered in detail in chapters 2 and 7. However, it should be emphasized that EEG practice has often involved the assumption of a so-called quiet reference without application of such simple tests of the veracity of this concept.

3 The Monopolar Source

If point $\mathbf{r}_2$ is a genuine reference and our recording electrode at $\mathbf{r}_1$ is placed close to the single point source (electrode A) but far from the sink (electrode B), the potential close to point A may be approximated as a monopole, that is

$$\Phi(r, t) \cong \frac{I(t)}{4\pi\sigma r} \qquad (5.3)$$

where $r = R_{A1}$ in this case. Equation (5.3) may be derived with a simple argument. Surround the point source with an imaginary surface of radius r. Since total current is conserved, the current density at this surface must be current/(surface area), all in the radial direction. Application of Ohm's law (3.4) to this current density yields (5.3).

In this example, local current from the source A is mostly in the radial direction away from point A. Here r is the radial coordinate in a spherical coordinate system with origin at point A. Equation (5.3) predicts that the potential in the tank becomes infinite if either the distance r or the water conductivity σ is zero. This physical impossibility results from two implicit assumptions used in deriving (5.3). First, we have assumed point electrodes, but genuine electrodes have nonzero size so r cannot actually be zero in (5.3). Also, various chemical processes can be expected near the metal−water interface. Thus, a small region near the electrode surface could have a conductivity that differs from the bulk water conductivity. It is then useful to imagine the source current emanating from a small spherical surface surrounding the electrode tip.

The second implicit assumption is that we are able to maintain constant current in the generating circuit independent of water conductivity. However, as water conductivity becomes progressively smaller, larger and larger generator voltages are required to maintain constant tank current. Thus, as water conductivity approaches zero ($R_W \to \infty$ in fig. 5-2), the current source I must also approach zero so that water potential remains finite.

Another source structure consists of uniformly distributed sources inside a saltwater-filled spherical volume. This might be simulated approximately in the tank with an electrode grid structure consisting of fine noninsulated wire. Figure 5-4 shows the case of moderate point source density within the sphere; the potential recorded by a small electrode (X) is expected to fluctuate substantially as the electrode is moved. However, when the electrode diameter is larger than the average space between point sources, we expect a relatively smooth change of potential with

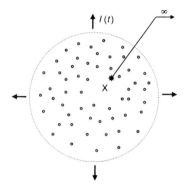

Figure 5-4 A distribution of current sources within a homogeneous spherical region is shown with a probe to record potential at point X. The total current exiting the sphere and flowing to distant sinks is $I(t)$. If the sources are continuously distributed, the potential may be calculated from (5.4). For this approximation of continuously distributed sources to be accurate, the probe diameter must be larger than the average space between sources, as indicated by the definition of coarse-grained potentials (5.30).

location because the electrode records a space-averaged potential. A possible electrophysiological analog involves small electrode measurements of extracellular potentials within the dense branches of a cortical dendritic tree or basket cell. If there are only sources (no sinks) within or near the spherical region of radius a, the potential inside the sphere (with respect to infinity) is predicted to vary with radial distance r from the center of the sphere according to

$$\Phi(r, t) \cong \frac{I(t)}{8\pi\sigma a}\left[3 - \left(\frac{r}{a}\right)^2\right] \tag{5.4}$$

Equation (5.4) is obtained by adding up (integrating over) the contributions from elemental point sources using (5.3), but here $I(t)$ is the total current generated in the entire sphere. (Sophomore physics students learn how to derive relations like (5.4) using the integral form of Gauss's law.) When $r = a$, the potential (5.4) equals that of a point source as expected. For locations $r > a$, (5.4) is not valid, but (5.3) still applies. In both examples of this section, local current is not conserved; that is, local current must enter sinks assumed to lie far outside the region of measurement. Obviously, such an assumption must be evaluated carefully in the context of any experiment, but these simple examples serve as building blocks that prepare us for studies of more representative source configurations.

4 Concentric Spherical Surfaces and Closed Fields

Here we present an example of what electrophysiological pioneer Lorente de No called a *closed field*. This simply means that sources and sinks have a certain symmetric geometric relationship so that currents and potentials

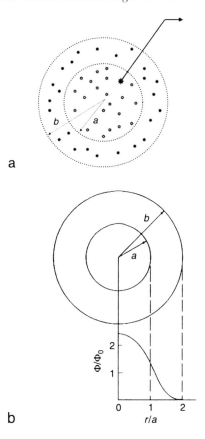

a

b

Figure 5-5   (a) An inner sphere of radius a containing a uniform distribution of current sources is surrounded by a spherical shell of radius b containing a uniform distribution of current sinks. All source current is accepted by the sinks so no current flows in the external region $r > b$. A probe (star) measures potential. (b) The internal (normalized) potential is plotted as a function of radial distance for the special case $b = 2a$ and $\Phi_0 = I/4\pi\sigma b$.

are nearly all confined to some local region. One configuration producing a closed field is a tissue volume with equal strengths of microsources and microsinks distributed uniformly throughout the volume, as discussed in chapter 4. Another example is a spherical volume of sources surrounded by a spherical shell of sinks, as indicated in fig. 5-5. Inner and outer sphere radii are given by a and b, respectively.

Possible electrophysiological applications include small electrode recordings of extracellular potentials generated by central sources, due for example to inhibitory synapses on a single cell body or central mass of cell bodies having a spherical distribution of dendrites. The surrounding dendrites provide the passive sinks. A single cortical *basket cell* having roughly spherical structure is one example. A larger brain structure that may approximate closed field geometry is the *hippocampus*, a portion of cortex in the subtemporal region with a single cell layer. Hippocampus, from the Greek word for seahorse, is essential to memory processing.

The structure is folded onto itself in a peculiar shape that may substantially limit the spread of currents and potentials outside its boundaries.

It is not necessary that the volumes of sphere and spherical shell in fig. 5-5 be equal for this source–sink structure to produce a closed field. It is only required that all the source current from the inner spherical volume enters sinks in the outer shell. While such perfect idealizations are not expected in genuine electrophysiological applications, they provide a useful framework supporting experimental studies. Separate expressions are required for the potential in the inner sphere and outer spherical shell, that is

$$\Phi = \frac{I}{8\pi\sigma b} \left\{ \frac{(b/a)^3}{(b/a)^3 - 1} [2b/a + (a/b)^2 - 3] - (r/a)^2 + 1 \right\} \quad 0 < r < a \quad (5.5)$$

$$\Phi = \frac{I}{8\pi\sigma b} \left[\frac{(b/a)^3}{(b/a)^3 - 1} \right] \left[2b/r + (r/b)^2 - 3 \right] \quad a < r < b \quad (5.6)$$

The potential is continuous across each interface as shown in fig. 5-5b. The potential at the outer surface $(r = b)$ and at every other external location $(r > b)$ is zero. That is, the spherically symmetric source–sink regions produce a closed external field. Equations (5.5) and (5.6) also satisfy boundary conditions (4.7) and (4.8). In this example, all three regions have the same conductivity so that the both the radial r and tangential (θ, ϕ) components of the electric field are continuous across both interfaces, that is

$$(\partial\Phi_1/\partial r)_{r=a} = (\partial\Phi_2/\partial r)_{r=a} \text{ and } (\partial\Phi_2/\partial r)_{r=b} = (\partial\Phi_3/\partial r)_{r=b} = 0 \quad (5.7)$$

$$(\partial\Phi_1/\partial\theta)_{r=a} = (\partial\Phi_2/\partial\theta)_{r=a} = (\partial\Phi_2/\partial\theta)_{r=b} = 0 \quad (5.8)$$

$$(\partial\Phi_1/\partial\phi)_{r=a} = (\partial\Phi_2/\partial\phi)_{r=a} = (\partial\Phi_2/\partial\phi)_{r=b} = 0 \quad (5.9)$$

Here $\Phi_3 = 0$ is the potential external to the outer shell. Note that we are free to add an arbitrary constant to the potential, as long as we do this consistently in each region. Such constant cannot change electric field or current patterns. It is customary to choose the constant so that theoretical potential goes to zero as $r \to \infty$. With this choice, potential is zero everywhere for $r > b$. The derivatives of potential must also be zero everywhere in this region (since external current is zero), thus the zeros in (5.7) through (5.9). With another choice for the arbitrary constant, the derivatives must still be zero. In chapter 6, we apply the appropriate (generally nonzero) boundary conditions at interfaces between regions having different conductivity.

Figure 5-5b shows the potential (5.5) and (5.6) as a function of radial location for the example of an outer shell with radius $b = 2a$. The volume of the shell is 7 times the volume of the inner sphere, and the density of outer sinks is $1/7$ that of inner sources. If the total current emanating from sources is a little larger than that entering sinks, some current will leak from the outer surface and the field will no longer be fully closed. If this leaking current is strictly radial, the potential in the region $r > b$ will be that of a monopole (5.3), except that the current I in this expression then refers to the excess (leaking) current. Departures from spherical symmetry can be expected to lead to such current leaks.

5 The Branched Dendrite Model: A Partially Closed Field

The *core-conductor model* outlined in chapter 4 makes use of the assumption that extracellular current is confined to a small region next to the fiber and flows only in the axial direction. Thus, the core-conductor model is most applicable to axons in fiber tracts. We also wish to model neurons of finite length with multiple dendritic branches. Several assumptions of the core-conductor model are replaced here with the condition that the neuron lies in an infinite homogeneous conductor. For this picture to correspond to realistic physiology, the external medium must be composed of a mixture of cells and extracellular fluid. Thus, the conductivity of this composite medium must be lower than that used in the core-conductor model. We expect that the extracellular potential predicted with this model will correspond in a semiquantitative way to small electrode recordings of extracellular potential.

Here we describe the branched dendrite model developed by Rall (1962), which like the core-conductor model is based on (4.5) and (4.6). The problem is to find the distribution of extracellular potential due to synaptic input to the soma. The dendritic membrane is assumed to be passive (linear) since the possibility of action potential propagation into the dendritic region is not considered. Rall solved this problem in two steps. First, he found the transmembrane potential as a function of time and location along the dendrites in a manner similar to the core-conductor model. Second, he used the calculated transmembrane potential to calculate the extracellular potential distribution. The extracellular potential can be viewed as generated by a distribution of current sources in the dendrites with strength proportional to transmembrane potential, plus a sink region at the soma.

A simple model neuron consisting of soma and cylindrical dendrite is shown in fig. 5-6. The isopotential labels correspond to a nondimensional potential, making the results more general. However, for the particular case of the cat motoneuron near its action potential threshold, the isopotential labels correspond roughly to millivolts. Potentials very close to the soma are in the -1 mV range, as measured with respect to a distant (reference) electrode. Positive potentials at one soma diameter distance from the single dendrite are typically in the 100 μV range. Thus, if an imagined small electrode (with tip diameter small compared to soma

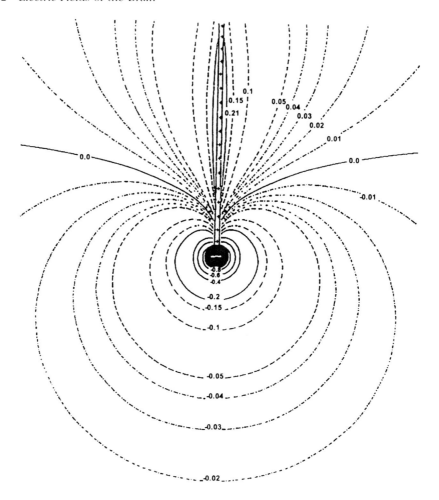

Figure 5-6   A simple model neuron consists only of soma and single passive cylindrical dendrite. The theoretical dendritic source distribution corresponds roughly to that of the peak action potential in the soma. Isopotential line labels are nondimensional potential. For the particular case of the cat motoneuron, the isopotential labels correspond roughly to millivolts. Reproduced with permission from Rall (1962).

diameter) were to be moved parallel to the neuron axis, the recorded extracellular potential (with respect to a distant reference) would change from positive to negative as the electrode tip approached the soma. The behavior is similar to that predicted by the standard core-conductor model (infinite cylindrical fiber).

As the number of dendritic branches increases, the surface area for source current increases, making current density through each source region smaller. A model neuron with seven dendritic branches is indicated in fig. 5-7, although only the three branches in the plane of the page are shown. The potential contours also apply to potentials in the plane of the page. The extracellular potential is negative everywhere within about eight soma radii of the soma, or about 0.3 mm for a typical soma radius of 35 μm. The positive potential is everywhere less than about 10 μV except

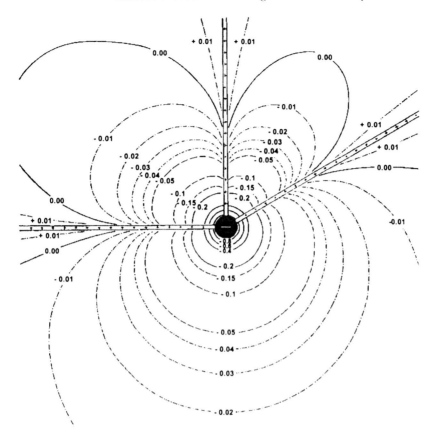

Figure 5-7 Isopotential map similar to fig. 5-6 except the model neuron has seven branches in three dimensions (only the three branches in the plane of paper are shown). The potential contours are drawn in the plane defined by these three dendrites. Reproduced with permission from Rall (1962).

for regions very close to each dendritic cylinder at intermediate distances from the soma. This model exemplifies to some extent the closed field of section 4. One similarity is that potential magnitudes fall off by factors of 100 to 1000 or more at relatively small distances. Another similarity is that if the source and sink regions of the idealized closed field model of section 4 are interchanged, the potential inside both the outer spherical shell and inner sphere are everywhere negative. Similarly, in the branched dendrite model all large potential magnitudes are negative.

Consider some of the experimental implications of Rall's theoretical work. If a small electrode were used to measure extracellular potentials near a neuron with many branches like those of fig. 5-7, the potential contours might look qualitatively different from potentials near a neuron with minor branching, as in the example of fig. 5-6. If the electrode is passed parallel to the axis of a neuron with only one branch, we may reasonably expect the sign of the potential to switch from positive to negative as the electrode passes close to the soma, as in fig. 5-6. However, a neuron with many branches might produce only very small positive potentials as in fig. 5-7. Such small positive potentials might easily be made negative by the additional effects of other neurons nearby. The electrophysiologist would then observe only a rise and fall of the magnitude of a negative potential as the electrode moved pass the soma.

Rall (1962) pointed out that this result contradicts earlier intuitive thinking by many experimental physiologists. It was once widely believed that an electrode must record a positive potential with respect to a distant (reference) electrode when placed near a portion of the membrane from which current flows into the extracellular medium. By contrast, fig. 5-7 shows that such reference potentials near the dendritic sources are negative within eight soma radii of the soma. With more branches, this distance from a soma source to a region of positive potential will generally be expected to increase. This kind of error can perhaps be avoided by keeping in mind that *current direction is determined by the local gradient of potential, as estimated by two closely spaced electrodes.* In the inner regions of the model neuron in fig. 5-7, current flows from places of small negative potential (with respect to distance reference) to places with negative potentials of larger magnitude near the soma surface. This occurs in accordance with Ohm's law (3.15) and the convention that current density direction is defined as the direction of positive charge movement, although both positive and negative ions contribute to electrolyte (or tissue) current. The branched dendrite provides an example of the pitfalls of imprecise concepts and associated language that place significance on labels such as "negativity" and "positivity" that sometime emerge from the lips of neuroscientists.

6 The Dipole Current Source

The usual *current dipole* consists of a point source I and sink $-I$, separated by a distance d, as shown in fig. 5-8a. The term "dipole" has two distinct meanings in this context. One interpretation is simply the two-monopole configuration shown in fig. 5-8a. This is perhaps the picture that comes to the minds of many physiologists and electroencephalographers when they hear the word "dipole." As a result, they may be quite skeptical of the relevance of neural dipoles because the complex source geometry associated with genuine neurophysiology looks nothing like two simple point sources. However, the word "dipole" has a second and more profound meaning that makes it generally applicable to nearly all complex source–sink configurations of interest in EEG. Perhaps it is unfortunate that physicists have adopted the same label for the two ideas, but we are stuck with this convention for historical reasons.

The dipole's importance in electrophysiology and in science generally far exceeds that of any other source configuration. The reason is that *nearly any source–sink region where the total source and sink currents are equal (local or*

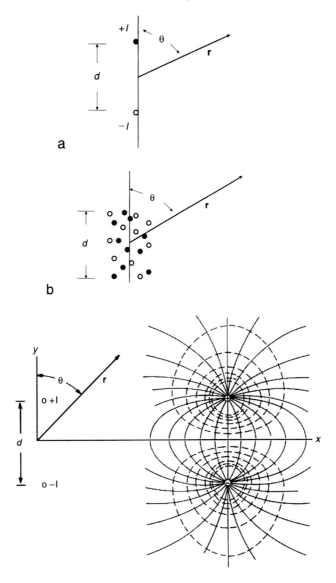

Figure 5-8 (a) The usual *current dipole* consisting of a point source $+I$ and a point sink $-I$, separated by a distance d. (b) A region of distributed sources and sinks. If local current is conserved, the potential at large distances is also dipolar, but with an effective pole separation d_{eff} smaller than d. With perfect source–sink symmetry, $d_{eff} \to 0$ and a so-called closed field is generated, as in fig. 5-5. (c) Dipole current lines (solid) and equipotentials (dashed) are plotted. These patterns occur in the saltwater tank if the tank walls and water surface are all located far from the dipole and both recording electrodes. Boundary surfaces tend to compress current lines and increase potentials.

regional current conservation) will produce an approximate dipole potential at distances large compared to the characteristic dimensions of the source–sink region. For example, the random collection of sources and sinks shown in fig. 5-8b produces a dipolar potential at distances r large compared to d. The branched dendrite models depicted in figs. 5-6 and 5-7 also produce dipole potentials at large distances, perhaps in the several millimeters to centimeters range in these examples. In other words, all source–sink configurations produce external potentials that can be expanded in *multipole expansions* as indicated in chapter 3. With local current conservation, the monopole contribution is zero. At sufficiently large distances, only the dipole term in the expansion makes a substantial contribution to the total potential at that point. Some special source geometries produce zero dipole moment so that only higher ordered terms contribute, but these require special symmetry not expected in genuine physiology.

The exact potential generated by the source–sink in fig. 5-8a in the surrounding medium is simply the sum of the two monopole contributions given by (5.1) in terms of the two distances between poles and measuring point. However, it is much more useful to express this potential in terms of a single radial coordinate r, measured from the midpoint of the two poles. That is, for distances r greater than about $3d$ or $4d$, the following dipole equation provides a reasonable approximation:

$$\Phi \cong \frac{Id\cos\theta}{4\pi\sigma r^2} \qquad (1.7)$$

where θ is the angle between the dipole axis and the vector **r** to the point of measurement, as shown in fig. 5-8a. The potential fall-off from the collection of sources and sinks shown in fig. 5-8b is also given by (1.7), but with an effective pole separation $d_{eff} < d$, as indicated by the examples in chapter 4. We emphasize that the potential due to the two monopoles in fig. 5-8a or the collection in fig. 5-8b may be generally expanded in a multipole expansion consisting of *dipole, quadrupole, octupole*, and higher order terms that are nonnegligible close to the sources. This fact may appear to be in conflict with our choice of language, that is, one might think that the physical dipole of fig. 5-8a would produce only a dipole term. Unfortunately, the "dipole" of conventional physics has led to some confusion in physiology.

Isopotential lines (dashed) and current lines (solid), which are identical to electric field lines in a linear conductor, are shown for the dipole in fig. 5-8c. In the case of the current dipole, the current density is highest where the lines are closest together. Potentials are maximum with respect to *orientation* along a line connecting the two poles ($\theta = 0°$). Potentials are zero at all locations in the plane perpendicular to this line and halfway between the poles ($\theta = 90°$). At locations above the upper (positive) pole or below the lower (negative) pole, potentials fall off rapidly with increased distance from the center of the poles. One can infer the special importance of dipoles normal to the scalp surface in producing relatively large scalp potentials because the dipole axis (of scalp surface normal dipoles) intersects the scalp surface at the shortest possible distance from the dipole center.

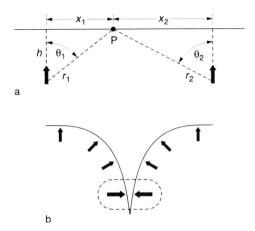

a

b

Figure 5-9 (a) Two dipole current sources located at depth h below a surface. (b) Rotated dipole sources in a cortical fissure are indicated. The potential at location P is due to the sum of contributions from each dipole. At locations large compared to the separation of the dipoles, these contributions tend to cancel. The net field is approximately quadrupolar at large distances.

7 Two Dipoles Below a Surface

Roughly 85% of cortical neurons are pyramidal cells oriented perpendicular to the local cortical surface (Braitenberg and Schuz 1991). Thus, it is of interest to consider the example of two synchronous dipole sources at equal depths h, as shown in fig. 5-9a. If the separation of the dipoles and their depths h are much smaller than the effective radius of the head, we may neglect scalp curvature in this semiquantitative argument. Also, we will first assume a homogeneous medium. Dipole 1 contributes a surface potential Φ_1 at horizontal distance x_1 as shown. Dipole 2 makes a similar contribution so that the potential at surface point P is $\Phi = \Phi_1 + \Phi_2$. From (1.5) it follows that the relative contribution of the two dipoles to surface potential is given by

$$\frac{\Phi_1}{\Phi_2} = \left(\frac{x_2^2 + h^2}{x_1^2 + h^2}\right)^{3/2} \quad \to 1 \quad h \to \infty$$

$$\to \left(\frac{x_2}{x_1}\right)^3 \quad h \to 0$$

(5.10)

The arrows indicate two limiting cases. When the dipoles are relatively deep (compared to surface separations x_1 and x_2), their contributions to surface potential are nearly equal. When they are shallow, the dipole closest to the surface point P makes the largest contribution. Although (5.10) was obtained for a homogeneous plane medium, similar qualitative behavior can be generally expected in an inhomogeneous nonplaner head medium.

This rough picture also allows us to provide a pretty good qualitative picture of surface potential due to dipoles in cortical fissures and sulci. If the upper poles are rotated towards each other, and the dipoles are close together, the dipole angles tend to satisfy the relation $\theta_1 + \theta_2 \approx \pi$ at all surface locations, as shown in fig. 5-9b. Thus, $\cos(\theta_1) \approx \cos(\pi - \theta_2) \equiv -\cos(\theta_2)$ in the two expressions of (1.7) for the two dipoles. Also, if the dipoles are close together, as in the case of equal depths in a fissure or sulci, $r_1 \approx r_2$. In this case, the surface potential from (1.7) for one dipole roughly cancels surface potential due to the other dipole; that is, net surface potential is very small. In other words, the dipole contribution to the multipole expansion becomes progressively weaker compared to the quadrupole contribution as the upper poles are rotated towards each other. If many synchronous dipoles on both sides of the fissure occur, a substantial cancellation effect also occurs. This cancellation effect applies to both EEG and MEG.

If only one side of a fissure is active, there is no cancellation effect. In this case, we may apply the following "rule of head" based on the 3 or 4-sphere model of the head (chapter 6). *The maximum scalp potential due to a tangential dipole is something like 1/2 to 1/3 the maximum potential of a radial dipole of the same strength and depth.* Of course, the potential maxima do not occur at the same location. The maximum surface potential due to a radial dipole occurs directly above the dipole on its axis. The maximum surface potential due to a tangential dipole occurs at a point intermediate between the surface intersection of the dipole axis and the point directly above the center of the dipole, typically several centimeters from a shallow tangential dipole. An additional effect that tends to reduce surface potential due to dipole sources in fissures and sulci is the increased distance between the dipoles and scalp surface as compared to dipoles in the crowns of cortical gyri. For example, a dipole in a cortical gyrus may be 1.0 to 1.5 cm from the nearest scalp location, whereas dipoles deep in sulci could be 2.0 to 3.0 cm from the local scalp. The combined effects of distance and orientation can be expected to decrease the relative contributions *of dipoles in fissures or sulci (compared to gyral dipoles) to* something like 1/2 to 1/6, other things (like source synchronization) being equal.

8 The Distributed Line Source

Here we consider the example of sources distributed uniformly over a distance d along a vertical axis, as shown in fig. 5-10. The source current all flows into a thin disk-shaped sink on the same axis. This source–sink geometry corresponds roughly to the case of extracellular current flow from a single vertical dendrite due to an *excitatory postsynaptic potential (EPSP)* at the soma. Of course, it is much more realistic to have the source current decrease with distance from the soma as in the Rall model neuron described in section 5. The actual manner in which source strength falls off

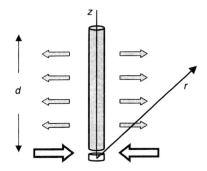

Figure 5-10   Current sources distributed over distance d along the z-axis flow into a thin sink region at $z = 0$. This source–sink geometry corresponds roughly to the case of extracellular current flow from a single vertical dendrite due to an *excitatory postsynaptic potential (EPSP)* at the soma.

with dendritic distance depends on capacitive-resistive membrane properties, as governed by the cable equation (4.16) or more complicated equations for branched dendrites. Nevertheless, our simple model reveals useful information about the extracellular (including scalp) potential using only elementary mathematics. As such it may be viewed as a first step toward more exact studies. By assuming a uniform distribution of sources along the z-axis and a thin sink at $z = 0$, (5.3) yields the following expression for *extracellular potential along the z-axis*:

$$\Phi_{\theta=0} = \frac{Id}{4\pi\sigma z^2}\left[\left(\frac{z}{d}\right)^2\log\left(\frac{z}{z-d}\right) - \frac{z}{d}\right] \tag{5.11}$$

The term in front of the square bracket is that of the dipole formula (1.5) with $(r, \theta) = (z, 0)$. The first and second terms inside the square bracket are contributed by the distributed sources and point sink, respectively. The more general expression for locations off the z-axis may be expanded in a Taylor series to obtain the multipole expansion:

$$\Phi(r, \theta) = \frac{Id}{4\pi\sigma r^2}\left\{\frac{\cos\theta}{2} + [1 + 3\cos(2\theta)]\frac{d}{12r} + \cdots\right\} \tag{5.12}$$

For distances $r \gg d$, the first term inside the brackets in (5.12) is much larger than the sum of all remaining terms. Thus, at relatively large distances, the potential is well-approximated by the dipole potential

$$\Phi(r, \theta) = \frac{Id\cos\theta}{8\pi\sigma r^2} \tag{5.13}$$

The next term in (5.12) is the quadrupole term; it falls off as r^{-3}. Equation (5.13) is identical to the usual dipole formula (1.7), but with the original pole separation d replaced by $d/2$. That is, *the effect of having sources uniformly distributed along the z axis ($0 < z < d$) rather than a point source at $z = d$ is to reduce the effective strength of the dipole to half its original value.* In more realistic cases of nonuniform source distributions over a distance d, the potential at large distances ($r \gg d$) will always be that of a dipole

(1.7), but with dipole moment (strength) less than Id. Generally, the larger the effective length constant of membrane and surrounding space (4.17) or (4.31), the larger the dipole moment created by the synaptic input to the soma. This is the basis for the low-pass filtering of membrane sources described in chapter 4; that is, *as the input frequency of synaptic action increases, the effective length constant shortens as a direct result of capacitive-resistive membrane properties.*

9 Source–Sink of Unequal Strength

The simple dipole consists of point source current (I) that flows into a point sink. By contrast, here we consider an example where only $\frac{1}{4}$ of the total sink current ($-4I$) originates at a local point source. The remaining current entering the sink originates from unspecified sources at "infinity." By this we mean that current originates from distances much larger than the source–sink separation. This could be demonstrated physically in a large spherical water tank (radius $\gg d$) with conducting walls by designing an external circuit such that the tank walls provide the missing source current $+3I$. In this case, local current is not conserved and the potential in the local region is not dipolar in nature. A Taylor expansion similar to (5.12) would include a monopole term in addition to the dipole and higher order terms. We avoid such expansion here, but rather express the potential in terms of two monopoles of unequal strength. That is, from (5.3)

$$\Phi = \frac{I}{4\pi\sigma}\left(\frac{1}{R_2} - \frac{4}{R_1}\right) \tag{5.14}$$

Here R_1 and R_2 are the distances between field point and the source and sink, respectively. The isopotential surface plot in fig. 5-11, obtained from a text on electromagnetic theory (Pugh and Pugh 1960), is based on two charges in a dielectric. Here we simply replace the charges by current sources since Poisson's equation governs the potential distribution in both instances. Note from (5.14) that the potential is negative at every location where R_2 is greater than $R_1/4$. As a result, the potential is negative everywhere in the medium except for a small region very close to the source, located at $(x, y) = (0, -d)$. For convenience, we define the non-dimensional potential $\Phi_0 = I/4\pi\sigma d$.

If one were to move a probe up along the negative y-axis in fig. 5-11, the measured potential would reach a local minimum $\Phi = -\Phi_0$ at $y = -2d$. This may be called an equilibrium point because all components of the electric field are zero here. The equipotential surface that passes through the equilibrium point actually consists of two completely closed surfaces, one inside the other and making contact only at the equilibrium point. The potential changes from negative to positive at $(x, y) = (0, -4d/3)$ and

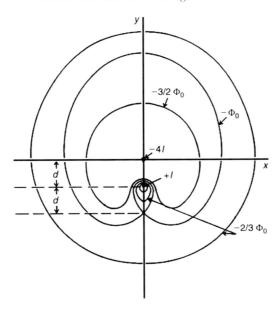

Figure 5-11 Isopotential surfaces for a point source $(+I)$ and sink $(-4I)$ of unequal strength. Local current is not conserved; that is, the sink must accept current $(+3I)$ from sources at infinity in addition to current $(+I)$ from the local source. Here "infinity" means any distance from the origin much larger than the local scale d. Modified from the corresponding electrostatic example in Pugh and Pugh (1960).

back to negative at $(x, y) = (0, -4d/5)$. As our imagined probe approaches the sink at $(0,0)$, larger magnitude negative potentials are observed. For distances from the origin that are large compared to the pole separation d (but still close enough to the origin to be far from the other sources at "infinity"), the potential is essentially that of a monopole of strength $(-3I)$.

This example source distribution demonstrates some of the complications that can confound attempts to map extracellular potentials from even relatively simple source geometry. Suppose, for illustrative purposes, that the required (balancing) distant source $+3I$ is located at $y = R$ (not shown). We can identify three distinct regions where potential is measured with an electrode of tip diameter ξ:

1. Close to the source–sink (say $r < 4d$), the potential map will generally be quite complicated. Each electrode records a space-averaged potential over the volume occupied by the electrode tip. If the potential changes rapidly over a distance of the order of ξ, the measured potential will generally be sensitive to changes in ξ, say as recorded from two different laboratories.

2. In the monopole region $(d \ll r \ll R)$, the potential may be approximated from (5.3), with total current $-3I$, that is

$$\Phi(x, y, z) = \frac{-3I}{4\pi\sigma\sqrt{x^2 + y^2 + z^2}} \tag{5.15}$$

3. In the dipole region $(r \gg R)$, the potential may be approximated from (1.7) with total current $+3I$ and pole separation R, that is

$$\Phi(x, y, z) = \frac{3IRy}{4\pi\sigma(x^2 + y^2 + z^2)^{3/2}} \tag{5.16}$$

In a genuine experiment, actual recorded potentials might differ substantially from those predicted by (5.14)–(5.16) depending on the radius of the electrode tip ξ, as discussed in section 16.

10 Distributed Source–Sink of Unequal Strength

When currents emanate from point sources, the basic monopole formula predicts infinite potentials at the sources. This is a consequence of idealizing current source regions as having zero size, but genuine physical or biological sources must be distributed over some volume. Here we consider a source–sink of unequal strength similar to that shown in fig. 5-11, except both are distributed over some volume. This might be expected, for example, if the source and sink regions each contain cell populations producing synaptic activity. The source $(+I)$ and sink $(-QI)$ are distributed over spherical volumes of radii a and b, respectively, with the sink region surrounding the origin as indicated in fig. 5-12 (left). For the sake of simplicity, we consider here only the potential and its derivatives along

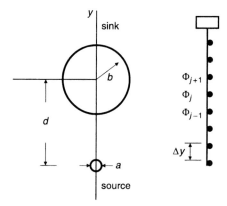

Figure 5-12 (*Left*) A source–sink of unequal strength similar to fig. 5-11 except here the source and sink regions are distributed over spherical volumes of radii a and b, respectively. Here d is the center-to-center source–sink separation. (*Right*) A probe with multiple electrode contacts of diameter ξ used to record closely spaced potential measurements at locations spaced by Δy in the cortical depths (or other tissue). The probe may be used to estimate second derivatives of potential in the axial direction y, an indicator of local current sources provided the sensor scales $(\Delta y, \xi)$ are sufficiently small compared to the source scales (a, b, d), and second derivatives of potential are sufficiently small in directions normal to the y-axis.

the y-axis. Such one-dimensional profiles might be of interest to physiologists recording extracellular potentials across the cortical depth, an important kind of study useful to establish the underlying causes of EEG. A probe to record such measurements is shown in fig. 5-12 (right).

There are five separate expressions for potential in the five regions along the y-axis. These follow directly from the expression for a monopolar source (5.3) and the equation for potential inside a spherical source region (5.4). To simplify the expressions, potentials are normalized with respect to $\Phi_0 = I/4\pi\sigma d$ and upper case letters indicate normalization with respect to the separation of the centers of the source and sink regions d, that is $Y = y/d$, $A = a/d$, and $B = b/d$.

Below the positive source region $y < -(d+a)$:

$$\frac{\Phi}{\Phi_0} = \frac{-1}{1+Y} + \frac{Q}{Y} \tag{5.17}$$

Inside the positive source region $-(d+a) < y < -(d-a)$:

$$\frac{\Phi}{\Phi_0} = \frac{1}{2A}\left[3 - \frac{(1+Y)^2}{A^2}\right] + \frac{Q}{Y} \tag{5.18}$$

Between the source and sink regions $-(d-a) < y < -b$:

$$\frac{\Phi}{\Phi_0} = \frac{1}{1+Y} + \frac{Q}{Y} \tag{5.19}$$

Inside the sink region $-b < y < +b$:

$$\frac{\Phi}{\Phi_0} = \frac{-1}{1+Y} - \frac{Q}{2B}\left[3 - \frac{Y^2}{B^2}\right] \tag{5.20}$$

Above the sink region $y > b$:

$$\frac{\Phi}{\Phi_0} = \frac{1}{1+Y} - \frac{Q}{Y} \tag{5.21}$$

It is easily verified that Φ and $\partial\Phi/\partial y$ are continuous across all interfaces between the five regions, as must be the case in a medium of constant conductivity as indicated by the general boundary conditions (5.7)–(5.9). By contrast, the second derivative $\partial^2\Phi/\partial y^2$ is discontinuous across these interfaces.

The potential Φ and its derivatives $\partial\Phi/\partial y$ and $\partial^2\Phi/\partial y^2$ are plotted verses vertical location y for the special case $(A, B, Q) = (0.1, 0.4, 4)$ in fig. 5-13. By choosing the sink strength $Q = 4$, this example is made similar to that of the point sources in fig. 5-11. Except for a very narrow region near the positive source, the potential is everywhere negative. An electrode probe sampling discrete locations in the cortical depth might easily miss this region. Furthermore, if measurements were made below a physiological source region of this kind, only negative potentials would be recorded, perhaps fooling the experimentalist by suggesting a nearby sink. As in the

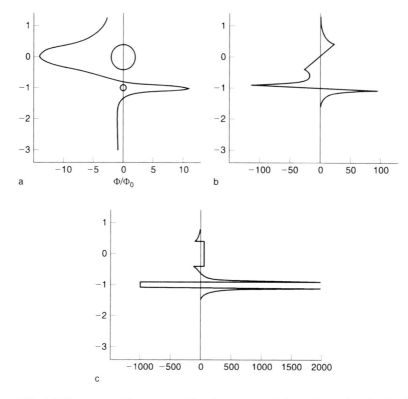

Figure 5-13 (a) The potential generated by the source–sink configuration in fig. 5-12 is plotted as a function of normalized vertical distance $Y = y/d$. Parameters are normalized such that $A = a/d$, $B = b/d$. All plots correspond to the case $\{A, B, Q\} = \{0.1, 0.4, 4.0\}$. (b) The first derivative $\partial \Phi / \partial Y$ is plotted versus Y. (c) The second derivative $\partial^2 \Phi / \partial Y^2$ is plotted versus Y. These analytic variables are defined at points rather than the experimental space-averaged potentials recorded by the probe in fig. 5-12.

examples of the Rall model neuron (section 5) and point sources (section 9), the sign of local potential does not necessarily match the sign of the nearest source or sink.

The presence of localized source or sink regions is more clearly indicated by the second spatial derivative of potential $\partial^2 \Phi / \partial y^2$, which is discontinuous in their vicinity, as indicted in fig. 5-13c. Negative second derivatives are associated with positive source regions. The second derivative at any vertical location y_i may be approximated by a variety of expressions, the simplest being

$$\left[\frac{\partial^2 \Phi}{\partial y^2} \right]_i \approx \frac{\Phi_{i+1} - 2\Phi_i + \Phi_{i-1}}{\Delta y^2} \tag{5.22}$$

where the Φ_i refer to potential measurements at successive vertical locations separated by Δy. Thus, second derivatives may be estimated from experimental potential profiles in cortical depth as shown in figs. 4-1 and

5-12. Experimentalists must, of course, be concerned with the sensor scales $(\Delta y, \xi)$ in comparison with the source scales (a, b, d). The theoretical depth profiles shown in fig. 5-13 can only be achieved experimentally when the former (recording) scales are much smaller than the source scales.

The second derivative measure obtained with this procedure is sometimes called *current source density* (CSD), but it should not be confused with scalp surface Laplacian estimates described in chapter 8, also sometimes referred to as current source density. Both methods involve estimation of second derivatives, but the underlying theoretical bases differ in important ways. For one thing, the utility of the scalp surface Laplacian depends on the presence of a poorly conducting skull layer to focus intracranial current in the direction normal to its surface. This current focusing property makes the outer skull surface act as a "source", but this is not a membrane source. By contrast, cortical depth recordings make use of second derivatives of potential in the direction of columnar axes, taking advantage of experimental observations (columnar morphology and electrophysiology) that derivatives in directions normal to columnar axes tend to be small. If axis-normal derivatives of potential are not small compared to axial derivatives, source location must be based on estimates of second derivatives in all three directions, a difficult, if not impossible, task in living tissue (Lopes da Silva et al. 1978; Petsche et al. 1984; review in Nunez 1995). The fact that the two approaches are both called "CSD" has led to some confusion in the EEG literature. We make additional efforts to clarify this distinction in chapters 2 and 8.

In order to obtain accurate estimates of second spatial derivatives from discrete measurements of potential as in (5.21), a number of closely spaced samples are required. If Δy is too large (fig. 5-12), large errors in estimates of the second derivative will occur even with accurate potential estimates. Discontinuity of the second derivative only occurs when there is a distinct boundary separating source from nonsource regions in the surrounding medium. Despite these experimental limitations, estimation of second derivatives of potential across the cortical surface has proven to be of considerable value in locating sources of activity evoked by nerve stimulation (Humphrey 1968), alpha rhythm in dogs (Lopes da Silva et al. 1978), spontaneous and evoked potentials in rabbit (Petsche et al. 1984), and evoked potentials in cat (Mitzdorf and Singer 1978) and macaque (Mitzdorf and Singer 1979). Generally, it is recommended that second derivative plots be presented together with potential and first derivative plots to make interpretations easier.

We again remind readers that any attempt to interpret experimental recordings in the brain depth must account for electrode size ξ. For example, if the electrodes shown in fig. 5-12 were to represent actual size relative to the indicated source distribution, only a smeared version of the potential profile of fig. 5-13 would be recorded, missing the small source region entirely.

11 The Quadrupole Source

Certain source–sink configurations with special symmetry produce potentials, that when expressed as *multipole expansions*, have both the monopole and dipole terms equal to zero. In such cases, the potential at intermediate and large distances is given approximately by the first nonzero term in the expansion, the *quadrupole term*. While such perfect symmetry of sources and sinks is not expected in genuine physiological systems, the quadrupole is worth consideration as a limiting case of physiologic source–sink configurations where the dipole term is relatively small over some range of distances.

Figure 5.14 shows two source–sink configurations that produce quadrupole potentials, the linear quadrupole (fig. 5-14a) and the two-dimensional quadrupole (fig. 5-14b). In both cases, the total source–sink current is zero. By contrast to the examples in sections 9 and 10, local current is conserved for both source–sink configurations so the monopole contribution to the potential is zero in both cases. The linear quadrupole

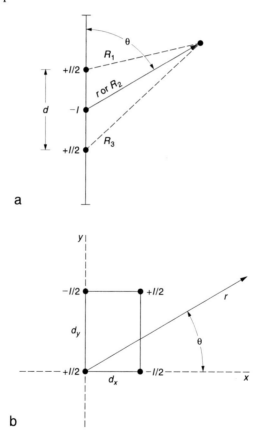

Figure 5-14   Two source–sink configurations that produce quadrupole potentials at large distances. (a) A linear quadrupole. Current $(+I/2)$ from two end points flows to a point sink $(-I)$ in the center. (b) A two-dimensional quadrupole. Current $(+I/2)$ at two corners flows into sinks $(-I/2)$ at the other two corners.

consists of two sources $(+I/2)$ and a sink $(-I)$ along a line with the two pole separations equal to d. As such, it bears some similarity to the *triphasic source distribution of the action potential*. The potential at any point in the surrounding conductive medium follows directly from the relation for the monopolar source (4.15) or (5.3):

$$\Phi = \frac{I}{4\pi\sigma}\left(\frac{1}{2R_1} - \frac{1}{R_2} + \frac{1}{2R_3}\right) \tag{5.23}$$

Here the three values of R are the three distances between sources and sink and measurement point as shown in fig. 5-14a. At intermediate or large distances, the potential may be expressed more simply in the spherical coordinate system (r, θ, ϕ). The first nonzero term in the multipole expansion is given by Panofsky and Phillips (1955)

$$\Phi \cong \frac{Id^2}{32\pi\sigma r^3}(3\cos^2\theta - 1) \tag{5.24}$$

The fact that the potential falls off as $1/r^3$ identifies it as a quadrupole potential. The potential is independent of the angle ϕ (longitude), but depends on the angle θ (latitude measured from north pole) between the quadrupole axis and vector $\mathbf{r}$ as shown. Unlike the dipole, the quadrupole potential is not zero on the horizontal axis passing half way between the two outer poles, rather zero potential occurs along two lines defined by $\cos^2\theta = 1/3$, or $\theta \approx 54.7°$, $125.3°$, $234.7°$, and $305.3°$. The potential of the two-dimensional quadrupole in fig. 5-14b is given by

$$\Phi \cong \frac{3Id_xd_y \cos\theta \sin\theta}{8\pi\sigma r^3} \tag{5.25}$$

The potential (5.25) also falls off as $1/r^3$, but with different angular dependence from that of the linear quadrupole.

A short intuitive explanation for the relationship between monopole, dipole, and quadrupole potentials follows. Monopoles produce a potential that falls off as $1/r$. When two monopoles of equal magnitude but opposite sign are combined, there is a large cancellation effect so that the net result is a dipole potential that falls off as $1/r^2$ at distances large compared to the pole separation. Similarly, when two dipoles are combined with certain perfect symmetries, the cancellation effect results in a quadrupole potential that falls of as $1/r^3$ at distances large compared to the pole separation. Octupoles with potential falling off as $1/r^4$ may be produced by combining quadrupoles, and so on. Multipoles are defined only in terms of their radial dependence on potential; the angular dependence depends on the actual configuration of sources and sinks and has no simple description. When local current conservation holds, the cancellation effect forcing the monopole contribution to zero is perfect. However, no equivalent biological principle is likely to force the dipole term to zero, although quadrupole sources have sometimes been proposed for the action potential. We suggest that this is generally a poor source model for the action potential in section 12.

12 A Crude Model for the Extracellular Action Potential

The *action potential* traveling along a single axon is *triphasic* if by "potential" one means *surface potential with respect to a distant reference electrode*. However, *transmembrane potential* is monophasic as shown in fig. 5-15. When membranes behave as linear conductors, current source distribution mimics transmembrane potential; however, active membranes are inherently nonlinear. This nonlinearity is immediately evident from the monophasic nature of the transmembrane potential. That is, the membrane source–sink distribution cannot be monophasic because membrane source current must have matching sinks somewhere along the membrane.

In order to calculate the extracellular potential of the single-fiber action potential, nonlinear membrane properties must be obtained as functions of location along the fiber, especially sodium and potassium conductances as nonlinear functions of transmembrane potential. Various theoretical and experimental analyses of action potential propagation have been studied extensively since the Nobel prize-winning work was first published

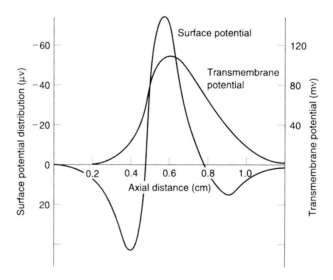

Figure 5-15 The (monophasic) transmembrane potential as a function axial location along the crayfish lateral giant axon was obtained from experiment. The (triphasic) surface potential (with respect to a distance reference) was computed from the experimental data. The peak magnitude transmembrane potential is of the order of 100 mV, whereas the surface potential peak is about 70 µV with respect to distant reference, or about a thousand times smaller. Reproduced with permission from Clark (1967).

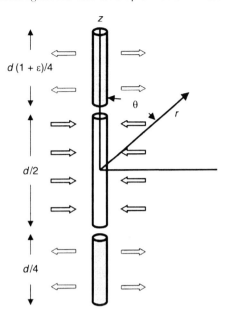

Figure 5-16 A crude model for the source distribution of the action potential. A triphasic line source similar to the linear quadrupole discussed in section 11 is proposed, except that the point sources and sink of fig. 5-14a are replaced here by distributed source and sink regions. The lower source region has total current $+I/2$ uniformly distributed over a region of length $d/4$, and the middle sink region has total current $-I$ uniformly distributed over a length $d/2$. An asymmetry not present in the discrete quadrupole is introduced by uniformly distributing the upper source $+I/2$ over a length $d(1+\varepsilon)/4$.

by Hodgkin and Huxley in 1952. Readers may be interested in excellent accounts by a leading electrophysiologist of the time, Cole (1968), or to a more recent summary by Malmivuo and Plonsey (1995). We do not repeat these analyses here. Rather, we focus on the general *triphasic* nature of the action potential current source distribution.

Figure 5.16 shows a triphasic line source similar to the linear quadrupole discussed in section 11, except here the point sources and sink of fig. 5-14a are replaced by distributed source and sink regions. The lower source region has total current $+I/2$ distributed over a region of length $d/4$, and the middle sink region has total current $-I$ distributed over a length $d/2$. We introduce an asymmetry not present in the discrete quadrupole by distributing the upper source $+I/2$ over a length $d(\varepsilon+1)/4$. Since total source current equals total sink current, the monopole contribution to extracellular potential must be zero. We may expect (correctly) that when there is perfect source–sink symmetry about the horizontal axis (the case $\varepsilon=0$), the dipole contribution is also zero and the extracellular potential at large distances $(r\gg d)$ from the fiber must be quadrupolar. This quadrupole potential is

$$\Phi(r,\theta) \cong \frac{Id^2(3\cos^2\theta - 1)}{64\pi\sigma r^3} \tag{5.26}$$

This is exactly half the potential (5.24) produced by the point quadrupole (fig. 5-14a). Both the fall-off with r and angular variation of potential are identical; only the strength is reduced by distributing the source regions.

In comparing the symmetric, idealized triphasic current source distribution of fig. 5-16 with the genuine source distribution of an action potential (Malmivuo and Plonsey 1995), we note two obvious differences. First, there is no physiological reason for the source distribution to be symmetric; that is, we expect $\varepsilon \neq 0$ for genuine action potentials. This is easily accounted for—the multipole expansion for the extracellular potential is obtained by integrating over the distributed source–sink regions in (5.16), that is

$$\Phi(r,\theta) \cong \frac{Id}{4\pi\sigma r^2} \left[\frac{\varepsilon \cos\theta}{4} + \frac{(3+5\varepsilon+4\varepsilon^2)(3\cos^2\theta-1)}{48}\left(\frac{d}{r}\right) + \vartheta\left(\frac{d}{r}\right)^2 \right]$$

(5.27)

The first term inside the square bracket of (5.27), which shows the characteristic $1/r^2$ dipole behavior, is zero for the special case when the line source is symmetric ($\varepsilon = 0$). The second term is that of the quadrupole (5.26). The symbol ϑ in the far right-hand term stands for standard mathematical jargon indicating multipole terms *of order* $(d/r)^2$ (and higher). When multiplied by the factor in front of the bracket, these are the *octupole* plus all other terms. Equation (5.27) reduces to (5.26) when $\varepsilon = 0$ as expected. When ε is not zero but small, *dipole, quadrupole, and higher order terms generally contribute to the potential at intermediate distances* with relative contributions dependent on the magnitude of ε and measurement location (r, θ).

Our motivation for expressing extracellular potential as multipole expansions is to produce analytic expressions that are easily interpreted intuitively, especially for applications where only one term, usually the dipole term, need be retained. However, when plotting the extracellular action potential, the exact expression is required because, in the case of myelinated fibers, we are interested in potentials at locations closer than the action potential length, that is, $r < d$. The exact expression is equivalent to a multipole expansion in which an infinite number of terms is retained. Figure 5.17 shows plots of extracellular potential as a function of radial distance (r/d) along the horizontal axis $(\theta = \pi/2)$ for symmetry parameter $\varepsilon = 0$ (lower curve) and $\varepsilon = 4$ (upper curve). The potential is normalized with respect to its value at $r/d = 0.0167$. If the action potential length is $d = 60$ mm, this normalization matches that used in the frog nerve experiment discussed in the next section. The qualitative behavior of extracellular potential close to the line source is relatively insensitive to the symmetry parameter ε. Of course, at very large distances, the symmetry parameter makes a big difference. However, in the case of genuine brain compound action potentials, such locations are typically far outside the head.

13 Experimental Measurement of the Extracellular Action Potential

Our idealized triphasic source is expected to differ from the genuine action potential in several ways. Genuine action potential source and sink

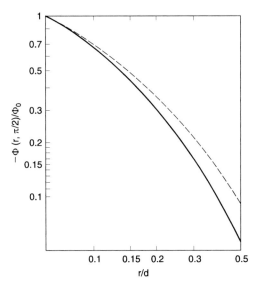

Figure 5-17   The theoretical extracellular potential of the triphasic line source of fig. 5-16 is plotted as a function of radial distance (r/d) along the horizontal axis ($\theta = 0$) for symmetry parameter $\varepsilon = 0$ (lower curve) and $\varepsilon = 4$ (upper curve). The calculation involves integrating the monopolar source function (5.3) over the line source with $I \to K dz$, where K is source current per unit length of "fiber." The behavior of the predicted extracellular potential near the axis is shown to be insensitive to the symmetry parameter ε. The potential is normalized with respect to its value at $r/d = 0.0167$. If the action potential length is $d = 60$ mm, this normalization matches the experimental plot in fig. 5-18b reasonably well.

current will vary with location within each source or sink region (Malmivuo and Plonsey 1995), rather than be constant over each region as assumed in fig. 5-16. While the actual source–sink distribution of the action potential may be of great interest to electrophysiologists working at cellular scales, such detailed information does not appear critical to EEG studies as suggested by the theoretical–experimental comparison of this section.

Additional complications to consider are action potentials in myelinated fibers and compound action potentials. The action potential length d, which is the nonlinear (active) analog of the neuron length constant, is much longer in myelinated than in nonmyelinated fibers. The extracellular potential from the compound action potential can then be expected to be considerably larger at large distances. If a nerve contains a mixture of myelinated and nonmyelinated axons, we expect the extracellular compound action potential to be due mainly to the myelinated fibers at centimeter-scale distances.

In support of these arguments, consider the following experiment to measure the extracellular potential generated by a compound action potential in the *frog sciatic nerve*, shown in fig. 5-18a (Flick et al. 1977). The compound action potential has a reported length $d \cong 6$ or 7 cm. The measured fall-off of potential with radial distance r, roughly along the horizontal direction $\theta = \pi/2$, is shown in fig. 5-18b. Extracellular potential varies from approximately 50 μV near the nerve surface ($\cong 1$ mm) to about

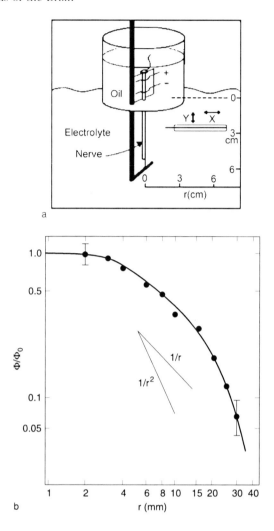

Figure 5-18 (a) Tank containing a frog sciatic nerve and probe used to measure the action potential as a function of distance r from the nerve axis. The compound action potential has a length of 60 or 70 mm. (b) Log–log plot of the potential (with respect to a distant reference) normalized with respect to its value at $r = 1$ mm. Reproduced with permission from Flick et al. (1977).

3 µV at a perpendicular distance of 3 cm. The experimental data in Fig. 5-18b and the idealized extracellular potential generated by the triphasic line source of figs. 5-16 and 5-17 are in semiquantitative agreement even though many details were omitted from the idealized model. For example, if the action potential length is $d = 60$ mm, the measurement at $r = 1$ mm (shown in fig. 5-18b) corresponds to the normalization used in fig. 5-17. Both theoretical and experimental potentials fall by about 95% as r is increased from 1 to 30 mm. More accurate calculations are required to determine the genuine action potential source distribution (Plonsey 1974) and the effect of the finite

Table 5-1 Action potential characteristics of several mammalian nerve fibers

Fiber type	A	B	C	drC
Diameter (μm)	1–22	≤ 3	0.1–1.3	0.4–1.2
Conduction velocity (m/s)	5–120	3–15	0.7–2.3	0.6–2.0
Spike duration (ms)	0.4–0.5	1.2	2.0	2.0
Action potential length (cm)	0.2–6.0	0.4–2.0	0.1–0.6	0.1–0.4

medium. For example, the free surface of the water (fig. 5-18a) can be expected to slow the fall-off of potential near the fiber.

Table 5-1 shows data for various mammalian nerve fibers (Rush et al. 1965). The action potential length d_{AP} is related to its duration T_{AP} (with respect to a fixed electrode) and propagation velocity v_{AP} by the relation

$$d_{AP} = T_{AP}v_{AP} \qquad (5.28)$$

The compound action potential of the auditory nerve has been suggested as a source of at least some components of the *brainstem auditory evoked response* (*BAER*) shown in Fig 1-17 (Jewett 1970; Jewett and Williston 1971). The theory and experiment discussed here suggest that axons generating long action potentials (implying myelinated fibers) can easily produce potentials in the few microvolt range at several centimeters distance from such axons. This picture is consistent with mammalian auditory nerve fibers, which are mainly myelinated.

Our idealized theoretical and experimental studies are limited to potentials generated in an infinite homogeneous medium, making our estimates of surface potential inaccurate. If we were to place a long nerve inside a homogeneous volume conductor (say to simulate the auditory evoked potential), potentials near the surface would be much larger than those predicted for an infinite medium. The multiplying factors due to confining the current inside an inhomogeneous medium like the head differ for each portion of the action potential. That is, chapter 6 indicates that multiplying factors for deep sources are greater than one (by compressing distant current lines), whereas multiplying factors for superficial sources will be less than one (due to dominant skull effects). Such effects will substantially distort action potential waveforms measured on the surface that travel between superficial and deep head locations, as in the auditory nerve. Additional waveform distortion is expected as an action potential passes between regions of different conductivity or when it passes a bent portion of axon (Stegeman et al. 1987). Because the auditory nerve does not follow a straight line, any theoretical prediction of scalp surface potential waveform must also account for this geometry as well as effects occurring when the action potential reaches the axon end.

Several of these issues were addressed in experiments with frog sciatic nerves placed in cylindrical (Deupree and Jewett 1988) and spherical tanks (Jewett et al. 1990). For example, extracellular potentials in the cylindrical tank showed no attenuation with axial distance over the tank dimensions. This may be explained by the compression of extracellular current lines by the nonconducting cylindrical walls. Action potentials recorded at the walls of the spherical tank were qualitatively consistent with the $\cos\theta$ dependence of the dipole term in (5.27).

Given the severe limitations on making realistic predictions of surface waveforms due to long action potentials in a genuine nerve fiber, readers can perhaps appreciate why we presented such an oversimplified action potential source model in this section. For purposes of predicting scalp potential waveforms, errors associated with the complications of genuine nerves and volume conductors outlined above are likely to be much larger than errors due to our oversimplification of the source model. Nevertheless, we argue here that predicted *scalp potential magnitudes due to compound action potential sources appear to be quite adequate to account for the brainstem auditory evoked potential*. In section 14 we suggest that *synaptic action along the auditory pathway may also produce scalp potentials of sufficient magnitude to contribute to the BAER*, although the case for action potential contributions appears to be much stronger because of the large size of the source–sink regions of compound action potentials.

14 Dipole Potentials Measured in the Superior Olive of Cats

In this section we discuss depth electrode measurements at various distances from a mass of neurons with known geometric structure: the superior olivary nucleus of cats, closely following the work of Biedenbach and Freeman (1964) and Freeman (1975). The anatomy of superior olive, the second relay station in the auditory pathway, has been described in detail (Stotler 1953). It has two major cell groups as pictured in fig. 5-19a. The medial segment of the superior olive is a flat plate of spindle-shaped cells. Their dendrites project in two directions, medially and laterally, perpendicular to the plate. The medial dendrites receive synaptic input from fibers from the contralateral cochlear nucleus, whereas the lateral dendrites receive input from the ipsilateral cochlear nucleus.

The potentials measured in the surrounding tissue due to synaptic activity in the superior olive are expected to be strongly influenced by the geometric arrangement of the cells. In the medial segment, the dendrites are oriented in parallel, and the afferent axons that are stimulated end on the same side of the cell layer. If these neurons are activated by synchronous input, the resulting evoked potentials of individual cells are expected to sum in accordance with the principle of linear superposition, discussed in chapter 4.

If local current is conserved, the potential at intermediate and large distances is expected to exhibit approximate dipolar behavior. We do not expect exact agreement for several reasons. First, the potential close to the

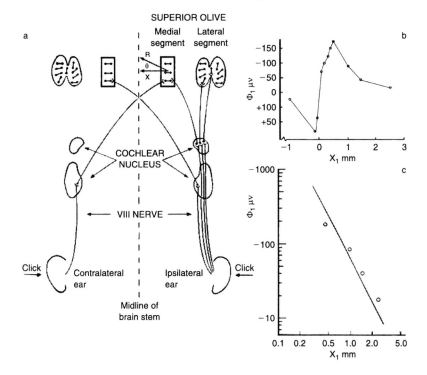

Figure 5-19 (a) The anatomy of the cat superior olive, the second relay station in the auditory pathway, is outlined. Cells in the medial segment are oriented in parallel, whereas cells in the lateral segment form an S-shaped plate. Modified from Stotler (1953). (b) Potential as a function of location along a tract through the superior olive, evoked by a contralateral ear click as recorded by Biedenbach and Freeman (1964). The origin is defined by the isopotential line. (c) Log–log plot of potentials recorded at the four most distant locations in plot (b). The line's slope is $n = -1.83$ corresponding roughly to the fall-off of potential from a dipole.

neural mass will be determined mostly by the three-dimensional shape of the cell plate, which partly determines the particular source-sink distribution. Second, the prediction of a dipolar fall-off of potential is based on the assumption of an infinite homogeneous medium.

The geometry of the lateral segment of the superior olive is quite different from that of the medial segment. The lateral segment is composed of a tightly curved S-shaped plate of cells receiving input from the ipsilateral cochlear nucleus. Thus, the synaptic current sources appear to consist of many small dipoles oriented in different directions. As a result, we expect a large cancellation effect. The net potential generated by the lateral segment should be much smaller than that generated by the medial segment at locations outside the neural mass. In other words the lateral segment should produce a reasonable approximation to a *closed field*.

The predictions outlined above were verified by the experiments of Biedenbach and Freeman. A series of click sounds were presented to the cat's ears to stimulate the superior olivary nucleus. Depth recordings were obtained a various locations, and spatial maps of the averaged evoked potential were constructed for various histological sections at a number of stereotaxic levels. Ipsilateral clicks cause EPSPs on the lateral side of the medial segment. This synaptic input causes current sinks on the lateral side that accept source current from the medial side of the medial segment. Thus, potentials recorded on the medial side are positive with respect to potentials on the lateral side. Medial side potentials are also positive with respect to a distant reference in this case because of the simple source–sink geometry. Contralateral clicks produce EPSPs on the medial side, producing sinks on the medial side and sources on the lateral side; the sign of all potentials is reversed from those of the ipsilateral clicks. In each experiment, there was a clear-cut zero isopotential. The S-shaped lateral segment apparently contributed very little to the potential as expected. That is, the potential of the lateral segment is approximately that of a *closed field*.

Potentials measured at multiple locations along a single electrode tract are plotted for the case of ipsilateral stimulation in fig. 5-19b. Position is measured from the isopotential line: positive is towards the medial side. The largest recorded amplitudes were in the 500 to 700 μV range; however, the plots shown here reflect clicks of submaximal intensity, producing maximum potentials in the 150 μV range. The precise spatial variation of potential within the nucleus must depend on source details; however, fig. 5-19b shows roughly the expected potential profile of a source–sink combination, involving either point or more realistically distributed line sources.

At relatively large distances, we expect the potential to fall off approximately as a dipole. Figure 5.19c shows a log–log plot of the four most remote potential measurements. At such distances, the potential is seen to fall off roughly as $1/r^n$, where $n \approx 1.83$ is the negative slope of the log–log plot. Within the limits of accuracy expected (from both the experiment and idealization of an infinite homogeneous medium), the potential fall-off is close to the expected dipolar behavior $n = 2$. The data suggest that the potential at even larger distances r can be estimated from the relation

$$\Phi \cong \Phi_0 \left(\frac{r}{r_0}\right)^2 \cos\theta \qquad (5.29)$$

Here Φ_0 is the maximum potential (recorded for $\theta = 0$) at an intermediate or relatively large distance r_0. The usual dipole angle θ is ambiguous at short distances because of the two-dimensional nature of the plate of cells forming the medial segment. However, at larger distances, the plate can be viewed as a single dipole so that θ is well defined as suggested by fig. 5-19a. In the case of the particular submaximal data shown in fig 5-19c, potentials in the 20 μV range were recorded at $r_0 \approx 2$ mm. The largest potentials at this distance were in roughly the 50 μV range. From

(5.28) we estimate that the corresponding potentials at locations $r \approx 1$ cm are 1 or 2 μV.

It was suggested in section 13 that the compound action potential of the human auditory nerve might produce potentials in the range of several microvolts or more at distances of several centimeters from the nerve. This is sufficient magnitude to be recorded on the scalp with appropriate averaging techniques. We can put forth a similar argument about synaptic potentials generated at the various relay stations along the auditory pathway. However, if such argument is to be based on the data shown in fig. 5-19, an appropriate extrapolation from cat to human anatomy is required. If cat and human brains scaled similarly, human pole separation in the superior olive would be about 3.5 times larger than the same structure in cat (Nunez 1995). This scale factor is simply the cube root of the ratio of the human to cat brain volumes. If this simple transformation were valid, human potentials due to a dipole in the superior olive would be 3.5 times larger than the equivalent cat potentials because dipole moment is proportional to pole separation. Anatomical reality is not so simple; the olfactory bulb of cat is actually about the same size as the human olfactory bulb, reflecting the much greater importance of cat's sense of smell.

An additional consideration is the effect of conductive inhomogeneity on these estimates, especially those of the high-resistance skull and finite size of the head. Whereas the skull acts to reduce scalp potentials due to internal sources, the effect of confining currents inside the head is to increase scalp potentials over estimates based on the assumption of an infinite, homogeneous volume conductor. It is shown in chapter 6 that, in the case of deep sources, the net result of skull and finite head size is to increase scalp potentials by roughly a factor of two over the homogeneous case. From these semiquantitative arguments, *we tentatively conclude that both synaptic and action potentials generated along the auditory pathway are capable of contributing to BAER component waveforms at the scalp, although the argument supporting action potential origins appears much stronger.*

15 Dipole Layers: The Most Important Sources of Spontaneous EEG

Dipole layers or "sheets" appear to be the most important source configurations for studies of spontaneous EEG. The reason is that nearly all scalp potentials recorded without averaging are believed to owe much of their origins to cortical dipole layers with differing locations, sizes, and shapes, perhaps generated mainly in the crowns of cortical gyri for reasons discussed below. Isolated cortical dipoles, often used as models for somatosensory evoked potentials and epileptic spikes, are simply special cases of dipole layers with very small dimensions. The single dipole description is appropriate when dipole layer sources occupy cortical regions with characteristic size much smaller than the local distance between cortex and scalp or about 1 cm.

The *mesosource vector* $\mathbf{P}(\mathbf{r}, t)$ of each tissue mass is defined as the dipole moment per unit volume in chapter 4. Cortical dipole layers occur when any of the components of $\mathbf{P}(\mathbf{r}, t)$ tend to line up in parallel and become synchronously active. As a result, the potentials generated by each tissue mass add by superposition. At any fixed time the potential above (or below) the dipole layer is due to the combined effect of all parts of the layer. While this combination of favorable geometry and timing of sources might occur in several brain structures, the crowns of contiguous cortical gyri appear capable of forming the largest dipole layers. Whereas the mesosources $\mathbf{P}(\mathbf{r}, t)$ in adjacent fissures and sulci may also exhibit synchronous synaptic action, cortical geometry is less favorable for lining up the $\mathbf{P}(\mathbf{r}, t)$ vectors from cortical folds. We do not claim that sources in fissures and sulci are unimportant, but they are more likely to be observed in MEG or time-averaged EEG as discussed in chapters 2 and 6.

Consider the case of a circular dipole layer of radius b placed in an infinite, homogeneous medium as shown in fig. 5-20. To be consistent with the other topics in this chapter, we first assume that brain, CSF, skull, scalp, and air space are infinite in extent and have equal conductivities. While

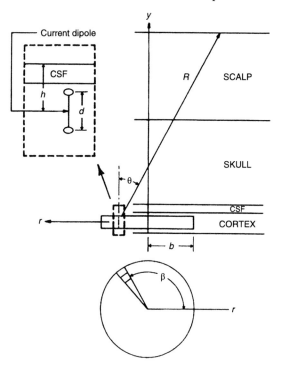

Figure 5-20 A circular dipole layer of radius b is placed in an infinite, isotropic, and homogeneous conductive medium. The effects of inhomogeneity (the separate layers indicating brain, CSF, skull, and scalp) are excluded from the calculations of fig. 5-21, but are included in figs. 1-20 and 8-1.

this assumption is quite unrealistic, it facilitates our discussion of the most important property of dipole layers in EEG studies. First, suppose that our dipole layer is "infinite" in extent. By this we mean that the field point y above the dipole layer is much smaller that layer radius b and the distance to the edge. In this case, the potential above (or below) the dipole layer is approximately constant as our imagined electrode is moved to larger vertical distances y. This result can be explained as follows. As we increase electrode position y, it moves progressively further away from dipoles directly underneath it, implying that potential due only to these relatively local dipoles falls off as $1/y^2$. This is correct, but we must remember that the *potential at any point is due to all dipoles in the layer*. When $y \ll b$, movement of electrode in the y direction has only minimal influence on contributions from more distant dipoles in the layer. Thus, minimal net fall-off in potential is experienced in this region.

The opposite limiting case occurs when the imagined electrode far above the dipole layer, that is, $y \gg b$. In this region the potential just falls off as a single dipole, $1/y^2$. In considering all the controversy concerning dipoles at EEG/MEG conferences observed by the authors over the past 30 years or so (perhaps second only to reference electrode controversies), we mention that the entire brain may be viewed as nothing but a single oscillating dipole if recorded by putative electric or magnetic field sensors (imagined to be very sensitive) from (say) the location of a distant laboratory door. Obviously, the issue of when a particular source configuration can be considered dipolar must be evaluated in the proper context. Our approach throughout this book is to view brain tissue as composed of small millimeter-scale volume elements. If these tissue elements are sufficiently large to contain all sources and sinks associated with a particular neural event, they will produce no monopole contributions to potential external to the elements. In addition, if their characteristic size is small compared the nearest scalp location, we may safely treat each such tissue mass as a *dipole mesosource* of strength $\mathbf{P}(\mathbf{r}, t)$.

In order to illustrate the importance of dipole layers in EEG, imagine that a disk-shaped "cortical" dipole layer is placed in an infinite homogeneous medium as indicated in fig. 5-20. Imagine further that potentials are recorded at a vertical distance y above (a disk-shaped) dipole layer of thickness d and radius b, roughly equivalent to sources in an (idealized) flat cortex. The plots in fig. 5-21 show the attenuation of potential above the center of dipole layers with different sizes. The vertical distance varies between $y = 2$ mm and 12 mm, roughly the distance between dura and scalp surfaces. In the case of the point dipole ($b \to 0$), the potential between (imagined) dura and scalp locations is reduced by a factor of $12^2/2^2 = 36$. The corresponding relative attenuations for dipole layer of radii $b = 0.5, 3, 10$, and 50 mm are $34.4, 10.8, 3.5$, and 1.3. In the case of larger dipole layers, minimal attenuation of potential occurs between dura and scalp locations. We have, of course, omitted the important effects of tissue inhomogeneity, especially those of the skull and air space above the

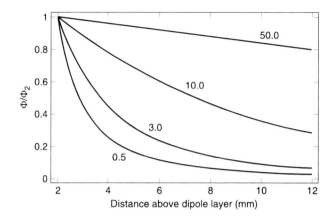

Figure 5-21 The attenuation of potential in an infinite, isotropic, and homogeneous conductive medium due to several dipole layers (shown in fig. 5-20) is plotted versus vertical distance y above the center of dipole layers of radii $b = 0.5$, 3, 10, and 50 mm. In order to emphasize the different fall-off rates, potentials Φ are normalized with respect to their separate values Φ_2 at $y = 2$ mm. The larger the dipole layer, the slower the fall-off of potential.

scalp. The net result of these effects is to cause faster attenuation, as discussed in chapter 6. However, an important qualitative point is made here: in order for the ratio of dura to scalp potential to be in the general range of about two to five (the general rule observed for most spontaneous EEG), cortical sources must form dipole layers with diameters much larger than cortical–scalp separations. This issue is discussed in the context of a much more realistic (layered) head model in chapters 1, 6, and 8. In particular, fig. 1-20, based on our standard 3-sphere model of the head, shows estimates of the ratio of dura to scalp potential directly above dipole layers of varying size, together with experimental data. This plot accurately predicts the observed ratio of cortical to scalp potential within the limits of available experimental data. Figure 6-9 shows the attenuation of dipole potential with radial location through CSF, skull, and scalp.

16 Summary

We have discussed potentials generated in an infinite, isotropic, and homogeneous volume conductor by various source–sink distributions. Physiological current sources, generated at membrane surfaces, are caused by synaptic input to cells or by action potentials. Membrane sources and sinks may be arranged in many different ways in three-dimensional space. Potentials measured inside a distribution of sources and sinks will generally be quite complicated as in the examples of cortical basket cells, the lateral segment of the superior olive, and any cells with many branched dendrites. Generally, if sources and their sinks are widely separated, external potentials will be relatively large as in the examples of cortical sources and sinks at remote surfaces of large pyramidal cells and the medial segment of the superior olive. By contrast, a mixing of sources and sinks within the same small region tends to produce small external fields as in the examples of cortical basket cells and the lateral segment of the superior olive.

In estimating the fall-off of external potentials generated within local source–sink regions, the issue of local current conservation is critical. If all local membrane sources are matched by local sinks, current is conserved locally and we expect external potentials to be roughly dipolar at large distances (with respect to the size of the local region), that is, to fall off as $1/r^2$. In contrast, if local sources in some region A are matched by distant sinks in another region B, the potential fall-off is expected to be roughly monopolar at locations close to either A or B, that is, potentials fall off as $1/r$.

The external potentials generated by distributed sources are discussed. At large distances, the potential is dipolar but with smaller effective pole separations (and effective source strength) that would have been generated by a pair of point sources. A crude model for the extracellular potential of the action potential is presented and shown to match experimental data to a reasonable approximation.

Multiple source–sink combinations in tissue masses, even when quite complicated, are often conveniently described as "dipoles," or more accurately as *dipole moments per unit volume* or *mesosources* $\mathbf{P}(\mathbf{r}, t)$ at intermediate and large locations from the generating tissue. Such approximations are especially useful in studies of the underlying sources of scalp potentials since the scalp typically lies "far" from intracranial tissue volumes in the millimeter or smaller ranges.

The large spatial extent of the many dipole layers that evidently generate EEG disqualifies them as single dipoles. In the case of dipole layers, we must add up individual dipole contributions in a manner similar to adding up contributions from multiple sources (superficial or deep) at any combination of brain locations. Compound action potential source–sink regions in myelinated fibers are apparently too large for the dipole approximation to be accurate at locations inside the head.

The study of potentials generated in the idealized infinite, homogeneous medium provides several useful estimates of physiological phenomena, including scalp potentials generated by synaptic and (in the case of the brainstem auditory evoked potential) action potentials. They also provide a necessary introduction to the study of potentials in inhomogeneous media of finite extent, presented in chapter 6.

Finally, we note that the theoretical functions of chapters 5 and 6 predict potentials at points. By contrast, experimental potentials are space-averaged potentials over electrode volumes. The potential recorded by a spherical electrode of radius ξ is related to theoretical point potentials by the (space-average) volume integral:

$$\Phi_{SA}(\mathbf{r}, t; \xi) = \frac{3}{4\pi\xi^3} \iiint\limits_{\text{Vol}(\xi)} \Phi(\mathbf{r}', t) d^3 r'$$ (5.30)

Given the fractal-like nature of cortical anatomy and the fact that experimental electrophysiology spans about five orders of magnitude of spatial scale, we expect the dynamic behavior of potentials inside the cranium to be very scale-sensitive. That is, the magnitude, spatial dependence, and time dependence of intracranial potentials Φ_{SA} depend critically on the scale ξ. Some experimental data supporting this view are reviewed in Abeles (1992) and Nunez (1995). By contrast, scalp potentials are severely space averaged between cortex and scalp; scalp potentials are mostly insensitive to electrode size. Nevertheless, we are able to observe dynamic behavior at somewhat smaller scales using the band-pass spatial filtering of high-resolution EEG discussed in chapter 8. As expected, somewhat different dynamic properties are observed on the scalp at different spatial scales as shown in chapter 10. Equation (5.30) is an example of experimental *coarse-graining* of a dynamic variable. The mesosource definition (4.26) and scalp potential expression (4.39) provide examples of theoretical coarse-graining of dynamic variables. Additional examples are discussed in chapter 11.

References

Abeles M, 1992, *Local Cortical Circuits*, New York: Springer-Verlag.

Biedenbach MA and Freeman WJ, 1963, Click evoked potential map from the superior olivary nucleus of cats. *American Journal of Physiology* 206: 423–439.

Braitenberg V and Schuz A, 1991, *Anatomy of the Cortex: Statistics and Geometry*, New York: Springer-Verlag.

Caldwell JA and Villarreal RA, 1999, Electrophysiological equipment and electrical safety. In: MJ Aminoff (Ed.), *Electrodiagnosis in Clinical Neurology*, 4th Edition, New York: Churchill Livingstone, pp. 15–33.

Clark J, 1967, *Bioelectric Field Interaction Between Adjacent Nerve Fibers*, Ph.D. Dissertation, Case Western Reserve University.

Cole K, 1968, *Membranes, Ions and Impulses*, Berkeley: University of California Press.

Deupree DL and Jewett DL, 1988, Far-field potentials due to action potentials traversing curved verves, reaching cut nerve ends, and crossing boundaries between cylindrical volumes. *Electroencephalography and Clinical Neurophysiology* 70: 355–362.

Ferree TC, Luu P, Russell GS, and Tucker DM, 2001, Scalp electrode impedance, infection risk, and EEG data quality. *Clinical Neurophysiology* 112: 536–544.

Flick J, Bickford RG, and Nunez P, 1977, Average evoked potentials from brain fiber tracts: a volume conduction model. *Proceedings of the San Diego Biomedical Symposium* 16: 281–284.

Freeman WJ, 1975, *Mass Action in the Nervous System*, New York: Academic Press.

Humphrey DR, 1968, Re-analysis of the antidromic cortical response: I. potentials evoked by stimulation of the isolated pyramidal tract. *Electroencephalography and Clinical Neurophysiology* 24: 116–129.

Jewett DL, 1970, Volume conducted potentials in response to auditory stimuli as directed by averaging in the cat. *Electroencephalography and Clinical Neurophysiology* 28: 609–618.

Jewett DL, Deupree DL, and Bommannan D, 1990, Far-field potentials generated by action potentials of isolated frog sciatic nerves in a spherical volume. *Electroencephalography and Clinical Neurophysiology* 75: 105–117.

Jewett DL and Williston JS, 1971, Auditory-evoked far fields averaged from the scalp of humans. *Brain* 94: 681–696.

Lopes da Silva FH and Storm van Leeuwen W, 1978, The cortical alpha rhythm in dog: the depth and surface profile of phase. In: MAB Brazier and H Petsche (Eds.), *Architectonics of the Cerebral Cortex*, New York: Raven Press, pp. 319–333.

Malmivuo J and Plonsey R, 1995, *Bioelectromagetism*, New York: Oxford University Press.

Mitzdorf U and Singer W, 1978, Prominent excitatory pathways in the cat visual cortex (A17 and A18): a current source density analysis of electrically evoked potentials. *Experimental Brain Research* 33: 371–394.

Mitzdorf U and Singer W, 1979, Excitatory synaptic ensemble properties in the visual cortex of the macaque monkey. A current source density analysis of electrically evoked potentials. *Journal of Comparative Neurology* 187: 71–83.

Nunez PL, 1995, *Neocortical Dynamics and Human EEG Rhythms*, New York: Oxford University Press.

Panofsky WKH and Phillips M, 1955, *Classical Electricity and Magnetism*, Reading, MA: Addison-Wesley.

Petsche H, Pockberger H, and Rappelsberger P, 1984, On the search for sources of the electroencephalogram. *Neuroscience* 11: 1–27.

Plonsey R, 1969, *Bioelectric Phenomena*, New York: McGraw-Hill.

Plonsey R, 1974, The active fiber in a volume conductor. *IEEE Transactions on Biomedical Engineering* 21: 371–381.

Pugh EM and Pugh EW, 1960, *Principles of Electricity and Magnetism*, Reading, MA: Addison-Wesley, p. 416.

Rall W, 1962, Electrophysiology of a dendritic neuron model. *Biophysics Journal* 2: 145–167.

Regan D, 1989, *Human Brain Electrophysiology: Evoked Potentials and Evoked Magnetic Fields in Science and Medicine.* New York: Elsevier.

Rush TC, Patton HD, Woodberry JW, and Towe AL, 1965, *Neurophysiology*, Philadelphia: WB Saunders.

Stegeman DF, van Oosterom A, and Colon EJ, 1987, Far-field evoked potential components induced by a propagating generator: computational evidence. *Electroencephalography and Clinical Neurophysiology* 67: 176–187.

Stotler WA, 1953, An experimental study of the cells and connections of the superior olive of the cat. *Journal of Comparative Neurology* 98: 401–431.

6

Current Sources in Inhomogeneous and Isotropic Media

1 General Considerations

This chapter considers the calculation of potentials in media having conductivity that varies with location, that is $\sigma = \sigma(\mathbf{r})$. In practice, we are normally concerned with layered media that are distinctly separated into two or more regions having different conductivities. Thus, the function $\sigma(\mathbf{r})$ is replaced by conductivities $\sigma_1, \sigma_2, \ldots \sigma_N$, which are constant within each of the N distinct regions. We limit our discussion to isotropic inhomogeneous media in which electrical properties are independent of current direction. All conductivities are assumed to be scalars. While the equation for potentials in anisotropic media is known, contemporary studies of volume conduction in the head are severely limited by a paucity of accurate data on anisotropic tissue properties.

Table 4-1 shows that the skull bone and the space surrounding the head are only two of the many kinds of inhomogeneity found in electrophysiology. The scalp, gray matter, white matter, blood, and cerebrospinal fluid (CSF) all have different conductivities. For EEG applications, the most important inhomogeneities are skull tissue and the external space (air) since both of these media have much lower conductivities than brain tissues, CSF, or scalp. Furthermore, the skull is actually a three-layered (sandwich) structure, with the middle layer substantially more conductive than the outer layers (see chapter 4). The introduction of these conductive inhomogeneities considerably complicates the picture of potentials due to current sources in comparison to the homogeneous (and isotropic) medium presented in chapter 5. In a homogeneous medium, potentials depend only on the magnitude and locations of the current sources. However, in an inhomogeneous medium, current paths and potentials are generally distorted because current follows the *path of least resistance*. In a homogeneous medium, the path of least resistance is the shortest path, but this need not be true if media conductivities vary with location.

The path of current flow in an inhomogeneous medium is, in fact, mathematically identical to current flow in a homogeneous medium but due to a different (but usually unknown) set of current sources. In most cases, it is difficult if not impossible to determine the magnitude and locations of these fictitious secondary sources (also called "virtual" or "image" sources). Instead, potentials generated in an inhomogeneous medium can be determined by the appropriate solution of Poisson's equation (4.12). These solutions depend on the magnitudes and locations of the current sources and the conductivities and the geometrical configurations of various regions of the medium.

Poisson's equation has been studied extensively in the physical sciences. Although the solutions can be computationally involved, our knowledge of potentials in an inhomogeneous medium due to known current sources is limited theoretically only by the availability of data on the conductive and geometrical properties of each region. This restriction can be quite severe in EEG studies since the brain and head are complex in both conductive and geometrical senses. Even though *exact* solutions are impractical, the fact that we can write a single, linear equation relating current sources to the resultant potential is an enormous advance. Not only does the equation give us a way to estimate the magnitudes of errors in our approximate theoretical solutions, it also provides critical guidelines for new experiments to check theory. The problem of volume conduction in the head is inherently far simpler than the problem of the origins of time-dependent EEG behavior, discussed in chapters 10 and 11, for which we are not even sure of the right equations.

As in the homogeneous case discussed in chapter 5, potentials in inhomogeneous media will normally fall off with distance from any source–sink configuration. In either instance, the nature of this spatial attenuation depends on the location of the sources and sinks. We can most easily understand how potentials behave in an inhomogeneous medium by separating the effects of the inhomogeneity from source characteristics. In order to simplify the discussion, we often express our solutions as the ratio of the potential in the inhomogeneous medium (Φ) to the potential generated by the same source when placed in an infinite homogeneous and isotropic medium (Φ_{II}). A summary of some general effects of conductivity inhomogeneity in head models is given at the end of the chapter.

The potential due to a number of point sources in a homogeneous medium is just the sum of the contributions of each source taken separately, and is given in terms of source strength and distance by (4.15). The validity of this expression is a direct consequence of the linearity of Poisson's equation (4.12). Recall from chapter 4 that Poisson's equation follows directly from the basic law of current conservation and Ohm's law. If a number of point sources are placed in inhomogeneous

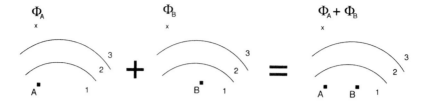

Figure 6-1 (*Left*) A current source placed at location A is "turned on" and generates potential Φ_A at location x. (*Middle*) Source A is turned off and source B is turned on and generates potential Φ_B at the same location x. (*Right*) The two sources at A and B are turned on simultaneously generating a potential at x given by $\Phi_A + \Phi_B$. The result follows from the linearity of Poisson's equation and remains valid in inhomogeneous and anisotropic volume conductors.

media, anisotropic media, or both, (4.15) is no longer valid; however, we can still exploit the linearity of Poisson's equation by summing the potentials due to each source. For example, consider a medium consisting of three different regions with different conductivities σ_1, σ_2, and σ_3 as shown in fig. 6-1. If a single source is placed at location A in region 1, a potential $\Phi_A(\mathbf{r})$ will be produced at location $\mathbf{r}$ (or x) in region 3, although not with the simple $1/r$ behavior characteristic of monopolar sources in a homogeneous medium. Similarly, if a source is placed at location B, a different potential $\Phi_B(\mathbf{r})$ will be produced at location $\mathbf{r}$. The linearity of Poisson's equation implies that if we now place the two sources at locations A and B, respectively, the potential at location $\mathbf{r}$ is simply the linear superposition $\Phi_A(\mathbf{r}) + \Phi_B(\mathbf{r})$.

Several of the expressions presented here have been obtained directly from the literature on electrostatics. In classic electrostatics, a charge q placed in an inhomogeneous dielectric medium consisting of several regions with permittivities $\varepsilon_1, \varepsilon_2, \varepsilon_3, \ldots$ produces a potential $\Phi(\mathbf{r})$. If instead a current source I is placed in an inhomogeneous conductive medium consisting of several parts with conductivities $\sigma_1, \sigma_2, \sigma_3 \ldots$ with identical geometrical configuration to the dielectric, we can use the classic electrostatic solutions for $\Phi(\mathbf{r})$. The procedure is simply to replace the charge source q by the current source I and replace permittivities $\varepsilon_1, \varepsilon_2, \varepsilon_3, \ldots$ with conductivities $\sigma_1, \sigma_2, \sigma_3 \ldots$, respectively. This simple formal substitution is possible because potentials in both kinds of media are governed by Poisson's equation, albeit with entirely different physical interpretation of the variables, as discussed in chapter 4.

2 The Two-Layered Plane Medium

We first consider the problem of a current source embedded in a medium with conductivity σ_1 (Jackson 1975). The source is located at a distance h below an interface with a second medium of conductivity σ_2 as pictured in fig. 6-2. Both media are assumed "semi-infinite," which in physics

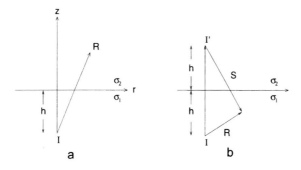

Figure 6-2 (a) Current source I located below an interface separating two regions having conductivities σ_1 and σ_2 produces a potential in the upper material. (b) The potential in the lower material can be pictured as due to a real source I plus a fictitious source I'.

parlance means that the media extend in both directions over distances much larger than the *characteristic scale h*. Of course, the current that flows away from the source must eventually pass into sinks. For the present discussion we assume that all sinks are also located at distances that are large compared to h. Once the effect of the inhomogeneity is understood, we can consider as many sources and sinks as needed.

If the medium were homogeneous ($\sigma_2 = \sigma_1$), the potential at any location would be given by (5.3). In the inhomogeneous medium, Poisson's equation (4.12) tells us that the potential in the upper material (or medium) is that which would have been produced by a different source I' located at the same point as I. This method of solution to Poisson's equation is called the "method of images" discussed in nearly any electrostatics text. The magnitude of the fictitious (image) source is such that the potential in the upper material ($z > 0$) is given by

$$\Phi = \frac{I}{2\pi(\sigma_1 + \sigma_2)R} \tag{6.1}$$

Here R is the distance between the source I and the field point, given in cylindrical coordinates by

$$R = \sqrt{r^2 + (h + z)^2} \quad z > 0 \tag{6.2}$$

and r is the perpendicular distance between the z-axis and the field point (not necessarily in the plane of the paper). Equation (6.1) tells us that the potential at any location in the upper material is simply obtained from the homogeneous formula (5.3) by replacing the homogeneous conductivity σ by the average conductivity of the two regions $\frac{1}{2}(\sigma_1 + \sigma_2)$. When there are n sources (or sinks) in the lower material, the potential in the upper material is then given by

$$\Phi_2 = \frac{1}{2\pi(\sigma_1 + \sigma_2)} \sum_{i=1}^{n} \frac{I_i}{R_i} \quad z > 0 \tag{6.3}$$

This is analogous to (4.15) for the case of a homogeneous medium. It should be noted that (6.3) does *not* apply if any sources are located in the upper material. Furthermore, the very direct procedure of replacing the conductivity of the homogeneous medium in (4.15) with the average conductivity of the inhomogeneous medium is *not* generally applicable to inhomogeneities with more complicated boundaries.

The potential in the *lower* material due to sources in the *lower* material is the potential due to two sources, as shown in fig. 6-2. One source is the real source I and the other source is a fictitious source $I' = I(\sigma_1 - \sigma_2)/(\sigma_1 + \sigma_2)$ located in the upper material at an equal distance h from the interface. The potential in the lower material due to n sources in the lower material is then given by

$$\Phi_1 = \frac{1}{4\pi\sigma_1} \sum_{i=1}^{n} \left[\frac{I_i}{R_i} + \left(\frac{\sigma_1 - \sigma_2}{\sigma_1 + \sigma_2} \right) \frac{I_i}{S_i} \right] \quad z > 0 \tag{6.4}$$

Here the R_i refer to the distances between the real sources I_i and the field point, and the S_i are the distances between the fictitious sources I_i' and the field point as indicated in fig. 6-2b. When $\sigma_1 = \sigma_2$, (6.4) reduces to the expression for the potential in a homogeneous medium, (4.15). When $R_i = S_i$ for every i, the field point is located at the interface between the two materials, and the potential calculated with (6.4) for the lower material equals the potential calculated with (6.3) for the upper material. Thus, the potential is shown to be continuous across the interface, as it must be in all conductive media.

We can make a few generalizations about the two-layered plane medium by comparing the potential Φ at a fixed location in the inhomogeneous medium with the potential Φ_{II} that would have been generated by the same sources in a homogeneous medium of conductivity σ_1. From (6.3), it is easy to show that the potential in the *upper* material due to a number of sources all in the lower material is always related to the equivalent homogeneous potential by the relation

$$\frac{\Phi_2}{\Phi_{II}} = \frac{2\sigma_1}{\sigma_1 + \sigma_2} \quad z > 0 \tag{6.5}$$

Thus, if the upper material is a *better* conductor than the lower material, the potential in the upper material is *reduced* in comparison to the case of a homogeneous medium composed entirely of the lower material. Conversely, if the upper material is a *poorer* conductor than the lower material the potential is *increased* in comparison to the homogeneous medium. When the upper material is a perfect insulator ($\sigma_2 = 0$), all of the current must be confined to the lower material. The potential in the upper material is then increased to twice its homogeneous value.

The ratio analogous to (6.5) for potentials in the *lower* material due to a number of sources in the *lower* material depends on the location of the field point. For example, if there is a single source in the lower material, the ratio analogous to (6.5) is given by

$$\frac{\Phi_1}{\Phi_H} = 1 + \left(\frac{\sigma_1 - \sigma_2}{\sigma_1 + \sigma_2}\right)\frac{R}{S} \quad z < 0 \tag{6.6}$$

Thus, if the upper material is a *better* conductor than the lower material ($\sigma_2 > \sigma_1$), the potential in the lower material will be *reduced* from its equivalent homogeneous value. In contrast, if the upper material is a *poorer* conductor than the lower material, the potential in the lower material will be *increased* from its equivalent homogeneous value. If the source is located far from the interface, and the field point is close to the source ($R \ll S$), the upper material will have negligible effect on the potential in the lower material.

3 Dipole Inside a Homogeneous Sphere

The potential due to a current dipole inside a conducting sphere of radius a and conductivity σ_1, surrounded by air ($\sigma_2 = 0$) is considered here. The potential on the surface of the sphere due to a dipole oriented along the radial direction, as measured from the center of the sphere, is given by

$$\Phi = \frac{Id}{4\pi\sigma_1 a^2}\left\{\frac{2(\cos\theta - f)}{(1 + f^2 - 2f\cos\theta)^{3/2}} + \frac{1}{f}\left[\frac{1}{(1 + f^2 - 2f\cos\theta)^{1/2}} - 1\right]\right\}$$
$$a \gg d \tag{6.7}$$

Here $f = r_z/a$ locates the dipole along the radial direction as shown in fig. 6-3. This expression is only valid for potentials measured on the surface of the sphere $r = a$. The general expression for the potential at any radial

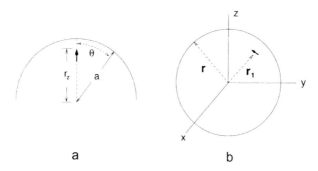

a   b

Figure 6-3 (a) A radial dipole inside a sphere of radius a. (b) A dipole with eccentric location and orientation inside a sphere.

location is given by Wilson and Bayley (1950). When the dipole is located at the center of the sphere, that is, in the limit $f \rightarrow 0$, this expression reduces to three times the potential due to the same dipole in an infinite homogeneous medium, given by (4.15). The increased potential over the homogeneous case is due to the fact that all current is confined inside the sphere.

Another limiting case of (6.7) occurs when f is close to 1, which means the dipole is just below the surface of the sphere. If we further restrict the expression to surface locations close to the dipole such that the angle θ is small, it can be shown that (6.7) reduces to the potential due to a dipole in a two-layered plane medium with the upper conductivity equal to zero. To show this, let $f = 1-\varepsilon$ and expand (6.7) in a double Taylor series about $\theta = 0$ and $\varepsilon = 0$. This value of potential on the surface of the sphere is twice that of the potential due to the same dipole in an infinite homogeneous medium, shown in section 2.

4 Dipole in Multilayer Plane Media

The problem of a dipole current source located below multiple interfaces that separate planar regions having different conductivities is indicated in fig. 6-4. Each layer is assumed to be semi-infinite in extent; that is, the layers extend to large distances in horizontal directions. This approximation may be reasonable in the case of the CSF, skull, and scalp. The problem of a source in a multilayered plane medium has been studied in detail (Stefanesco and Schlumberger 1930; Zhadin 1969). Expressions for the potential in each of the three regions is typically given in terms of integrals of the form

$$\Phi(r, z) = \int_0^\infty A_i(k) J_0(kr) e^{\pm kz} dk \qquad (6.8)$$

where the $A_i(k)$ are coefficients that depend on the magnitudes and locations of the current sources, $J_0(kr)$ is the zeroth order Bessel function, and (r, z) refers to a cylindrical coordinate system, with z as the vertical coordinate. The details of the calculation are provided in appendix F.

Figure 6.4 shows a five-layered model representing the five principal tissue compartments of the head: brain, CSF layer, skull, scalp, and surrounding air. Here we consider a simpler case of three layers by assuming skull conductivity equal to zero ($\sigma_3 = 0$). This example corresponds to calculating the potential on the surface of the CSF; that is, the potential inside the cranium is expected to be minimally influenced by small skull currents. (When calculating scalp potentials, this approximation obviously fails.) When $\sigma_1 = \sigma_2$, the problem reduces to that of two layers, and the ratio of the potential Φ to the potential at the same location in an

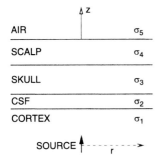

Figure 6-4 Five-layered plane medium used to model surface potentials due to a cortical dipole located at $z = 0$, $r = 0$. The solution for potential on the surface is outlined in appendix F (but with layers 1–5 numbered from the top down).

infinite homogeneous medium Φ_0 equals two. If $\sigma_2 > \sigma_1$ this potential ratio is decreased. The effect of confining current to the region below the top of the CSF (by the zero-conductivity skull) is to increase Φ. By contrast, the effect of the CSF layer, having higher conductivity than the brain, is to reduce Φ. Example values of parameters are $\sigma_2/\sigma_1 \sim 5$ (CSF conductivity is five times higher than brain conductivity) and $s/h = 1$ (CSF thickness = 0.5 mm and dipole center located 0.5 mm below cortical surface). For these parameters $\Phi/\Phi_H \sim 1$. Thus, the two effects nearly cancel one another at locations directly above the dipole source, so that the potential is roughly the same as that which would have occurred if the same source were placed in an infinite homogeneous medium of conductivity σ_1.

5 Dipole Inside Concentric Spherical Surfaces

A radial dipole is shown inside a model consisting of three concentric spherical shells (scalp, skull and CSF) and an inner sphere (brain) in fig. 6-5. We refer to this standard head model as the *4-sphere model*. When the CSF layer is omitted, we call this the *3-sphere model*. This model captures several of the critical features of volume conduction in the head, and is used extensively in theoretical developments and simulation studies in chapters 7, 8, and 9. For mathematical convenience, we orient the coordinate system such that the dipole is located on the z axis. The dipole may be located arbitrarily within the spheres since we can always rotate the coordinate system such that the z axis passes through the center of the dipole axis. In fig. 6-5, the dipole is located at position r_z along the z axis with dipole axis oriented normal to the spherical surfaces. In section 6 dipoles oriented tangential to the spherical surfaces are considered. Any arbitrarily oriented dipole on the z axis of the coordinate system can be replaced by two tangential dipoles oriented along the x and y axes and one (radial) dipole along the z axis, with relative magnitudes depending on the orientation of the dipole source.

The 4-sphere model consists of an inner sphere representing the brain ($r_1 \sim 8.0$ cm), surrounded by a thin shell of CSF layer ($r_2 \sim 8.1$ cm), a skull layer ($r_3 \sim 8.6$ cm), and scalp layer ($r_4 \sim 9.2$ cm). Scalp and brain are soft tissues assumed to have approximately equal conductivities ($\sigma_1/\sigma_4 \sim 1$).

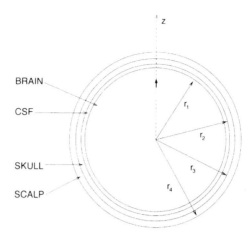

Figure 6-5 A dipole is shown in the inner sphere of our standard 4-sphere head model consisting of the inner sphere (brain) and three spherical shells representing CSF, skull, and scalp. The parameters of model are the radii (r_1, r_2, r_3, r_4) of each shell and the conductivity ratios (σ_1/σ_2, σ_1/σ_3, σ_1/σ_4). Typical values for the radii are (8, 8.1, 8.6, 9.2 cm) and the conductivity ratios (0.2, 40, 1). Surface potential magnitudes due to a fixed current source depend on the individual radii and conductivities; however, relative potentials as functions of surface location depend only on the ratios.

The spherical layer representing the skull has conductivity much lower than that of the brain, σ_1/σ_3 is perhaps in the range of 20 to 80. As discussed in chapter 4, the brain-to-skull conductivity ratio is not well known, but the most important predictions of the model depend only on the fact that skull tissue has a much lower conductivity than brain tissue. The thin layer representing the CSF has higher conductivity than brain tissue, something like $\sigma_1/\sigma_2 \sim 0.2$. The 3-sphere model is obtained by excluding the CSF layer, either by setting $\sigma_2 = \sigma_1$ or forcing the CSF thickness to zero. The outer spherical shell (scalp) is surrounded by a medium of zero conductivity (air). All such multisphere models can be reduced to a single homogeneous sphere by setting all the conductivity ratios to one.

The 4-sphere model is clearly only a rough approximation to genuine heads in both the geometric and conductive senses, but it provides a useful way to gain insight on the general effects of the conductive inhomogeneities. The potential in any such volume conductor model is given by the appropriate solution of Poisson's equation, which in spherical geometry involves the Legendre polynomials rather than the Bessel functions characteristic of the planar medium (section 4). The methods of obtaining solutions to Poisson's equation in n-sphere models have been widely published (Rush and Driscoll 1969; Nunez 1981; Srinivasan et al. 1996, 1998); they are outlined in appendices F, G, and H.

In order to define a standard potential for normalization purposes, suppose that a dipole is placed in the center of the inner sphere (conductivity σ_1). We define the *homogeneous potential* as the potential in an

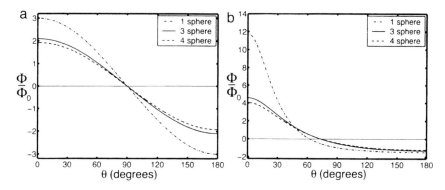

Figure 6-6 The potential on the surface of the outer spherical shell due to a radial dipole in three n-sphere models is plotted as a function of the polar angle θ measured from the z axis. (a) The dipole is located at the center (outer sphere radius is 9.2 cm). (b) The dipole is located at a radius of 5 cm (4.2 cm below the surface of the outer sphere). The three curves in each figure correspond to the 1-sphere, 3-sphere, and 4-sphere models with $\sigma_1/\sigma_3 = 80$.

infinite medium that would be generated at the radial coordinate corresponding to the outer sphere ($r = r_4$). From (1.7), the homogeneous potential due to a central dipole falls off with angular distance θ from the dipole axis according to

$$\Phi_H = \frac{Id\cos\theta}{4\pi\sigma_1 r_4^2} \tag{6.9}$$

In fig. 6-6, the scalp potential Φ in the 4-sphere model has been scaled by the potential $\Phi_0 = \Phi_H(r_4, 0)$. Figure 6.6a shows the fall of the potential ratio Φ/Φ_0 with angle θ for a dipole source at the center of the spheres in 1-sphere, 3-sphere, and 4-sphere models. In all three spherical volume conduction models, the surface potential above the dipole is larger than the potential that would have been produced by the same source in an infinite homogenous medium. This occurs because of *confinement of current flow entirely within the spherical conductive volume*. That is, current lines are compressed, especially near the outer surface resulting in larger current densities and, by implication, larger potentials. The introduction of the poorly conducting skull in the 3-sphere model decreases the ratio of inhomogeneous to homogeneous potential from three to about two by confining substantial current inside the skull. The consequence of including the CSF layer (4-sphere model) is an additional small decrease in surface potential. In each example shown in fig. 6-6a, the potential falls off with angular distance at the same rate as in the infinite homogenous medium Φ_H. When a dipole is placed at the center of a homogeneous sphere, the potential at *any* angular location on the surface of a homogeneous sphere is exactly three times larger than that which would have been produced by the same dipole in an infinite homogeneous medium Φ_H.

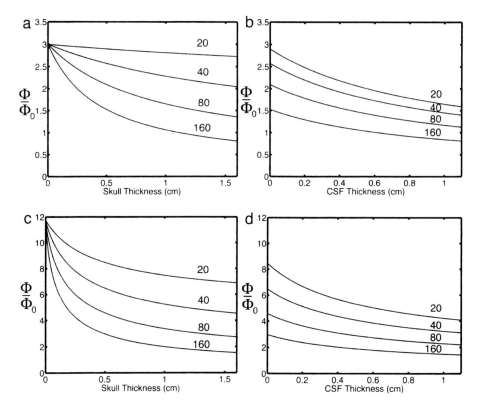

Figure 6-7 The dependence of maximum surface potential on skull and CSF thickness in the 4-sphere head model. In each plot, the four curves correspond to the brain-to-skull conductivity ratios 20, 40, 80, and 160. Scalp potential directly above the radial dipole is normalized with respect to potential at the same location due to the same source placed in the center of an infinite homogeneous medium. (a, b) Central dipole. (c, d) Dipole at radial location $r_z = 5$ cm. (a, c) Variation of maximum potential with skull thickness when CSF thickness is zero. (b, d) Variation of maximum potential with CSF thickness when skull thickness is fixed at 0.5 cm.

Figure 6.6b shows the surface potential due to a dipole oriented in the radial direction located at an intermediate radius $r = 5$ cm. The potential directly above the dipole ($\theta = 0$) in the 4-sphere model is now four times larger than the homogeneous potential produced by a dipole at the center of the spheres, $\Phi_0 = \Phi_H(r_4, 0)$. Scalp potential is doubled by moving the dipole from $r = 0$ to 5. By contrast, this same dipole movement in a homogeneous sphere increases surface potential by a factor of four from $3\Phi_0$ to $12\Phi_0$. The smearing of the potentials, mainly by the skull, is also evident. The surface potentials in the 3-sphere and 4-sphere models fall off much more slowly with angular location in comparison to the surface potential on a homogeneous sphere.

In the n-sphere models, the potential ratio Φ/Φ_0 is determined by the conductivity ratios and relative radii of the spherical shells. Figure 6.7 shows the dependence of the surface potential on skull conductivity and thickness for the 3-sphere model with a central dipole (fig. 6-7a) and a radially oriented dipole at $r = 5$ cm (fig. 6-7c). In both cases, the potential ratio Φ/Φ_0 decreases as skull thickness increases as expected. In the idealized (but unrealistic) case of a homogeneous skull, the skull resistance per unit area is proportional to the ratio between skull thickness and skull conductivity. For example, a 50% increase in skull thickness and 50% decrease in skull conductivity have roughly the same influence on the potential ratio Φ/Φ_0. The effect of the skull on surface potential is stronger when the dipole is closer to the scalp surface than when the dipole is located at the center of the spheres. Figure 6.7b and d show similar plots for increasing CSF thickness in the 4-sphere model assuming a skull of fixed thickness equal to 0.5 cm. As CSF thickness increases, the potential ratio Φ/Φ_0 decreases gradually due to shunting of currents in directions tangent to the inner skull surface.

The effects of variation in the brain-to-skull conductivity ratio become stronger as the source is located closer to the surface of the inner sphere (brain). Figure 6.8 shows the fall-off of the potential ratio Φ/Φ_0 with angular distance on the outer sphere (scalp) of a 4-sphere model when the dipole is moved progressively closer to the surface. For the case of a dipole at the center of the spheres (fig. 6-8a), the potentials fall off similarly with angular distance (minimal smearing) and show less than 25%

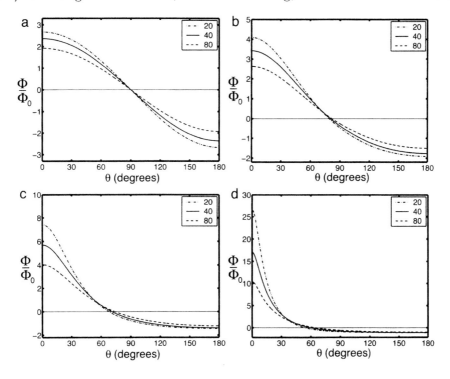

Figure 6-8 Potential on the outer surface of the 4-sphere head model as a function of polar angle θ. The four figures correspond to different radial locations (r_z) of the radial dipole: (a) 0 cm, (b) 2.5 cm, (c) 5 cm, (d) 7.5 cm. In each, the three curves correspond to brain-to-skull conductivity ratios of 20, 40, and 80.

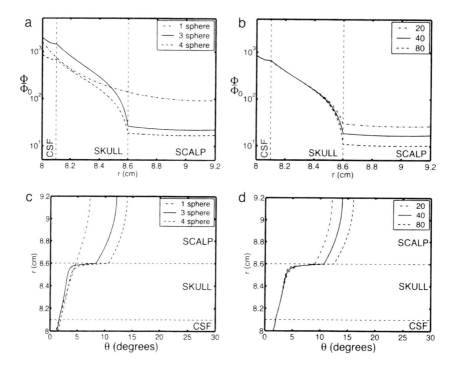

Figure 6-9 Potential inside the n-sphere models generated by a radial dipole located at $r_z = 7.0$ cm. (a) Fall-off of potential directly above the dipole (radial direction along the z axis) through the thickness of the CSF, skull, and scalp. The three curves correspond to the 1-sphere, 3-sphere, and 4-sphere models. Note the logarithmic scale. (b) Fall-off of potential directly above the dipole (radial direction along the z axis) through the thickness of the CSF, skull, and scalp in the 4-sphere model. Similar to (a) except the three curves correspond to brain-to-skull conductivity ratios 20, 40, and 80. (c) Angular spread of potential in the skull and scalp in 1-sphere, 3-sphere, and 4-sphere models. The curves represent the angular distance at which potential is 50% of its maximum directly above the dipole ($\theta = 0$), shown for each radial location. (d) Similar to (c) except the angular spread of potential in the 4–sphere model is shown for different values of the brain-to-skull conductivity ratio, 20, 40, and 80.

variation in the potential directly over the source ($\theta = 0$) for the labeled range of conductivity ratios (20 to 80). In the cases of fig. 6-8b, c, and d, as the radial location of the dipole increases within the brain sphere, the surface potential becomes more sensitive to the brain-to-skull conductivity ratio. For smaller values of the brain-to-skull conductivity ratio (better skull conductor), the magnitude of the potential is larger over the dipole source and falls off more rapidly with tangential distance.

The solution to the 4-sphere model presented in appendix G can be used to compute potential anywhere in the volume conductor. Figure 6.9a shows potential as a function of radial position above a radial dipole source (located at $r = 7$ cm) in a homogeneous sphere (1-sphere model), 3-sphere, and 4-sphere models. In the homogenous sphere (1-sphere model), the potential gradually falls off towards the boundary of the outer sphere

$(r = r_4 = 9.2$ cm). Within the thickness of the skull, the potential in the 3-sphere or 4-sphere models fall off by more than an order of magnitude because of low skull conductivity. By contrast, the potential change across the thickness of the scalp is negligible in both 3-sphere and 4-sphere models. The addition of a CSF layer (the 4-sphere model) causes a reduction in surface potential directly above the dipole, an effect also demonstrated with the three-layered planar model of section 4. This occurs because of tangential current shunting by the relatively high-conductivity CSF layer. For the same value of the brain-to-skull conductivity ratio $(\sigma_1/\sigma_3 = 40)$, the potential in the 3-sphere model is larger than the potential in the 4-sphere model throughout the thickness of the skull and scalp.

Figure 6.9b shows the fall-off in potential with radial position above the source in the 4-sphere model for different values of the brain-to-skull conductivity ratio. For all three cases the potential decreases in an identical manner through the CSF and most of the thickness of the skull, but decreases more rapidly at the skull-scalp boundary if the skull has lower conductivity (higher brain-to-skull conductivity ratio).

Figure 6.9c shows the distribution of potentials with radial position and angular distance to the dipole axis θ within the homogeneous sphere (1-sphere model) and 3-sphere and 4-sphere models. In these examples, the same radial dipole source is located at $r_z = 7.0$ cm. At each radial location r, the potential at each angular position is normalized with respect to the potential directly above the dipole. The contour lines indicate the angular distance at which the potential is 50% of the peak potential at each radial position directly above the dipole in each head model. Within the CSF layer and skull, potentials are only slightly smeared as radial position increases. The main spreading of potentials occurs near the skull-scalp boundary. A similar but much smaller effect occurs in the 4-sphere model at the brain-CSF boundary and partly accounts for the greater angular spread of potentials in the 4-sphere model in comparison to the 3-sphere model. This spreading effect is small in this simulation because the CSF layer is only 1 mm thick. In both 3-sphere and 4-sphere models, the main factor that determines the spatial smearing of scalp potentials is the poor conductivity of the skull in comparison to scalp and brain tissue. Figure 6.9d shows that the effect of lower skull conductivity (higher brain-to-skull conductivity ratio) is to increase the tangential spread of potentials in addition to reducing the peak potential magnitude over the dipole.

6 Relative Magnitudes of Potentials Generated by Radial and Tangential Dipoles

The location and orientation of cortical dipole mesosources $\mathbf{P}(\mathbf{r}, t)$ are constrained by the geometry of the folded cortical surface with dipole axis expected to be everywhere normal to the local cortical surface. That

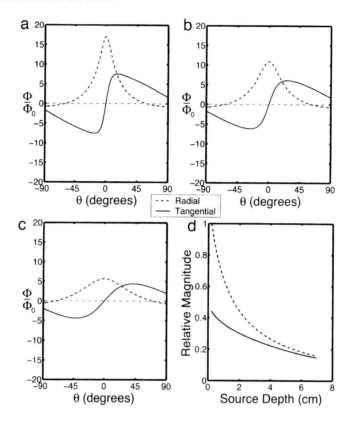

Figure 6-10 The potential at the scalp sphere versus polar angle due to a radial and tangential dipole at the same radial location r_z in the 4-sphere model. Model parameters are provided in the caption to fig. 6-5. (a) $r_z = 7.8$ cm, (b) $r_z = 7.0$ cm, (c) $r_z = 5.0$ cm. (d) Relative magnitude of the potential due to a radial and tangential dipole normalized with respect to the potential due to a radial dipole 2 mm below the brain surface ($r_1 = 8.0$). The plot is presented versus source depth ($r_1 - r_z$).

is, local normal dipole axes are expected as a result of the parallel arrangement of pyramidal cells in cortical columns as indicated in fig. 5-9b. Because of irregular cortical folding, cortical current sources can have all possible orientations with respect to scalp surface. When n-sphere head models are used, any arbitrary dipole orientation can be modeled by three equivalent dipoles: one oriented radial to the interfaces between spherical surfaces and two oriented tangential to the surfaces. The solutions for radial and tangential dipoles are derived in appendices G and H, respectively. For a radial dipole with axis aligned in the z-direction of a standard spherical coordinate system, spherical symmetry allows for solutions to be expressed as a single sum over Legendre polynomials $P_n(\cos\theta)$, thereby avoiding the more cumbersome double sums over the spherical harmonic functions. In the case of a tangential dipole located on the z axis and oriented in the x y plane, the sum is taken over the (first-order) associated Legendre functions $P_n^1(\cos\theta)$ When the source consists of only a single dipole, the coordinate system can always be rotated so that the dipole is located on the z axis. In this case the potential due to any arbitrarily oriented dipole can be obtained as the weighted sum of the potentials generated by two tangential dipoles oriented along the x and y axes and a radial dipole oriented along the z axis. When multiple sources occur, the potential at any location can be calculated separately for each single dipole using rotated coordinates and the solutions combined by linear superposition.

Tangential dipoles generally make a smaller contribution to scalp potentials than radial dipoles of the same strength and depth. Figure 6-10a-c shows scalp potentials due to a pair of dipoles (one radial and one tangential with equal strengths) at different radial locations r in the 4-sphere head model. For simplicity, we selected an x-oriented tangential dipole and plot the normalized potential versus the spherical coordinate θ (see figure caption). Unlike the radial dipole, the potential due to a tangential dipole is antisymmetric about the polar (z) axis and reaches its peak magnitude at a distance of 10 or more degrees from the dipole center, depending on dipole depth. Figure 6-10a shows scalp potentials due to superficial dipoles (one radial and one tangential) located 2 mm below the surface of the brain sphere at $r = 7.8$ cm. The maximum potential directly above the radial dipole is more than twice the maximum potential generated by the equivalent tangential dipole at an angular distance of about $10°$.

Superficial gyral surfaces are expected to produce dipoles with larger radial components. By contrast, sulcal walls are expected to produce dipoles with larger tangential components, although the irregularity of cortical surfaces limits the accuracy of this generalization. Consequently, tangential cortical dipoles are expected to be at deeper locations more often than radial dipoles and generate even smaller relative potentials than indicated in fig. 6-10a. Figure 6-10b shows that a radial dipole 1 cm below the surface of the brain sphere produces maximum potentials about twice as large as the maximum potential due to a tangential dipole at the same depth. At a depth of 3 cm the radial dipole produces slightly higher maximum potentials than the tangential dipole, as shown in 6-10c. Equal maximum potentials occur when both dipoles are placed in the center of the spheres.

Figure 6-10d shows the relative peak magnitude of radial and tangential dipoles normalized with respect to the peak potential generated by a superficial radial dipole considered in fig. 6-10a. Radial dipoles produce larger potentials than tangential dipoles at any depth above the center of the sphere (where they are equivalent). This effect is more pronounced for superficial sources that generate larger potentials than deeper sources. The effect of source orientation is expected to be even larger than these comparisons imply since radial dipole sources in gyral surfaces may generally be located more superficially than tangential dipoles in (even superficial) sulcal walls. Still another advantage of radial dipoles is the apparent cortical ability to produce synchronous sources in many gyral crowns that have nearly parallel dipole axes. This advantage of radial over tangential dipoles can be large. Tangential dipoles can certainly make important contributions to scalp potential measurements. However, *when a mixture of radial and tangential dipole sources contribute to the scalp potential, radial sources are normally expected to make the largest contributions.*

7 Scalp Potentials due to Dipole Layers

We have considered examples of single dipole sources in n-sphere models representing the head volume conductor. To determine the potential due to several current sources, the coordinate system can be successively rotated so that the z axis passes through each dipole and the single dipole potentials summed at any scalp location. Our simulations in this chapter suggest that superficial radial dipole sources generate larger scalp potentials than deeper radial sources or tangential dipoles at any depth in the n-sphere models. However, a single dipole source can only be used to describe the current source activity in a volume of tissue much smaller (of the order of a few millimeters) than the distance between superficial cortex and scalp (about 1 cm). Thus, sources in the superficial cortical gyri are better described as dipole layers, consisting of synchronous dipole sources oriented mainly perpendicular to the cortical surface. As discussed in chapter 5, the most important sources of EEG apparently consist of *dipole layers* or sheets of aligned radial dipoles in crowns of the cortical gyri. When these dipole layers occur in contiguous gyral crowns, widespread alignment of radial sources can produce large scalp potentials.

Figure 6-11 shows the potential over the center ($\theta = 0$) of a dipole layer (or spherical cap) of transcortical potential equal to 100 μV and located at a fixed depth ($r = 7.8$ cm) in the 4-sphere models. The size of the

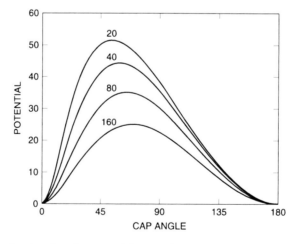

Figure 6-11 The simulated scalp potential over the center of a dipole layer (or spherical cap) of radial sources at a fixed depth ($r_z = 7.8$ cm) in the 4-sphere model. The four curves correspond to brain-to-skull conductivity ratios 20, 40, 80, and 160.

dipole layer (or cap angle) is varied for different values of the brain-to-skull conductivity ratio. In each case, the potentials increase up to a cap angle of about 60° (which roughly corresponds to 2/3 of the upper hemisphere) and then decrease as the sources at the edge of the cap begin to contribute negative potential at the measurement location above the center of the cap. It is clear from fig. 6-11 that scalp potentials progressively increase as the sizes of the dipole layers increase up to a size larger than the superficial surface of a cerebral hemisphere. Thus, a reasonable conclusion is that scalp potential magnitudes are strongly influenced by the sizes of underlying dipole layers. The scalp potential generated by a large, synchronous dipole layer with radius greater than 3 or 4 cm can be 50–100 times larger than potentials due to dipole layers with radii smaller than 1 cm. However, one caveat is appropriate here: larger layers may be less likely to exhibit as much synchrony over their surfaces.

Radial dipole layers covering a larger extent of the superficial cortex will make a much larger contribution to scalp potentials than smaller dipole layers. Since deeper dipole layers (for instance, in the thalamus) make much smaller contributions to scalp potentials due to the greater distance between sources and electrodes, we can generally conclude that most spontaneous EEG is generated by large dipole layers, and that larger synchronous dipole layers generate larger EEG signals. Although averaging (including Fourier methods) can be used to extract signals possibly generated by smaller dipole layers from the background spontaneous EEG, *averaged signals are as sensitive to dipole layer size as spontaneous EEG.*

8 Spatial Transfer Functions for n-Sphere Models

In this section we investigate properties of potentials generated on the external surface (scalp) of the head model for the general case of complex source patterns distributed spatially within the inner sphere (brain). Again, we adopt the 4-sphere head model. Since superficial radial dipoles produce larger potentials than other sources, we consider spherical layers composed of radial dipoles all at the same radial location. We develop the concept of a spatial transfer function, originally suggested by Katznelson (1982), to summarize how the *distribution* of source strength over the spherical layer of sources is represented in the scalp potential.

The potential distribution on the surface of the outer sphere $r = r_4$ due to a radial dipole at an arbitrary location (r', θ', ϕ') in the innermost sphere $(r' < r_1)$ can be expressed as sum over the spherical harmonics $Y_{nm}(\theta, \phi)$, that is

$$G(\theta, \phi, r', \theta', \phi') = \frac{Id}{4\pi\sigma_1(r')^2} \sum_{n=1}^{\infty} \frac{4\pi}{2n+1} H_n(r') \sum_{m=-n}^{n} Y_{nm}(\theta, \phi) \cdot Y_{nm}(\theta', \phi')$$

(6.10)

The spherical harmonics form an orthogonal basis set for functions defined on a spherical surface. Appendix I provides mathematical background and example plots of spherical harmonics. They are the natural functions typically used to describe nearly any static or dynamic behavior on the surface of a sphere or in a spherical shell. The coefficients H_n depend on the radial position of the dipole source r' and the radii and conductivities of the spherical layers. The formula for H_n in the 4-sphere model is given in appendix G. In (6.10), the Green's function G is expressed for the case of potentials on the outer sphere due to radially oriented sources in the innermost sphere. For any instantaneous mesosource distribution composed of radial dipoles in the inner sphere, $P(r', \theta', \phi')$, the potential on the outer sphere can be obtained by first multiplying the source distribution by the Green's function and then integrating over the volume of the inner sphere, that is

$$\Phi(r, \theta, \phi) = \int_0^{r_1} \int_0^{\pi} \int_0^{2\pi} P(r', \theta', \phi') \cdot G(r, \theta, \phi; r', \theta', \phi') r'^2 \sin \theta' dr' d\theta' d\phi'$$

$$(6.11)$$

Here we introduce a spherical source distribution at a fixed depth $r' = r_z$. With $r_z = 7.8$ cm and $r_1 = 8$ cm, $P(r_z, \theta', \phi')$ is a useful approximation to superficial gyral sources 2 mm below the cortical surface. This distribution can also be expressed as a sum over spherical harmonics:

$$P(r_z, \theta', \phi') = \delta(r - r_z) \sum_{n=1}^{\infty} \sum_{m=-n}^{n} P_{nm} Y_{nm}(\theta', \phi') \qquad (6.12)$$

Here, $\delta(r - r_z)$ is the usual delta function indicating that all sources are located at the same depth and the expansion coefficients P_{nm} are calculated as described in appendix I. The potential on the outer sphere due to a dipole layer $P(r_z, \theta', \phi')$ is calculated by substituting (6.12) and (6.10) into (6.11) and integrating to obtain (Srinivasan et al. 1998)

$$\frac{\Phi(r_4, \theta, \phi)}{\Phi_0} = \sum_{n=1}^{\infty} \sum_{m=-n}^{n} \Phi_{nm} Y_{nm}(\theta, \phi) = \sum_{n=1}^{\infty} \sum_{m=-n}^{n} \frac{4\pi}{2n+1} H_n(r_z) \cdot P_{nm} Y_{nm}(\theta, \phi)$$

$$(6.13)$$

Here the potentials have been normalized by the homogeneous potential above the dipole Φ_H obtained by evaluating Φ_H at $r = r_4$ and $\theta = 0$, as in (6.9). Each component of the source distribution P_{nm} is multiplied by the transfer function T_{nm} to obtain the corresponding component of the scalp potential:

$$T_{nm} = \frac{\Phi_{nm}}{P_{nm}} = \frac{4\pi}{2n+1} H_n(r_z) \qquad (6.14)$$

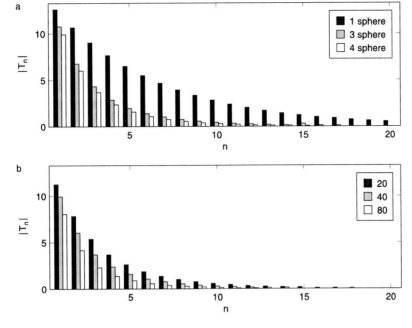

Figure 6-12 The magnitudes of the spatial transfer functions (6.14) for the n-sphere models are plotted versus surface spatial frequency index n (degree of the spherical harmonic function). The transfer functions are based on dipole layer sources at fixed depth $r_z = 7.8$ cm. (a) Spatial transfer function for 1-sphere, 3-sphere, and 4-sphere models. (b) Spatial transfer function for the 4-sphere model with brain-to-skull conductivity ratios 20, 40, and 80.

The transfer function depends only on the degree n of each component of the spherical harmonic expansions, that is, $T_{nm} \rightarrow T_n$. This allows for concise expression of spatial filtering by the head volume conductor in terms of the n index.

The dependence of the transfer function on the spherical harmonic degree n is closely related to the dependence of the transfer function on one-dimensional spatial frequency. Latitudinal wavenumber or spatial frequency k on a spherical surface is approximately related to the (n, m) indices and sphere radius R by

$$k \approx \frac{n}{(2\pi)R} \tag{6.15}$$

Here spatial frequency is expressed in cycles/cm, analogous to Hz (cycles/sec) for temporal frequencies by including the factor (2π) in the denominator. This approximation is valid only if the index m is small. The index n is a measure of the "overall spatial frequency" of each spherical harmonic Y_{nm}, involving a sort of "average" over the m indices. On a spherical cortex of 8 cm radius, $n = 8$ corresponds to a wavenumber $k \cong 1/2\pi$ cycles/cm or a spatial wavelength of 2π cm.

Figure 6-12a shows the magnitude of the transfer function $|T_n|$ for the homogeneous sphere (1-sphere model), 3-sphere model, and 4-sphere model. Introducing the skull in the 3-sphere and 4-sphere models has the effect of attenuating the potentials generated by source components at all spatial frequencies with a greater reduction at higher degrees n. Thus, *the skull acts as a low-pass spatial filter of cortical source activity*. Large dipole layers distributed over the brain surface contain low spatial frequencies and contribute large scalp potentials. Smaller dipole layers have more relative energy at higher spatial frequencies and are selectively attenuated. The 4-sphere model introduces a CSF layer, which slightly increases the spatial low-pass filtering effect. Figure 6-12b shows that this spatial low-pass filtering characteristic is very similar over the relatively wide range of assumed brain-to-skull conductivity ratios. The main effect of increasing the brain-to-skull conductivity ratio is to decrease potential magnitudes, but such relative decreases are fairly uniform over the spatial frequency spectrum.

In chapter 8 we show that the spatial filtering properties associated with the (spline) surface Laplacian are more band-pass than low-pass, generally allowing for more accurate estimates of small superficial dipole layers. The concept of spatial filtering is also used in chapter 9 to understand the influence of head volume conduction on statistical properties of EEG time series measures such as coherence.

9   Comparisons of n-Sphere Models with More "Advanced" Head Models

The next four chapters of this book make extensive use of n-sphere head models that consist of concentric spherical shells representing tissues with different conductivity: brain, CSF, skull, and scalp. These idealized models have obvious shortcomings: genuine heads are not spherical, tissue layers have nonuniform thicknesses and conductivities, bulk skull and white matter are anisotropic, and so forth. Nevertheless, the layered spherical models apparently include the most important features of large-scale volume conduction in genuine heads—the large conductivity changes that occur at three critical interfaces: CSF-skull, skull-scalp, and scalp-air.

Examples of the robust nature of 3-sphere and 4-sphere head models are provided here and in chapter 8. These models have also been useful to test and develop source localization algorithms. Dipole localization algorithms based on n-sphere models typically provide location accuracy in the 1 to 2 cm range in both simulations and physical experiments when the source is known to consist of only a single dipole. The accuracy of these algorithms in simulations with n-sphere models is limited only by sampling density (number of electrodes) and noise. This feature sharply distinguishes 3-sphere or 4-sphere models from models based on a homogeneous sphere (1-sphere model).

The 3-sphere and 4-sphere models have also provided a means to develop and test high-resolution EEG methods. The spline-Laplacian and dura imaging algorithms discussed in chapter 8 work well in simulations provided that brain conductivity in forward solutions is greater than about five times skull conductivity, thereby forcing skull currents to be mostly radial. Although published estimates of the brain-to-skull conductivity ratio vary considerably as discussed in chapter 4, all the various estimates all satisfy this criterion.

If the 3-sphere model is much better than a 1-sphere model, does this automatically imply that the 4-sphere model is even better? Taking this idea even further, would we expect even more accuracy from models with realistic tissue boundaries, perhaps *finite element* or *boundary element* models using data from MRI images? In practice, these questions do not have simple answers. The main reason is that accurate tissue conductivities are just as important as accurate geometric information to the construction of accurate head models. That is, the resistance of current paths depends on the product of distance with tissue resistivity as given by (1.6). Several tissue conductivities (notably skull) are poorly known and may (apparently) vary by 50 to 100% or more between subjects (and perhaps within the same subject). Furthermore, both bulk skull (with three distinct layers) and white matter are substantially anisotropic, meaning that each tissue conductivity is an inhomogeneous tensor (or 3×3 matrix), whose individual components are poorly known. Data indicating that bulk skull plug resistance is apparently uncorrelated to thickness are reported in chapter 4. This is apparently a consequence of different conductivities in each skull layer; that is, thicker skulls may occur largely with thicker middle layers having the largest conductivity.

Figure 6-13 demonstrates that the 3-sphere model (no CSF) with a particular brain-to-skull conductivity ratio is essentially equivalent to the 4-sphere model with a smaller brain-to-skull conductivity ratio. This near equivalence occurs because the CSF layer provides an additional low-resistance pathway for tangential current spread. That is, the high-resistance skull and inner layer of low-resistance CSF conspire to spread out scalp potentials due to a local source, thereby confounding localization efforts. In the comparison presented in fig. 6-13a, the solid curve was calculated from the 4-sphere model with a brain-to-skull conductivity ratio of 40, CSF-to-brain conductivity ratio of 5, and a CSF thickness of 2 mm. The lower (dashed) curve was calculated using a 3-sphere model (no CSF) and a brain-to-skull conductivity ratio equal to 80. The two curves are nearly identical except directly above the dipole. In fig. 6-13b, the lower curve (dashed) was calculated using a 4-sphere model with 1 mm CSF thickness and brain-to-skull conductivity ratio equal to 30. The upper (solid) curve was calculated with a three-sphere model with no CSF (layer added to brain) and a brain-to-skull conductivity ratio equal to 40. These simulations indicate that *effective value of skull conductivity is model dependent*. It can differ substantially from actual skull conductivity depending critically on CSF thickness (which typically depends on age of subject) and other assumed features of the volume conductor model.

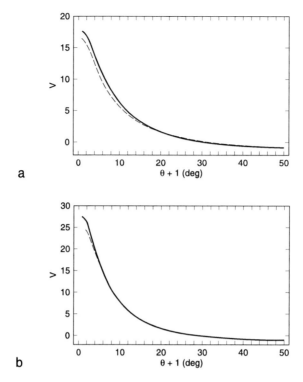

a

b

Figure 6-13 The predicted fall-off of scalp surface potential as a function of spherical coordinate θ (degrees) from similar head models is compared. Each degree corresponds to 0.157 cm of surface distance. The horizontal axis spans 50° or 7.86 cm on a 9.0 cm radius sphere. (a) The solid curve was calculated from the 4-sphere model with a brain-to-skull conductivity ratio of 40, CSF to brain conductivity of 5, and radial locations of the spherical shells given by [dipole, brain, CSF, skull, scalp] = [7.8, 7.801, 8.0, 8.5, 9.0 cm]; that is, a CSF thickness equal to 2 mm. The lower (dashed) curve was calculated using the 3-sphere model with a brain-to-skull conductivity ratio of 80 and the radial locations of the spherical shells given by [dipole, brain, skull, scalp] = [7.8, 8.0, 8.5, 9.0 cm]. (b) The dashed curve was calculated using the 4-sphere model with a 1 mm CSF thickness and brain-to-skull conductivity ratio of 30. The solid curve was calculated with the 3-sphere model with no CSF (space added to brain) and a brain-to-skull conductivity ratio of 40.

The development of progressively more accurate head models can be expected to continue into the foreseeable future. More accurate impedance imaging using scalp current injection (Nunez 1987; Ferree et al. 2000) or relations between tissue conductivities and MRI-based diffusion coefficients (Ueno and Iriguchi 1998) can eventually lead to more accurate head models. In the meantime, the most obvious application of finite element models is in directed studies of specific n-sphere model defects. For example, one finite element model indicates that differences in predicted scalp potential between spherical and realistic head models are typically in the 10 to 20% range (Yan et al. 1991). This finite element model cannot claim to be more accurate than a similarly layered spherical model because of the large uncertainty of the tissue conductivities. Finite element or boundary element models can provide a rough idea of the magnitude of inaccuracy of spherical models due only to approximating the surface geometry with a sphere.

10 Effects of Variable Skull Conductivity

The n-sphere models discussed in the previous sections account for each tissue compartment as a spherical shell of uniform thickness and conductivity. The low skull conductivity in comparison to scalp and brain tissue largely determines the magnitude and spatial extent of potentials measured on the outer sphere (scalp). Variations within a spherical layer such as openings in the skull or very thin skull regions (for example, the eye sockets) are not included in symmetric spherical models. Such skull regions can provide preferential current paths that can strongly influence scalp potentials. These effects may be particularly important in infants. Infant skulls are only partly closed; skull openings known as *fontanelles* are found over both anterior and posterior regions of the head. Even in the completely formed adult skull, skull thickness varies over its surface (Law 1993). However, evidence to support the idea that thicker skull has lower conductance is lacking, as discussed in chapter 4. Thus, although the details about head shape and spatial variations in skull thickness can be obtained from MRI or CT, skull conductivity variations cannot be surmised from the geometric information. Variation in skull conductivity is likely to have greater impact on scalp potentials than geometric features such as irregular head shape.

In order to model some effects of variable conductivity in a portion of the skull, we make use of an earlier 2-sphere approximation to the 3-sphere model (Plonsey 1969; Nunez 1987). The solution involves new boundary conditions applied across the skull layer. We call this head model the *two spheres with skull (TSS) model*. The two regions are the inner sphere (brain conductivity σ_1) and outer spherical shell (scalp conductivity $\sigma_3 = \sigma_1$). In between the two regions is the shell representing the skull, with conductivity dependent on angular position about the z axis, that is, $\sigma_2 = \sigma_2(\theta)$. In order to preserve symmetry with respect to the spherical coordinate ϕ, our solution is restricted to the case of a radial dipole on the z axis, that is, directly below the region of skull inhomogeneity.

The essential approximations of TSS are that the skull is very thin and that current flow through the poorly conducting skull is assumed to be strictly radial across the thickness of the skull; that is, tangential skull current is assumed to be zero, as shown in fig. 6-14. Boundary conditions are then applied between brain and scalp regions (across the skull) so that no explicit solution for potential inside the skull region is required. By dropping the skull solution Φ_2 we lose the two associated sets of coefficients in the expansion (see appendix G) and the four boundary conditions at the brain–skull and skull–scalp interfaces, given by (4.7) and

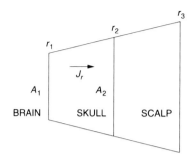

Figure 6-14 An elemental volume of the two sphere with skull (TSS) model is shown. The essential assumption of the TSS model is that current flow in the skull is only in the radial direction as indicated by the vector $\mathbf{J}_r$. In the elemental volume shown, total current entering the inner surface of the skull at r_1 through the area A_1 equals the total current leaving the outer surface of the skull at r_2 through area A_2. See text for details.

(4.8). Thus, we require two additional relations between solutions Φ_1 and Φ_3 to solve for the required coefficients in the solution expansion.

 If all skull current is radial, the total current entering an area A_1 at the inner surface of skull ($r = r_1$) must equal the total current passing through area A_2 at the outer skull surface ($r = r_2$). This requires skull potential Φ_2 to vary according to $1/r$ over the (assumed) very thin skull. The two new relations between brain and scalp potentials are

$$\Phi_3(r_2) - \Phi_1(r_1) = (r_2 - r_1)\left(\frac{r_2\sigma_3}{r_1\sigma_2}\right)\left(\frac{\partial\Phi_3}{\partial r}\right)_{r=r_2} \qquad (6.16)$$

$$\left(\frac{\partial\Phi_1}{\partial r}\right)_{r=r_1} = \left(\frac{r_2}{r_1}\right)^2\left(\frac{\sigma_3}{\sigma_1}\right)\left(\frac{\partial\Phi_3}{\partial r}\right)_{r=r_2} \qquad (6.17)$$

These new boundary conditions, applied across the skull, allow for solutions for scalp potential when skull conductivity varies over spherical cap regions centered on the z axis, that is, $\sigma_2 = \sigma_2(\theta)$.

 To validate the solution, first consider the case where skull conductivity is constant, that is, $\sigma_2(\theta) = \sigma_2$. In this case, TSS model should closely approximate the 3-sphere model if the approximation of radial current flow in the skull is valid. Figure 6-15a shows the potential above a superficial radial dipole in standard 3-sphere model with identical radius and conductivity parameters. The TSS model overestimates the potential directly above the dipole, but its accuracy is within about 7% of the solution to the three-sphere model when the brain-to-skull conductivity ratio is 80. Figure 6-15b shows the error in the TSS model estimate of the potential directly above the dipole as a function of the brain-to-skull conductivity ratio. When conductivity ratio is sufficiently large (>20), scalp potentials obtained with the TSS model provide a reasonable approximation to the standard three-sphere model. This constraint limits the

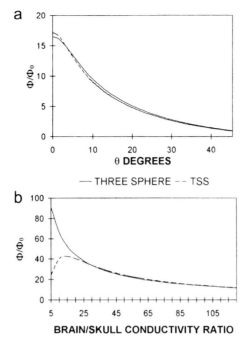

Figure 6-15 Approximation of the 3-sphere model by the TSS model under conditions of uniform skull conductivity. Scalp potentials are normalized by the surface potential due to a central dipole in an infinite homogeneous medium. (a) Scalp potential as a function of spherical coordinate θ in the 3-sphere model (solid) and TSS model (dashed). The radii of the brain, skull, and scalp layers are 8.0, 8.5, and 9.0 cm, respectively, and the radial dipole source is placed at $r_z = 7.8$ and $\theta = 0$. The brain-to-skull conductivity ratio is 80. (b) Scalp potential directly above the dipole source ($\theta = 0$) is plotted versus brain-to-skull conductivity ratio in the 3-sphere model (solid line) and TSS model (dashed). Other model parameters are identical.

range of allowed brain-to-skull conductivity ratio in simulations of variable skulls.

The main factor that determines the spatial smearing of scalp potentials is low skull conductivity in comparison to brain and scalp conductivities. To investigate the effects of variable skull conductivity, the TSS model was used to examine a spherical cap having either higher or lower conductivity than the remaining skull. The spherical cap is located (symmetrically) directly above a radial dipole source on the z axis. A smooth transition between higher and lower conductivity (near the edge of the spherical cap) was obtained with a sigmoid function to ensure convergence of the solution. Figure 6-16a (upper) shows four profiles of the functional dependence of conductivity ratio on angular position for a spherical cap of higher skull conductivity (lower ratio) directly above the radial dipole source located at $\theta = 0$. The profiles indicate a lower brain-to-skull conductivity ratio of 20 directly above the dipole; the remaining skull has a constant ratio of 80. For a skull radius of 8.25 cm (at the midpoint of the skull thickness), these profiles correspond to skull caps of radii along

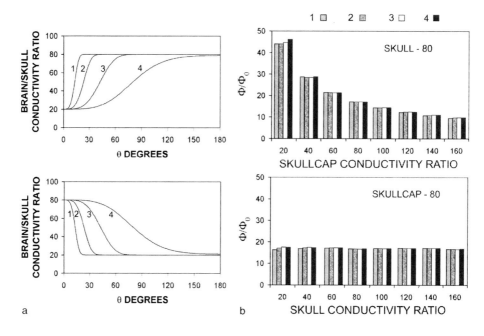

Figure 6-16   (Column a) Example profiles of variable skull cap conductivity were constructed using a sigmoid function. Each profile labeled 1–4 is characterized by a half-width (radius) where the brain-to-skull conductivity ratio is halfway between the ratio for the local skull cap and the remainder of the skull. Assuming a skull radius of 8.25 cm at the midpoint of the thickness of the skull, the half-width for each profile shown is (1) 1.9 cm, (2) 3.4 cm, (3) 6.1 cm, (4) 11.6 cm. (*Upper row, column a*) A higher skull cap conductivity (local brain to skull conductivity ratio = 20) than the remaining homogeneous portion of the skull (brain-to-skull conductivity ratio = 80) is shown. (*Upper row, column b*) Effects of near and distant skull layer on scalp potential above a radial dipole source. The horizontal axis is the skull cap conductivity ratio (only one example ratio of eight is shown in the upper part of (a)) with the ratio over the remaining skull fixed at 80. Other TSS head model parameters are fixed with brain, skull, and scalp radii of 8, 8.5, and 9 cm, respectively. Scalp potentials are generated by a dipole source at $(r_z, \theta) - (7.8 \text{ cm}, 0)$ and normalized with respect to the potential generated by the same source at the same location in an infinite homogeneous medium. In each figure the bars correspond to the four different widths of variable skulls as shown in (a). (*Lower row, a*) Lower skull cap conductivity (brain-to-skull cap conductivity ratio = 80) than the remainder of the skull (brain-to-skull conductivity ratio = 20). (*Lower row, b*) Skull cap conductivity ratio is held fixed at 80 while this ratio for the remainder of the skull is varied from 20 to 160. Note that scalp potential above the skull cap region is not influenced by the conductivity of distant (or even nearby) skull.

the surface of (1) 1.9 cm, (2) 3.4 cm, (3) 6.1 cm, and (4) 11.6 cm. Figure 6-16a (lower) shows four profiles of the dependence of conductivity ratio on angular position for a spherical cap with lower skull conductivity directly above the dipole (conductivity ratio of 80 compared to the constant value of 20 over the remainder of the skull).

Figure 6.16b (upper) shows normalized scalp potential directly above ($\theta = 0$) a radial dipole in the TSS model for four spherical skull caps of varying size with brain-to-skull cap conductivity ratios ranging from 20 to 160. In each case, the homogeneous parts of the skull have a brain-to-skull conductivity ratio of 80. As is our usual practice, scalp potential is normalized with respect to the potential generated at the same location by a central dipole in an infinite homogeneous medium. The scalp potential is strongly influenced by local skull cap conductivity, but is not substantially influenced by the spatial extent of the skull cap over this range of skull cap sizes. Obviously, if the skull cap is smaller than these examples, cap size will also have an effect on surface potential.

Figure 6-16b (lower) shows the normalized scalp potential directly above a radial dipole in the TSS model for four spherical skull caps of varying size and a fixed brain-to-skull cap conductivity ratio of 80, with brain-to-skull conductivity ratio of the larger homogeneous portion of the skull varying from 20 to 160. In all four cases scalp potential above the dipole is not influenced by the value of brain-to-skull conductivity ratio in the homogeneous portion of the skull.

These simulations suggest the following. (i) If the local skull conductivity is high, scalp potentials due to local sources will be substantially increased over those in a homogeneous skull as expected. In the case of a source directly below the center of this "hole," the size of the hole (above a certain minimum size) has minimal influence on scalp potential. (ii) If local skull conductivity is very low, scalp potentials due to local sources will be minimally influenced if the rest of skull is also a relatively poor conductor. These results are, of course, severely limited by our requirement that the dipole source be placed directly below the center of the inhomogeneous region. This model is perhaps most useful as a check on finite element models that allow for variable skull conductivity and arbitrary source placement.

11 Summary of Effects in the Inhomogeneous Models

In chapter 5, the homogeneous potential Φ_H due to a number of current source–sink distributions (or in more concise language, simply "sources") is given. Different sources produce potentials that fall off differently with distance r. This chapter focuses on dipoles and dipole layers and estimates the effects of various kinds of inhomogeneity on surface (scalp) potential generated in spherical head models. This focus is justified because of the relatively large distance of scalp from cortical sources, thereby allowing the convenient treatment of cortical sources in terms of dipole moment per unit volume or cortical *mesosources* $\mathbf{P}(\mathbf{r}, t)$ defined in chapter 4.

The simplest inhomogeneity of interest in EEG is the *confinement of current inside a volume conductor of finite size*, thereby compressing current lines near the inner surface and increasing potential over the

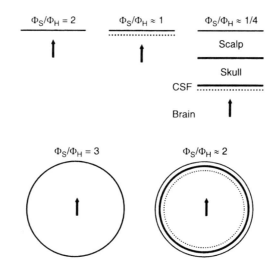

Figure 6-17 A summary of some general effects of head model inhomogeneity. In each example, the arrow represents a current dipole of fixed strength in a linear, isotropic conductive medium. Surface potentials Φ_S are normalized with respect the potentials Φ_H that would have been generated at the same locations if the same dipole had been placed in an infinite, homogeneous medium. Dashed lines indicate lower boundaries of cerebrospinal fluid (CSF). In all examples the conductivity outside (or above) the volume conductor is zero. Φ_S/Φ_H generally depends on the conductivity ratios and material boundaries; however, in two cases (semi-infinite plane and homogeneous sphere) the conductivity ratio is infinite and Φ_S/Φ_H is exact.

homogeneous case. One example is the potential due to a dipole at the center of a homogeneous sphere of radius R (Plonsey 1969; appendix H):

$$\Phi(r,\theta) = \frac{Id\cos\theta}{4\pi\sigma r^2}\left(1 + \frac{2r^3}{R^3}\right) \tag{6.18}$$

The term multiplying the expression in parenthesis is the usual dipole potential for a homogeneous medium Φ_H, given by (1.7). Near the dipole the inhomogeneous and homogeneous potentials are nearly identical, but as the measuring point approaches the surface, the ratio Φ/Φ_H becomes progressively larger reaching exactly 3.0 at $r = R$.

The second major inhomogeneity emphasized here is the *low skull conductivity compared to brain and scalp conductivities*, a property that is especially important in EEG applications. Addition of the poorly conducting skull layer reduces the surface ratio Φ_S/Φ_H to approximately two (depending on the actual tissue conductivity ratios) as summarized in fig. 6-17.

The 4-sphere model can be used to construct estimates of scalp potentials based on measured conductivities and thicknesses of brain, CSF, skull, and scalp. Using this model, we find that scalp potentials are preferentially sensitive to large dipole layers and much less sensitive to smaller dipole layers. The effect of volume conduction can be summarized by a transfer function, which has low-pass spatial filtering characteristics. Sources distributed over larger regions will generate larger potentials over the scalp than focal sources.

The 3-sphere or 4-sphere models are approximate models of the head in both geometric and electrical (conductivity) senses. We emphasize that *an exact geometric model is still an approximate electrical model*, an inconvenient fact of EEG science that severely limits the efficacy of advanced computer head models. Better estimates of tissue properties are required to improve volume conduction models. For example, variation of skull conductivity over its surface appears to be a potentially significant issue for EEG. As suggested by the TSS model, local scalp potentials depend strongly on skull conductivity in the region directly above their associated sources.

The appropriate range of skull conductivity variations in living heads is not well known at this time. Furthermore, effective skull conductivity can be quite different from the actual conductivity depending on head model details. Thus, we cannot easily evaluate the overall importance of variable skull effects on measured potentials in EEG experiments. However, one preliminary conclusion is that *normalized measures like phase and coherence may be more effective indicators of cortical source dynamics than simple amplitude or power measures*, the latter being more obviously influenced by local skull properties.

References

Ferree TC, Eriksen KJ, and Tucker DM, 2000, Regional head tissue conductivity estimation for improved EEG analysis. *IEEE Transactions on Biomedical Engineering* 47: 1584–1592.

Jackson JD, 1975, *Classical Electrodynamics*, 2nd Edition, New York: Wiley.

Katznelson RD, 1982, *Deterministic and Stochastic Field Theoretic Models in the Neurophysics of EEG*, Ph.D. Dissertation, La Jolla: University of California at San Diego.

Law SK, 1993, Thickness and resistivity variations over the upper surface of the human skull. *Brain Topography* 6: 99–110.

Nunez PL, 1981, *Electric Fields of the Brain: The Neurophysics of EEG*, 1st Edition, New York: Oxford University Press.

Nunez PL, 1987, A method to estimate local skull resistance in living subjects. *IEEE Transactions on Biomedical Engineering* 34: 902–904.

Plonsey R, 1969, *Bioelectric Phenomena*, New York: McGraw-Hill.

Rush S and Driscoll DA, 1969, EEG electrode sensitivity: an application of reciprocity. *IEEE Transactions on Biomedical Engineering* 16: 15–22.

Srinivasan R, Nunez PL, and Silberstein RB, 1998, Spatial filtering and neocortical dynamics: estimates of EEG coherence. *IEEE Transactions on Biomedical Engineering* 45: 814–825.

Srinivasan R, Nunez PL, Tucker DM, Silberstein RB, and Cadusch PJ, 1996, Spatial sampling and filtering of EEG with spline-Laplacians to estimate cortical potentials. *Brain Topography* 8: 355–366.

Stefanesco S and Schlumberger CM, 1930, Sur la distribution electrique potentielle autour d'une prise de terre ponctuelle dans un terrain a couches horizontals, homogenes et isotropes. *Journal de Physique* 1: 132–140.

Ueno S and Iriguchi N, 1998, Impedance magnetic resonance imaging: a method for imaging impedance distributions based on magnetic resonance imaging. *Journal of Applied Physics* 83: 6450–6452.

Wilson FN and Bayley RH, 1950, The electric field of an eccentric dipole in a homogeneous spherical conducting medium. *Circulation* 1: 84–92.

Yan Y, Nunez PL, and Hart RT, 1991, Finite element model of the human head: scalp potentials due to dipole sources. *Medical and Biological Engineering and Computing* 29: 475–481.

Zhadin MN, 1969, Mechanisms of the origin of synchronization of biopotentials in the cerebral cortex: I. Model of independent sources. *Biophysics* 14:732–743.

7

Recording Strategies, Reference Issues, and Dipole Localization

1 EEG Recording Systems

EEG recordings from the scalp provide an indirect means to extract information about brain current sources. In this chapter we focus on certain aspects of experimental design and EEG recording that have been only sparsely covered in other publications. The more conventional recording issues in EEG are mostly left to the references (Regan 1989; Fisch 1999; Picton et al. 2000; Niedermeyer and Lopes da Silva 2005). We make extensive use of the analyses in chapter 6, which is concerned with the distribution of the electric potentials due to known configurations and locations of current sources and sinks in n-sphere models of volume conduction in the head. Here, the head models of chapter 6 are recruited to assess impacts of different experimental strategies on information obtained from scalp recordings. We are concerned with determining the location and dynamic behavior of the mesosources $\mathbf{P}(\mathbf{r}, t)$ that cause observed potentials. In order to address such questions, information about the dynamic distribution of potential over the scalp is required. Recorded scalp potentials generally depend on three factors: the spatial extents and locations of the mesosources, head volume conduction, and the specific experimental methods adopted to record these potentials.

Figure 7-1 indicates both similarities and contrasts between today's EEG systems and the systems in common use in the 1970s. The upper photograph shows cup electrodes being pasted on the scalp with collodion and dried with an air gun. After attachment, the scalp was abraded and conductive gel injected through a hole in the cup. In this laboratory, EEG was displayed on a 16-channel paper chart on a Grass EEG machine and stored on a PDP-12 computer. Later, fast Fourier transforms (FFTs) were calculated on the PDP12, which could only be programmed in

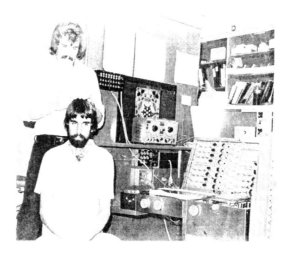

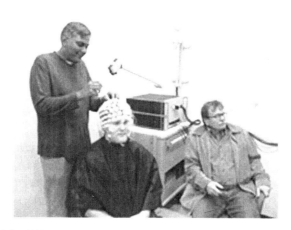

Figure 7-1 (*Upper*) Paul Nunez pastes electrodes on assistant Larry Reid in a study to check the postulated negative correlation between brain size and peak alpha frequency (1976, see Chapter 11). EEG was recorded and displayed by paper and ink chart with the 16-channel Grass EEG machine in the background. FFT was accomplished with machine language programming on the PDP12 computer. This laboratory, headed by Reginald Bickford, was located at the Medical School of the University of California, San Diego (*Lower*) Ramesh Srinivasan fits a Geodesic Sensor Net (Electrical Geodesics, Inc., Eugene, Oregon) with 128 channels to assistant Sam Thorpe's head in his laboratory at the University of California, Irvine while Paul Nunez checks computer traces in a SSVEP experiment (2005). Data reported in this book were recorded either with the geodesic net (128 electrodes, 2.7 cm average spacing) in Irvine or an electrode cap (Electro-Cap International, Inc., Eaton, Ohio; 131 electrodes, 2.2 cm average spacing; see fig. 10-1) at the Brain Sciences Institute, then headed by Richard Silberstein, in Melbourne, Australia.

cumbersome assembly language. More advanced data analyses strategies (like spatial-temporal Fourier transforms or PCA) required a special purpose tape drive to convert the PDP12 tape to an IBM-compatible tape (in this case only available at a remote laboratory). Once the EEG data were stored on the IBM mainframe, advanced data analyses were accomplished with Fortran programs. Such studies were limited by finite budgets

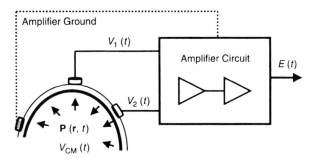

Figure 7-2 Brain mesosources $\mathbf{P}(\mathbf{r}, t)$ generate scalp potential differences $V_2(t) - V_1(t)$. The potentials at scalp locations 1 and 2 are $V_1(t) + V_{\mathrm{CM}}(t)$ and $V_2(t) + V_{\mathrm{CM}}(t)$, respectively, where the common-mode potential $V_{\mathrm{CM}}(t)$ is typically due mostly to capacitive coupling with power line fields. The amplifier circuit may contain several amplifier stages plus external circuit elements. The EEG system is designed to reject the common-mode potential $V_{\mathrm{CM}}(t)$ and amplify the potential difference between pairs of scalp locations such that the output voltage is proportional to scalp potential differences, that is, $E(t) \cong A[V_2(t) - V_1(t)]$, where A is the total system *gain*. The amplifier system makes no distinction between recording electrodes and the so-called EEG "reference electrode." By contrast, the (internal) ground electrode placed on the scalp, nose, or neck provides a reference voltage to the amplifier to prevent amplifier drift and to facilitate better common mode rejection.

as mainframe computer time was expensive. The lower photograph shows a much more convenient modern system using a Geodesic net containing 128 electrodes that can be applied and impedance checks completed in about 20 minutes. Raw traces and processed data can be readily displayed on a fast (and relatively low-cost) computer.

Figure 7-2 depicts EEG recording from a human subject (conductively) isolated from the ground of the power supply. The amplifier (internal) ground is also isolated from the ground of the power supply. Brain mesosources $\mathbf{P}(\mathbf{r}, t)$ (current dipole moments per unit volume) and biological artifacts generate scalp potential differences $V_2(t) - V_1(t)$. Environmental electric and magnetic fields also generate scalp potentials typically due mostly to capacitive coupling of body and electrode leads to power line fields. The potentials with respect to an external ground ("infinity") at scalp locations 1 and 2 are given by $V_1(t) + V_{\mathrm{CM}}(t)$ and $V_2(t) + V_{\mathrm{CM}}(t)$, respectively, where the *common-mode potential* $V_{\mathrm{CM}}(t)$ is typically caused mostly by power line fields, but can also have cardiac (EKG) and other contributions. This EEG system is designed to reject the (spatially constant) common-mode potential $V_{\mathrm{CM}}(t)$ and amplify the potential difference between pairs of scalp locations such that the output voltage is proportional to scalp potential differences generated within the body, that is

$$E(t) \cong A[V_2(t) - V_1(t)] \tag{7.1}$$

where A is the total system *gain* often due to several amplifier stages. The amplifier system makes no distinction between recording electrodes and the so-called EEG "reference electrode." By contrast, the (internal) amplifier ground electrode placed on the scalp, nose, or neck provides a distinct reference voltage to the amplifier to prevent amplifier drift and facilitate better common mode rejection. The internal ground is isolated from true ground.

One study of a practical differential amplifier system by Ferree et al. (2001) found the following approximate relationship between amplifier output $E(t)$, scalp potential difference $[V_2(t) - V_1(t)]$, recording electrode contact impedances (Z_1 and Z_2), and amplifier input impedance Z_{IN}:

$$E(t) = \left(1 - \frac{Z_1 + Z_2}{2Z_{IN}}\right)[V_2(t) - V_1(t)] + \left(\frac{Z_1 - Z_2}{Z_{IN}}\right)V_{CM}(t) + \vartheta\left(\frac{1}{Z_{IN}^2}\right)$$

(7.2)

The approximations leading to (7.2) are based on the assumption of large amplifier input impedance typical of modern EEG systems. The first term on the right-hand side is proportional to the desired scalp potential difference, but with reduced amplitude. It may be amplified in a later stage provided that signal loss in this first stage is not too severe. The unwanted contribution from the common-mode signal (second term on the right-hand side) is due mainly to an imbalance of recording electrode contact impedances. When using modern amplifiers with large input impedances (say 200 MΩ), relatively large electrode contact impedances (compared to traditional guidelines, say >50 kΩ) can easily be tolerated. While (7.2) is independent of the amplifier (internal) ground electrode impedance, a separate analysis of environmental fields induced in electrode leads suggests the importance of the (internal) ground electrode (Ferree et al. 2001). More details about EEG amplifier systems may be found in the references (see also Simpson 1998 and Kamp et al. 2005).

Figure 7-3 shows a simple schematic diagram of a generic EEG recording system. The system records potential differences between electrode pairs placed on the scalp. The goal is to record potentials due only to brain sources (arrows), but biological artifact can never be completely eliminated by the amplifiers and filters. That is, any current source in the body (EKG, muscle, tongue movement, and so forth) that produces scalp potential differences in frequency bands that overlap EEG will contribute to the recorded signal. The amplifier–filter system cannot, in principle, distinguish such artifact from brain sources. Rejection of *obvious artifact* is accomplished by visual inspection and, in some cases, computer analysis. But rejection of *subtle artifact* is another matter entirely.

Typically one electrode is singled out as the "reference electrode"; the remaining electrodes are characterized as "recording" electrodes. However, electrode *pairs* are always required to measure scalp potentials because such recording depends on current passing through a measuring circuit analogous to the fish tank example of fig. 5-1. The (internal) ground

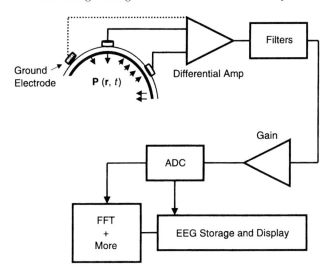

Figure 7-3 The major components of a typical EEG recording system. Electrodes record scalp signals due to brain current sources (arrows) that are passed through differential amplifiers sensitive to potential differences between electrode pairs and insensitive to the (generally much larger) spatially constant potentials over the scalp (common modes). Modern EEG systems record simultaneously from about 32 to 131 scalp locations. Analog filters low pass the input signal, typically removing substantial EEG power above about 50 to 100 Hz. High-pass analog EEG filters typically remove substantial power below about 0.5 Hz, depending on application and filter roll-off characteristics. A notch filter may or may not be used to remove power line frequencies (60 Hz in the US). The scalp potential difference signal is substantially boosted by amplifier gains. In modern EEG systems, the analog signals are sampled and numbers assigned to each part of the waveforms (ADC, analog to digital conversion). This step requires measuring ADC output produced by a calibration signal. EEG waveforms may then be displayed on a paper chart or computer screen and stored for additional processing, typically starting with application of fast Fourier transforms (FFT) to each data channel. Adapted from Cadwell and Villarreal (1999) and Fisch (1999).

serves as a reference for the differential amplifier as shown in figs. 7-2 and 7-3. The measured signal is then amplified and filtered by analog circuits to remove both low- and high-frequency noise plus power at frequencies greater than the Nyquist limit established by the sampling rate of the analog to digital converter (ADC). The analog signal from each channel is sampled at perhaps 200 to 1000 times per second, assigned numbers proportional to instantaneous amplitude (digitized), and converted from ADC units to volts.

Choice of filter settings requires some care. For example, EEG systems typically have notch filters to remove power line interference (60 Hz in the US; 50 Hz in other countries). However, the presence of power line noise in the recorded EEG signal can provide an excellent "canary in the mine shaft" test to detect electrodes that develop high contact impedances (or come off entirely) during the recording as shown by (7.2) when one of the contact impedances becomes very large, that is $(Z_1 \text{ or } Z_2) \rightarrow Z_{IN}$. If EEG processing is based on FFT analysis, the presence of moderate 60 Hz noise will have no practical effect on results at lower frequencies. Thus, it may be better engineering practice to avoid the notch filter in many instances. Another issue concerns the low-pass analog filter. Clearly, this filter must be set to ensure removal of power at the very high frequencies greater than the Nyquist limit. However, severe low-pass filtering runs the risk of removing obvious muscle artifact (data that would normally be discarded), while passing subtle muscle artifact that can be easily mistaken for EEG (Fisch 1999). To take an extreme example, imagine using an analog filter to remove most power at frequencies greater than 30 Hz, thereby obtaining a much cleaner-looking signal. However, muscle artifact is broad band so that the remaining signal might well contain subtle but significant muscle artifact in roughly the 15–30 Hz range, where genuine EEG power is typically low. Such subtle artifact could substantially reduce signal-to-noise ratio in the beta band.

In most EEG practice, one electrode location is chosen as the reference location and the potentials at all the other electrode sites are recorded with respect to the reference by exploiting the properties of the differential amplifiers. This reference point is largely arbitrary; it is special only because we choose to record potential differences with respect to one fixed location. We have the option of changing the effective reference to another recording site further down the processing chain of fig. 7-3 by simple subtraction. That is, the original N-channel recording with respect to reference location r yields the signals

$$V_n - V_r \quad n = 1, N \tag{7.3}$$

We are free to re-reference to any one of the original recording sites y by the transformation

$$V_n - V_y \equiv (V_n - V_r) - (V_y - V_r) \tag{7.4}$$

where the potential difference inside the second parenthesis is obtained in the original recording. This transformation can be applied to any recording location y other than one with noisy data. Other simple linear transformations are often useful, including the nearest-neighbor (Hjorth) Laplacian and common average reference discussed in this chapter.

The old EEG myth that makes a sharp distinction between *reference* and *recording* electrodes is exposed here, extending the discussions in chapters 1, 2, and 5. *There are no monopolar recordings in EEG; all recordings are bipolar.* Every EEG recording depends on the location of both recording and "reference" electrodes; any particular choice of reference placement offers possible advantages and disadvantages depending on actual source locations. However, in general, we do not know the location of the sources prior to recording EEG so no ideal reference location is likely to be found in advance. Reference strategies have often been adopted in

EEG laboratories without a clear understanding of the attendant biases imposed on the recording. The linked-ears or linked-mastoids reference, a historically popular reference choice with cognitive scientists, is one such idea with minimal theoretical justification, but nevertheless persists in a number of laboratories. Another popular choice is the common average reference. We consider the properties of these two approaches in detail in this chapter.

Another important practical question is how closely electrodes must be spaced in order to obtain accurate representations of continuous potential distributions on the scalp. We consider this problem in terms of the familiar Nyquist theorem: *to represent a continuous signal by discrete sampling, the sampling rate must exceed twice the highest frequency in the signal.* In other words, at least two samples per cycle are required to avoid aliasing. This requirement is quite familiar to scientists who digitally sample EEG time series. The spatial sampling of scalp potentials is subject to a similar requirement. To assess this issue, we provide estimates of the highest spatial frequencies that can be expected to contribute significantly to EEG recordings and consider the number of electrodes required to discretely sample the scalp potentials.

Let us first pose the fundamental question of EEG. Can we use the potential distribution over the scalp to obtain reasonably accurate estimates of the locations and dynamic behaviors of the underlying current sources? As discussed in this and earlier chapters, this basic question cannot be answered satisfactorily in the absence of some knowledge of the sources. An effectively infinite number of possible source distributions can give rise to the same scalp potential distribution. Despite this fundamental limitation on our knowledge of current source locations and dynamics, we are able to obtain nearly unique estimates of the dynamic behavior of potentials on the dura surface as discussed in chapter 8. In many EEG applications, this is all the information we need. That is, the establishment of robust relationships between dura potential dynamics and brain state is, of itself, an important achievement. Often, we can reasonably assume that the most dominant sources are located in cortical gyri, in which case the cortical mesosource function $\mathbf{P}(\mathbf{r}, t)$ and dura potential behavior are nearly identical.

The *n-sphere models* discussed in chapter 6 satisfactorily predict important properties of volume conduction in the head. We make extensive use of these models to investigate aspects of EEG recording in this chapter. Of course, real heads are not spherical shells, and skulls have openings and irregularities that cause deviations from our idealized models. Such deviations from our idealized head models may be quite important in some applications and unimportant in others. Generally, skull openings or regions with lower resistance tend to distort scalp potentials because current follows paths of lowest resistance. The ratio of skull resistivity to brain or scalp resistivity (perhaps 20 to 80) is the same order of magnitude as the ratio of the circumference to thickness of the skull. Hence, the effective resistance of a long current path through a distant skull opening is comparable to the effective resistance through the thickness of a local portion of the skull. As a result, EEG electrodes may record substantial scalp currents due to generators located far from the recording site. These and other considerations such as signal-to-noise ratio and electrode density must be accounted for when assessing the advantages and drawbacks of the recording methods discussed in this chapter.

2 The Quest for an Ideal Reference

One of the most important issues in any EEG recording strategy is the choice of reference electrode location. Figure 7-4 shows examples of a visual evoked potential (VEP) recorded at a right occipital electrode (O_2 in the 10/20 electrode system) with the reference mathematically shifted by (7.1) to different electrode positions. Since the occipital cortex contains striate and extrastriate visual areas, the VEP is expected to include signals generated by sources in occipital cortex. The upper figure (fig. 7-4a) shows the VEP with reference shifted to three different electrodes within 2.7 cm of the vertex electrode (C_Z), which was the reference electrode position chosen for recording. The VEP is often characterized in terms of the magnitudes of positive and negative voltage peaks. The first positive peak (approximately 100 ms poststimulus) has its amplitude reduced by 33% as the reference site is changed from the midline position (1) to either of the other two positions. Amplitude differences are also evident at other peaks in the evoked potential waveform. The middle figure (fig. 7-4b) shows the same VEP with the reference site shifted to three midline frontal locations separated by less than 2.7 cm. The first positive peak is reduced in comparison to reference positions near the vertex shown in fig. 7-4, a and the shape of the evoked potential is considerably altered between 100 and 350 ms poststimulus. The VEP is dominated by a faster oscillation when the reference is located at frontal sites in comparison to the waveform obtained when the reference is close to the vertex. The lower figure (fig. 7-4c) shows the VEP with the reference site mathematically shifted to the left mastoid (1) and temporal electrodes (2 and 3) separated by approximately 3 cm. The positive peak 100 ms poststimulus is no longer distinguishable from noise, and the first distinct peak occurs 200 ms poststimulus. Thus, we find that both the amplitude and temporal structure of the VEP recorded at a channel over the occipital lobe (O_2) can be altered considerably by the choice of reference site, even though the dominant VEP sources are expected to be close to the occipital electrode.

Is there an ideal or "correct" reference position? The EEG folklore suggesting that an "inactive" electrode is the ideal reference electrode stems from the idea that if the recording electrode is near a "generator" (mesosource) and the reference electrode is "far" from the generator, the reference electrode can be thought of as being at an infinite distance.

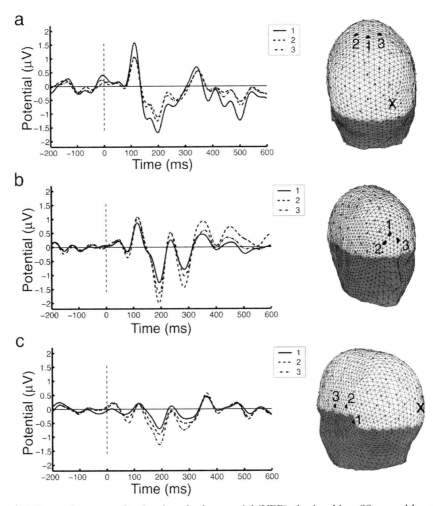

Figure 7-4 Example traces of a visual evoked potential (VEP) obtained in a 22-year-old male using different references. The visual stimulus was a circular Glass pattern formed by superimposing a rotated random dot pattern on itself (Murias 2004). The EEG data were sampled at 1000 Hz with a hardware high-pass filter at 0.1 Hz and low-pass filter at 100 Hz. The traces of EEG were then low-pass filtered at 30 Hz using a 10th order Butterworth filter, and averaged over 100 repetitions of the stimulus. The VEP was recorded at a channel over right occipital cortex (X or O_2) with respect to a vertex reference. The reference was shifted by subtracting the potential recorded at the new reference location (with respect to the vertex) from the potential at the occipital channel (with respect to the vertex) as in (7.1). The head plots locate the recording electrode (X) and three reference sites (1–3) for each plot. (a) Three near-vertex references (one recorded and two transformed). (b) Three frontal references (transformed from vertex recording). (c) Three left mastoid references (transformed from vertex recording).

In this idealized picture, one could truly record potentials with respect to a standard zero-potential reference. However, the so-called inactive electrode may or may not be a good reference depending partly on the size of the generator region. Consider a single-unit recording electrode close to a neuron a few hundred microns in length. With a reference electrode located at a distance of (say) 5 cm, the distance between reference electrode and recording electrode is about 100 times the size of the generator region. If the reference electrode were moved to any distance greater than 5 cm from the generator region, we would expect no perceptible difference in the recording since both locations of the reference are, for practical purposes, at infinity. By contrast, the examples of an occipital electrode recording the VEP in fig. 7-4 suggest that no point on the upper surface of the head is "far" from the generators (mesosources) of the VEP.

Dipole layers of synchronous and partly aligned cortical neurons extending over large areas of the cortical surface (multiple gyri) are apparently the primary generators of scalp EEG as discussed in chapter 6. Hence, generator dimensions can be as large as tens of centimeters whereas head diameters are on the order of 20 cm. Thus, for the common case of large generator (source) regions, it is not generally possible to find a point on the head at a sufficiently large distance from the generator regions (*compared to their sizes*) to be considered at "infinity." *The requirement that the electrode be located at a place where there is no underlying generator is not sufficient for it to be considered at infinity.* An example simulation illustrating this point is given in fig. 2-1. Furthermore, low-resistance current paths in an inhomogeneous or anisotropic head can make electrical distances shorter than actual distances as discussed in chapter 3. For a reference to be considered "at infinity," the *electrical distance* between reference and recording electrodes must be very large in comparison to the generator region, even if there is no generator activity directly beneath the reference electrode. These ideas are also illustrated in fig. 2-1 by simulations with several thousand sources in a head model (Nunez and Westdorp 1994).

Is it possible for an EEG scientist to use a sufficiently distant reference on the body to approximate a reference at infinity? Figure 7-5a illustrates a reference on a portion of the body below the head, in this case the hand. Because all sources and sinks of interest in EEG are located in the head, which is partly isolated (electrically) from the body except for a path through the neck, the current produced by brain sources is expected to be mostly confined to the head (Katznelson 1981). We expect minimal current flow through the more narrow neck region. If the neck geometry did not severely restrict neck currents, scalp potentials would likely be more contaminated by EKG sources, which are about 100 times stronger than EEG sources.

It follows from Ohm's law that the potential difference between points A and B in fig. 7-5a is nearly zero for generators located only in the head. Thus, the effective reference is not distant at all, but is essentially located on the neck (Katznelson 1981). This is illustrated by fig. 7-5b which shows the equivalent circuit for the layout in fig. 7-5a. The body resistance from point A to B is roughly several thousand ohms, which is very small compared to the input impedance of the EEG amplifiers. Thus, the effect

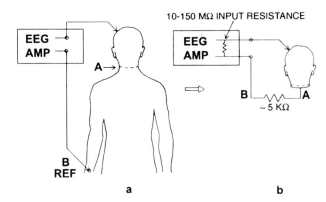

Figure 7-5 This figure addresses the general question—Can a "distant" reference for scalp EEG be found? (a) The physically distant reference at the hand (B) is electrically equivalent to a reference at the neck (A) with respect to sources in the head. The hand reference can be expected to pick up more EKG and other artifact. (b) The circuit equivalent to (a), but ignoring non-brain sources. Reproduced with permission from Katznelson (1981).

of the body resistance (from A to B) is negligible, and the EEG record will be practically identical to that obtained by using point A as the reference except for the probable addition of new artifact. A similar situation occurs for a reference placed on any "distant" part of the body like the toe, for example. The effective reference location for all lower body locations is essentially the neck with minimal additional series resistance due to the lower body.

A simple test of EEG will reveal if any putative reference location can be considered a true reference; that is, a reference at infinity. Suppose, for example, that we suspect localized (epileptic) spike activity in right temporal cortex. If this assumption of a localized generator region is correct, any location on the left side of the head may qualify as a suitable reference. We might, for example, choose a putative reference over left frontal cortex. The critical reference test is to see if the essential dynamic behavior of the spike activity remains constant as we change the reference location from left frontal to (say) left temporal or left mastoid or left neck. If the spike timing, waveform and amplitude are unchanged with change of trial reference, then *the true reference test is passed*. If, however, the recorded spike dynamics changes with choice of trial reference location, *the true reference test fails*, probably because the postulate of a localized source region is incorrect. For example, unexpected sources in mesial (underside) cortex have been known to confound clinical electroencephalographers investigating epileptic discharges.

The examples of a VEP recorded at an occipital channel shown in fig. 7-4 indicate that none of the reference sites examined meet the true reference test. The peak amplitudes and temporal waveforms both depend on the so-called reference location. At each reference location (fig. 7-4a–c), shifting the reference locally among three closely spaced electrodes produces substantial effects on peak amplitudes. The implication is that with every reference location, the potential difference between recording and reference electrode are sensitive to different sets of sources. The source distribution underlying this example VEP may be sufficiently large and distributed to prevent any location on the head from qualifying as a true reference.

To summarize the ideas of this section, the unavoidable conclusion is that no "distant" reference point is generally available in EEG recording. We rarely know in advance where such sources are located (or if they are indeed localized at all) so as to know where to place the so-called reference. Even in cases where the sources (generators) are truly localized, the reference electrode concept is meaningless if we do not know source locations in advance. Thus, we are forced to face the (perhaps) painful truth about EEG references—there is essentially no difference between recording and reference electrodes. *In EEG, potential differences between pairs of locations on the head are measured, and these differences depend on both electrode locations, as well as all brain generator configurations and locations.*

3 Reciprocity and EEG Lead Fields

We have suggested that the sharp distinction between recording and reference electrode is a myth that has often obscured EEG studies. The reference issue has also been addressed by making use of the reciprocity theorem and lead fields associated with EEG electrodes (Plonsey 1969; Rush and Driscoll 1968, 1969; Katznelson 1981; Malmivuo and Plonsey 1995).

The basic approach of the reciprocity theorem is that knowledge of the current density (or electric field) through a volume conductor caused by an injection of current between two stimulating electrodes (placed on the scalp, for example) completely specifies how those same electrodes, when serving as recording electrodes, pick up potentials caused by dipole sources in the volume conductor. Suppose that a pair of stimulating electrodes is placed at locations A and B on the scalp as indicated in fig. 7-6. An external current source will cause current to flow from electrode B through the brain, cerebrospinal fluid (CSF), skull, and scalp to electrode A. The total current I_{AB} passing through electrode A must equal the total current through electrode B. However, because of the geometry, inhomogeneity, and anisotropy of the head, there will be considerable variation of the *current density* with location. For example, there will be some tendency for current to flow only through the scalp rather than through the low-conductivity skull. The fraction of the current that actually passes through the brain depends critically on the spacing of the electrodes: the closer the electrodes, the lower the brain currents (Rush and Driscoll 1968). The electric field at various locations can be determined theoretically or experimentally in a saline filled skull or

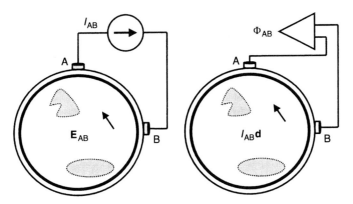

Figure 7-6 (*Left*) Current I_{AB} is injected into the surface of the (general) linear volume conductor using electrodes at A and B. As a result, current passes through the volume conductor, and the electric field $\mathbf{E}_{AB}$ (arrow) at any inner location is proportional to local current density (Ohm's law). The dashed grey areas represent regions with different conductivity than the remainder of the inner material, emphasizing that the reciprocity theorem applies to volume conductors of arbitrary shape and consisting of material that may be inhomogeneous and anisotropic. (*Right*) The identical volume conductor containing a dipole current source ($\mathbf{p} = I\mathbf{d}$) is shown. The surface potential difference Φ_{AB} is recorded with electrodes placed at identical locations (A and B). The reciprocity theorem provides a simple relationship between this potential difference Φ_{AB} and the lead field $\mathbf{E}_{AB}$ given by (7.5).

animal brain. Let this electric field be denoted $\mathbf{E}_{AB}$ with corresponding current density $\mathbf{J}_{AB}$ given by Ohm's law.

If we double the injected current, the current density doubles at each location due to linearity of the volume conductor. The electric field normalized by the injected current $\mathbf{L}_{AB} = \mathbf{E}_{AB}/I_{AB}$ is independent of the strength of the external current source and depends only on the geometry and electrical properties of the volume conductor and electrode placement. This normalized *lead field* characterizes a kind of "electrical access" property of a pair of electrodes to any point in the volume conductor. *The reciprocity theorem states that this access applies equally when these same electrodes are used to record potentials generated from brain sources instead of being used for stimulation. We emphasize that the reciprocity theorem is valid in any linear conductive medium; for example, it is valid in inhomogeneous and anisotropic media.*

The reciprocity theorem played an important role in the early development of n-sphere models of the head described in chapter 6. The 3-sphere model was used to predict current flow in the brain due to injected surface current. The validity of this model was tested using an electrolytic tank containing a human skull and by comparison with in vivo data recorded within the brain of a monkey and on the surface of the human head (Rush and Driscoll 1968, 1969). Good agreement between theory and measured currents in the tank experiment was obtained if the skull had an effective resistivity of about 80 times that of the fluid inside. The theoretical model was also reported to be capable of predicting measured potentials of the human scalp and potentials measured within a monkey brain due to current introduced at the surface of the scalp. These data, together with the reciprocity theorem, have encouraged use of n-sphere models with skull conductivity of the order of 80 times lower than brain or scalp to predict scalp potentials due to dipole sources. More recent experiments suggest that this ratio for living skull may be lower, perhaps closer to 40 or even 20 as discussed in chapter 4.

The reciprocity theorem can be written mathematically in terms of the potential difference between recording electrode A and B due to a dipole source:

$$\Phi_B - \Phi_A = \frac{\mathbf{E}_{AB} \cdot I\mathbf{d}}{I_{AB}} = \mathbf{L}_{AB} \cdot \mathbf{p} \qquad (7.5)$$

where $\mathbf{p} = I\mathbf{d}$ is the dipole moment vector of a mesosource, essentially the product of $\mathbf{P}(\mathbf{r}, t)$ with its tissue volume element. I_{AB} is the current flowing between source and sink poles and $\mathbf{d}$ is the direction vector between the poles. The dot product between lead field vector and dipole vector means that the location of the dipole source alone does not fully specify the sensitivity of the electrodes to that dipole. Dipole orientation is also needed for this purpose. Imagine that we somehow knew the lead field at every location within the volume conductor (for a given electrode placement). Then any dipole placed at locations where the lead field is large and oriented parallel to the local lead field will generate relatively large potential differences between the given elec-trodes. By contrast, any dipole oriented perpendicular to the local lead field vector (regardless of magnitude) will produce zero potential differ-ence between the same electrode pair. Thus, the reciprocity theorem provides a very convenient intuitive feeling for the probable surface potentials expected from internal dipole sources.

Malmivuo and Plonsey (1995) carried out calculations of lead fields for different EEG electrode configurations in n-sphere models of the head. For a fixed pair of electrodes, the lead field vectors can be calculated as a function of position throughout the volume conductor. In n-sphere models, the lead field vectors are of equal length but opposite direction in the brain volume beneath stimulating and reference electrode positions. This distribution of lead field vectors is essentially the sensitivity of the same electrode pair to dipole sources as a function of their location and orientation in the volume conductor. Thus, at each location, the orientation of the lead field vector $\mathbf{L}_{AB}$ is the orientation of the dipole source that produces the largest potential difference between the electrodes.

The actual sensitivity of any electrode pair depends on the orientation of the dipole source, which is expected to be determined by the local orientation of the folded cortical surface. In actual heads, complex source orientations (typically along the folded cortex), inhomogeneity, and anisotropy of tissue conductivities further complicate the picture. In such cases, we can expect more complex forms of the sensitivity distribution for any pair of electrodes than in the idealized case of a spherical head model. However, our main point is that we cannot *in principle* distinguish sources near the recording electrode from sources near the reference electrode, given only the information provided by the measured potential difference between two locations. *Reversing the conceptual role of "recording" and "reference" electrodes only reverses the sign of recorded potentials.*

4 Bipolar Recordings

The notion that every EEG recording is a *bipolar recording* is made obvious by the above analysis of EEG lead fields. Of course, the term "bipolar recording" in EEG often refers to the special case where the potential difference between two electrodes that are relatively closely spaced is measured. Bipolar recording is more popular in clinical work than in cognitive studies. As demonstrated in more detailed papers (Srinivasan et al. 1996; Nunez et al. 1997), bipolar recordings with very close electrodes (say 1 to 3 cm) typically offer much better spatial resolution than conventional reference recordings. Of course, raw EEG data may be recorded with respect to a fixed reference and later converted to bipolar recording provided that electrodes are sufficiently close together to provide the desired estimate.

As the electrodes of any pair are moved closer together, they provide progressively better estimates of the local gradient of the potential (or electric field) along the scalp surface, in the direction (along the scalp) between the electrodes. By Ohm's law, the electric field is proportional to current density along the scalp surface. When the two electrodes are placed close together, the recorded potential difference is roughly proportional to the current density tangential to the scalp. The direction of this current is from higher to lower potentials.

Bipolar recordings (with close electrodes, say less than 3 cm) are better localized than recordings with fixed reference at some "far" distance at least for idealized superficial generators. *The use of bipolar electrode pairs to estimate local tangential electric fields is an improvement over reference recordings in the sense that both recording and reference electrode are explicitly acknowledged and the reference issue becomes moot.* If the bipolar pair is placed across isopotential lines, the bipolar pair is sensitive to current flow from regions of higher to lower potential. However, if the bipolar pair is placed along an isopotential line, zero potential is recorded. Clinical electroencephalographers often make use of different bipolar pairs to emphasize different sources, and make qualitative judgments of their orientation and

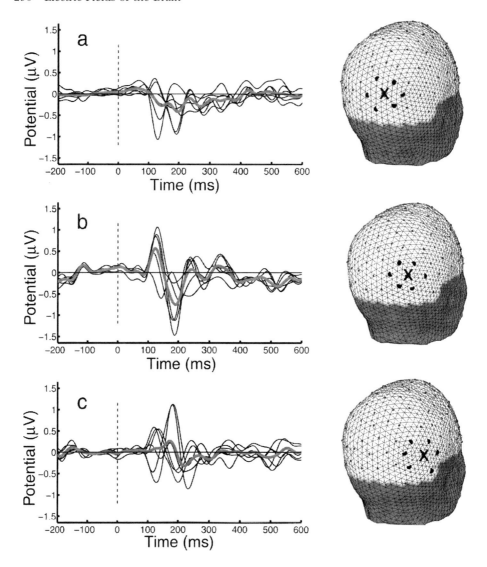

Figure 7-7 Example bipolar potentials for a visual evoked potential (VEP). The details of the recording are given in the caption of fig. 7-3. Bipolar potentials are calculated by taking the difference between the potential recorded at the central electrode (with reference at the vertex) and the potential at each of six surrounding electrodes (with reference at the vertex). The separation distance between electrode pairs is 2.7 cm. Each plot (a–c) corresponds to the center electrode X in a different location in the right posterior area. The six black lines in each plot correspond to each bipolar evoked potential. The thick gray lines are the average of the six bipolar evoked potentials in each plot (a–c).

localization based on long experience with such methods (Pilgreen 1995; Fisch 1999).

Figure 7-7 provides three additional examples of the VEP shown in fig. 7-4 using bipolar pairs obtained using one fixed (central) recording electrode with the second electrode mathematically shifted to six surrounding positions all at roughly 2.7 cm distance. In each plot, the six black curves indicate the bipolar potentials while the thick gray line is the mean of all six bipolar potentials. The temporal structure of the bipolar potentials is considerably different from the "distant" reference potentials shown in fig. 7-4. Peaks are still evident at 100 and 200 ms poststimulus, but the slower oscillation evident in fig. 7-4a and potentials at 300 ms or later are reduced in each set of bipolar pairs shown in fig. 7-7. The positive peak 100 ms poststimulus is most clear in fig. 7-7b, where five of six bipolar pairs exhibit a positive peak. The potential at this central electrode is larger than any surrounding potential for almost all bipolar pair directions, which suggests that some of the source activity is localized to tissue beneath the recording electrode. In fig. 7-7 a and c, individual bipolar pairs show peaks but with opposite polarity, which average to near zero at the 100 ms peak poststimulus. This indicates that tangential current passing from regions of higher potential to lower potential at the central electrodes mostly passes to other regions of even lower potential than the central electrode. This comparison of all bipolar pairs involving one central electrode is closely related to the nearest-neighbour estimate of the surface Laplacian discussed in chapter 8. A small signal estimated by the nearest-neighbor Laplacian is indicated by the average gray line in fig. 7-7a and c and a large signal is indicated by the average gray line in fig. 7-7b. Thus we have strong evidence of a local source under the central electrode in fig. 7-7b, and little evidence of sources near the central electrodes for the arrays of fig. 7-7a and c.

The analysis of EEG recorded with close bipolar pairs can be an effective strategy to identify local generators. By placing the "reference" electrode nearby rather than at a distant location on the head, the sensitivity of each pair of electrodes is mainly limited to local sources. *With a limited number of electrodes, bipolar recordings are perhaps the best option available to improve the spatial resolution of the EEG.* Closely related to this strategy is the nearest-neighbor Laplacian or Hjorth Laplacian. If enough electrodes are available, better estimates of local sources are obtained with spline Laplacians, discussed in chapter 8.

5 Linked-Ears or Linked-Mastoids Reference

The linked-ears or linked-mastoids reference is a popular choice, apparently mostly for historical reasons. The origins of this reference choice appear obscure; its common use in many laboratories today seems to be an historical epiphenomenon given the minimal theoretical basis supporting this approach. As shown below, there is no compelling reason to believe that the linked-ears approach approximates reference-free potentials (potentials with respect to infinity). Furthermore, the apparent symmetry of the method that has apparently seduced so many EEG scientists is largely an illusion.

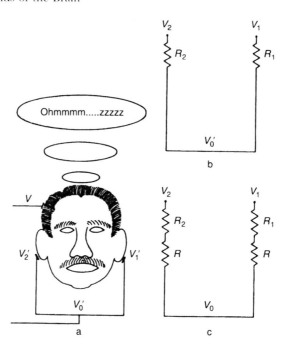

Figure 7-8 Schematic of the physically linked-ear or linked-mastoid reference. (a) The physically linked ear reference imposes a new boundary condition forcing the two sites to essentially the same potential, thereby generally changing the potential distribution over the head. The magnitude of this effect depends on the source distribution and the contact resistances R_1 and R_2. (b) The link between electrodes has a resistance that is equal to the combined resistance of the two ear contacts, $R_1 + R_2$. (c) The problem of current flowing in the wire can be minimized by adding a large series resistance R, but this may result in a substantial rise in noise level depending on the imbalance between this linked-reference and the contact resistances of the recording electrodes (Ferree et al. 2001). This implies that as the effective resistance of the linked-reference varies during an experiment, the corresponding noise level also varies.

There are two ways in which the linked-ears/linked-mastoids reference has been implemented in published studies. One approach is to physically link the ears (or mastoids) by a wire to serve as the reference as shown in fig. 7-8. We label this *the physical linked-ears reference*. Alternatively, with the *mathematical linked-ears reference* all scalp potentials are recorded with respect to a reference placed at one ear $(V - V_1)$, with the second ear potential measured with respect to the first ear $(V_2 - V_1)$. The mathematically linked-ears reference is calculated by subtracting half this potential difference from all the measured potentials, creating an artificial reference at the average potential of the two ears or mastoids, that is

$$(V - V_1) - \frac{V_1 - V_2}{2} \equiv V - \frac{V_1 + V_2}{2} \tag{7.6}$$

The mathematically linked-ears reference has grown in popularity principally because it is now more widely (but not universally) recognized that the physical linked-ears reference suffers from serious problems detailed below.

The first possible problem is that the physical linked-ears reference illustrated in fig. 7-8 imposes a new *boundary condition* on head volume conduction (Katznelson 1981). In chapter 6 the potential due to a dipole source was calculated in the 4-sphere model with the boundary condition forcing zero radial current flow from the scalp surface. Physically linking the ears or mastoids provides a low resistance path for current to flow out of the scalp at one location and back into the scalp at another location. Let V be the potential with respect to infinity at some scalp location, and let V_1 and V_2 be the left and right ear (or mastoid) potentials, respectively. When the ears are linked, some current will flow through the wire connecting the ears. *Thus, the potentials V, V_1, and V_2 all change from their values before linkage. This generally means that all potentials on the scalp also change.* As illustrated in fig. 7-8b, the properties of the current path between ears depend on the electrode contact resistances R_1 and R_2 at each ear. The magnitude of change in the natural distribution of potential depends on the magnitude of contact resistance relative to head tissue resistance and on the locations of the current sources relative to the ears. The resulting distortion of potential may be negligible in many or even most cases (Miller et al. 1991), but it is difficult to estimate this effect without knowing the orientation and location of the sources; *the lower the contact resistance the larger the distortion of the surface potential.* Thus, the experimenter must aim for contact resistances that are low compared to the amplifier input impedances, but not so low that significant current flows in the wire between the ears. One suggested strategy to minimize current flowing in the wire is to add a series resistance much larger than R_1 or R_2 to the wire and using the midpoint of the resistor as the reference, as shown in fig. 7-8c, although this procedure may add substantial noise to recordings.

The second problem afflicting the physically linked-ears reference is probably more serious than the first in many applications. Even if the contact resistances are in the right range to prevent shorting the two sides of the head, balancing the contact resistances to create a symmetric reference is a remaining problem (Nunez 1991). The potential across the wire connecting the ears or mastoids is given by

$$V_{12} = \frac{R_2 V_1 + R_1 V_2}{R_1 + R_2} \tag{7.7}$$

If the ear contact resistances are equal, $R_1 = R_2$, the linked-ears reference potential is simply the average potential of the two ears as in (7.6). The opposite limit occurs when one of the electrodes comes off making its contact resistance infinite (say $R_2 \rightarrow \infty$), in which case the reference potential is the potential at the opposite ear ($V_{12} \rightarrow V_1$). In actual EEG practice, neither of these limiting cases is likely to occur so that the actual reference is unbalanced to one side or the other. Thus, one of the common motivations for using a linked-ears reference, to achieve a "balanced" (symmetric) reference for studies of lateralization of brain function, is self-defeating. To make the physical linked-ears reference symmetric, we must ensure that ear contact resistances are equal, rather than the common practice of checking only to see if they are less than (typically) 10 or 20 kΩ. We note that the implementation of modern amplifiers with very high input impedances (>200 MΩ) has allowed for good recordings with contact impedances of 50 kΩ or more (Ferree et al. 2001). However, this technical advance has the potential to make the physically linked-ears imbalance (7.7) even worse. For example, with 3 kΩ left electrode and 30 kΩ right electrode resistances, the effective reference is the left ear. If electrode resistances change, either during individual recording sessions or from subject to subject, *the physically linked-ears reference may become a random reference*, switching back and forth from ear to ear.

The mathematical linked-ears or linked-mastoids reference may seem to provide a "solution" to these problems associated with the physical linked reference. However, does the original goal of using the average potential of the two ears as the reference make sense? The motivation for this procedure is not based on any physical properties of head volume conduction. The measured potential difference between a pair of electrodes depends on sources located near both electrode positions. *With the mathematical linked-ears reference, the recorded potential depends on sources at three different locations.* This approach may further complicate the interpretation of scalp potentials and possible source locations rather than simplifying it. One rationalization often argued to support the linked-ears or linked-mastoids reference is its purported tendency to be a "symmetric" reference with respect to both brain hemispheres, thereby providing a tool for characterizing hemispheric asymmetries in EEG studies. However, this is not generally true; the effect of the average mastoids reference is artificially to correlate data from recording electrodes near the two mastoids (Srinivasan et al. 1998), potentially reducing estimates of dynamic hemispheric source asymmetries. We will consider several simulations in the next section where we introduce the average reference and compare it to the mathematical linked-ears reference.

6 The Average Reference

The average reference (also called the common average reference) has become commonplace in EEG studies and has some theoretical justification (Bertrand et al. 1985). As has been emphasized throughout this chapter there is essentially no difference between recording electrode and reference electrode. Thus, when one records EEG data from N

electrodes, the measured potentials V_n ($n = 1, 2, \ldots N$) are related to the scalp potential $\Phi(\mathbf{r})$ with respect to "infinity" by

$$V_n = \Phi(\mathbf{r}_n) - \Phi(\mathbf{r}_R) \tag{7.8}$$

where $\mathbf{r}_n$ is the position of the nth electrode and $\mathbf{r}_R$ is the reference electrode site. Note that the average of these measured potentials can be written in terms of the scalp potentials as

$$\frac{1}{N} \sum_{n=1}^{N} V_n = -\Phi(\mathbf{r}_R) + \frac{1}{N} \sum_{n=1}^{N} \Phi(\mathbf{r}_n) \tag{7.9}$$

Rearranging the terms, scalp potential at the reference location is

$$\Phi(\mathbf{r}_R) = \frac{1}{N} \sum_{n=1}^{N} \Phi(\mathbf{r}_n) - \frac{1}{N} \sum_{n=1}^{N} V_n \tag{7.10}$$

The first term on the right-hand side of (7.10) is the average of the scalp surface potential at all recording sites. Theoretically, this term vanishes if the electrodes are positioned such that the mean of the potentials approximates a surface integral over a closed surface containing all current within the volume. As noted in section 2, apparently only minimal current flows from the head through the neck even with reference electrode placed on the body, so a reasonable approximation considers the head to be a closed volume that confines all current. The surface integral of the potential over a volume conductor containing dipole sources must be zero as a consequence of current conservation (Bertrand et al. 1985). In this case, the surface integral can be estimated by the second term on the right-hand side of (7.10); that is, by averaging the measured potentials and changing the sign of this average. This potential $\Phi(\mathbf{r}_R)$ can be added to each measurement V_n using (7.8), thereby estimating the reference-free potential (potential with respect to "infinity") at each location $\Phi(\mathbf{r}_n)$.

Since we cannot measure the potentials on a closed surface surrounding the brain, the first term on the right-hand side of (7.10) will not generally vanish. The distribution of potential on the underside of the head (within the neck region) cannot be measured. Furthermore, the average potential for any group of electrode positions, given by the second term on the right-hand side of (7.10), can only approximate the surface integral over the volume conductor. For example, *this is expected to be a very poor approximation if applied with the standard 10/20 electrode system.* As the number of electrodes increases the error in the approximation is expected to decrease. Thus, like any other choice of reference, the average reference provides biased estimates of reference-independent potentials.

Nevertheless, when used in studies with large numbers of electrodes (say 128 or more), we have found that the average reference often performs reasonably well as an estimate of reference-independent potentials in simulation studies (Srinivasan et al. 1998).

Figure 7-9 illustrates a simulation of scalp potentials generated by two dipole sources, one radial and one tangential in the 4-sphere model. The radial source is located at a depth approximating superficial gyral surfaces, while the tangential dipole is located somewhat deeper approximating a sulcal wall. Figure 7-9a shows the location of the two sources and the reference independent potentials (with respect to infinity) obtained on the surface of the outer sphere in a 4-sphere model at 111 electrode locations. The average nearest-neighbor (center-to-center) separation between these electrodes is 2.7 cm. The topographic maps were interpolated from the potentials calculated at the electrode positions. The positive and negative lobes of the potential distribution associated with the tangential dipole are readily apparent, reversing over the midline, while the radial dipole generates a more restricted potential distribution close to the mastoid electrode. Figure 7-9b shows the potential distribution with reference electrode placed at the vertex, indicated by an X. Directly above the center of the tangential dipole, the potential generated by the tangential dipole is zero and a small positive potential is contributed by the radial dipole. This results in an apparent asymmetry in the potential distribution due to the tangential dipole, with a reduced magnitude of the positive peak on the right-hand side of the array, and an increase in the magnitude of the negative peak. Figures 7-9c and 7.9d show the potential distribution with the reference placed at the left and right mastoid, respectively. The left-mastoid reference produces little change in the potential distribution, as the potential at the left mastoid is close to zero. By contrast, placing the reference electrode at the right mastoid (fig. 7-9d) significantly distorts potentials by adding a positive potential to all locations. This effect is also present but with smaller magnitude when a mathematical linked-ears reference is used, as shown in fig. 7-9e. The average reference was computed from 110 electrodes using the vertex-referenced potentials. In this particular case, the average reference provides a reasonable estimate of reference independent potentials as shown in fig. 7-9f.

The redistribution of recorded potential resulting from changing the reference location makes intuitive sense since this approach involves subtracting the potential at one location on the head from all the other potentials. This will impact not only the estimated spatial properties of the EEG but also temporal properties since the potential at the reference location generally varies over time. This essential idea is evident in fig. 7-5 where the time course of the VEP depends on the reference electrode position. The main point is that any specific reference, including the mathematical linked-ears or linked-mastoids reference, contributes potentials from distant sites to each so-called recording electrode.

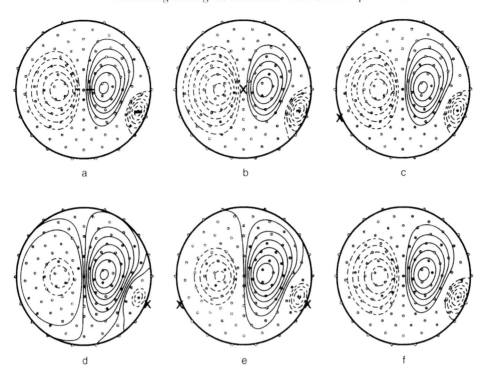

Figure 7-9 Potential maps on the surface of the 4-sphere head model due to two dipole sources – one radial at lower right and one tangential in the center. The tangential source is located 3.2 cm below the scalp; it has twice the strength of the radial dipole located 1.4 cm below the scalp. The four concentric spheres model parameters are given in fig. 6-5. Potentials were calculated at 111 surface sites, with nearest-neighbour separation of about 2.7 cm and subtending an angle of 109 degrees from vertex. The simulated electrode positions are indicated by small gray circles. Topographic maps of the potential distribution were obtained from a spline interpolation as discussed in chapter 8. (a) Potential map with respect to infinity. (b) Potential map with reference indicated by an X located at the vertex. (c) Potential map with reference X at the left mastoid. (d) Potential map with reference to a right mastoid electrode. (e) Potential map with respect to the mathematically linked (averaged) mastoids. (f) Average reference potential map obtained by first calculating the potentials at 110 electrode sites with respect to the vertex and then calculating the average reference using (7.10) with the first sum set to zero.

The specific effects of any choice of reference will depend on the configuration of generators. *The point that we have made repeatedly is that with any reference strategy we record the potential at one head location with respect to some other head location.* By definition, this potential difference is the result of integration of the electric field over any path connecting the reference point and the point in question. We say any path because electric potentials are fundamentally path-independent. The average reference can provide a good estimate of reference-independent potentials because it integrates many possible paths to the point, depending on the number of electrodes.

One concern often expressed about the average reference is that the presence of strong sources deep in the brain may result in major misinterpretations of recorded data. In typical EEG recording, there are few if any electrodes on the lower surface of the head. Thus a dipole near the center of the head contributes more positive potential to the array of electrodes than negative potential. By taking the average reference, we force the potential distribution to have zero mean over the portion of the head covered by the electrodes (typically 50–70% of the head surface). The average reference recording will certainly distort the potentials generated by these deep sources. However, the size of this effect depends on the relative strength of deep sources versus superficial sources. In EEG practice, the effectiveness of the average reference also depends on the number of electrodes used to record the potentials and on the nature and number of sources. While the average reference offers theoretical as well as practical advantages, it is effective only if there are a sufficient number of electrodes (perhaps 64 to 128 or more) distributed over the entire scalp, including (if practical) samples on the lower surface of the head. Practical considerations that limit information from the lower surface of the head include muscle sources and other artifacts. The average reference is probably a poor choice for use with the standard 10/20 system (Fein et al. 1988). That is, the first term on the right-hand side of (7.12) is expected to yield very inaccurate estimates of the surface integral of potential when sparse electrode arrays are used.

7 Spatial Sampling of EEG

Topographic mapping of scalp potentials is now commonplace in clinical and research laboratories. The brain's current sources generate potential distributions that are continuous over the scalp and lower surface of the head. In this section we consider the number of electrodes needed to map accurately surface potentials in order to interpret the measured potentials at discrete locations as a continuous function of surface location. The discrete sampling of continuous signals is a well-characterized problem in time series acquisition and analysis (Bendat and Piersol 2001). The central concept is the *Nyquist criterion:* $f_{dig} > 2f_{max}$ where f_{dig} is the digitization rate or sampling rate and f_{max} is the highest frequency present in the time series. For instance, if the highest frequency in a signal is 20 Hz (cycles/second), a minimum sampling rate of 40 Hz (one sample every 25 ms) is required to record the signal discretely without *aliasing*. Aliasing is the misrepresentation of a high-frequency signal as a low-frequency signal because the sampling rate used during analog-to-digital conversion is lower than the Nyquist limit. If a time series has been aliased by under-sampling, no digital signal processing method can undo the aliasing because the necessary information has been lost. In conventional digital EEG practice, a sampling rate is selected and the aliasing error is avoided by applying a low-pass filter to the analog signal, thereby eliminating power at frequencies greater than the maximum frequency determined by the Nyquist limit (fig. 7-3). The low-pass filter is typically applied with a cut-off frequency 2.5 times smaller than the sampling rate. This more restrictive limit, known as the *Engineer's Nyquist criterion*, accounts for the possibility of phase locking between the sampling and high-frequency components of the signal (Bendat and Piersol 2001).

The Nyquist criterion for discrete sampling of any analog signal applies to spatial sampling as well as temporal sampling. The scalp surface potential at any point in time is a continuous field variable over the surface of the head. The EEG electrode array provides a discrete sampling of this field, and is therefore subject to the Nyquist criterion. Unlike the time series of a single amplifier channel, the spatial signal is acquired discretely. The temporal signal can be easily low-pass filtered to meet the Nyquist criterion implied by the sampling rate. However, the raw spatial signal cannot be treated in the same manner because no continuous representation of the spatial signal is ever available. As a consequence of this limitation, any aliasing due to under-sampling cannot be prevented; adequate sampling of the potentials must be accomplished from the outset. The electrode density (assuming relatively uniformly distributed electrode placements) and electrode size determine the highest spatial frequency that can be observed without aliasing. If the EEG contains signals with spatial frequencies that are too high, they will be *spatially aliased*; that is, they will appear in topographical maps or spatial spectra as signals of lower spatial frequency, thereby distorting spatial maps of potential, and other dynamic measures. We note in this context that when the EEG is under-sampled spatially (for example, with only one recording electrode and one reference electrode), the measured time series is a valid measurement of the potential difference between the two sites, but the spatial distribution of the potential is unknown.

To illustrate spatial sampling issues, we consider the problem of discrete sampling of the potential distribution on a spherical surface containing dipole current sources. As discussed in chapter 6, any distribution (or function) on a spherical surface can be expressed as a sum of *spherical harmonics* Y_{nm}, mathematical functions analogous to the sine and cosine functions used in spectral analysis of EEG time series (see chapter 9). The n and m indices of the Y_{nm} functions denote spatial frequencies in the two surface directions. The surface coordinates are the angles θ (essentially latitude, but measured from the north pole) and ϕ (longitude). Any potential distribution due to dipole sources in a spherical head model may be represented by a double sum of spherical harmonic functions, called a *generalized Fourier series*.

Examples of spherical harmonics of degree $n = 4, 5, 7$, and 9, with order m fixed at -3 are shown in each column of fig. 7-10. The first column (fig. 7-9a) shows each spherical harmonic under assumptions of perfect sampling, while the successive rows show the same spherical harmonic,

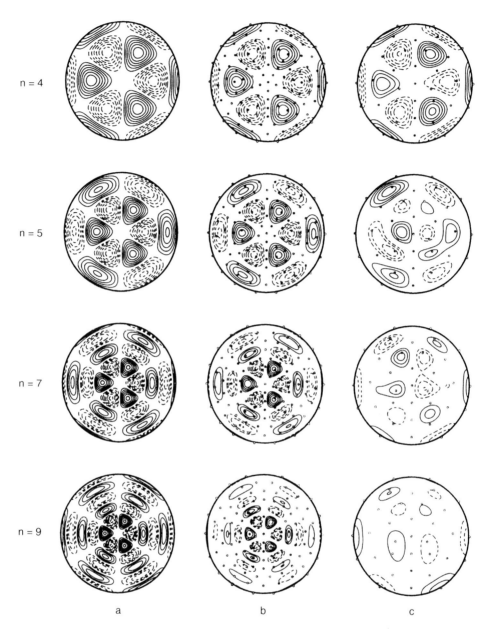

Figure 7-10 Spatial sampling of spherical harmonics. Each row corresponds to a different spherical harmonic of degree $n = 4, 5, 7,$ and 9 with order fixed at $m = -3$. These functions are plotted on a sphere as viewed from the north pole with latitude angle (measured from the pole) in the range $0° < \theta < 109°$. The spatial patterns contain progressively higher spatial frequencies as the degree n increases down the plot. (a) The *gold standard*, that is, the functions are plotted with infinite or perfect sampling. (b) The map obtained by sampling each spherical harmonic with 111 electrodes (2.7 cm spacing) and spline-interpolation. (c) The map obtained by sampling each spherical harmonic with 36 electrodes (5.8 cm spacing) and spline interpolation. Small gray circles indicate the electrode positions.

discretely sampled with 111 (simulated) electrodes (fig. 7-9b) and 36 electrodes (fig. 7-9c). The samples are assumed to cover the upper sphere to a maximum "latitude" somewhat below the equator ($0 < \theta < 109$). With these 111 assumed electrode positions the average (center-to-center) nearest-neighbor separation between electrodes is 2.7 cm, while with 36 electrode positions the average separation is 5.8 cm (similar to the spacing of the 10/20 system). The topographic maps in fig. 7-10 were produced by interpolation. It is clear that discrete sampling distorts the spherical harmonics of higher degree as the index (n) increases. In this simulation, aliasing appears as the erroneous appearance of low spatial frequencies (broad, smooth spatial distributions). The spherical harmonic of degree 4 is accurately represented using both 36 and 111 electrode arrays, but serious aliasing of the spherical harmonic of degree 5 takes place with 36 electrodes. With 111 electrodes the spherical harmonic of degree 7 is well represented, but loss of spatial detail is evident in the spherical harmonic of degree 9.

From these examples it is evident that the highest spatial frequency present in the scalp potential determines the required sampling density to accurately sample the spatial signal. Scalp potentials are believed to be generated by dipole layers mainly from upper regions of cortex. Here we use information gained from the 4-sphere model in chapter 6 to investigate spatial sampling. We restrict our attention to columnar source regions confined to a smooth model cortex at fixed radial location in an idealized spherical head model. The vector dipole moment per unit volume $\mathbf{P}(\mathbf{r}, t)$ is assumed to have only a radial component (although this approximation is not required for most of this description). Any distribution of this scalar mesosource strength $P(\theta, \phi, t)$ over the smooth part of cortex may be expanded in a series of spherical harmonic functions, that is

$$P(\theta,\phi,t) = \sum_{n=0}^{\infty} \sum_{m=-n}^{n} p_{nm}(t)\, Y_{nm}(\theta,\phi) \qquad (7.11)$$

Equation (7.11) is a generalized Fourier series where the basis functions are the (orthogonal) spherical harmonics $Y_{nm}(\theta, \phi)$ replacing sine and/or cosine terms of common Fourier series (Morse and Feshbach 1953; Jackson 1975). The double sum in (7.11) is over *spatial frequencies* in the (θ, ϕ) directions with the indices (n, m) defined such that larger indices indicate higher spatial frequencies.

The (unknown) functions $p_{nm}(t)$ are determined by the dynamic properties of neocortical sources. Regardless of the nature of the underlying neocortical dynamics, (7.11) is general in the sense that it applies to localized sources, distributed sources, or anything in between. Furthermore, (7.11) applies just as well to nonlinear as to linear dynamic processes. The $p_{nm}(t)$ are functions that weigh different parts of the spatial spectrum differently. Widespread synchronous sources are generally described accurately by a relatively small number of terms in (7.11), that is, the $p_{nm}(t)$ tend to be small for moderate and large n and m. More focal sources require more terms in the sums, that is, more contributions from higher spatial frequencies.

Scalp potential in the 4-sphere model can then be expressed by substituting (7.11) into (4.39), that is

$$\Phi(\theta,\phi,t) = \sum_{n=0}^{\infty} \sum_{m=-n}^{n} p_{nm}(t) g_{nm}(\mathbf{r}_z) Y_{nm}(\theta,\phi) \qquad (7.12)$$

Here the functions $g_{nm}(\mathbf{r}_z)$ involve integrals of the Green's function. They depend only on the properties of the volume conductor and the radial location of the source distribution r_z as discussed in chapters 4 and 6. As suggested in fig. 6-12 the functions g_{nm} decrease rapidly as the index n increases. Source activity with spatial frequency corresponding to a spherical harmonic of degree $n = 10$ will generate less than 10% of the potentials due to source activity corresponding to a spherical harmonic of degree $n = 1$. While it is evident that the smearing of potentials by volume conduction is "bad" because it severely limits the spatial resolution of the EEG, it actually makes the problem of discrete sampling of scalp potentials more manageable. The effect of the skull is to spatially low-pass filter cortical potentials as demonstrated with n-sphere models of the head. Thus, it is possible to achieve valid spatial sampling of the scalp potentials with a reasonable number of electrodes. *Nature has conveniently provided us with an anti-aliasing spatial filter in the form of the poorly conducting skull.* This filter is absent in cortical arrays, thereby adding (perhaps substantially) the problem of spatial aliasing to mapping ECoG in animal and epileptic patient studies.

There does exist one method to (analog) filter EEG signals spatially that will prevent spatial aliasing of signals with power at high spatial frequencies. It is analogous to analog filtering in the time domain. In our simulations, we have assumed that potentials are measured at discrete points, but this is not strictly true. Each electrode forces the contiguous scalp tissue to constant potential, essentially averaging the potential over the scalp region under that electrode, or over a somewhat larger region due to spread of electrode gel or other conductive interface under the electrode. Space averaging of potentials by electrodes of nonzero size provides an analog filter, thereby eliminating spatial frequencies with wavelengths approximately shorter than electrode diameters from the recorded data (Nunez et al. 1988).

Figure 7-11 considers simple examples of one-dimensional spatial signals that are discretely sampled over a spatial extent of 30 cm. In the first case (fig. 7-11a), the spatial signal has wavelength of 15 cm, which is discretely sampled using (point) electrodes separated by 1.9 cm (circles) and 3.8 cm (triangles). Both electrode arrays capture the essential spatial variation of the signal. Figure 7-11b shows a spatial signal of higher spatial frequency

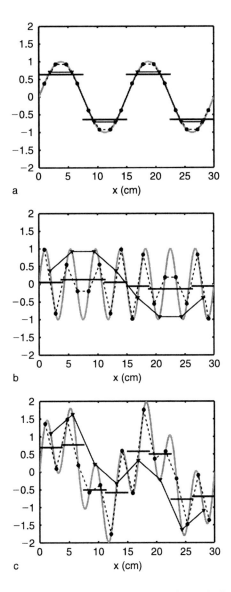

Figure 7-11 Several examples of aliasing of spatial signals. Each figure has plots of spatial signals composed of sine functions along the horizontal coordinate x. Each sine function is discretely sampled at points spaced by 1.9 cm (circles) and 3.8 cm (triangles); samples are linearly interpolated. The horizontal lines represent extended disk electrodes of width $\Delta x = 3.8$ cm and 3.8 cm center-to-center spacing (full spatial coverage). Note that edges of extended electrodes are close together. (a) Sine wave of wavelength 15 cm. Both the point electrodes and extended electrodes reasonably represent this spatial sine function. (b) Sine wave of wavelength 3.3 cm. With coarse point samples (triangles) the signal is spatially aliased and appears (falsely) as a signal of wavelength 30 cm. Note that even at the finer sampling with point electrodes (circles) some spatial aliasing takes place. When sampled with disk electrodes of width 3.8 cm, the signal averages towards zero. (c) The simulated signal consists of the sum of waveforms in (a) and (b). In this case, point electrode measures are severely aliased. Spatially extended disk electrodes accurately indicate the longer wavelength (15 cm) sine wave and filter out the short wavelength (3.3 cm) sine wave.

which is aliased by both arrays. The coarse array (triangles) falsely represents the signal as having spatial wavelength of 30 cm (one oscillation over 30 cm). The aliasing is less severe in the case of the finer array with a spacing of 1.9 cm. Figure 7-11c shows that the sum of the two signals is also severely aliased by sampling with a spacing of 3.8 cm.

Consider an electrode array consisting of electrodes of diameter D (including the extent of spreading of conductive gel) and uniform center-to-center spacing d. The Nyquist criterion requires at least two spatial samples per spatial wavelength λ. With spatially extended sampling, we apply this criterion to the edge-to-edge distance between adjacent electrodes, that is, $d - D < \lambda/2$. However, space averaging by electrodes ensures that recorded data will have most of the power in wavelengths $\lambda > 2D$. This filtering occurs because shorter wavelengths present mixtures of positive and negative potentials to electrode surfaces leading to signal canceling. (This is essentially the reason that a ship tends not to be rolled by waves shorter than its width nor pitched by waves shorter than its length.) Thus, by choosing the electrode diameter $D > d/2$ (edge-to-edge spacing less than or equal to electrode diameter), spatial aliasing is largely avoided.

Consider the extended disk electrodes indicated by horizontal lines in fig. 7-11 with center-to-center spacing $d = 3.8$ cm, which equals the point electrode spacing indicated by triangles. These extended electrodes average the potential over a width Δx equal to the center-to-center electrode separation, $\Delta x = d$. Figure 7-11a shows that for a signal of longer wavelength, the use of a large electrode has little effect on the measured signal. Figure 7-11b shows that a signal that is severely aliased by point electrodes has magnitude close to zero with the disk electrodes. In the combined signal shown in fig. 7-11c, the point electrodes indicated by triangles are severely aliased, while the disk electrodes reflect mainly the long-wavelength signal, but with reduced magnitude. *Spatial aliasing can be largely avoided if electrode diameter is chosen to equal the edge-to-edge distance between electrodes (or spread of the gel layer), or fully half the upper portion of the scalp covered by electrode contact!*

This is probably a very counterintuitive experimental strategy for many electroencephalographers who may equate smaller electrodes with increased accuracy. However, we do not have to worry about implementing this extreme strategy. That is, we expect spatial filtering by the head volume conductor generally to eliminate most spatial aliasing effects when more than about 64 electrodes are distributed uniformly over the scalp (approximately 3 cm center-to-center spacing). However, we note that many topographical EEG maps have been published based on the standard 10/20 montage (about 6 to 7 cm center-to-center spacing). Needless to say, the accuracy of such maps is in serious question.

In conclusion, we note that strict application of the Nyquist criterion to EEG requires a priori knowledge of spatial spectra of EEG, implying prior knowledge of source distributions. Such information is not generally available, in part because knowledge of the adequate number of electrodes for a specific EEG signal would first require over-sampling of the potential distribution to determine that the highest spatial frequencies present in the data. Our simulations using head models suggest that in most applications, spatial aliasing is minimal with modern EEG systems using 64–256 electrodes (Spitzer et al. 1989). Using the example of the VEP shown in figs. 7-4 and 7-7, we can ask how much information is present at any particular electrode site that is absent at neighboring sites. Figure 7-12 shows the average reference potential at the identical three central electrodes X shown in fig. 7-7. In each plot, the measured (average reference) potential is compared to the average potential at the six electrode sites that entirely surround the central electrode (all 6 are average-reference potentials). The positive potential 100 ms poststimulus is well estimated by the average of potentials recorded at neighboring electrode sites in the examples of fig. 7-12a and fig. 7-12c. However, in the example of fig. 7-12b the potential at this electrode site 100 ms poststimulus is underestimated by neighboring electrodes. Other peaks in the evoked potential waveforms may fall in either category. These data suggest that the optimal number of electrodes remains somewhat of an open question that deserves further attention, especially in the context of the potential information yield in high-resolution EEG methods discussed in chapter 8.

8 Addressing the Inverse Problem with Dipole Localization

The forward problem in EEG is the task of obtaining solutions to Poisson's equation (2.1) for surface potential due to known sources as discussed in chapter 6. A convenient form of this solution is (4.39) expressed as a cortical surface integral for exclusively cortical sources, or more generally, a volume integral over the whole brain. In this manner, the volume *microsources* $s(\mathbf{r}, t)$ are replaced by the *mesosources* $\mathbf{P}(\mathbf{r}, t)$, *the dipole moments per unit volume*, and our description is moved up one level in the brain's hierarchy. The potential at any location in the volume conductor may be expressed as the following volume integral in which the mesosources are a function of location $\mathbf{r}'$ and all electrical and geometric properties of the volume conductor are given by the volume Green's function $\mathbf{G}(\mathbf{r}, \mathbf{r}')$:

$$\Phi(\mathbf{r}, t) = \iiint_{\text{Brain}} \mathbf{G}(\mathbf{r}, \mathbf{r}') \cdot \mathbf{P}(\mathbf{r}', t)\, d\Re(\mathbf{r}') \qquad (7.13)$$

The integral is over the entire brain volume $\Re$ because any mesoscopic tissue mass containing synaptic or action potential activity can be expected to produce a dipole moment per unit volume $\mathbf{P}(\mathbf{r}, t)$, even though the contributions of most brain regions to surface potential may be negligible because of smaller weighting by $\mathbf{G}(\mathbf{r}, \mathbf{r}')$ or smaller magnitude of $\mathbf{P}(\mathbf{r}, t)$. The *forward problem* in EEG involves solving (7.13) using a head model, that

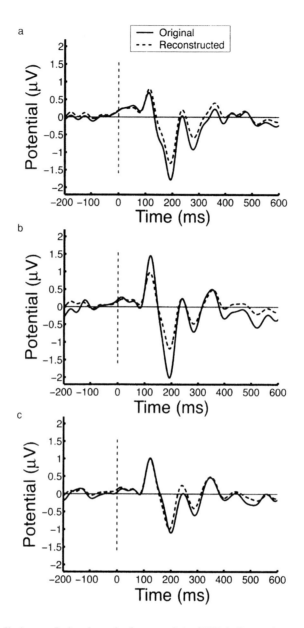

Figure 7-12 Predictions of visual evoked potentials (VEPs) from the average potential recorded by six nearest-neighbor electrodes. The VEP data here are identical to the data shown in fig. 7-4a–c. Each plot corresponds to a different central electrode as indicated in fig. 7-7 by the X. The average reference potentials at each electrode site are shown as solid lines, based on a full 111-channel recording (labeled "Original"). The dashed line shows the average potential of 6 surrounding electrodes located at an average distance of 2.7 cm. All 6 electrodes are average-referenced potentials. These electrode positions are shown in the corresponding plot (a–c) in fig. 7-7. In cases (a) and (c) the early evoked potential component 100 ms poststimulus can be estimated from the (average reference) potentials recorded at the surrounding electrode sites. However, in case (b), the actual recorded potential is larger than the average potential of the surrounding electrodes. Some evoked potential components are well represented by the local average; others are less well represented.

is, a Green's function $\mathbf{G}(\mathbf{r}, \mathbf{r}')$ and some (assumed known) mesosource distribution $\mathbf{P}(\mathbf{r}, t)$. This is formally the approach outlined in chapters 5 and 6 to obtain solutions for surface potential distribution due to known sources.

The basic *inverse problem* in EEG is to use experimental estimates of the potential distribution at the scalp surface $\Phi(\mathbf{r}_S, t)$ to "invert" (7.13), that is, to solve the integral equation (7.13) for the function $\mathbf{P}(\mathbf{r}, t)$ using a head volume conductor model to specify the function $\mathbf{G}(\mathbf{r}, \mathbf{r}')$. Our description of the inverse problem in EEG is based on the fundamental integral equation (7.13). Alternative formulations of this problem and many possible algorithms used to find solutions of one kind or another are available, but none of these computational methods can alter the physical fundamentals presented here. *Thus, if 22nd century scientists armed with vastly improved algorithms, computer power, and perfect head models choose to estimate inverse solutions using only surface potentials, they will be bound by these same fundamentals.*

The basic inverse problem is nonunique, that is, there are a very large number of functions $\mathbf{P}(\mathbf{r}, t)$ that will yield the same surface distribution $\Phi(\mathbf{r}_S, t)$ for any fixed volume conductor as discussed in chapters 1 and 2. Note that this source indeterminacy in EEG and MEG is fundamental; that is, it results not from imperfect head models or noise, but occurs whenever the data are limited to surface potentials $\Phi(\mathbf{r}_S, t)$ rather than potentials throughout the volume $\Phi(\mathbf{r}, t)$. Given the nonuniqueness of the inverse problem, *any inverse solution must depend partly on added information, the solution constraints.* The origins of these required constraints in published works have included plausible conjectures based on physiology, independent anatomical information perhaps obtained from MRI, fMRI, or PET data, hopeful assumptions, or combinations of these constraints. Common constraints are listed as follows:

1. The mesosource function $\mathbf{P}(\mathbf{r}, t)$ is negligible at all but a few discrete locations. In other words, the sources consist of one or perhaps several dipoles. This constraint is, of course, quite appropriate for implanted sources. It may also apply approximately to some fMRI and PET co-registration studies, to some epileptic discharges, and to some evoked potentials (EPs), notably early or mid-latency sensory EPs. However, this is clearly not the appropriate constraint for most spontaneous EEG and late EPs.

2. *All mesosources are located in neocortical tissue*, perhaps with tissue boundaries located with MRI. Actually, this constraint by itself is not sufficiently restrictive to ensure a unique solution because of the difficulty of distinguishing superficial gyral mesosources from mesosources in fissures and sulci. The more restrictive constraint of *confining all assumed mesosources to the crowns of cortical gyri* can be expected to yield an inverse solution that will closely match dura image estimates (obtained with either dura image or spline-Laplacian algorithms discussed in chapter 8).

3. *Placing spatial smoothness criteria on the mesosource function* $\mathbf{P}(\mathbf{r}, t)$, or perhaps finding the inverse solution that maximizes the smoothness of $\mathbf{P}(\mathbf{r}, t)$. We can think of no physiological justification for employing the spatial smoothness assumption generally in brain tissue. However, arguments supporting such spatial smoothness appear much stronger when $\mathbf{P}(\mathbf{r}, t)$ is doubly constrained by assuming that mesosources are both smooth and located in neocortex. This follows from the high density of excitatory intracortical connections presumably facilitating smooth spatial behavior of the mesosource function, although the effects of lateral inhibition may counter this effect by sharpening functional boundaries.

4. *Placing temporal smoothness criteria on the mesosource function* $\mathbf{P}(\mathbf{r}, t)$ (Scherg and von Cramon 1985). The justification for this constraint is that mesosources are unlikely to turn on and off abruptly. EEG (and ECoG) power in mammals tends to fall off sharply above 50 or 100 Hz, apparently reflecting cortical cell time constants in the 10 ms range as indicated in chapter 4. That is, we expect minimal changes in the mesosource function $\mathbf{P}(\mathbf{r}, t)$ over mesoscopic "relaxation times" in the range of 10 ms or perhaps several tens of milliseconds. Thus, this temporal constraint appears to rest on solid physiological ground, at least if applied with relatively short relaxation times. Given this basis, we outline an example application using this temporal smoothing constraint in the following paragraphs, showing that it substantially improves the prospects for locating multiple dipoles.

Consider an EEG experiment where potential is recorded at K scalp locations at I discrete times. Typically, an average reference is used; this is more justified if the number of electrodes is large (say > 64). We assume N dipole sources that have fixed locations $\mathbf{r}_n$ and vector orientations $\mathbf{\theta}_n$ over some (short) chosen time interval $(i = 1, I)$. For convenience, we make the notation change $\Phi(\mathbf{r}_k, t_i) = \Phi_{ki}$ ($k = 1, K$ and $i = 1, I$). Given the assumption of N discrete dipoles, the mesoscopic source function is

$$\mathbf{P}(\mathbf{r}, t) = \sum_{n=1}^{N} g_n(t)\delta(\mathbf{r} - \mathbf{r}_n)\mathbf{a}_n(\mathbf{r}) \qquad (7.14)$$

Here the delta functions $\delta(\mathbf{r} - \mathbf{r}_n)$ locate each mesosource (dipole) at the vector locations $\mathbf{r}_n$, $\mathbf{a}_n(\mathbf{r})$ is the location-dependent unit vector pointing in the axial direction of each dipole, and the functions $g_n(t)$ provide the time courses of dipole moments (strengths). Substitution of (7.14) into (7.13) yields a set of KI equations of the form

$$\Phi_{ki} = f(P_{1i}, \mathbf{r}_1, \mathbf{\theta}_1; P_{2i}, \mathbf{r}_2, \mathbf{\theta}_2; \ldots P_{Ni}, \mathbf{r}_N, \mathbf{\theta}_N) \quad k = 1, K; i = 1, I \qquad (7.15)$$

That is, each potential measurement Φ_{ki} at surface location k and time point i yields a separate equation relating the dipole moments (mesosource strengths) P_{ni}, their locations r_n, and the angles of their two axes θ_n to the surface potential. We have separated the mesosource strengths P_{ni} from their locations and orientations because only the strengths are allowed by the chosen smoothness constraint to vary over the assumed relaxation time, indicated by the time period $i = 1, I$. Dipole locations and axis orientations are assumed fixed within this time period. Each dipole (n) is defined by five time-independent scalar parameters (r_n, θ_n) plus I time-dependent parameters P_{ni}. Thus, (7.15) represents KI equations and $N(I + 5)$ unknowns.

These ideas may be illustrated by a hypothetical study of some evoked potential over the latency range (from the stimulus) 20 to 200 ms using $K = 64$ surface electrodes (plus reference). Suppose waveforms are digitized at 250 Hz (every 4 ms) and we apply our basic constraint to each 20 ms block of data separately. Thus, a different set of dipoles may be obtained for each of the 9 data blocks. In each 20 ms data block there are $I = 5$ time slices. Assume that $N = 5$ mesosources (dipoles) can adequately represent the surface potential over any 20 ms data block. In this example, (7.15) yields 320 equations for the 50 unknown dipole parameters. These dipole parameters may be obtained by standard optimization algorithms, in which a least squared error measure is minimized to obtain the "optimal" solution to the 320 equations. Another option is to obtain many different solutions using different subsets of the 320 equations, thereby allowing for variance estimates on the optimal solution. This is just one of several important issues associated with choice of computer algorithm that we avoid here; however, such operational issues do not change the fundamental physics underlying dipole localization.

In practice, many spatial patterns of EEG can be reasonably fit (in a least squares sense) by a few equivalent dipoles. Of course, as the number of dipoles (and hence parameters) increases, the confidence intervals on the solutions become broader. Other than in cases where the experimenter has independent evidence that only a few dipole sources generate the EEG, such as in the case of early sensory evoked potentials, equivalent dipole solutions are suspect. For example, these equivalent dipoles may (at best) reflect "centers" of complex patterns of activity distributed throughout many regions of the brain. In many applications, it may make more sense to replace the constraint of one or two equivalent dipoles by the constraint that all sources are cortical. This approach is to seek distributed solutions, by using thousands of dipole sources whose positions and orientations are fixed by the folded cortical surface, and solve this under-constrained (but linear) problem of determining the moments (strength) of the dipole sources (Russell et al. 1998).

The limited evidence available from intracranial recordings in humans does not support the contention that only a few sites in the brain are active in generating most EEG signals (Aoki et al. 2001; Ragavachari et al. 2001; Menon et al. 1996). Theoretical arguments developed in chapter 6 also support the notion that the sources of the EEG are dipole layers rather than point dipole sources. Although evidence from other methods (fMRI or PET) is often provided as support for inverse solutions, or even used to seed these inverse solutions, there may be only minimal theoretical bases to make such connection (Nunez and Silberstein 2000; Horowitz and Poeppel 2002). Thus, *there remains considerable motivation to approach the problem of locating the generators of the EEG by making improvements to spatial resolution rather than making assumptions about the nature or number of sources.* High-resolution EEG methods that provide reference-independent estimates of the dura surface (inner skull surface) potential from scalp potentials are discussed in the next chapter. Unlike the inverse problem, which effectively has an infinite number of possible solutions, *the scalp potential distribution is closely related to the dura surface potential.* The relationship is unique if there are no sources between the dura and the scalp, and the (noise free) potential on an entire outer closed surface is known perfectly.

9 Summary

The spatial information available in EEG is severely limited. EEG electrodes are separated from current sources in the brain by CSF, skull, and scalp resulting in the smearing of potentials and poor spatial resolution as discussed in chapter 6. In this chapter, we find that every EEG measurement depends on the locations of both the recording and so-called reference electrode. The measured potential difference is a property of the path between the electrode pairs. Every EEG recording is a bipolar recording, an idea that appears more widely appreciated in clinical EEG than in cognitive science.

This basic fact applies to any choice of reference including linked-ears or linked-mastoid reference. The physical linked-ears reference poses two possible problems. First, by imposing a new boundary condition, the scalp potential distribution may be changed. Second (and probably more importantly), it provides an unbalanced "random" reference. The mathematical linked-ears reference avoids the problems associated with physically linking the ears, but offers no obvious advantages over other references. The average reference enjoys some advantages in approximating reference independent potentials if used with a large number of electrodes. However, like any reference strategy, the average reference method has inherent biases, mainly as a consequence of limited sampling of the potentials over the lower surface of the head.

Modern EEG systems with 64–256 channels of EEG have facilitated spatial mapping of scalp potentials. Are these number of electrodes sufficiently large to accurately represent continuous potential distributions over the scalp? The answer depends on the properties of head volume conduction and source configurations. The effect of volume conduction is to reduce potentials at higher spatial frequencies, which allows the potentials to be spatially sampled without aliasing. No matter the nature of the sources, the EEG is low-pass filtered spatially, making discrete sampling of the potential distribution feasible.

Any potential distribution on the scalp can be fit (in a least-squared sense) by an equivalent dipole distribution by solving the inverse problem. However, these solutions are far from unique: they require additional assumptions about the sources. By contrast, the high-resolution EEG methods considered in chapter 8 offer improved spatial resolution compared to conventional EEG methods, without making assumptions about the underlying neural sources.

References

Aoki F, Fetz EE, Shupe L, Lettich E, and Ojemann GA, 2001, Changes in power and coherence of brain activity in human sensorimotor cortex during performance of visuomotor tasks. *Biosystems* 63: 89–99.

Bendat JS and Piersol, A, 2001, *Random Data: Analysis and Measurement Procedures,* 3rd Edition, New York: Wiley.

Bertrand O, Perrin F, and Pernier J, 1985, A theoretical justification of the average reference in topographic evoked potential studies. *Electroencephalography and Clinical Neurophysiology.* 62: 462–464.

Cadwell JA and Villarreal RA, 1999, Electrophysiological equipment and electrical safety. In: MJ Aminoff (Ed.), *Electrodiagnosis in Clinical Neurology,* 4th Edition, New York: Churchill Livingstone, pp. 15–33.

Fein G, Raz J, Brown FF, and Merrin EL, 1988, Common reference coherence data are confounded by power and phase effects. *Electroencephalography and Clinical Neurophysiology* 69: 581–584.

Ferree TC, Luu P, Russell GS, and Tucker DM, 2001, Scalp electrode impedance, infection risk, and EEG data quality. *Clinical Neurophysiology* 112: 536–544.

Fisch BJ, 1999, *Fisch & Spehlmann's EEG Primer*, Amsterdam: Elsevier, 1999.

Horowitz B and Poeppel D, 2002, How can EEG/MEG and fMRI/PET be combined? *Human Brain Mapping* 17: 1–3.

Jackson JD, 1975, *Classical Electrodynamics*, 2nd Edition, New York: Wiley.

Kamp A, Pfurtscheller G, Edlinger G, and Lopes da Silva FH, 2005, Technological basis of EEG recording. In: E Niedermeyer and FH Lopes da Silva (Eds.), *Electroencephalography. Basic Principals, Clinical Applications, and Related Fields*, 5th Edition, London: Williams and Wilkins, pp. 127–138.

Katznelson RD, 1981, EEG recording, electrode placement, and aspects of generator localization. In: PL Nunez (Au.), *Electric Fields of the Brain: The Neurophysics of EEG*, 1st Edition, New York: Oxford University Press.

Malmivuo J and Plonsey R, 1995, *Bioelectromagnetism*, New York: Oxford University Press.

Menon V, Freeman WJ, Cutillo BA, Desmond JE, Ward MF, Bressler SL, Laxer KD, Barbaro N, and Gevins AS, 1996, Spatio-temporal correlations in human gamma band electrocorticograms. *Electroencephalography and Clinical Neurophysiology* 98: 89–102.

Miller GA, Lutzenberge W, and Elbert T, 1991, The linked-reference issue in EEG and ERP recording. *Journal of Psychophysiology* 5: 273–276.

Morse PM and Feshbach H, 1953, *Methods of Theoretical Physics*, Vols 1 and 2, New York: McGraw Hill.

Murias M, 2004, *Oscillatory Brain Electric Potentials in Developmental Psychopathology and Form Perception*, Ph.D. Dissertation, University of California, Irvine.

Niedermeyer E and Lopes da Silva FH (Eds.), 2005, *Electroencephalography. Basic Principals, Clinical Applications, and Related Fields*, 5th Edition, London: Williams and Wilkins.

Nunez PL, 1988, Spatial filtering and experimental strategies in EEG. In: D Samson-Dollfus (Ed.), *Functional Brain Imaging*, Paris: Elsevier, pp. 196–209.

Nunez PL, 1991, Comments on the paper by Miller, Lutzenberger and Elbert. *Journal of Psychophysiology* 5: 279–280.

Nunez PL and Silberstein RB, 2000, On the relationship of synaptic activity to macroscopic measurements: does co-registration of EEG with fMRI make sense? *Brain Topography* 13: 79–96.

Nunez PL, Srinivasan R, Westdorp AF, Wijesinghe RS, Tucker DM, Silberstein RB, and Cadusch PJ, 1997, EEG coherence: I. Statistics, reference electrode, volume conduction, Laplacians, cortical imaging, and interpretation at multiple scales. *Electroencephalography and Clinical Neurophysiology* 103: 516–527.

Nunez PL and Westdorp AF, 1994, The surface Laplacian, high resolution EEG and controversies. *Brain Topography* 6: 221–226.

Picton TW, Bentin S, Berg P, Donchin E, Hillyard SA, Johnson Jr. R, Miller GA, Ritter W, Ruchkin DS, Rugg MD, and Taylor MJ, 2000, Guidelines for using human event-related potentials to study cognition: recording standards and publication criteria. *Psychophysiology* 37: 127–152.

Pilgreen KL, 1995, Physiologic, medical and cognitive correlates of electroencephalography. In: PL Nunez (Au.), *Neocortical Dynamics and Human EEG Rhythms*, New York: Oxford University Press, pp. 195–248.

Plonsey R, 1969, *Bioelectric Phenomena*, New York: McGraw-Hill.

Ragavachari S, Kahana MJ, Rizzuto DS, Caplan JB, Kirschen MP, Bourgeois B, Madsen JR, and Lisman JE, 2001, Gating of human theta oscillations by a working memory task. *Journal of Neuroscience* 21: 3175–3183.

Regan D, 1989, *Human Brain Electrophysiology*, New York: Elsevier.

Rush S and Driscoll A, 1968, Current distribution in the brain from surface electrodes. *Anesthesia Analgesia* 47: 717–723.

Rush S and Driscoll A, 1969, EEG electrode sensitivity: an application of reciprocity. *IEEE Transactions on Biomedical Engineering* 16: 15–22.

Russell GS, Srinivasan R, and Tucker DM, 1998, Bayesian estimates of error bounds for EEG source imaging. *IEEE Transactions on Medical Imaging* 17: 1084–1089.

Scherg M and von Cramon D, 1989 Dipole source potentials of the auditory cortex in normal subjects and in patients with temporal lobe lesions In: M Hoke, F Grandori, GL Romani (Eds). *Auditory Evoked Magnetic Fields and Potentials, Advances in Audiology*, vol 6, Basel: Karger.

Simpson DG, 1998, Instrumentation for high spatial resolution steady state visual evoked potentials. Brain Sciences Institute & Biophysical Sciences and Electrical Engineering, Swinburne University of Technology, Melbourne, Australia.

Spitzer AR, Cohen LG, Fabrikant J, and Hallett M, 1989, A method for determining the optimal interelectrode spacing for cerebral topographic mapping. *Electroencephalography and Clinical Neurophysiology* 72: 355–361.

Srinivasan R, Nunez PL, and Silberstein RB, 1998, Spatial filtering and neocortical dynamics: estimates of EEG coherence. *IEEE Transactions on Biomedical Engineering* 45: 814–826.

Srinivasan R, Nunez PL, Tucker DM, Silberstein RB, and Cadusch PJ, 1996, Spatial sampling and filtering of EEG with spline Laplacians to estimate cortical potentials. *Brain Topography* 8: 355–366.

8

High-Resolution EEG

1 Improved Spatial Resolution versus Source Localization

Spatial information in EEG is limited by uncertainty of head current patterns (volume conduction, chapter 6) and reference electrode effects (chapter 7). Spatial EEG patterns may often be fit accurately to a few equivalent dipoles in the sense of minimizing mean-square errors between predicted and actual scalp potential distribution; however, the physiological basis for fitting spatial patterns to just a few isolated dipoles is often lacking. The putative dipoles could easily reflect "centers" of complex patterns of synaptic activity distributed in multiple brain regions. It is also possible that best-fit dipoles have no relation at all to genuine brain sources. They might, for example, occur in deep tissue when the actual sources occupy cortical surface areas ranging from a few to hundreds of squared centimeters as discussed in chapters 2 and 6. Clearly, any interpretation of equivalent dipoles depends critically on the spatial extent of these sources. Although evidence from methods like fMRI or PET may provide additional support for inverse dipole solutions, or may be used to explicitly bias inverse solutions, the theoretical bases for such connections has yet to be established (Nunez and Silberstein 2000; Horowitz and Poeppel 2002).

This background on EEG spatial analysis provides substantial motivation to *improve EEG spatial resolution rather than making (often) unsupported assumptions about the nature or number of sources.* High-resolution EEG methods have been developed to estimate dura surface (or the CSF/skull boundary) potentials from scalp potential recorded at multiple locations. Unlike estimating the location of brain sources, an exercise with an effectively infinite number of possible solutions, the procedure of estimating dura potentials from scalp potentials has solutions that are theoretically unique, subject to engineering limitations associated with sampling, noise, and head model uncertainty.

Two distinct high-resolution EEG methods have been developed independently: (i) skull current density estimates obtained by means of surface Laplacian algorithms (Perrin et al. 1987, 1989; Nunez 1988, 1989, 1990, 1995; Nunez et al. 1991, 1994; Law et al. 1993; Babiloni et al. 1996; Srinivasan 1999; Srinivasan et al. 1996, 1998) and (ii) estimates of dura surface potential using dura imaging algorithms (Gevins et al. 1991, 1994; Sidman 1991; Cadusch et al. 1992; Edlinger et al. 1998). Estimates obtained by dura imaging (also known as *spatial deconvolution, deblurring,* or *cortical imaging*) require no assumptions about EEG sources, but do require a volume conductor head model, typically 3-sphere or 4-sphere models. All high-resolution analyses in this book are based on either the Melbourne dura imaging algorithm or the New Orleans spline-Laplacian. We expect that similar estimates are obtained with (apparent) equivalent algorithms developed in other laboratories, but we have no direct confirmation of this expected similarity. We have, however, confirmed the practical equi-valence of Melbourne dura imaging and New Orleans spline-Laplacian algorithms when used with a 131-electrode array.

The surface Laplacian of scalp potential (or second spatial derivative in two surface coordinates) is an estimate of current density entering (or exiting) the scalp through a local region of the skull. The Laplacian method requires only that the outer surface shape of the volume conductor be specified; typically a best-fit spherical surface is adopted. Despite the independent theoretical bases of the two high-resolution methods, both yield robust estimates of (relative) spatial distribution of dura surface potentials in simulation studies and in applications to EEG data (Nunez et al. 1994, 2001). The surface Laplacian algorithm requires less detailed information about volume conduction in the head and is emphasized in this chapter.

Laplacian estimates are independent of the choice of reference electrode. One of the complicating factors in interpreting scalp EEG involves reference electrode effects as discussed in chapter 7. At any instant, the potential recorded at the reference electrode is subtracted from potentials recorded at all the other electrodes. Since the surface Laplacian is a second spatial derivative, the potential common to all electrodes is automatically removed in the surface Laplacian estimate. Thus, the reference electrode can be moved to any position on the head without influencing the surface Laplacian. Since the surface Laplacian requires estimates of derivates of the potential along the scalp surface, high *spatial sampling* of scalp potentials, using 64–131 (or more) closely spaced electrodes, is recom-mended to obtain good spatial resolution.

The theory and examples presented in this chapter demonstrate that *the surface Laplacian algorithm acts as a band-pass spatial filter that tends to isolate effects due to sources localized in superficial cortex,* with typical resolu-tion in the 2 to 3 cm range in surface tangential directions. The portion of the EEG signal removed by the surface Laplacian filter is not as easily localized; it may be generated by very deep sources or, more likely, by coherent sources distributed over large cortical areas on the lobeal or even larger scales. In the latter case, the question of EEG source localization is essentially meaningless, since the underlying phenomena are regional or global (Nunez 2000). A more useful approach is to characterize the spatial and temporal dynamics of EEG signals by spectra, coherence, and other dynamic measures as discussed in chapters 9 through 11.

This chapter begins by briefly reviewing the nature of EEG sources and their associated scalp potential and surface Laplacian signatures. The relationships between the surface Laplacian, dura imaging algorithms, skull current density, dura surface potential, and the underlying source distribution are investigated using a 4-sphere model of volume conduction in the head. We use the term *surface Laplacian* to refer to a theoretical estimate, which is usually obtained analytically from the 4-sphere model with known sources. The practical engineering issues associated with EEG experimental design, such as electrode density and choice of surface Laplacian algorithm, are considered here in the context of real EEG data. We use the term *spline Laplacian* to refer to the surface Laplacian estimates using a spline interpolation of potentials measured (or simulated with the 4-sphere model) at a set of discrete electrode locations; this refers specifically to the New Orleans spline Laplacian estimate. In our example applications to genuine EEG data, the abbreviated term *Laplacian* is often used. Finally, we present several caveats appropriate for implementation and interpretation of high-resolution EEG. Appendix J presents details of the New Orleans three-dimensional spline Laplacian algorithm and MATLAB (Natick, MA) source code for convenient implementation of this high-resolution method.

2 Spatial Properties of EEG Sources

Localized generators are not a general property of EEG data. In some cases, such as short-latency sensory evoked potentials or focal epileptic discharges, the assumption that a single localized cortical region is the main EEG generator may justify modeling signals with a single dipole source. However, most EEG signals are evidently generated regionally or even globally, involving neural populations acting in concert and distributed throughout several brain regions (Nunez 2000). The underlying sources of most EEG phenomena are generally unknown; however, EEG signals related to cognitive processes probably involve distributed cortical tissue, perhaps often in multiple, widely separated brain regions. Large-scale theoretical models suggest that mixtures of local, regional, and global sources is the most likely picture (Nunez 1989, 1995, 2000, 2001).

In this context, the issue of the multiple spatial scales of brain dynamics and EEG sources is discussed in chapters 1, 10, and 11.

The dipole approximation to cortical current sources provides the basis for most source localization algorithms. It is based on the idea that at large distances, any complex current distribution in a region of the cortex can be approximated by a "dipole" or, more accurately, a dipole moment per unit volume (see chapters 1, 4, and 5). A "large distance" in this case is at least three or four times the effective pole separation of the dipole. Superficial gyral surfaces are located at roughly 1.5 cm from scalp electrodes. In this context, the dipole approximation appears valid only for superficial cortical tissue with a maximum extent in any dimension of roughly 0.5 cm or less. If we choose tissue at this scale or smaller to describe single dipoles, there can be multiple active dipole sources within a 2 cm^2 gyral crown; that is, the crown actually forms a small dipole layer. Macrocolumns (of approximately 3 mm diameter) provide a convenient scale to picture dipoles. In this case, the sources of many (if not most) EEG phenomena may then be pictured as thousands (or even tens of thousands) of cortical dipoles, mainly oriented perpendicular to the cortical surface forming dipole layers (or folded dipole sheets). We emphasize that the word "dipole" is actually just convenient jargon for the continuously varying dipole moment per unit volume or mesosources $\mathbf{P}(\mathbf{r}, t)$ defined generally by (4.26).

If we assume that EEG sources consist of thousands of dipoles oriented perpendicular to the cortical surface, "localization" can be defined approximately in terms of dipole layers of nonzero spatial extent and *relatively segregated from the surrounding areas of cortex*. In the context of EEG dynamics, segregation of a dipole layer implies that the time-dependencies of dipole source strengths in the layer are temporally correlated to each other and relatively uncorrelated to other dipoles in the surrounding cortex. In general, we expect that EEG signals are generated by multiple contributions from many dipole layers of different sizes and locations, perhaps overlapping in location. Thus, localizing the so-called generators of EEG is only meaningful in this context. For instance, EEG signals may be generated in one region of the brain by both strongly correlated dipole sources at a small spatial scale (say a dipole layer of about 1 cm diameter) and moderately correlated dipole layers at larger spatial scales (say 5–10 cm). The usual dipole localization approach may be meaningful for locating the smaller source regions, but is inappropriate for larger source regions.

High-resolution EEG methods are based on a quite different conceptual framework from that pertaining to source localization. As discussed in chapters 2 and 7, the EEG signal recorded at each electrode is a spatial average of active current sources distributed over a volume of brain space. The size and shape of this volume depends on a number of factors including the volume conduction properties of the head and choice of reference electrode location. *The contribution of each source to this spatial average depends on the electrical distance between source and electrode, source orientation, and source strength.* When two electrodes are very closely spaced, similar signals are recorded because they record the average activity in largely overlapping volumes of tissue. High-resolution EEG methods, such as the surface Laplacian, have the effect of reducing the effective volume that each electrode averages, thereby improving spatial resolution. As discussed in this chapter, the surface Laplacian emphasizes certain types of source activity: mainly superficial, localized sources (as defined above). At the same time, the surface Laplacian deemphasizes other kinds of activity- deep sources and widespread coherent superficial sources.

3 Physical Basis for Surface Laplacian Estimates

The dominant properties of volume conduction in real heads are due to the poorly conducting skull layer located between the much more highly conductive brain and cerebrospinal fluid (CSF) layers and the scalp. The 4-sphere model of chapter 6 incorporates this critical feature and can be used to compute potential anywhere in the volume in order to further develop our intuition about potentials and current paths in the head. The upper part of fig. 8-1 shows potential as a function of radial location above a radial dipole in the 4-sphere model consisting of brain, CSF, skull, and scalp. The potential falls off by two orders of magnitude within the thickness of the skull because of its poor conductivity. By comparison, the potential fall-off across the thickness of the scalp is negligible. The lower part of fig. 8-1 shows the potential fall-off from the dipole axis in tangential directions, indicating very little tangential current spread within most of the skull layer. The main spreading of current in tangential directions occurs near the skull/scalp boundary. Within the (idealized) skull layer minimal tangential current occurs; most current flows in the radial direction through the skull into the scalp.

From these simulations we can develop an intuitive picture of current flow in the scalp due to dipole sources in the brain as shown schematically in fig. 8-2. In brain regions with dense source activity, current flows mainly in the radial direction through the skull into the scalp and spreads tangentially, while in other regions with less source activity current converges and flows through the skull into the brain. With mesosources $P(r, t)$ oscillating in time, the current direction reverses every half cycle. There can also be regions that neither inject nor accept much scalp current. Thus, different surface regions of the skull behave as skull "sources," "sinks," or "quiet regions" with respect to the scalp current injection, as a consequence of genuine physiological source activity within the brain. In genuine heads the picture is more complicated because the conductivity and thickness of the skull and scalp are not uniform. Also, holes or regions of low skull resistance may act as preferential current paths, but the general qualitative idea expressed by fig. 8-2 is valid.

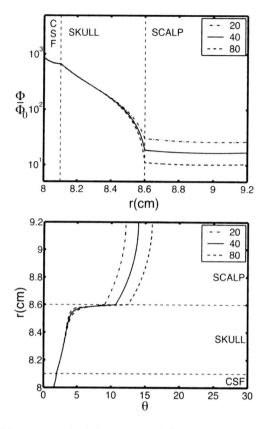

Figure 8-1 Potential in our standard 4-sphere model due to a radial dipole source in the inner sphere (the model brain). The model consists of four spherical layers: sphere radii are (brain, CSF, skull, scalp) = (8.0, 8.1, 8.6, 9.2). Brain and scalp are assumed to have the same conductivity; CSF conductivity is five times brain conductivity. Three brain-to-skull conductivity ratios are plotted (20, 40, 80). (*Upper*) Fall-off of potential in the radial direction through the thickness of the skull and scalp. Potential is plotted on a logarithmic scale. (*Lower*) Angular spread of potential in the skull and scalp. Each curve represents the distance at which potential is 50% of its maximum directly above the dipole ($\theta = 0$).

Total scalp current passing a particular scalp region can change only as a result of a skull "source" or "sink" of current directly below the local scalp. In order to determine whether a given skull location serves as a source or sink for scalp currents, the change in current density ($\mathbf{J}_S$) along the two-dimensional scalp surface may be evaluated. Ohm's law for linear conductors indicates that current density in the scalp is proportional to the spatial gradient of the potential (3.15). The divergence of current density along the scalp is then equivalent to the surface Laplacian (∇_S^2) of the scalp potential Φ_S:

$$\nabla_S \cdot \mathbf{J}_S = \nabla_S \cdot \sigma_S \nabla_S \Phi_S = \sigma_S \nabla_S^2 \Phi_S \qquad (8.1)$$

where σ_S is the (assumed constant) conductivity of the scalp. Note that the gradient operator ∇_S is the derivative along the scalp surface S,

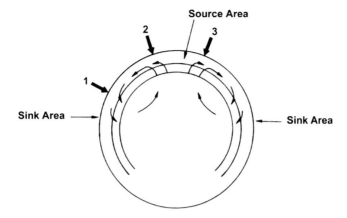

Figure 8-2 Schematic view of cortical dipole layer sources and volume-conducted currents. For the temporary purposes of this description, we may define a scalp "source" as the scalp region into which current is injected by brain current sources and a scalp "sink" as that scalp region in which current is flowing back into the skull. Reproduced with permission from Katznelson (1981).

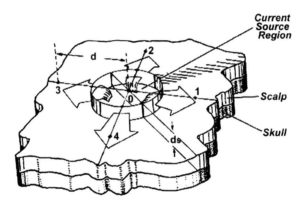

Figure 8-3 Scalp source region. EEG scalp currents are indicated by the flat arrows. The cylinder through the thickness of the scalp d_S indicates the basis for the nearest-neighbor Laplacian estimate (8.5). Reproduced with permission from Katznelson (1981).

expressed in the two surface coordinates that define the local geometry of the scalp. The surface Laplacian operator $L_S = \nabla_S^2$ is the second spatial derivative along the two surface coordinates. On a planar surface with x and y coordinates:

$$L_S = \nabla_S^2(\Phi_S) = \frac{\partial^2 \Phi_S}{\partial x^2} + \frac{\partial^2 \Phi_S}{\partial y^2} \tag{8.2}$$

In spherical or ellipsoidal geometries, the expression for the surface Laplacian can be written as derivatives in the corresponding system coordinates (See appendices G and H and Law et al. 1993). The surface Laplacian can also be calculated for an arbitrary surface geometry, for instance a realistic scalp geometry derived from MRI images (Babiloni et al. 1996) by making use of local surface normals and electrode positions.

Any change in tangential current flow in the scalp must be due to the emergence of current into the scalp from the skull or the convergence of current into the skull. *Thus, the surface Laplacian can be used to detect sources and sinks of current flow between the scalp and skull.* We expect that within the skull, most current flows in the radial direction with minimal flow in tangential directions. Simulations using a spherical model with a poorly conducting skull layer shown in fig. 8-1 suggest that this intuition is quite reasonable. Very little smearing of the potential distribution takes place within most of the skull, suggesting minimal tangential skull current.

Consider a small cylinder of scalp tissue of thickness d_S with principal axis perpendicular to the scalp surface, as shown in fig. 8-3. Since no current passes across the scalp-air boundary, the current entering (or exiting) this cylinder from (or to) the skull at the base of the cylinder must equal the total current exiting (or entering) the cylinder walls. The total current exiting the cylinder walls into the nonlocal scalp is

$$I_S = \iint_C \mathbf{J}_S \cdot \mathbf{ds} = \sigma_S \iint_C \mathbf{E}_S \cdot \mathbf{ds} \tag{8.3}$$

We have used Ohm's law (3.15) to express tangential current density in the skull in terms of the tangential (surface) components of the electric field ($\mathbf{E}_S$). To estimate this integral, five electrodes, labeled 0–4 in fig. 8-3, may be used. Electrode 0 is located on the principal axis of the cylinder of scalp tissue, and electrodes 1 through 4 are equally spaced at a tangential distance d as shown. To estimate the integral in (8.3) we partition the cylinder wall surface into four equal sections, and estimate the electric field $\mathbf{E}_S$ at the center of each section by the potential gradients halfway between the electrodes:

$$\iint_C \mathbf{E}_S \cdot \mathbf{ds} \approx \sum_{j=1}^{4} \left(\frac{\Phi_0 - \Phi_j}{d} \right) \frac{S_C}{4} \tag{8.4}$$

where the surface area of the cylinder wall is $S_C = \pi d d_S$. Rearranging terms, the total current exiting the cylinder walls can be rewritten as

$$I_S \approx \frac{\pi \sigma_S d_S}{4} [4\Phi_0 - \Phi_1 - \Phi_2 - \Phi_3 - \Phi_4] \tag{8.5}$$

The current entering the cylinder can also be approximated by the radial current density at the outer surface of the skull (J_K) multiplied by the surface area of the cylinder face at the skull-scalp interface. By dividing

I_S by the surface area of the base of the cylinder we obtain an approximation for the current density entering the scalp from the skull through the cylinder base:

$$J_K \approx \frac{I}{\pi(d/2)^2} = \sigma_S d_S \frac{[4\Phi_0 - \Phi_1 - \Phi_2 - \Phi_3 - \Phi_4]}{d^2} \qquad (8.6)$$

The ratio in the right-hand term in (8.6) is a finite difference approximation to the negative surface Laplacian of Φ_S at the location of electrode 0. Hence, we can approximate (8.6) as

$$J_K \sim -\sigma_S d_S L_S \qquad (8.7)$$

That is, the radial current density in the skull that enters or exits the scalp under an electrode is approximately proportional to the surface Laplacian of the potential at the electrode.

The physical basis for relating the surface Laplacian of the scalp potential to the dura (inner skull) surface potential is based on Ohm's law, the assumptions that the skull is very thin, and that most current flows in the radial direction through the skull into the scalp. In this case, the potential difference between the inner and outer surfaces of the skull is given approximately by (6.16). In order to keep the notation consistent within this chapter, we use corresponding symbols

$$\{\Phi_1(r_1), \Phi_3(r_2), J_3(r_2), \sigma_2, (r_2 - r_1)\} \rightarrow \{\Phi_C, \Phi_K, J_K, \sigma_K, d_K\}$$

and rewrite (6.16) in terms of (outer surface) skull current density J_K, that is

$$\Phi_K - \Phi_C \approx d_K \left(\frac{r_K}{r_C \sigma_K}\right) J_K \qquad (8.8)$$

Here Φ_C is the potential on the outer surface of the CSF (or the inner surface of the skull), Φ_K is the potential on the outer surface of the skull, and skull thickness is given by d_K.

Substitute (8.7) into (8.8) to obtain the following approximate expression for the surface Laplacian L_S in terms of the inner skull (or outer CSF) surface potential Φ_C, outer surface skull potential Φ_K, and surface Laplacian L_S:

$$L_S \approx \left(\frac{1}{d_K d_S}\right)\left(\frac{r_C}{r_K}\right)\left(\frac{\sigma_K}{\sigma_S}\right)(\Phi_K - \Phi_C) \qquad (8.9)$$

Figure 8-1 indicates that for a single dipole, the potential on the inner surface of the skull is two or three orders of magnitude larger than the potential on the outer surface of the skull (or scalp). Thus, in the case of a single dipole (or small dipole layer), the magnitude of the outer skull surface potential Φ_K is negligible in comparison to the inner skull surface potential Φ_C. It then follows from (8.9) that *in the case of localized cortical sources, the (negative) surface Laplacian (L_S) is roughly proportional to the potential on the inner surface of the skull Φ_C (or equivalently the outer surface of the CSF).* In high resolution EEG we adopt the label "surface Laplacian" to indicate the negative surface Laplacian. Whereas the derivation of (8.9) is based on physical arguments (Nunez et al. 1994), it has recently been derived mathematically (Kramer and Szeri 2004), thereby allowing for analytic error estimates, which appear to be minimal.

This close correspondence between surface Laplacians and dura potential does not occur for broadly distributed sources, for which the ratio of cortical to scalp potential is typically in the range of two to four (see fig. 1-20). That is, Φ_C and Φ_K are in the same general range for broadly distributed sources. As indicated by (8.9), the surface Laplacian is then no longer proportional to cortical potential for such broad source distributions, and raw scalp potentials may provide better estimates of cortical potential distribution. In summary, *the surface Laplacian provides good estimates of dura surface potential when the underlying source regions are relatively localized*, with areas smaller than perhaps 10 or 20 cm^2. By contrast, very broadly distributed sources cause the surface Laplacian to underestimate substantially dura surface potentials. Expressed another way, the surface Laplacian is relatively insensitive to very low spatial frequency source activity. It tends to filter out such sources, along with low spatial frequency potentials due only to volume conduction. The surface Laplacian filters out potentials due to genuine brain sources that are not localized in addition to unwanted contributions from current spreading due to volume conduction.

To test the validity of the rough approximations leading to (8.9), scalp potential Φ_S, scalp surface Laplacian L_S, radial skull current density J_K, and dura surface potential Φ_C due to a dipole source in a 4-sphere model are simulated here. The surface Laplacian may be calculated using the 4-sphere model by applying the Laplacian operator in spherical coordinates to the solution for scalp potential (Srinivasan et al., 1998). Figure 8-4 demonstrates the fall-off of these quantities with tangential distance measured along the outer spherical surface. The two sets of plots correspond to brain-to-skull conductivity ratios of 80 and 20, roughly consistent with reported ranges of tissue impedance measurements (see chapter 4). With either a radial or tangential dipole source, scalp potential falls off very slowly with tangential distance. By contrast, the surface Laplacian, dura surface potential, and radial skull current density fall off much more rapidly—all three measures have much tighter point-spread functions than scalp potential. The approximation of dura potential by surface Laplacian improves somewhat if these quantities are averaged over the nonzero electrode surface area (Srinivasan et al. 1996), consistent with the large-scale approximation inherent in assuming purely radial current flow in the skull.

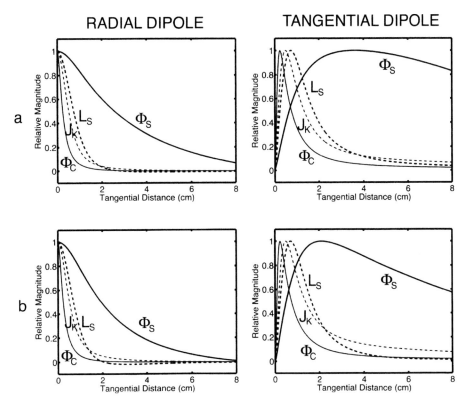

Figure 8-4 Simulations of scalp potential and analytic scalp Laplacian are used to verify the theoretical basis for the surface Laplacian method. Scalp potential Φ_S, scalp Laplacian L_S, radial skull current density J_K (evaluated here in the middle of the skull layer), and cortical surface potential Φ_C due to a radial dipole source (left column) and tangential dipole source (right column) in our standard 4-sphere model. Each variable is normalized with respect to the peak value. *Row* (a): brain-to-skull conductivity ratio $= 80$. *Row* (b): brain-to-skull conductivity ratio $= 20$. In each example, the surface Laplacian provides a biased estimate of cortical potential, but the estimate is far more accurate than raw scalp potential (even when ignoring the attendant reference problem with raw potential).

This approximation of dura potential by surface Laplacian is even better for deeper dipoles, but surface Laplacian magnitudes are sharply reduced as source depth increases. Figure 8-5 shows magnitudes of potential and surface Laplacian due to radial and tangential dipoles as a function of source depth. The most superficial position shown is 2 mm below the surface of the brain sphere; the deepest position is 1 cm above the center of the brain sphere. The two plots correspond to brain-to-skull conductivity ratios of 80 and 20. The plots for the potential show that at any depth, radial dipoles generate larger scalp potentials than tangential dipoles. This relative sensitivity to radial dipoles increases for dipoles placed superficially in the brain sphere. The surface Laplacian shows the same advantage for recording radial dipoles over tangential dipoles, but the surface Laplacian falls off rapidly as source depth increases for both dipole orientations. At depths greater than 3 cm below the surface of the

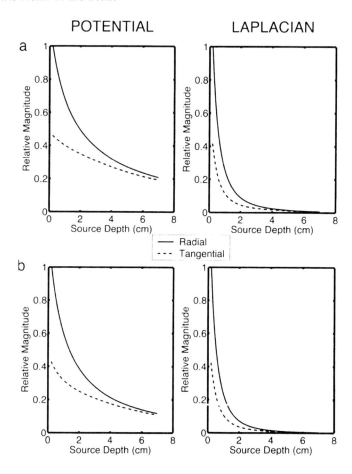

Figure 8-5 Maximum scalp potential generated by a radial (solid line) and tangential dipole (dashed line) as a function of depth in the brain sphere. (*Left column*) Scalp potential. (*Right column*) surface Laplacian. *Row* (a): brain-to-skull conductivity ratio = 80. *Row* (b): brain-to-skull conductivity ratio = 20.

brain sphere, the surface Laplacian due to either source configuration falls to less than 5% of the surface Laplacian generated by a superficial source (2 mm brain depth). In other words, deeper sources produce more broadly distributed cortical potentials, and the surface Laplacian is relatively insensitive to very low spatial frequency activity.

At the macrocolumn scale, dipoles (*mesosources*) in the cortex are generally oriented perpendicular to the cortical surface, implying that tangential dipoles are located mainly in sulci and fissures; that is, further from EEG electrodes than radial dipoles in the gyri. Thus for most EEG phenomena, the ratio of scalp potential generated by radial dipoles to scalp potential generated by tangential dipoles is generally expected to be larger than indicated in fig. 8-5. Dipole orientation contributes a factor of about two to the ratio, and fissure or sulci depth contributes factors of about one to three, yielding a crude estimate for the ratio of two to six. This greater sensitivity to radial dipoles is also evident in the surface

Laplacian. Furthermore, the surface Laplacian reduces the contribution of deep sources relative to superficial sources. These combined effects indicate that *the surface Laplacian is likely to be dominated by cortical sources oriented in the radial direction, and these dominant sources probably occur mostly in the superficial gyral surfaces of neocortex.*

This selective sensitivity of the surface Laplacian may be of substantial importance when the objective is source localization, as in the example of focal epilepsy. Without making any assumptions about the underlying sources, the surface Laplacian provides estimates of local source activity in superficial areas of the brain, which can be compared to estimates obtained with source localization algorithms. In the more general use of EEG data in cognitive and clinical studies, the surface Laplacian provides a spatial filtering of the EEG that limits electrode sensitivity to more local sources (within a few centimeters of each electrode), thereby revealing source dynamics at smaller spatial scales than scalp potentials. Estimates of the spatial resolution of the surface Laplacian are obtained in the next section.

4 The Surface Laplacian as a Band-Pass Spatial Filter

Here we compare the sensitivity of conventional EEG potentials to surface Laplacians in the general case of complex patterns of cortical source activity. In chapter 6 a spatial transfer function based on the 4-sphere model is introduced. We use this transfer function to demonstrate low-pass spatial filtering by tissue layers between cortex and scalp. This same approach is extended here to surface Laplacians. The surface Laplacian operator is a high-pass spatial filter. For any well-behaved function defined on the surface of a sphere, this high pass operation may be written

$$L_S[\Phi_S(\theta, \phi)] = L_S\left(\sum_{n=1}^{\infty} \sum_{m=-n}^{n} \Phi_{nm} Y_{nm}(\theta, \phi)\right) = \sum_{n=1}^{\infty} \sum_{m=-n}^{n} n(n+1)\Phi_{nm} Y_{nm}(\theta, \phi)$$

(8.10)

Here we have represented the potential Φ_S on the outer surface (scalp) in terms of an expansion in the spherical harmonic basis functions Y_{nm} with weights given by the coefficients Φ_{nm}. The *spherical harmonics form a set of basis functions on a spherical surface,* analogous to the sine and cosine basis functions used in the usual Fourier series in the time domain (see appendix I). Equation (8.10) shows that the surface Laplacian is a spatial high-pass filter, with increasing weight given to each term in the spherical harmonic expansion by a factor roughly equal to the square of the spatial frequency index (n).

If we assume a source distribution at a fixed depth (say in an idealized smooth cortex), the potential on the outer sphere (scalp) is a spatially low-pass filtered representation of underlying source distribution, that is, from the arguments of chapter 6

$$T_{nm} = \frac{\Phi_{nm}}{P_{nm}} = \frac{4\pi}{2n+1} H_n(r_z)$$ (6.14)

Here T_{nm} is the transfer function relating the (radial) source distribution $P(\theta, \phi)$ to scalp potential; both are expanded in spherical harmonic series. The transfer function relating sources and potentials depends only on the degree n of the spherical harmonic expansion, which provides a convenient index of the overall spatial frequency "averaged" over the m indices. The formula for $H_n(r_z)$ depends on the 4-sphere model parameters (conductivities and sphere radii) and the source layer's radial location (r_z) as provided in appendix G. The potential transfer function (6.14) is plotted for different values of the brain to skull conductivity ratio in the upper portion of fig. 8-6. The low-pass filtering characteristics of the layered spherical model are due mostly to the poor conductivity of

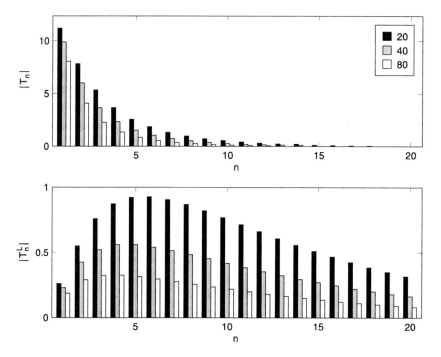

Figure 8-6 (*Upper*) Spatial transfer function for scalp potential $|T_{nm}| \rightarrow |T_n|$ obtained from (6.14). (*Lower*) Spatial transfer function for surface Laplacian $|T_{nm}^L| \rightarrow |T_n^L|$ obtained from (8.11). Each transfer function relates the strength of a radial dipole of fixed depth (1.2 cm below the scalp) to the corresponding scalp variable: potential or surface Laplacian. The horizontal axis n is the degree of the corresponding spherical harmonic function, essentially the spatial frequency index. The rapid fall-off of $|T_n|$ with n (upper histograms) shows that high (and even moderate) spatial frequency source activity in the cortex is sharply attenuated at the scalp. By contrast, the surface Laplacian transfer function $|T_n^L|$ (lower histograms) falls off slowly at large n.

the skull compared to brain, CSF, and scalp tissue and the physical separation between sources and scalp.

If we similarly expand the surface Laplacian of the scalp potential in a series of spherical harmonics with coefficients L_{nm}, the transfer function relating the source distribution to the surface Laplacian may be expressed as

$$T_{nm}^L = \frac{L_{nm}}{P_{nm}} = \frac{4\pi n(n+1)}{2n+1} H_n(r_z) \qquad (8.11)$$

The surface Laplacian transfer function (8.11) is expressed in terms of the spatial frequency index n. It involves the product of low-pass filtering by the 4-sphere model given in (6.14) with the $n(n+1)$ term, which indicates the high-pass filtering of the surface Laplacian operator. The combined effect is a band-pass filter of the source distribution as shown in the lower portion of fig. 8-6. *Given a spherical source distribution uniformly distributed over spatial frequencies (spatial white noise) in the 4-sphere model, the surface Laplacian selectively passes the influence of the source distribution over the middle range of spatial frequencies.* It suppresses both high spatial frequencies (due to low-pass filtering by the head volume conductor) and low spatial frequencies (due to the high-pass filtering of the surface Laplacian operator on a sphere). By contrast, unprocessed scalp potentials strongly emphasize low spatial frequency components of the source distribution, as shown in the upper plot in fig. 8-6. We emphasize that this limitation of raw scalp potentials occurs in addition to reference electrode issues.

Of special note is that the *relative magnitudes* of different spatial frequencies passed by surface Laplacian spatial filtering do not depend strongly on brain-to-skull conductivity ratio. *Absolute magnitudes* of the surface Laplacian do depend strongly on the conductivity ratio. Thus, surface Laplacian magnitudes are influenced by small changes in tissue properties (in a manner similar to influences on the potential), but relative spatial properties are not as strongly influenced. Of course, if tissue properties vary spatially (in tangential directions) more complex effects can be expected in both potential and surface Laplacian, as discussed in the context of a skull with variable resistance in section 10 of chapter 6.

In comparison to unprocessed potentials, band-pass filtering of cortical source distributions by the surface Laplacian operator tends to reduce the surface contribution of very large dipole layers (more power at low spatial frequencies) in favor of smaller dipole layers (more power at higher spatial frequencies). The upper part of fig. 8-7 shows scalp potential as a function of dipole layer size (expressed as a % of transcortical potential). In these simulations, source distributions consist of radial dipole layers located 1.4 cm below the outer scalp surface, forming spherical caps of uniform transcortical potential V_C. As shown in chapter 4, V_C is a measure of the strength of sources in the dipole layer. The ratio of scalp potential to transcortical

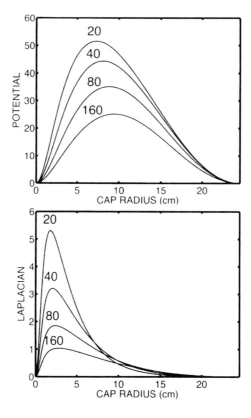

Figure 8-7 (*Upper*) Maximum scalp potentials due to dipole layers of varying angular extent, forming superficial spherical caps in the 4-sphere model. Each curve shows the ratio of scalp potential to transcortical potential V_C (expressed as %). (*Lower*) The surface Laplacian due to the same dipole layers. The four curves shown in each figure correspond to four different ratios of brain-to-skull conductivity as indicated by the labels. Note that potentials are primarily sensitive to broad dipole layers while surface Laplacians are sensitive to smaller dipole layers, as implied by figs. 8-6 and 8-8.

potential is maximum for a dipole layer with angular extent of approximately 60 degrees, expressed here as cap "radius" (measured along the spherical cap surface). The cap radius that generates the maximum scalp potential lies between about 7 and 10 cm depending on brain-to-skull conductivity ratio. The lower part of fig. 8-7 shows the surface Laplacian as a function of dipole layer size. This ratio is maximum for a spherical cap of angular extent equal to about 20 degrees, corresponding to a cap radius of less than 2.5 cm.

These simulations emphasize that the surface Laplacian is preferentially sensitive to source activity at spatial scales substantially smaller than the preferential scale of raw scalp potentials. The surface Laplacian selectively measures activity within short distances (less than about 2–3 cm) of the electrode both in depth and in tangential directions. By contrast, unprocessed potentials are maximally sensitive to the very large scale source distributions over tangential directions and to deeper sources

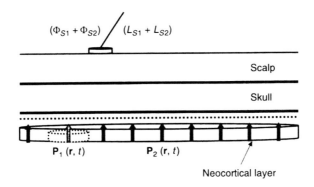

Figure 8-8 The scalp potential and surface Laplacian depend on the mesosource functions $P_1(r, t)$ and $P_2(r, t)$ integrated over the surfaces of their respective regions as given by (4.39). Here we picture two cortical dipole layers (generally representing multiple gyral crowns) defined as follows. The mesosource functions $P_1(r, t)$ and $P_2(r, t)$ are synchronous over their respective regions and asynchronous with other cortical tissue. The scalp potential and surface Laplacian are due to the sum of contributions from each dipole layer, given by $\Phi_{S1} + \Phi_{S2}$ and $L_{S1} + L_{S2}$, respectively. However, the relative contributions of the individual regions (dipole layers) can differ substantially. For example, if the small and large regions have diameters in the 2 cm and 10 cm ranges, respectively, we expect $|\Phi_{S1}/\Phi_{S2}| \ll |L_{S1}/L_{S2}|$. That is, smaller regions tend to make larger relative contributions to the surface Laplacian while larger regions contribute more to potential. If the two regions generate dynamics with different dominant temporal frequencies, scalp potential spectra will differ from surface Laplacian spectra, as demonstrated with alpha rhythm data in chapter 10.

(see fig. 8-5). This sensitivity distinction has several important implications as indicated in fig. 8-8. *A large superficial dipole layer generating a large scalp potential may contribute only minimally to the surface Laplacian. By contrast, a small dipole layer (possibly overlapping spatially with the larger dipole layer) tends to make a larger relative contribution to the surface Laplacian, while contributing only small signals to the potential.*

Based on these arguments, time series of unprocessed potentials and surface Laplacians may differ substantially. To picture some expected effects of this preferential spatial filtering on temporal waveforms, imagine that different sized dipole layers contribute mainly to different frequency bands as suggested in fig. 8-8. The surface potential and Laplacian are sums of the contributions from each dipole layer, given by $\Phi_{S1} + \Phi_{S2}$ and $L_{S1} + L_{S2}$, respectively. Based on the simulations in fig. 8-7, we expect $\Phi_{S2} \gg \Phi_{S1}$ and $L_{S1} \gg L_{S2}$—the scalp potential is due mostly to the large dipole layer and the scalp Laplacian is due mostly to the small layer. For purposes of this general argument, it does not matter if multiple dipole layers overlap as in fig. 8-8 or are spatially separated in neocortex. In the case of multiple dipole layer source regions, different frequency bands may be expected to make different contributions to cortical potentials, scalp potentials, and surface Laplacians. We will examine these issues first using simulations and then by examining EEG data in section 9 of this chapter and again in chapters 9 and 10.

5 Simulation Studies

Here several example simulations of the surface Laplacian as an estimate of dura potential are presented. The simulations are in two categories. The first examples are based on a small number of dipole sources; the second and third example sets consist of distributed source configurations with more than a thousand dipoles. The term "dipole" indicates a discrete version of the local dipole moment per unit volume or mesosource $\mathbf{P}(\mathbf{r}, t)$ defined in chapter 4. We have carried out several thousand simulations to test the surface Laplacian method using both spherical and more realistic shape volume conduction models (Nunez et al. 1991; Law et al. 1993; Yan et al. 1993; Nunez et al. 1994; Srinivasan 1994, 1999; Srinivasan et al. 1996, 1998). In addition, multiple comparisons of the New Orleans spline Laplacian algorithm with the Melbourne dura imaging algorithm have yielded consistent estimates of dura surface potential in both simulations and experimental studies (Nunez et al. 1994, 2001).

Figure 8-9 shows a simple example of three superficial dipole sources as indicated on the source map. Two radial dipoles are located at a depth of 1.4 cm below the scalp surface, corresponding to sources in cortical gyri. One dipole is oriented with the positive pole up (solid contour lines) and one is oriented with the negative pole up (dashed contour lines). The third dipole is tangential, as indicated by the positive (+) and negative (−) poles, and located at a depth of 2.2 cm below the scalp, corresponding to synaptic action in a sulcal wall. The three examples correspond to different strengths of the tangential source. In the case of fig. 8-9a the three dipoles have the same dipole moment; in fig. 8-9b the tangential dipole moment is twice that of the radial dipoles; and in fig. 8-9c the tangential dipole moment is four times the radial dipole moment. The scalp potential, surface Laplacian, and dura surface potential were calculated using the 4-sphere model (see caption for details). Each of the topographic maps has been normalized by its peak magnitude, and the contour lines are plotted in steps of 10% of the peak value with solid lines indicating positive values and dashed lines indicating negative values.

In the example of fig. 8-9a, radial and tangential dipoles have equal strength; the two radial dipoles provide much stronger contributions to potential than the tangential dipole, with only a weak positive region evident over the right side of the map. The potential generated by the negative radial dipole appears to fall off with tangential distance more slowly than the positive dipole and have larger magnitude, due to the influence of the tangential dipole. The surface Laplacian and cortical potential maps are nearly identical, revealing positive and negative radial dipoles with nearly equal magnitudes, but these maps fail to indicate the presence of the tangential dipole.

In fig. 8-9b, tangential dipole strength is twice radial dipole strengths; the broad field of the tangential dipole becomes evident over the right side of potential map, while a complex distribution is apparent over the left,

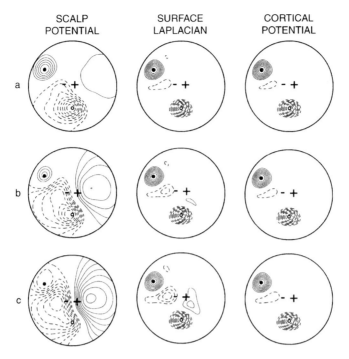

Figure 8-9 Simulation of scalp potential, cortical potential, and surface Laplacian due to multiple isolated dipole sources in the 4-sphere model of the head. The model consists of four spherical layers with parameters given in the caption for fig. 8-1, with brain-to-skull conductivity ratio equal to 40. Two radial dipole sources, one positive (solid contours) and one negative (dashed contours), are located at spherical coordinates $(r, \theta, \phi) = (7.8, 20, 180)$ and $(7.8, 45, 270)$ degrees. The tangential dipole is oriented along the x axis $(\phi = 0)$ as indicated by the positive $(+)$ and negative $(-)$ poles. The maps have been normalized with respect to the maximum value of each variable in order to display relative values. The three examples correspond to the same dipole locations, but different strengths of the tangential dipole source. (a) Dipole moment of the tangential dipole equals the radial dipole moments. (b) Dipole moment of the tangential dipole is twice the radial dipole moments. (c) Dipole moment of the tangential dipole is four times the radial dipole moments.

reflecting a mixture of the potentials due to both radial and tangential dipoles. The scalp potential is strongly influenced by the positive pole of the tangential dipole and the negative radial dipole. The potential fields generated by the negative pole of the tangential dipole and the positive radial dipole partly cancel. The net effect is a reversal of the field over the lower right portion of the sphere, an area that contains no source. The surface Laplacian and cortical potential again identify the two radial sources with magnitude unaffected by the tangential dipole.

In fig. 8-9c, tangential dipole strength is four times radial dipole strengths; the potential distribution is dominated by the broad positive and negative potentials over the left and right parts of the map. To first approximation, this is the scalp potential of a single tangential dipole. The surface Laplacian again reveals the radial dipoles, but also detects a much smaller field that appears to have the structure of a tangential dipole,

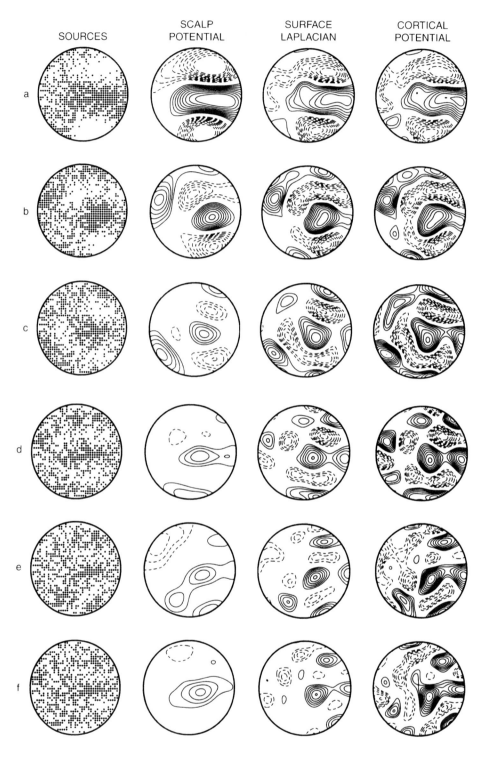

	SOURCES	SCALP POTENTIAL	SURFACE LAPLACIAN	CORTICAL POTENTIAL
a				
b				
c				
d				
e				
f				

Figure 8-10 Simulations of scalp potential, cortical potential, and surface Laplacian due to distributed radial sources. Here, 1600 radial dipole sources are uniformly spaced in the upper surface of the brain sphere, located in a spherical shell 1.2 cm below the scalp surface. The 4-sphere model parameters are identical to those used in fig. 8-1, with brain-to-skull

332

with sharp inversion of the sign of the field over the center of the map. However, this field is much smaller than the surface Laplacian field generated by the more superficial radial dipoles, even though the tangential dipole has four times the strength of the radial dipoles. Interestingly, the simulated cortical potentials, corresponding to recordings on the brain surface (ECoG), are even less sensitive to the deeper, stronger tangential source than the surface Laplacian.

These simulations show that the effectiveness of the surface Laplacian as a tool to identify EEG sources depends strongly on the spatial properties (depth and orientation) of the sources. The surface Laplacian is a spatial filter that emphasizes the contributions of superficial radial sources. The unprocessed EEG signal is expected to contain more relative contributions generated by deeper sources like tangential dipoles. As suggested by fig. 8-5, superficial sources produce surface Laplacian magnitudes that are much larger than those produced by sources that are only 1 or 2 cm deeper. Given that tangential dipoles produce smaller potentials at the outset, it follows that the surface Laplacian detects primarily superficial radial sources with good spatial resolution in tangential directions. *If superficial radial sources are not the primary contributors to a particular EEG signal, the surface Laplacian will simply filter out most of the signal!* As noted in chapter 2, MEG may be a useful adjunct to high-resolution EEG since it is mainly sensitive to the tangential sources (that tend to be deeper). Thus, MEG can perhaps be used to clarify the presence of deeper tangential sources (producing broad scalp potentials) that contribute minimally to the surface Laplacian.

In general, the source configurations underlying the EEG are expected to be complex and distributed over large regions. In fig. 8-10 we present simulations of 1600 radial dipoles sources uniformly distributed over the upper surface of a hemispherical "cortex" in the 4-sphere model. Thus, each surface voxel (and corresponding dipole) represents cortical tissue at the scale of several macrocolumns. The left-hand column of fig. 8-10 shows six different source distributions. In these plots a filled space (voxel) indicates a radial dipole source with positive pole up; an empty space indicates a negative pole up. In these simulations every location in the

conductivity ratio equal to 40. However, here every dipole source has equal strength but possibly unequal sign. The left column shows source distributions. In each small region (voxel) positive pole is indicated by a filled space and negative pole is indicated by an empty space. The source configurations differ only in their dominant spatial frequency or effective correlation length. The source distributions were obtained by randomly averaging the set of $2n + 1$ spherical harmonics of fixed degree (n) and adding random noise of equal magnitude to each average. Source strength at each location is expressed in terms of an assumed transcortical potential $V_C = \pm 250\ \mu V$, consistent with cortical depth experiments (reviewed in Nunez 1995) Contour line intervals are as follows: (scalp potential, surface Laplacian, cortical potential) = (6 μV, 3 $\mu V/cm^2$, 30 μV). (a–f) Spatial frequencies $n = 4$ through 9, respectively, where n is the degree of the spherical harmonic.

(simulated) smooth cortex contains a source of equal magnitude. Figure 8-10a–f have source configurations generated with equal numbers of positive and negative sources, but with *decreasing effective correlation lengths*. That is, the sources become progressively less clumped from fig. 8-10a to f. Large dipole layers are evident in fig. 8-10a; only small dipole layers are evident in fig. 8-10f.

Scalp potential, surface Laplacian, and cortical potential maps corresponding to each source distribution are shown in fig. 8-10. A fixed contour interval for each measure has been adopted in order to compare maps across fig. 8-10a–f. Comparing the highest peak in each potential map, we notice a dramatic reduction in scalp potential extrema as the source correlation length is decreased. By contrast, the average cortical potential magnitude is approximately constant across all cases. This indicates that the cortical potentials are influenced mainly by local sources and much less by the size of the dipole layers. In each example, the major features of the source distribution are evident in cortical potential maps and appear with matching magnitudes. In fig. 8-10a–d, surface Laplacian maps closely approximate corresponding cortical potential maps, but unlike cortical potential maps, surface Laplacian magnitudes decrease as the dipole layer size decreases. Even in the case of relatively small dipole layers (fig. 8-10e and f), the main features of source distributions are still captured by the surface Laplacian.

These simulations with known sources demonstrate that the surface Laplacian can often provide excellent estimates of cortical potential. When the sources are superficial radial dipoles, even very complex patterns of cortical source activity can be reasonably estimated by the surface Laplacian. By contrast, very little information about deeper tangential sources is available in the surface Laplacian. Thus, the surface Laplacian provides an effective means to estimate exclusively superficial radial sources, and can do so with remarkable spatial resolution, comparable in these simulations to the cortical potentials. Of course, these idealized simulations avoid several practical issues that are addressed in the following sections: surface Laplacian estimates with limited spatial sampling of (possibly) noisy data and errors due to local variations in skull resistance.

6 Methods to Estimate Surface Laplacians from EEG Data

Thus far our demonstrations of surface Laplacian properties have been based only on an analytic calculation of the surface Laplacian, a variable that cannot be measured directly. Methods to estimate the surface Laplacian from scalp potentials have evolved considerably since the simple nearest-neighbor Laplacian was first suggested (Hjorth 1975; Nunez 1981; Gevins et al. 1983; Gevins and Cutillo 1986). A simple nearest-neighbor Laplacian algorithm follows closely from fig. 8-3 suggesting a finite-difference approximation to the second spatial derivative of scalp-recorded potential. The Laplacian may be estimated (crudely) at each electrode location by averaging potential differences between a central location and four surrounding electrode locations as given by the ratio on the right-hand side of (8.6). Although we may now characterize these simple nearest-neighbor Laplacian methods as "crude," they were very useful when most EEG was recorded with only a small number of electrodes (fewer than 21). The nearest-neighbor Laplacian often provided a more accurate picture of local cortical source distributions than conventional EEG by eliminating volume conducted signals from distant regions and removing reference electrode effects (Nunez and Pilgreen 1991). The nearest-neighbor Laplacian remains a practical and easily implemented method to improve spatial resolution in EEG recorded with a small number of electrodes, provided its limitations are appreciated.

Surface Laplacian algorithms designed for multichannel EEG systems with (approximately) 64 or more electrodes are based on fitting instantaneous scalp potentials to spline functions and then evaluating surface Laplacians of spline functions at each time step. If waveforms are not required, it is not necessary to spline each time slice of multichannel data. Alternatively, spline functions may be obtained for real and imaginary parts of Fourier transforms representing (say) one second of data as discussed in chapter 10. Mathematical splines are smooth interpolations through fixed points, the electrode locations in EEG applications. The general concept originated in the ship and aircraft industries in which thin wooden planks were held at fixed points while plank curvature between these points assumed shapes of minimum strain energy.

Various spline functions have been applied to this task, including spherical splines $\Phi_{SS}(\theta, \phi)$ for interpolation of recorded potential on an (assumed) spherical scalp surface (Wahba, 1981), two-dimensional splines $\Phi_{2D}(u, v)$ (Perrin et al. 1989) for interpolating projections of the scalp surface onto a plane, and splines $\Phi_{3D}(x, y, z)$ for which interpolation of potential occurs in three-dimensional Cartesian coordinates (Law et al. 1993; Nunez et al. 1994; Srinivasan et al. 1996; Srinivasan 1999). The three-dimensional spline involves interpolation of potential in space, independent of scalp surface shape. The spline functions employ a regularization parameter to smooth the data, allowing matrix inversion to fit the spline, prior to the surface Laplacian calculation. The value of the regularization parameter is somewhat arbitrary (over a small range) in this algorithm. One of the main factors determining this choice of smoothing is the electrode separation, which fixes the upper limit on spatial information available in the EEG record (see chapter 7 and Srinivasan et al. 1996). Essentially, we try to avoid showing more detail in the surface Laplacian estimate than is warranted by the spatial sampling density.

The three-dimensional spline function developed for EEG interpolation and surface Laplacian estimates offers at least one advantage over the spherical spline method (Law et al. 1993; Nunez et al. 1994;

Srinivasan et al. 1996; Srinivasan 1999). The main motivation for using the three-dimensional spline is that it can be used to fit the scalp potential on any surface that passes through the electrodes. That is, the function $\Phi_{3D}(x, y, z)$ is constructed from recorded data and is expected to be accurate for a small range of locations near the scalp surface. An estimate of the potential at location (x_s, y_s, z_s) on a surface of any shape is given by $\Phi_{3D}(x_s, y_s, z_s)$. By contrast to this three-dimensional interpolated potential, the surface Laplacian calculation depends on the local surface geometry: a sphere or prolate spheroid, for example (Law et al. 1993).

Theoretically, the regularization parameter in the spline function is mostly fixed by the effective electrode diameter, including gel or saline interface with the scalp (Srinivasan et al. 1996). This reflects the fact that recorded potential is a space average over the electrode rather than a point measure. The details of this spline function are presented in appendix J.

In order to compare three-dimensional splines to spherical splines (Perrin et al. 1989), the three-dimensional spline has been expressed in a spherical harmonic expansion for the case of electrodes on a best-fit spherical surface (Srinivasan et al. 1996). The three-dimensional spline intrinsically smooths the data at high spatial frequencies above the Nyquist limit implied by the electrode size and spacing (Srinivasan et al. 1996). In applications with fewer electrodes, more smoothing may be necessary to avoid spatial aliasing. Thus, both electrode size and electrode spacing determine the amount of smoothing to be applied. In simulations, improvements in surface Laplacian estimates are obtained if center-to-center electrode spacing is about 2 cm or less, corresponding to more than 180 electrodes on the upper surface of the head. Spatial aliasing of scalp data is generally believed to be small because of spatial filtering by the head volume conductor. It may be eliminated entirely by spatial filtering by choosing electrode plus gel diameters equal or larger than edge-to-edge electrode spacing as discussed in chapter 7.

The three-dimensional spline functions have been used to calculate the surface Laplacian along best-fit spherical and ellipsoidal surfaces, showing similar results (Law et al. 1993). In principle, the three-dimensional spline can be used to interpolate the potential along any realistic scalp surface if electrode positions and scalp surface position are accurately known. Some improvement in the accuracy of surface Laplacian estimates is expected if scalp surface is extracted from MRI so that spatial derivatives in local surface coordinates may be more accurately estimated (Babiloni et al. 1996). However, our comparisons of spherical and ellipsoidal surface Laplacians (Law et al. 1993) suggest that the surface Laplacian based on a spherical surface is relatively insensitive to the variations in local geometry of the scalp.

We have carried out extensive tests of the New Orleans three-dimensional spline surface Laplacian estimate (Nunez et al. 1993, 1994, 2001; Law et al. 1993; Srinivasan et al. 1996; Srinivasan 1999). These simulations have mainly tested the effects of spatial sampling and noise using a wide range of local and distributed cortical sources. To a more limited extent, we have also used finite element models to test the effects of surface geometry and local variations in skull resistance. Examples comparing analytic calculation of the surface Laplacians to calculation of spline Laplacians with a finite number of samples (electrodes) are presented in appendix J.

7 Comparison of Spline Laplacian and Dura Imaging Estimates

Dura imaging (also known as *spatial deconvolution, cortical imaging,* or *deblurring*) provides an alternative approach to obtaining high-resolution EEG estimates from scalp potential recordings. Dura imaging methods are theoretically distinct from surface Laplacian estimates. Surface Laplacians provide estimates of radial current flux through local skull. It so happens that this local current is closely related to local cortical surface potential as shown by (8.9) and fig. 8-4. This close relationship (which is not obvious) is a direct consequence of the large brain-to-skull conductivity ratio. In this sense, surface Laplacian-based high-resolution EEG is independent of any specific volume conductor model. Variations in skull resistance over its surface will, of course, introduce distortions in dura potential estimates obtained with Laplacians or any other method that fails to account for such inhomogeneous tissue properties.

By contrast to surface Laplacians, dura imaging methods provide an inward continuation solution of scalp potential to the dura surface by explicit use of a volume conductor model, usually one of the familiar 3-sphere or 4-sphere models. The basis for this approach is as follows: if the potential everywhere on the outer surface of a volume conductor is known perfectly, the potential on any inner closed surface may be calculated uniquely, without knowledge of the location or number of sources, provided no sources are located between the two surfaces, in this case outer scalp and inner CSF. Of course, in practice we are only able to sample part of the outer surface (scalp) and only at discrete locations. Nevertheless, because the inner surface of interest (dura) is close to the outer surface, these limitations do not appear overly severe. *Thus, the potential on the inner surface of the skull can be estimated directly from the scalp potential, given a volume conductor model of the head.* We note that dura imaging and surface Laplacians estimate different physical quantities, dura potential and radial skull current density, respectively, both of which are closely related to cortical surface potential and superficial cortical source distribution in simulations as suggested by the rough approximation (8.9).

We do not know the potential on the scalp surface perfectly due to finite spatial sampling primarily restricted to the upper surface of the head. Furthermore, all volume conduction models, including finite element models derived from MRI, are only approximate due to minimal knowledge of tissue conductivities. In spite of these limitations, our simulations show that the Melbourne dura imaging algorithm (Cadusch et al. 1992), which uses a 3-sphere model, provides estimates of cortical potential patterns that are very similar to those obtained by the New Orleans spline-Laplacian based on a spherical surface. Correlation coefficients between cortical patterns generated by the two algorithms are typically in the 0.80−0.85 and 0.95 ranges for 64 and 131 surface samples, respectively. These cross correlation ranges comparing the two high-resolution methods apply approximately to both simulated and genuine EEG data. If a perfect head model were used with dense spatial sampling, one might expect dura imaging to provide more accurate estimates of dura potential than spline Laplacian estimates. However, with 131 electrodes on the upper surface of the head (approximately 2.3 cm center-to-center spacing of electrodes), the two methods yield essentially identical estimates as indicated below.

A number of simulation and experimental studies of the high-resolution EEG estimates obtained with spline Laplacian and dura imaging are outlined here (Nunez et al. 1994, 2001). These studies have tested the effects of noise, limited spatial sampling, and (to a lesser degree) head model errors. The results are summarized in table 8-1. Group 1 simulations show correlation coefficients between high-resolution EEG estimates obtained from 100 simulated cortical source distributions, each consisting of 3602 randomly clumped radial dipole sources as demonstrated in fig. 8-11a The head volume conductor model used to create forward solutions is our standard 4-sphere model. For each source

Table 8-1 Correlation coefficients for simulated and genuine EEG

Measurement	Correlation coefficient
Group 1 simulations: 100 source distributions with perfect skull model, imperfect CSF	
Spline-Laplacian/inner surface	0.965 ± 0.010
Dura Image/inner surface	0.957 ± 0.012
Spline-Laplacian/dura image	0.986 ± 0.006
Group 2 simulations: 100 source distributions with skull resistivity variations (40 to 120)	
Spline-Laplacian/inner surface	0.963 ± 0.010
Dura Image/inner surface	0.957 ± 0.014
Spline-Laplacian/dura image	0.983 ± 0.007
Group 3 simulations: 100 source distributions with 15% noise added to surface potentials	
Spline-Laplacian/inner surface	0.736 ± 0.082
Dura Image/inner surface	0.692 ± 0.087
Spline-Laplacian/dura image	0.970 ± 0.006
Group 4 EEG data: 600 time slices of alpha rhythm	
Spline-Laplacian/dura image	0.950 ± 0.017
Group 5 EEG data: 20 one-second epochs. Phase estimates obtained with and without 15% noise added to genuine data	
Spline-Laplacian clean/noise	0.950 ± 0.040
Dura Image clean/noise	0.952 ± 0.032

distribution, outer surface potentials were calculated at 131 locations corresponding to the electrode positions of genuine EEG data studied separately. Inner skull surface potentials estimated from the dura image and spline Laplacian algorithms were compared with actual (computed) inner skull surface potential at 131 "dura" locations. Each table entry in Group 1 is a correlation coefficient calculated by comparing the two high-resolution estimates (point by point) with calculated dura potential and with each other at 131 dura surface locations. Estimates of the variance of the correlation coefficient were obtained from 100 different simulations.

A typical source distribution used to construct table 8.1 is shown in fig. 8-11. The simulated scalp potential calculated from the 4-sphere model is shown in fig. 8-11b. The spline Laplacian estimate of dura potential (obtained only from the 131 scalp potential samples) is shown in fig. 8-11c and the corresponding dura imaging estimate is shown in fig. 8-11d (also obtained only from the 131 scalp potential samples). These figures are printed in large size to demonstrate the practical equivalence of spline Laplacian and dura image methods when applied to 131-channel simulations (or EEG data). Note that the performances indicated in fig. 8-11 do not represent a "best case" simulation: rather it is a typical example. We emphasize again that the two estimates of dura potential were obtained "blind"; that is, by submitting only the 131 surface potentials to the two algorithms. Algorithm outputs were then normalized with respect to individual maxima so that dura potential maps (μV) and spline Laplacian maps (μV/cm^2) could be compared directly. The spline Laplacian estimates are independent of both head model (except for the assumption of a spherical surface) and reference location. The dura image estimates depend only weakly on spherical head model parameters provided that skull conductivity is much lower than brain and scalp conductivity.

The dura image estimates were calculated by first converting scalp potentials (simulated or genuine EEG data) so the potential at each sampled location is referenced to the average potential of the 131 surface locations (the *common average reference* discussed in chapter 7). Correlation coefficients were obtained by electrode-by-electrode comparisons of the calculated dura potential (not shown) at 131 locations to simulated scalp potential (0.627), spline Laplacian (0.974), and dura image (0.954) at corresponding surface locations. In all similar simulations high-resolution methods provide much more accurate representations of dura potential distribution than maps obtained from unprocessed scalp potentials. The spline Laplacian is slightly more accurate in this particular example, but this is a coincidence. The two methods are operationally identical when electrode arrays are sufficiently dense.

In Group 1 simulations of table 8-1, the brain-to-skull conductivity ratio used by the 4-sphere model in forward solutions was fixed at 80. The dura imaging algorithm used a 3-sphere model (no CSF), also with a brain to skull conductivity ratio of 80. As shown in chapter 6, the 4-sphere model

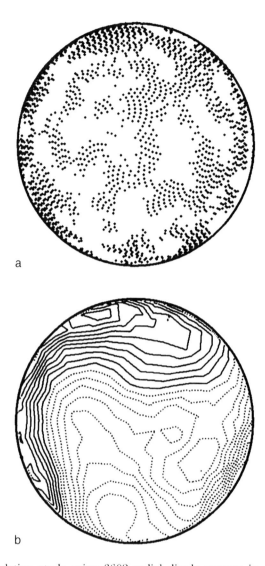

a

b

Figure 8-11 A simulation study using 3602 radial dipole sources in the 4-sphere model with radii (brain, CSF, skull, scalp) = $(8.0, 8.2, 8.7, 9.2)$ cm. Relative shell layer conductivities are $(1, 5, 1/80, 1)$. (a) A moderately clumped source distribution in a thin spherical shell centered at 7.8 cm radius. Filled and empty spaces indicate positive and negative dipole moments, respectively. Magnitudes vary randomly in contrast to fig. 8-10. (b). The scalp surface potential map calculated from the forward solution at 131 discrete scalp locations with subsequent interpolation (2.2 cm average spacing between samples). These locations match the electrode locations used in our experiments in Melbourne (see chapter 10). The correlation coefficient between scalp and cortical potential (not shown) is 0.627, obtained by comparing the two variables at the 131 discrete angular locations. (c) The New Orleans spline-Laplacian calculated "blind"; that is, by using only potentials at the 131 sampled locations. The spline Laplacian/cortical potential correlation coefficient is 0.974. (d) The Melbourne dura imaging estimate (based on a three-sphere model) was calculated from the same 131 sampled potentials. The dura image/cortical potential correlation coefficient is 0.954.

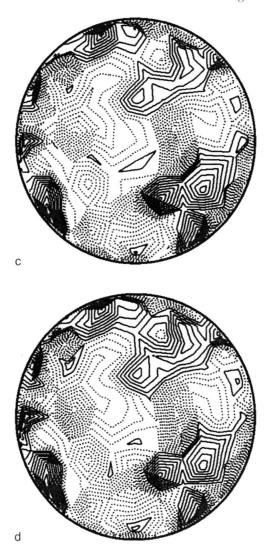

Figure 8-11 Continued.

is roughly equivalent to a 3-sphere model with a lower brain-to-skull conductivity ratio (depending on CSF conductivity and thickness). In any case, simulations in table 8-1 indicate that dura image estimates are insensitive to these parameters.

Correlation coefficients are shown in Group 1 of table 8.1 for three electrode-by-electrode comparisons: spline Laplacian/cortical potential, dura image/cortical potential, and spline Laplacian/dura image. The smoothing parameter in the dura imaging algorithm was set to zero for all calculations shown in table 8-1. The agreement between cortical potential, spline Laplacian, and dura imaging is excellent. In Group 2 simulations, the brain-to-skull conductivity ratio used in the forward solutions (4-sphere model) was drawn from a uniform distribution on the interval (40, 120) while the dura imaging algorithm (3-sphere model) was based on a fixed ratio of 80. The correlations for Group 2 simulations are just as strong as in Group 1, indicating that the correlations are insensitive to brain-to-skull conductivity ratios over a broad range. Only absolute magnitudes are sensitive to this ratio. In Group 3 simulations, a perfect head model was used with 15% (RMS) uncorrelated noise added to each surface potential calculated with forward solutions. In this case, dura potential estimates obtained with both methods are much less accurate as shown by reduced correlations with inner skull surface potential. Nevertheless, the spline Laplacian and dura imaging estimates remain in close agreement (0.970 correlation). These correlations are based on single slices, but time averages are often employed in actual EEG practice. In many such cases, noise distortions can be substantially reduced as shown in Group 5 simulations of table 8-1.

In Group 4 EEG studies of table 8-1, correlation coefficients were obtained by comparing spline Laplacian and dura image predictions of dura potential using 131-channel EEG data (eyes closed alpha) recorded in two human subjects. The average correlation (0.950) is based on 600 individual time slices, taken at one-second intervals without consideration of EEG amplitude. That is, spatial maps of surface Laplacian and potential were obtained for each time slice, and correlation coefficients for each pair of maps calculated from electrode-by-electrode comparisons. Thus, the two high-resolution methods agree closely when applied to genuine data recorded with 131 electrodes.

In Group 5 EEG studies of table 8-1, correlation coefficients were obtained from 20 one-second epochs of alpha rhythm as follows. First, the Fourier transform of each one-second epoch at each of the 131 surface locations was calculated. For each epoch, we passed the 131 complex Fourier coefficients (real and imaginary parts separately) corresponding to the peak alpha frequency (10 Hz) through dura image and spline Laplacian algorithms. High-resolution phase estimates of this 10 Hz signal at each of the 131 electrode sites were then calculated. Phases were rotated so that all were expressed with respect to zero phase at electrode Cz. (This later step is required for studies described in chapter 10 in which phase structure in successive epochs is compared.) Each high-resolution phase estimate was obtained twice: first from the recorded scalp potentials and second from the same potentials with noise added to the raw EEG data (15% of RMS potentials). Correlation coefficients were obtained by comparing the two cosine phase sets (zero noise and 15% noise) at each of the 131 locations for both dura image and spline Laplacian phase estimates.

The correlations are all greater than 0.95 showing that noise of this magnitude had minimal influence on phase estimates, which are much more sensitive to noise than amplitude estimates. Note that correlations obtained by passing the raw potential data (at individual time slices) through high-resolution algorithms before Fourier transformation are identical to those shown here, but the computation time is several hundred times longer. This computational time difference occurs because each second of data requires up to 500 passes through the dura imaging algorithm (500/3 passes if 3 successive time slices are averaged). By contrast, each second of Fourier transformed data requires only two passes through the algorithm for each frequency component (real and imaginary parts). Of course, if we were to calculate phases over broad frequency ranges, computational times would be similar.

The addition of uncorrelated noise to the actual data (Group 3) substantially reduced the accuracy of single time slice high-resolution EEG. However, the addition of uncorrelated noise presented minimal problems for frequency domain measures. The reason is clear. Fourier transforms of one-second epochs involved 500 time points, thereby reducing the noise effect by the factor $500^{-1/2}$. Thus, the effect of noise on phase estimates is minimal as shown in Group 5 of table 8-1; the corresponding effect on amplitude is even smaller (not shown). The possibility of such enormous reduction in noise effects (especially biological artifact) provides one strong motivation to use frequency-domain measures in the EEG and steady-state visually evoked potential (SSVEP) studies, as discussed in chapters 9 and 10.

Accuracy of high-resolution EEG is determined by signal-to-noise level, electrode density, and volume conductor model. Remarkably, these two distinct high-resolution EEG algorithms (having different theoretical bases) produce very similar estimates of cortical potentials across all the simulations summarized in table 8-1. In several parts of this book we emphasize the spline Laplacian algorithm for high-resolution EEG estimates rather than dura imaging. This choice is based partly on the surface Laplacian's independence of head model, but mostly on our longer experience with the New Orleans spline Laplacian algorithm presented in appendix J. In any case, the two methods yield nearly identical estimates of dura potential maps when applied to 131-channel data. It should be noted, however, that the spline Laplacian is more computationally intensive than dura imaging, but speed is an important issue only in some applications.

Dura image methods require an electrical head model. In principal, MRI can be used to construct accurate geometrical head models. Tissue boundaries can be estimated for individual subjects, and may be used to construct computer models that incorporate the geometry of the cortical surface, inner and outer skull surfaces, and scalp surface (Gevins et al. 1994). However, no matter how sophisticated the geometric model, the corresponding volume conductor model will be severely limited by the current lack of detailed information on tissue conductivity.

The effective resistance of each compartment in numerical models depends on the product of tissue resistivity with thickness. Thus, for example, a 50% uncertainty in conductivity is generally just as critical as a 50% uncertainty in geometry. In chapter 4 we cited several studies indicating rather large uncertainties in skull conductivity (perhaps 50 to

100%). Furthermore, both radial and tangential conductivity variations appear to be large. For example, the resistance of 1 cm diameter skull plugs (in vitro) was found to be independent of their thickness (Law 1993), apparently because of their three-layered structure, as discussed in chapter 4. If these *in vitro* experimental results are valid in living skulls, MRI methods used to determine the thickness of tissue compartments could easily yield head models that are less accurate than those based on a uniform skull layer. In the absence of better information about human heads, the surface Laplacian appears to provide a relatively robust approach to high-resolution EEG. Of course, surface Laplacian methods have their own limitations, as outlined in sections 6 and 9. Should detailed information about tissue conductivity become available in the future, perhaps by impedance imaging techniques (Nunez 1987; Ferree et al. 1999) or from MRI data (Ueno and Iriguchi 1998), dura imaging methods offer the possibility of highly accurate estimates of dura surface potential, thereby dramatically improving EEG spatial resolution.

It should be emphasized, however, that advances of volume conduction models will do nothing to overcome the fundamental nonuniqueness of the inverse problem as discussed in chapter 2. By comparison, high-resolution EEG methods (dura imaging and surface Laplacians) yield estimates of dura surface potential that are "unique" in the sense discussed here. Despite this obvious advantage, practitioners of EEG source localization have rarely made use of information available with high-resolution EEG methods. We suspect that part of the reason is that *source localization methods lend themselves naturally to local views of brain function*, where a small (or even just one) location in the brain is assumed to generate the measured potentials, whereas *high-resolution EEG is neutral with respect to any specific model (local versus distributed) of the underlying sources*. When the assumption of a small number of sources is warranted, for instance in early sensory evoked potentials, high-resolution EEG can provide a useful check on source localization methods. More importantly, high-resolution EEG can provide a means to test the validity of the basic assumption of a small number of sources.

8 Applications to Spontaneous EEG

The accuracy and spatial resolution achieved by the spline Laplacian depends mainly on electrode density and signal-to-noise ratio: both are crucial experimental conditions. The spline Laplacian algorithm is most effective when signal-to-noise ratio is high, since the underlying opera-tion of taking spatial derivatives will not only emphasize local sources, as discussed in this chapter, but will also emphasize the noise signals present at each electrode site. In general, averaging (in the time domain as in evoked potentials or by Fourier methods described here and in chapter 9) is an important step to obtain signals suitable for surface Laplacian analysis. This step can substantially reduce the effect of noise that is uncorrelated between electrode sites.

The issue of optimal electrode density for surface Laplacians may be considered theoretically. In practice, we expect that beyond some limiting electrode density no additional information can be obtained from adding more electrodes (Srinivasan et al. 1996). This expectation is based on the spatial filtering properties of the head volume conductor, which severely limits the power in short spatial wavelengths that can be recorded on the scalp. These issues are considered in detail for scalp potential recordings in chapter 7. As in the case of sampling in the time domain, the Nyquist criterion requires two spatial samples per cycle. A 1 cm effective electrode diameter (including conductive gel) and a 2 cm center-to-center electrode spacing ensures than any signal power not removed by the volume conductor with wavelengths shorter than 1 cm will be removed as a result of spatial averaging by individual electrodes (in a manner analogous to the action of analog filtering of EEG time series). Simulations using a 4-sphere model suggest that a center-to-center electrode spacing of about 2 cm is sufficient to record the highest spatial frequencies likely to be recordable in EEG data (Srinivasan et al. 1996; Srinivasan et al. 1998). The actual limiting electrode density for genuine heads may be a little different, but in any case, measurements of a variety of EEG signals in different heads would be required to obtain a more comprehensive estimate. In this context, we again emphasize that without high-resolution algorithms, the information yield of dense electrode arrays (64–128 or more) appears to be quite limited.

In order to demonstrate the effect of the surface Laplacian on EEG data, we applied the spline-Laplacian algorithm to eyes closed resting spontaneous EEG data using a best-fit sphere to 111 electrode positions (2.7 cm center-to-center electrode spacing, with 1 cm effective diameter electrodes). Experimental conditions were chosen to generate alpha oscillations, which have large amplitudes and high signal-to-noise ratio without averaging. Figure 8-12a shows two seconds of average-referenced EEG potentials at nine midline electrodes. Not surprisingly, with this dense electrode array neighboring electrodes show very similar potentials. Two dashed vertical lines are drawn on each time plot to direct the reader to two common time slices. At these two times electrode sites over occipital cortex (electrodes 1–3) show a peak positive potential of the alpha rhythm while electrode sites near the frontal pole (electrodes 8 and 9) show a peak negative potential at the same time slice. The back-to-front spatial distribution of the alpha rhythm gives the appearance of very low spatial frequency (long wavelength) source activity, with minimum potential magnitude at electrodes near the vertex.

Figure 8-12b shows the spline Laplacian at these nine midline electrodes. The Laplacian-transformed alpha oscillations demonstrate maximum amplitude (among these electrodes) at two electrode sites near the vertex (electrodes 5, and 6). The dashed vertical lines indicate the

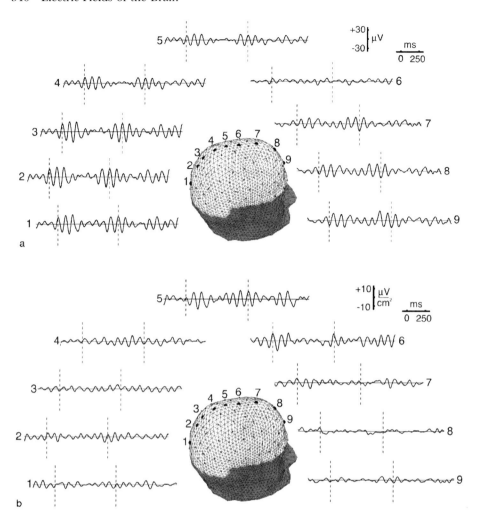

Figure 8-12 EEG (alpha rhythm) waveforms recorded along the midline (with respect to the average reference). Nine out of a total of 111 channels (electrodes) are shown. The two dashed lines on each waveform indicate fixed time slices and phase differences between oscillations recorded from different locations. (a) Potential waveforms. (b) Spline-Laplacian waveforms calculated from the entire 111-channel array. The combined information from (a) and (b) suggests both global and local (near electrodes 5 and 6) source contributions to alpha rhythm, as depicted conceptually in fig. 8-8.

same time slices as the potential plots in fig. 8-12a. Note that the alpha burst has a different time course at these two electrodes, with a peak occurring at the first marked time slice (vertical line) in electrode 6 with no corresponding peak at electrode 5. The distinctness of the time course of Laplacians at these two electrodes is also evident just prior to the second time slice (vertical line) where a strong alpha oscillation is evident at electrode 5 but not at electrode 6. The electrodes over occipital and frontal areas show the strongest alpha signal in the potential plots, but much smaller amplitude Laplacian signals.

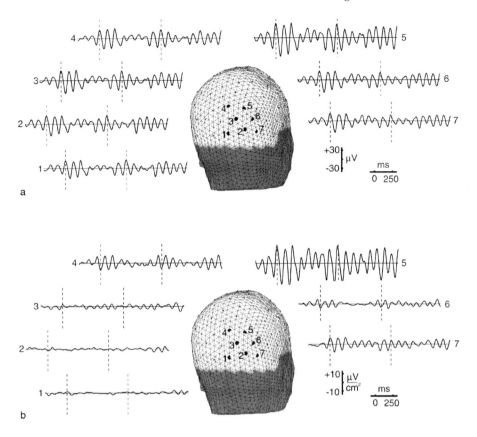

Figure 8-13 Same data epoch shown in fig. 8-12, but electrode positions over right posterior regions are shown. (a) Potential waveforms. (b) Spline-Laplacian waveforms calculated from the entire 111-channel array. The combined information from (a) and (b) suggests both global and local (near electrode 5) source contributions to alpha rhythm, as depicted conceptually in fig. 8-8.

The striking difference between potentials and Laplacians reflects the fact that the potentials and Laplacians are sensitive to different spatial bandwidths of sources as discussed in section 4. The potentials are dominated by long-wavelength source activity that extends from frontal to occipital poles. By contrast, the Laplacian is insensitive to this low spatial frequency source activity, but rather emphasizes (apparent) local sources near the two electrodes close to the vertex. Such local sources are masked in the potential plots apparently due to the dominant contribution from the low spatial frequency (global) source distribution.

Figure 8-13 shows potentials (fig. 8-13a) and Laplacians (fig. 8-13b) for the same recording of alpha rhythm from seven electrodes over the right occipital cortex. Very similar results were obtained for electrodes over left occipital cortex (not shown). Note that electrodes at the edge of the array have been excluded in producing these plots. Laplacian estimates are relatively inaccurate at the edge of the array because the spline estimates are not well constrained. Figure 8-13a shows alpha rhythm potentials that are very similar at all seven right occipital electrodes. At both marked time slices (vertical lines), the potential reaches a positive peak at all electrode locations shown. The largest potentials were recorded at electrode 5, which is closer to parietal cortex. Figure 8-13b shows the Laplacian at these same electrode sites. A strong Laplacian signal is evident at electrode 5; smaller signals are present at electrodes 4, 6, and 7, and much weaker signals at electrodes 1–3. Note that the marked time slices (vertical lines) elicit a positive peak in the alpha rhythm at electrode 5 and a peak with lower magnitude at electrode 7. By contrast, electrodes 4 and 6 show a negative peak at the same time slice.

Again, we can interpret the scalp potential distribution shown in figs. 8-12 and 8-13 as generated partly by a low spatial frequency source distribution, which appears relatively uniform under these electrodes. This can be pictured as a large dipole layer. The larger potential magnitude at electrode 5 suggests that local source activity is also contributing to potentials recorded by this electrode. This local activity is confirmed by the Laplacian plot at electrode 5 that places more emphasis on this local source activity. We emphasize that *the source activity identified by the surface Laplacian does not generally represent all the sources that generate the EEG potentials*. Rather, the surface Laplacian identifies a subset of sources that are more superficial and tangentially local (within 2–3 cm of an electrode). By contrast, the potential map includes signals generated by sources that are broadly distributed and, perhaps in some cases, deep sources. *Thus, surface Laplacian and dura image estimates should be used to complement, but not replace, raw scalp potentials.* Contrasting potential and Laplacian signals can clarify the nature of EEG generators. Neither measure is as informative when used in isolation.

9 Conclusions and Caveats

Most EEG phenomena are apparently generated by coherent neural sources organized at macroscopic (centimeter) scales in the neocortex (Nunez, 1995, 2000; see chapter 11). The source distribution underlying any particular EEG waveform need not be generated by a single dipole source located in a restricted cortical area. Such a simple model can explain very few EEG phenomena and typically down-plays dynamic interactions between the densely interconnected cortex and thalamic input from sensory stimuli. Such interactions apparently take place at many spatial and temporal scales including macroscopic scales observable with EEG, as discussed in chapters 2, 4, 10, and 11. In this case, source localization obtained by fitting dipoles to measured scalp potentials is neither technically feasible nor physiologically realistic.

High-resolution EEG methods apply spatial filters rather than fitting the data to a source model. This offers a number of advantages for EEG analysis. The results of such spatial filtering can be evaluated objectively since the operation does not depend on assumptions about the sources. Instead, high-resolution filters isolate those aspects of the EEG that are associated with superficial cortical tissue in the immediate neighborhood surrounding the electrode (typically 2–3 cm). *Signals that are removed by applying this spatial filter can be eliminated as local source candidates.* Thus, the surface Laplacian acts to increase the sensitivity of each electrode to superficial cortical sources near the electrode. Such Laplacian-identified sources are likely to be mainly radial dipoles in the proximal gyral surfaces.

High-resolution EEG offers the advantage of viewing cortical dynamics at smaller spatial scales than is possible with raw scalp potentials. In this chapter, we demonstrate theoretically that the surface Laplacian is a band-pass filtered representation of source activity, as compared to scalp potentials which are dominated by very low spatial frequencies in the source distribution. Thus, the surface Laplacian allows examination of the dynamics of more localized sources than do raw potentials. In the next chapter, we discuss methods to characterize EEG dynamics. The information yield of methods used to study spatial properties (such as EEG coherence) is greatly enhanced by high-resolution methods.

The alpha rhythm data of figs. 8-12 and 8-13 demonstrate how potential and Laplacian measures may complement each other to provide plausible explanations for the underlying mechanisms. Our tentative conclusions from these data are that this alpha rhythm(s) is generated by a combination of global activity represented by a large dipole layer covering most or all of the electrode array and more local activity represented by multiple smaller dipole layers as depicted conceptually in fig. 8-8. This interpretation is fully consistent with the cortical surface recordings of Grey Walter and Penfield and Jasper cited in chapter 1. The oscillations produced by smaller dipole layers can have similar (but not necessarily identical) temporal frequencies within the alpha band. *Humans generate multiple alpha rhythms over a range of spatial and temporal frequencies. Both the magnitudes and strengths of interaction between these rhythms is expected to vary with brain state.*

We conclude this chapter with several caveats concerning high-resolution EEG:

(i) The surface Laplacian is a spatial filter: it emphasizes some sources and suppresses the effects of others. Thus, this approach represents an alternative to source localization in the sense that it does not attempt to account for all the sources of the EEG potentials. Even when (apparent) localized superficial sources are identified using Laplacian or dura imaging methods, more widely distributed sources are probably making substantial contributions to scalp potential.

(ii) The surface Laplacian estimate is distorted by variations in local skull properties. Similar distortions occur with raw EEG, dura imaging, or any source localization method that assumes uniform tissue properties. No method of analysis is perfect (or even close to perfect). Since different strengths and weaknesses characterize different analysis methods, physiological interpretations of EEG are most convincing when based on multiple methods. It follows that *Laplacian or dura imaging estimates should be used to complement, but not replace, raw scalp potentials.*

(iii) The Laplacian can be distorted by noise and can be inaccurate when applied to un-averaged potentials (single time slices). A substantial improvement in accuracy can be obtained by using averaging over N samples (either in the time or frequency domains) to obtain $N^{-1/2}$ reductions in uncorrelated noise effects.

(iv) All simulations and EEG data analyses involving high-resolution methods presented in this book are based on specific algorithms: the *New Orleans spline-Laplacian* and *Melbourne dura imaging*. Algorithms developed in other laboratories that are based on the same physical principles should, in theory, provide similar estimates. If discrepancies between algorithms developed in different laboratories are identified, multiple tests using identical sets of simulated data should help to resolve such discrepancies.

References

Babiloni F, Babiloni C, Carducci F, Fattorini L, Onaratti P, and Urbano A, 1996, Spline Laplacian estimate of EEG potentials over a realistic magnetic resonance-constructed scalp surface model. *Electroencephalography and Clinical Neurophysiology* 98: 204–215.

Cadusch PJ, Breckon W, and Silberstein RB, 1992, Spherical splines and the interpolation, deblurring, and transformation of topographic EEG data, *Brain Topography* 5: 59.

Edlinger G, Wach P, and Pfurtscheller G, 1998, On the realization of an analytic high-resolution EEG. *IEEE Transactions on Biomedical Engineering* 45: 736–745.

Ferree T, Eriksen K, and Tucker DM, 2000, Regional head tissue conductivity estimation for improved EEG analysis. *IEEE Transactions on Biomedical Engineering* 47: 1584–1592.

Gevins AS and Cutillo BA, 1986, Signals of cognition. In: FH Lopes da Silva (Ed.), *Handbook of Electroencephalography and Clinical Neurophysiology*, Vol. 2, Amsterdam: Elsevier, pp. 335–381.

Gevins AS, Le J, Brickett P, Reutter B, and Desmond J, 1991, Seeing through the skull: advanced EEGs use MRIs to accurately measure cortical activity from the scalp. *Brain Topography* 4:125–131.

Gevins AS, Le J, Martin N, Brickett P, Desmond J, and Reutter B, 1994, High-resolution EEG: 124 channel recording, spatial enhancement and MRI integration methods. *Electroencephalography and Clinical Neurophysiology* 90: 337–358.

Gevins AS, Schaffer RE, Doyle JC, Cutillo BA, Tannehill RL, and Bressler SL, 1983, Shadows of thought: rapidly changing asymmetric brain-potential patterns of a brief visuo-motor task. *Science* 220: 97–99.

Horowitz B and Poeppel D, 2002, How can EEG/MEG and fMRI/PET be combined? *Human Brain Mapping* 17: 1–3.

Hjorth B, 1975, An on line transformation of EEG scalp potentials into orthogonal source derivations. *Electroencephalography and Clinical Neurophysiology* 39: 526–530.

Katznelson RD, 1981, EEG recording, electrode placement and aspects of generator localization. In: PL Nunez (Au.), *Electric Fields of the Brain: The Neurophysics of EEG*, 1st Edition, New York: Oxford University Press, pp. 176–213.

Kramer MA and Szeri AJ, 2004, Quantitative approximation of the cortical surface potential from EEG and ECoG measurements. *IEEE Transactions on Biomedical Engineering* 51: 1358–1365.

Law SK, 1993, Thickness and resistivity variations over the upper surface of human head. *Brain Topography* 6: 11–15.

Law SK, Nunez PL, and Wijesinghe RS, 1993, High-resolution EEG using spline-generated surface Laplacians on spherical and ellipsoidal surfaces. *IEEE Transactions on Biomedical Engineering* 40: 145–152.

Nunez PL, 1981, *Electric Fields of the Brain: The Neurophysics of EEG*, 1st Edition, New York: Oxford University Press.

Nunez PL, 1988, Spatial filtering and experimental strategies in EEG. In: D Samson-Dollfus (Ed.), *Functional Brain Imaging*, Paris: Elsevier, pp. 196–209.

Nunez PL, 1990, Localization of brain activity with EEG. In S Sato (Ed.), *Advances in Neurology, Vol. 54, Magnetoencephalography*, Raven Press, New York, pp. 39–65.

Nunez PL, 1995, *Neocortical Dynamics and Human EEG Rhythms*, New York: Oxford University Press.

Nunez PL, 2000, Toward a quantitative description of large-scale neocortical dynamic function and EEG. *Behavioral and Brain Sciences* 23:371–437.

Nunez PL and Pilgreen KL, 1991, The Spline-Laplacian is clinical neurophysiology: a method to improve EEG spatial resolution. *Journal of Clinical Neurophysiology* 8: 397–413.

Nunez PL and Silberstein RB, 2000, On the relationship of synaptic activity to macroscopic measurements: does co-registration of EEG with fMRI make sense? *Brain Topography* 13: 79–96.

Nunez PL, Pilgreen KL, Westdorp AF, Law SK, and Nelson AV, 1991, A visual study of surface potentials and Laplacians due to distributed neocortical sources: computer simulations and evoked potentials. *Brain Topography* 2: 151–168.

Nunez PL, Silberstein RB, Cadusch PJ, Wijesinghe RS, Westdorp AF, and Srinivasan R, 1994, A theoretical and experimental study of high resolution EEG based on surface Laplacians and cortical imaging. *Electroencephalography and Clinical Neurophysiology* 90: 40–57.

Nunez PL, Wingeier BM, and Silberstein RB, 2001, Spatial-temporal structure of human alpha rhythms: theory. micro-current sources, multi-scale measurements, and global binding of local networks. *Human Brain Mapping,* 13: 125–164.

Perrin F, Bertrand O, and Pernier J, 1987, Scalp current density mapping: value and estimation from potential data. *IEEE Transactions on Biomedical Engineering* 34: 283–289.

Perrin F, Pernier J, Bertrand O, and Echalier JF, 1989, Spherical splines for scalp potential and current density mapping. *Electroencephalography and Clinical Neurophysiology* 72: 184–187.

Sidman RD, 1991, A method for simulating intracerebral fields: the cortical imaging method. *Journal of Clinical Neurophysiology* 8: 432–441.

Srinivasan R, 1999, Methods to improve the spatial resolution of EEG. *International Journal of Bioelectromagnetism* 1: 102–111.

Srinivasan R, Nunez PL, and Silberstein RB, 1998, Spatial filtering and neocortical dynamics: estimates of EEG coherence. *IEEE Transactions on Biomedical Engineering* 45: 814–826.

Srinivasan R, Nunez PL, Tucker DM, Silberstein RB, and Cadusch PJ, 1996, Spatial sampling and filtering of EEG with spline Laplacians to estimate cortical potentials. *Brain Topography* 8: 355–366.

Ueno S and Iriguchi N, 1998, Impedance magnetic resonance imaging: a method for imaging impedance distributions based on magnetic resonance imaging. *Journal of Applied Physics* 83: 6450–6452.

Wahba G, 1981, Spline interpolation and smoothing on a sphere. *SIAM Journal on Scientific and Statistical Computing* 2: 5–16.

Yan Y, Nunez PL, and Hart RT, 1991, Finite element model of the human head: scalp potentials due to dipole sources. *Medical and Biological Engineering and Computing* 29: 475–481.

9

Measures of EEG Dynamic Properties

1 Computer Analyses of EEG Data

Here we are concerned with computer analyses used to reveal EEG dynamic properties that are difficult or impossible to discover by looking only at unprocessed data. Several signal processing methods are outlined and demonstrations using simulated data are provided. These same computer methods are applied to genuine EEG data in chapter 10. A wide range of computer methods have been applied successfully in the physical sciences by scientists, mathematicians, and engineers, but perhaps only a few of these methods are useful in EEG analysis. EEG scientists must be especially wary of mathematics in search of applications—after all, the number of ways to transform data is infinite. In evaluating new methods, *the central question is not what EEG can do for mathematics, but rather what mathematics can do for EEG.*

Several complementary issues motivate the methods outlined in this chapter. First, we may wish simply to reduce data to a more manageable form. Clinical or research EEG records often occupy many pages (or computer screens) containing information that is both redundant and difficult to interpret. A natural question is—how can we compress this information into more convenient formats? Because the spatial and temporal properties of EEG can vary widely, no universal answer to this question is expected. Research and clinical applications benefit from spectral analysis in which temporal waveforms are decomposed into their discrete frequency components. One reason is that *complex systems,* for which human brains provide the preeminent examples, typically exhibit distinct dynamic behavior at multiple spatial and temporal scales. Thus, if all we knew about EEG data are their origins in complex systems, we could plausibly conjecture several general properties of EEG dynamics. We might expect that different frequency ranges would be associated with different brain functions. We might also guess that dynamic measures recorded at different spatial scales differ substantially. Indeed, these predictions have substantial experimental support. By transforming raw data in ways suggested by our guesses about EEG properties, we attempt to establish new relationships between the transformed data and brain state that would be difficult or impossible with only the raw data.

Several general methods are emphasized here because they seem to be effective in our quest to understand the physiological bases for EEG. We focus on spectral analysis and mostly avoid some of the more esoteric transformations like correlation dimension estimates. While such methods have potential applications in EEG, we suggest they should normally be used to complement rather than replace more traditional time series analyses. One reason is that the application of multiple methods to the same data set facilitates both its interpretation and communication to the EEG community. This is especially true when unfamiliar methods are adopted. We do not attempt to evaluate specific algorithms that may find application in specific clinical or psychophysical settings. We take the approach that spectral analysis is the obvious entry point for studying EEG dynamics. While spectral analysis is widely used in EEG time series analysis, proper interpretation of EEG spectra in terms of the source dynamics does not consist of simply assigning one source to each frequency band (as is occasionally suggested). Analyses of spatial properties of the EEG spectrum are required—measures of phase synchronization between different brain regions appear especially promising. Such phase synchronization may be anticipated if we view cell assemblies (or networks) as structures underlying cognitive events. Chapters 9 and 10 emphasize coherence, a method to estimate phase synchronization based on Fourier analysis, but also consider other methods of spatial analysis, including principal components analysis, frequency–wavenumber spectra, and estimates of propagation velocity across the scalp.

A second reason for adopting these data analysis methods is to provide more direct links between the underlying physiology and experimental EEG. That is, mathematical models based on genuine physiology make predictions of EEG dynamics that can be tested in the laboratory. Many such predictions involve subtleties that are not readily observed in raw data. Our choice of analysis methods must depend partly on the imagined theoretical model (either explicit or implicit) so an iterative process is often required. We try hard to *avoid the pitfall of becoming stuck in local psychological minima*, that is, tied only to one method of analysis in any given experiment. If one type of data transformation suggests genuine brain properties, we should be able to find supplementary computer methods that yield similar physiological or cognitive conclusions. Otherwise, we run the well-known scientific risk that our *conclusions are no more than the summation of assumptions made in the process of choosing experimental and analysis methods*. For example, some physiological interpretations have depended on the unwarranted assumption that a few isolated sources generate EEG. Another example is the implicit assumption that the brain is a system with only a few degrees of freedom when interpreting measures of chaotic dynamics.

Thus far, computer analyses have played mostly minimal roles in clinical EEG as compared to cognitive science applications. The varied reasons for this omission include time constraints in clinical environments, problems with artifact, and limitations of local technical expertise. Misguided attempts by some mathematicians or physical scientists to sell computer methods high on sophistication but low on practical benefits may cause clinicians to be wary of new computer analyses, thereby erecting obstacles to the adoption of truly beneficial methods. Given these caveats, this chapter focuses on research methods that appear to be especially illuminating of dynamic properties. Some of these methods are currently used in clinical settings; others may later find their way to clinical practice.

Choice of analysis methods to study complex EEG dynamics requires grasps of the interactions between several issues specific to EEG—volume conduction, dynamic theory, and signal processing methods are of special importance. Experimental methods can either reveal or obscure dynamic behavior due to physical aspects of EEG recording, introduced in chapter 7. The n-sphere models of chapter 6 are adopted to *investigate theoretical limitations on EEG dynamic properties as estimates of brain dynamics*. The resulting mathematical models provide a conceptual framework for understanding EEG data that should guide experimental design and physiological interpretation. Improved communication between clinicians, experimental neuroscientists, and theoreticians is required for successful implementation of these new methods of analysis. The central goal of this chapter is to facilitate such communication.

2 Synaptic Action Generates EEG

Our choice of analysis methods must depend partly on our conceptual framework supporting brain function as outlined in fig. 1-8. Like many neuroscientists, we view higher brain functions as originating with *cell assemblies* that develop, disconnect, and reform on roughly 10 to 100 ms timescales. Cell assemblies (or probably less accurately *neural networks*) can apparently range from local networks to networks distributed over regions with sizes varying up to brain dimensions. These cell assemblies are immersed in a brain environment that (we conjecture) may facilitate interactions between such networks, thereby potentially providing a solution to the *binding problem* (Habeck and Srinivasan 2000). EEG is a very large-scale measure of brain source activity, apparently recording some mixture of cell assembly and global activity organized over macroscopic (centimeter) and even whole-brain spatial scales. Tentative adoption of this general conceptual framework does not appear restrictive of our choice of data analysis methods. For example, localized source activity like focal epilepsy or short-latency evoked potentials (for example, from primary sensory cortex) are just special cases where isolated cell assemblies generate the dynamic properties of EEG signals.

Large-scale cortical and scalp potentials are believed to be generated by *millisecond-scale modulations* of synaptic current sources at the surfaces of neocortical neurons (Lopes da Silva and Storm van Leeuwen 1978; Nunez 1981, 1995, 2000a,b; Lopes da Silva 1999). We distinguish these short-time modulations of synaptic current sources about background synaptic action from the chemical actions of *neurotransmitters*, which act as *neuromodulators* over much longer time scales. For example, we might imagine a 40 Hz natural frequency in a local neural network (due to millisecond synaptic source modulations) to change as network parameters vary over relatively long timescales (seconds to minutes) because of neurotransmitter action. A physical analog may help to distinguish modulation time scales. Ordinary sound waves are short-timescale pressure modulations about background air pressure, analogous to short-time-scale modulations of synaptic action in neocortex. Sound properties (say propagation speed) may be changed by external influences like long-time scale modulations in air temperature, analogous to the actions of chemicals (neuromodulators) in neocortex.

While cortical and scalp potentials are generated by the microsources $s(\mathbf{r}_n, t)$ associated with synaptic action, potentials are more conveniently described in terms of the intermediate-scale *mesosource function* $\mathbf{P}(\mathbf{r}, t)$ or *dipole moment per unit volume* defined in terms of the microsources by (4.26). The potential anywhere in the brain or scalp surface is then expressed as a weighted sum (or integral) of contributions from all mesosources as indicated generally by (2.2), or by (4.39) in the case of exclusively cortical sources. For convenience of this discussion, the brain volume may be parceled into N tissue masses or voxels of volume ΔV, each producing its own time-dependent mesosource strength $\mathbf{p}_n(t) \cong \mathbf{P}(\mathbf{r}_n, t) \Delta V(\mathbf{r})$ as in (2.3). Expressing this relation in a more simplified form, scalp potential at any location is given by

$$\Phi_S(t) = g_1 p_1(t) + g_2 p_2(t) + \cdots + g_{3N} p_{3N}(t) \tag{9.1}$$

Each weighting coefficient g_n depends on the properties of the volume conductor and the location of nth source and measurement location; it is essentially the *inverse electrical distance* between source and surface location. We might, for example, parcel a 1400 cm^3 brain into $N =$ one million (1.4 mm^3) voxels. Equation (9.1) has three million terms in this case because each voxel generates three scalar dipole moments. As discussed throughout this book, most of the terms in (9.1) will generally be negligible because the coefficients are small. Thus, although scalp potential is theoretically generated by all brain voxels, (excluding ventricles or tissue with no source activity) only the voxels "close" to the surface make substantial contributions. Thus, the existence of millisecond modulations of $\mathbf{P}(\mathbf{r}, t)$ does not guarantee that corresponding scalp (or even cortical) surface potentials will be observed. Calling on our physical analog, the presence of sound waves in a room does not guarantee that they will be heard outside the room.

The ability to record potentials on the scalp surface requires sufficient modulation of synaptic action, that is, relatively large changes in meso-source strengths $p_n(t)$ with time. These can be measured indirectly as potential differences between deep and superficial cortex, typically in the several hundred microvolt range for spontaneous EEG (Lopes da Silva and Storm van Leeuwen 1978; Petsche et al. 1984). A second requirement, discussed above, is that the mesosources must be *electrically close* to scalp electrodes. The so-called *electrical distances* are defined by the inverse coefficients g_n^{-1} in (9.1). Often, this favors cortical sources generally and sources in cortical gyri in particular. A third requirement for recordable scalp potentials (obtained without averaging) is that cortical mesosources $p_n(t)$ must be approximately "synchronously active" at scales of at least several centimeters (Cooper et al. 1965; Delucchi et al. 1975; Nunez 1981; Ebersole 1997) as indicated by fig. 1-20.

3 Fourier Analysis

Since the first recording of human EEG in the mid-1920s, temporal waveforms have often been characterized by counting zero crossings. This was even more common before spectral analysis came to more use in EEG in the 1970s. If a signal is near sinusoidal, the number of zero crossings accurately indicates the frequency of the signal. For example, a 10 Hz sine wave has 20 zero crossings per second. However, when the signal contains a broad mix of frequencies, the zero crossing measure can yield a misleading picture.

Some of the advantages of using Fourier analysis as opposed to simply counting zero crossings are illustrated by the following simulations. A short (2 s) simulated waveform composed of many frequency components and its amplitude spectrum (based on 62 s of data) are shown in fig. 9-1a and b. There are 878 zero crossings in the 62 s record (not shown). If this waveform were to be characterized only by zero crossings, it would be classified as a theta rhythm of 7.1 Hz. However, its amplitude spectrum shown in fig. 9-1b reveals broad frequency contributions from the delta, theta, and alpha bands. The peak frequency actually occurs in the alpha band. Another simulated waveform is shown in fig. 9-1c. In this example, there are 1875 zero crossings in the 62 s record. If this waveform were to be characterized only by zero crossings, it would be classified as a beta rhythm of 15.1 Hz. However, its amplitude spectrum shown in fig. 9-1d reveals broad frequency contributions from the alpha and beta bands. The peak frequency again occurs in the alpha band.

In these examples, Fourier analysis reveals much more accurate information about the underlying dynamic properties of the signal than

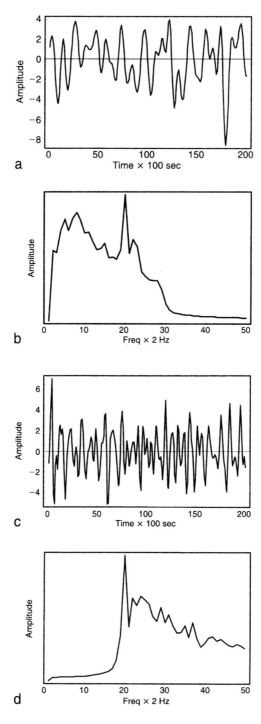

Figure 9-1 (a) A two-second simulated waveform composed of many frequency components producing an average of 14.2 zero crossings per second (7.1 Hz). (b) The amplitude spectrum of waveform (a) obtained by averaging the spectra of 31 two-second epochs. (c) A two-second simulated waveform producing an average of 30.2 zero crossings per second (15.1 Hz). (d) The amplitude spectrum of waveform (c) obtained by averaging the spectra of 31 two-second epochs.

the number of zero crossings. The power spectrum (squared amplitude) provides a measure of the energy (or variance) in the signal as a function of temporal frequency. In many brain states, the EEG is characterized by power spectra (or amplitude spectra) with peaks at multiple frequencies. These frequency peaks are modulated by changes in brain state (for example, sleep versus awake), by sensory stimulation, and so forth. We do not expect most EEG phenomena to be purely sinusoidal, although many examples such as the alpha rhythms consist of oscillations concentrated over a narrow frequency range. Nearly pure sinusoidal oscillations can appear in the EEG when forced by a periodic external input such as flicker (see section 11). However, Fourier analysis of the EEG signals can be accomplished whether or not the signals are sinusoidal, but will be most useful when near-sinusoidal signals occur in the record, thereby providing spectra that are simpler than the raw waveform. Perhaps the most important point is that when strongly oscillatory activity is concurrent in different frequency bands, they can be separated by spectral analysis and estimates of the energy in each frequency band can be obtained.

Any sinusoidal function is fully described by three parameters: amplitude A, frequency f, and phase ϕ, that is

$$E(t) = A \sin(2\pi f t + \phi) \tag{9.2}$$

Fourier analysis is concerned with expressing any arbitrary time series, such as an EEG signal, as a sum of sine waves with different frequencies:

$$V(t) = \sum_n A_n \sin(2\pi f_n t + \phi_n) \tag{9.3}$$

Many texts cover the theory and application of Fourier analysis. In addition there are several ways to obtain the representation (9.3) given a time series $V(t)$. We focus here on the fast Fourier transform (FFT), the most widely used Fourier analysis method in EEG and readily accessible as packaged software. The FFT algorithm accepts time series sampled at discrete times $t_n = n\Delta t$, $n = 1, 2, \dots N$ for a total duration $T = N\Delta t$. The appropriate choice of sampling interval Δt is essential. As shown in fig. 9-2, the appropriate Δt depends on the frequency content of the underlying signal. In the example shown in fig. 9-2a, the sum of two sinusoids of equal amplitude but distinct frequencies (1 and 3 Hz) is sampled with an interval of $\Delta t = 40$ ms or a sampling rate $f_{\text{dig}} = 1/\Delta t = 25$ Hz capturing the oscillation (fig. 9-2c). But if the time series also contains a 19 Hz sinusoid as in fig. 9-2b, sampling the time series at 25 Hz is inadequate and significant *aliasing* takes place (fig. 9-2d). Aliasing refers to the misrepresentation of a high-frequency signal by a lower-frequency signal due to under-sampling. In this example, the 19 Hz sinusoid is aliased into a 6 Hz sinusoid. No signal analysis method can undo aliasing once it has occurred because the appropriate information has been lost. To avoid aliasing, the discrete

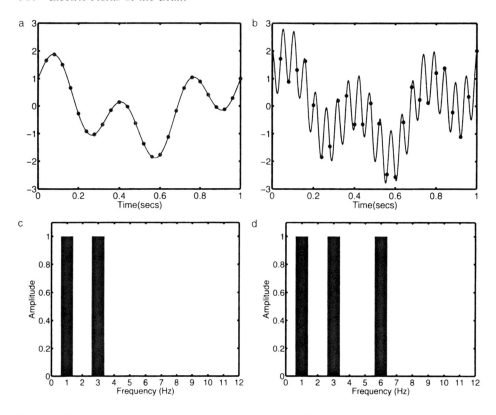

Figure 9-2 (a) A 1 s simulated waveform composed of 1 and 3 Hz sine waves of equal amplitude. The composite waveform is sampled every 40 ms as indicated by the gray dots. (b) A 1 s simulated waveform composed of a 1 Hz, 3 Hz, and 19 Hz sine waves of equal amplitude. Sampling every 40 ms (gray dots) aliases the signal because peaks and troughs of the 19 Hz oscillation are missed. (c) Amplitude spectrum obtained by applying the FFT to the signal (a) sampled every 40 ms. The 1 Hz and 3 Hz components have amplitude 1. (d) Amplitude spectrum obtained by applying the FFT to the signal of example (b) sampled every 40 ms. This aliased signal has an additional component at 6 Hz due to aliasing of the 19 Hz component.

sampling of the signal must take place at a sampling rate more than twice the highest frequency present in the unprocessed signal. This is known as the *Nyquist criterion* for discrete sampling of a continuous signal (Bendat and Piersol 2001). In essence this criterion expresses the idea that without at least two samples per cycle, it is not possible to detect the time course of a sinusoidal function. In practice, a more rigorous test known as the *Engineer's Nyquist criterion* is recommended, that is

$$f_{\text{dig}} > \tfrac{5}{2} f_{\text{max}} \tag{9.4}$$

where f_{max} is the highest frequency in the signal. Equation (9.4) accounts for the experience that power in frequencies close to the theoretical Nyquist limit is typically underestimated (Bendat and Piersol 2001). The

EEG machine should apply analog filtering to the raw signal in order to remove frequencies that are too high to be sampled accurately at the selected sampling rate.

Given the time series $V(t_n)$ as its input, the FFT algorithm calculates the amplitude A_n and phase ϕ_n of the frequencies:

$$f_n = \pm n \Delta f \quad n = 0, 1, \ldots (N/2) \tag{9.5}$$

The frequency resolution Δf depends on the epoch length T submitted to the FFT:

$$\Delta f = \frac{1}{T} = \frac{1}{N\Delta t} \tag{9.6}$$

At each frequency f_n, the Fourier coefficient F is usually calculated in complex-valued form as

$$F(f_n) = A_n e^{j\phi_n} = \frac{1}{N} \sum_{n=1}^{N} V(t_n) e^{j2\pi f_n} \tag{9.7}$$

Each Fourier coefficient has a real and imaginary part; together these contain the amplitude and phase information in the signal at each frequency. This complex-valued formulation of the Fourier coefficient is mathematically convenient and is used throughout this chapter. Note that both positive and negative frequencies from 0 to Nyquist limit are included in (9.5); frequencies f_n above $n = 2N/5$ (the Engineer's Nyquist frequency) are poorly estimated (Bendat and Piersol 2001) and should be discarded. The coefficient F_0 at the lowest frequency $f_0 = 0$ is the mean of the signal, that is, the DC component. In practice, the mean and any linear trend are usually removed from the signal before calculating the FFT. Since our time series is real valued, the Fourier coefficients at positive and negative frequencies are complex conjugates. Following convention, only positive frequencies are retained by doubling estimates (Bendat and Piersol 2001).

Equations (9.6) and (9.7) express the basic ideas of Fourier analysis. By multiplying the time series by sine and cosine functions of frequency f_n and averaging over all N samples, estimates of the real and imaginary parts of the corresponding Fourier coefficient are obtained. The estimates are obtained only at the discrete frequencies f_n given in (9.5). To apply the Fourier transform, which is defined over the interval $t = [-\infty, \infty]$ to a short time series over the interval $t = [0, T]$, we *require* the observed signal recorded on this interval to be *periodic*, that is, $V(t) = V(t + T)$. Some texts claim that the signal is "assumed" to be periodic, implying a fundamental limitation on FFT applications, but this may be misleading terminology. When a signal is recorded on $[0, T]$, we do not care how the associated function behaves outside the recording interval. We always force the function to be periodic with period T, in order to characterize the signal only on the interval $[0, T]$. Proper interpretation of spectral estimates obtained on finite intervals requires scrutiny as discussed below.

The use of a finite interval T restricts f_n to frequencies which complete an integer number of periods within the interval T as given by (9.5), that is, $Tf =$ integer. Any other frequencies in the signal will fail to meet this periodicity condition, leading to power spillage into sidebands in the estimated spectra. A_n and ϕ_n are estimates of the amplitude and phase over the bandwidth Δf centered on frequency f_n. In the examples shown in fig. 9-2, $T = 1$ s and $\Delta f = 1$ Hz. Figure 9-2c shows the amplitude spectrum A_n corresponding to the time series plotted in fig. 9-2a, indicating unit amplitude at frequencies of 1 and 3 Hz corresponding to the original signal. Figure 9-2d shows an additional peak at 6 Hz corresponding to the aliased 19 Hz signal plotted in fig. 9-2b. With a 1 Hz bandwidth, when we refer to the 3 Hz component, we are actually referring to a band of frequencies 2.5–3.5 Hz.

In all the examples of fig. 9-2 the center frequencies f_n are exactly equal to the frequencies of each oscillation. In general, oscillations in an EEG record will take place with different center frequencies and bandwidths. When the FFT is applied to the same epoch ($T = 1$ s), but the signal includes a 9.5 Hz component (fig. 9-3) in addition to the 1 and 3 Hz components, the energy of the 9.5 Hz oscillation is mainly divided between the frequency bands centered on 9 and 10 Hz, with lower power distributed in other frequency components, as shown by the amplitude spectrum in fig. 9-3b. That is, the spectrum of the 9.5 Hz sinusoid is smeared across the spectrum because this signal is aperiodic over $T = 1$ s. Multiplying the original signal by a window function as shown in fig. 9-3c reduces this smearing of the aperiodic signal at 9.5 Hz. The window function forces the data towards zero at the boundaries of the epoch, artificially making the signal closer to periodic. Figure 9-3d shows the amplitude spectrum of the windowed epoch. The 9.5 Hz oscillation contributes only to the 8–11 Hz band. However, the use of this window function effectively reduces frequency resolution, and the two peaks at 1 and 3 Hz become smeared. In practice, window functions become increasingly more important as epoch length T is reduced.

A number of important issues in practical FFT analysis are detailed in several texts (for example, Bendat and Piersol 2001). For our purposes, the estimation of the Fourier coefficients for each epoch is the starting point for the development of various statistical tools based on *spectral analysis*. A number of new approaches to Fourier analysis including wavelet analysis (Lachaux et al. 2002), multi-taper analysis (Percival and Walden, 1993), autoregressive models (Ding et al. 2000), and Hilbert transforms (Bendat and Piersol 2001; le van Quyen et al. 2001) have potential applications in EEG, particularly in the analysis of short data epochs. For example, these may be used to obtain estimates of the temporal evolution of spectra following an external sensory stimulus. All such methods yield estimates

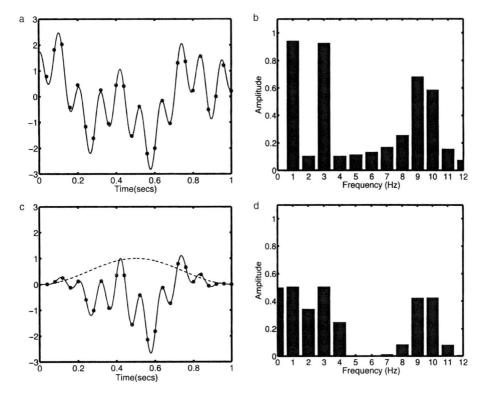

Figure 9-3   (a) A 1 s simulated waveform composed of 1 Hz, 3 Hz, and 9.5 Hz sine waves of equal amplitude sampled every 40 ms as indicated by the gray dots. (b) Amplitude spectrum of the signal shown in (a). The 1 Hz and 3 Hz sine waves are clearly identified, but the 9.5 Hz signal appears mainly at 9 and 10 Hz and is smeared throughout the spectrum. (c) A Hanning window function, shown by the dashed lines, is applied to the data of (a). The windowed data are shown by the solid lines. (d) The amplitude spectrum after windowing shows that the 9.5 Hz oscillation appears mainly in the 8–11 Hz bins. However, the 1 Hz and 3 Hz oscillations are now smeared due to loss of frequency resolution.

of "Fourier coefficients" that reflect the amplitude and phase of the oscillations within one frequency band (and perhaps for one window in time). Any of these Fourier coefficients can support spectral analysis of time series. However, interpretations using different techniques depend on the assumptions and parameter choices built into the specific methods chosen to estimate Fourier coefficients. These limitations are probably not as widely appreciated as those associated with conventional FFT methods, again suggesting advantages of comparing multiple methods applied to the same data.

4 Time Domain Spectral Analysis

In EEG applications, spectral analysis provides a means to assess *statistical properties* of oscillations in different frequency bands. It is customary to view any experimental data record as one *realization of a random process* (or *stochastic process*) (Bendat and Piersol 2001). In this context, the word "random" does not imply lack of statistical structure or possibly deterministic origins of the signals, only that its statistical properties are yet to be discovered. For, example, a casino "experiment" with loaded dice can be considered a random process even though there may be a simple mechanical explanation for the bias. Because the word "random" may carry some misleading baggage for some readers, we emphasize the word "stochastic" in this text. The amplitude spectrum obtained by applying the FFT to a single EEG epoch provides information about the frequency content of that particular epoch. Any observed time series is just one physical realization (sample) of the underlying stochastic process, but is not sufficient to *represent* the stochastic process. Thus, the amplitude spectrum of one epoch of EEG is an exact representation of the frequency content of that particular signal epoch, but only provides one observation about the stochastic process. An ensemble of K observations $\{V_k(t)\}$ must be used to make a statistical estimate the *power spectrum* (*auto spectral density function*) of an EEG signal. The power spectrum provides a decomposition of the *variance* of the signal as a function of frequency.

In engineering applications of spectral analysis it is often useful to assume that the stochastic process is a Gaussian random process. In this case, the ensemble mean of observations

$$\mu(t) = \frac{1}{K} \sum_{k=1}^{K} V_k(t) \tag{9.8}$$

and the *power spectrum* provide all that is required to estimate the signal probability density function (Bendat and Piersol 2001). However, even if the stochastic process is non-Gaussian, the EEG power spectrum provides an estimate of the signal variance as a function of frequency.

A more important assumption in spectral analysis is stationarity. A stochastic process is weakly stationary if the mean (9.8) and the power spectrum are invariant to shifts in the time at which the sample records are obtained. Thus, the mean (9.8) is assumed to be constant, $\mu(t) = \mu$, and the power spectrum of the stochastic process is assumed to be independent of the starting point of the epoch. Many studies have contrasted the EEG in different brain states such as eyes closed resting, eyes open resting, during mental calculations, and different sleep stages under the assumption that within these states the EEG power spectrum can be reasonably assumed to be stationary. By contrast, EEG data collected following a sensory stimulus clearly violate the stationarity assumption since the mean of the ensemble of signals given by (9.8) is the evoked potential (EP) or event-related potential which varies as a function of time over the epoch. We can still use spectral analysis in this case but the interpretations of the results may be more difficult. We consider the use of spectral analysis in experiments with external stimuli in the specific case of steady-state evoked potentials in section 11.

In EEG and many other fields, the *auto spectral density function* or in the more common parlance "power spectrum" of a time series is of special interest. The *amplitude spectrum*, the square root of the power spectrum, places more emphasis on nondominant spectral peaks and is often our measure of choice for visualization. As in the case of any other statistical measure, we can never know the *actual* power spectrum of a stochastic process. Rather, we find *estimates* of the power spectrum. The *power spectrum* may be estimated from an ensemble of observations by averaging over K epochs, that is

$$P(f_n) = \frac{2}{K} \sum_{k=1}^{K} F_k(f_n) F_k^*(f_n) = \frac{2}{K} \sum_{k=1}^{K} |F_k(f_n)|^2 \quad n = 1, 2, \ldots N/2 - 1 \quad (9.9)$$

For each sample epoch $V_k(t_n)$, Fourier coefficients $F_k(f_n)$ can be obtained using the FFT procedure indicated by (9.7). The factor of two occurs because we use only the positive frequencies defined in (9.5) here; note that we have excluded the DC signal at f_0 and the Nyquist frequency $f_{N/2}$ in (9.9) for convenience of notation. The form of the power spectrum estimate in (9.9) does not depend on the specific algorithm used to estimate the Fourier coefficients. The power spectrum summed over all positive and negative frequencies (including f_0 and $f_{N/2}$) is equal to the variance in the signal, a relationship known as *Parseval's theorem* (Bendat and Piersol 2001). If the EEG time series is recorded in units of microvolts, (9.9) provides a definition of the EEG power spectrum in units of μV^2 with magnitudes that depend on the bandwidth Δf. The power spectrum is sometimes normalized with respect to Δf to express power in units of $\mu V^2 / Hz$.

Implementation of (9.9) forces tradeoffs involving frequency resolution, statistical power, and putative stationarity. For example, consider the choices involved in analyzing a 60-second EEG record. Figure 9-4 demonstrates power spectra of two EEG channels, one occipital and one frontal, recorded with the subject's eyes closed and at rest. The power spectral estimates were obtained using an epoch length $T = 60$ s ($\Delta f = 0.017$ Hz) and no epoch averaging ($K = 1$). With this choice, the exact spectra of the two EEG signals (FFT of the entire record) is obtained, but no information about the statistical properties of the underlying stochastic process is gained. Note that the power spectrum of the occipital channel (fig. 9-4a) contains two peaks, one below 10 Hz and a larger peak above 10 Hz. The frontal channel (fig. 9-4b) shows a larger peak below 10 Hz. By examining the other channels it was found that the two peaks have distinct spatial distributions over the scalp, suggesting they have different source distributions. Each peak is surrounded by power in sidebands (adjacent frequency bins) of the two peak frequencies. *The signals are stochastic processes occupying relatively narrow bands in the frequency spectrum.*

To analyze the 60 s signal properly, we must decide how to divide the record into epochs to implement (9.9). The choice is a compromise between the advantage of good frequency resolution yielded by long epochs (large T and small K) and the statistical power of our estimate gained by using a larger number of epochs (small T and large K). If a frequency resolution of $\Delta f = 0.5$ Hz is chosen, the record is segmented into $K = 30$ epochs of length $T = 2$ s. If frequency resolution is reduced to $\Delta f = 1$ Hz, we divide the record into $K = 60$ epochs of length $T = 1$ s. Figures 9-4c and d show the power spectra of the frontal and occipital

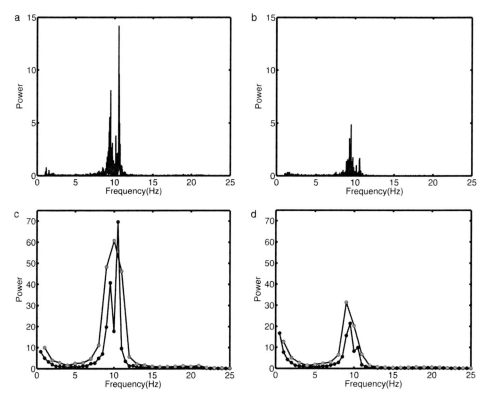

Figure 9-4 Example EEG power spectra from a single subject (female, 22 years). The subject is at rest with *eyes closed*. (a) Power spectrum of a midline occipital channel with epoch length $T = 60$ s and $K = 1$ epochs. The power spectrum appears to have two distinct peaks, one below 10 Hz and one above 10 Hz. (b) Power spectrum at a midline frontal channel with epoch length $T = 60$ s and $K = 1$ epochs. Here only the peak below 10 Hz is prominent. (c) Power spectra of a midline occipital channel calculated with two different choices of epoch length T and number of epochs K. The gray circles indicate the power spectrum with $T = 1$ s and $K = 60$ epochs. The black circles indicate the power spectrum with $T = 2$ s and $K = 30$ epochs. (d) Power spectra of a midline frontal channel calculated as in (c).

channels with $\Delta f = 1$ Hz (gray circles) and $\Delta f = 0.5$ Hz (black circles). The power spectra at the occipital and frontal channels are both dominated by alpha rhythm oscillations. At the occipital electrode (fig. 9-4c) two separate peak frequencies at 9.5 and 10.5 Hz are evident with $\Delta f = 0.5$ Hz, but this is not revealed with $\Delta f = 1$ Hz, where only a single peak frequency at 10 Hz is evident. Lowering frequency resolution has a similar effect at the frontal channel (fig. 9-4d), but since there is very little power at 10.5 Hz, the only clear peak appears at 9 Hz. By choosing lower frequency resolution we produce a signal representation having different (single) peak frequencies at the two sites, while choosing higher frequency resolution results in pairs of frequency peaks at both sites but with different relative magnitudes.

By examining the power spectra for the occipital (fig. 9-5a) and frontal sites (fig. 9-5b) for individual epochs with $\Delta f = 0.5$ Hz, support for two different oscillations within the alpha band is obtained. At the occipital channel individual epochs display two distinct peaks at 9.5 Hz and 10.5 Hz. The first 15 epochs show a strong response at 10.5 Hz but the later epochs show a stronger response at 9.5 Hz. The dominant frequency in each epoch is summarized in the peak power histograms in fig. 9-5c showing that individual epochs displayed peak frequencies at both 9.5 Hz and 10.5 Hz. By contrast, very few epochs have a peak frequency of 10.5 Hz

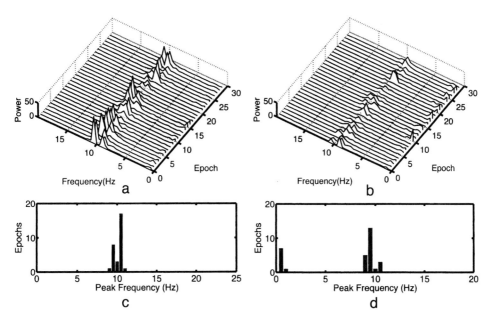

Figure 9-5 EEG power spectra and peak power histograms. (a) Plots of 30 (individual epoch) power spectra for the occipital channel shown in fig. 9-4a and c. (b) Plots of the same 30 individual epoch spectra for the frontal channel. (c) Peak power histograms show the distribution of peak frequencies for the 30 epochs shown in (a). (d) Peak power histograms for the 30 epochs shown in (b).

at the frontal site; most epochs have peak frequencies either at 9.5 Hz or in the delta band (<2 Hz). Note that during most epochs with strong delta activity in fig. 9-5b the alpha peaks are attenuated.

In summary, estimating the *power spectrum* from an ensemble of epochs provides a decomposition of the variance of the signal as a function of frequency. This is a particularly useful approach because EEG contains oscillatory activity in distinct frequency bands that are associated with different brain states. In the simple example we presented here of the alpha rhythm in figs. 9-4 and 9-5, electrodes at different locations show different magnitudes of two distinct oscillations with center frequencies at 9.5 Hz and 10.5 Hz. In the next section, factors that determine the magnitude of peaks in the EEG power spectrum are considered. In later sections, methods to quantify spatial properties of EEG rhythms, which are evidently different for the two peak frequencies in this example, are investigated.

5 The Impact of Source Synchrony and Spatial Filtering on EEG Power Spectra

Scalp potential amplitude at any frequency can change for several reasons related to "*synchrony.*" The large changes in scalp amplitude that occur when brain state changes are believed to be due mostly to such synchrony changes; thus EEG scientists and clinicians have adopted the label *desynchronization* to indicate large amplitude reductions, particularly in the alpha band (Pfurtscheller and Lopes da Silva 1999). However, the so-called synchrony so often discussed in the EEG literature may actually refer to several distinct phenomena. For example, synchrony may occur in different directions and at different spatial scales, and may occur with zero phase lag or with substantial phase differences.

For convenience, we can divide the brain into perhaps a million voxels (or essentially mesosource elements) each having a dipole moment per unit volume $\mathbf{P}(\mathbf{r}, t)$. There are several (possibly overlapping) means by which synchrony can influence the power spectrum. We first note that microscale changes in synaptic source synchrony across cortical columns change mesosource strength $\mathbf{P}(\mathbf{r}, t)$ by changing the effective pole separation of the equivalent dipoles as discussed in chapter 4. By this mechanism, the source strength can change, and such changes can be observed using intracranial electrodes by recording potential differences across local cortex as discussed in chapter 4. As the mesosource strength increases, we expect scalp potential to increase proportionately if there are no other changes. As the dipole layer enlarges with diameters in the approximate range 1 to 3 cm, large increases in scalp potential magnitudes are expected based on the exponential parts of the curves in fig. 1-20. Finally, even larger increases in dipole layer diameter (from about 3 cm to more than 10 cm), corresponding to the flatter parts of the curves in fig. 1-20, result in only modest increases in scalp magnitudes. Scalp potential magnitudes may actually begin to decrease when dipole layer diameters become larger than about 10 cm due to the canceling effects of the curved scalp surface as shown in fig. 8-7.

Figure 9-6 shows examples of simulated scalp potentials due to a single dipole and dipole layers of diameter ranging from 3 to 5 cm composed only of radial dipole sources. Each dipole layer is composed of dipole sources with time series that are constructed by adding a 6 Hz sinusoid of fixed amplitude $A = 15$ μV to a Gaussian random processes with mean $μ = 0$ and standard deviation $σ = 150$ μV. The 6 Hz components are phase locked across the dipole layers, whereas all other components have random phases. Each source signal is an independent stochastic time series representing transcortical potential across the dipole layer. The source time series of a single dipole source (dipole layer of very small size) is plotted in fig. 9-6a and the corresponding power spectrum is plotted in fig. 9-6b. The power spectrum shows that the source signal is broadband, with some power at 6 Hz but even higher power at other frequencies. The power of the 6 Hz sinusoid is only 1% of the total power of each dipole source, and does not stand out in either the time series or the power spectrum. Figure 9-6c and d show the estimated potential on the scalp directly above the center of a superficial dipole layer of diameter 3 cm, based on our standard 4-sphere model. The time series shows considerably less power at higher frequencies because of cancellation of potential from asynchronous sources and exhibits a smooth appearance compared to the source time series. The corresponding power spectrum (fig. 9-6d) shows a clear peak at 6 Hz and no other peak frequencies. As the diameter of the dipole layer is increased from 3 to 4 to 5 cm, the calculated surface potential becomes more obviously sinusoidal (fig. 9-6e–h). The power substantially increases at 6 Hz, but the power distributed across the rest of the spectrum is essentially unchanged.

Clearly, source synchrony is as important as source size in the generation of scalp potentials. Most (99%) of the source activity in these examples is uncorrelated; as a result, the uncorrelated sources contribute minimally to scalp potential even as the size of the source region increases. By contrast, relatively small-magnitude (1%) source activity that is synchronous across all sources in the dipole layer generates a large scalp potential that increases dramatically as dipole layer diameter increases by a few centimeters. In chapter 6, we quantified this effect of the size of a dipole layer on scalp potential which results from spatial filtering by volume conduction. *One important implication of fig. 9-6 is that spatial filtering by volume conduction can lead to temporal filtering of source activity in the scalp EEG.* If synchronous source activity in different frequency bands takes place in dipole layers of different sizes, frequency bands that are synchronized broadly over the cortical surface can easily generate higher power in the scalp potentials than a stronger but smaller dipole layer. The power at any frequency in the spectrum of scalp EEG is

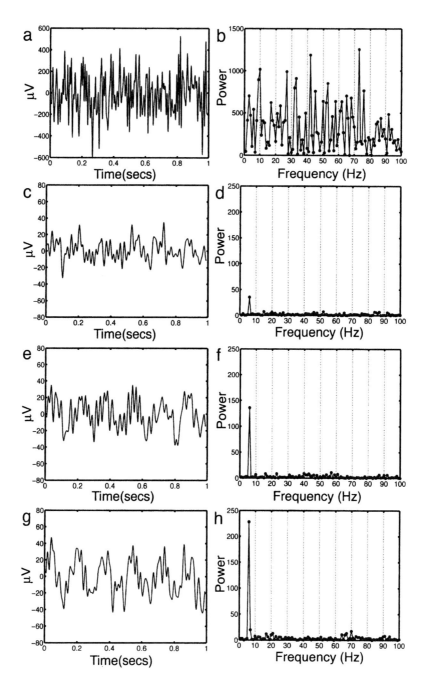

Figure 9-6 Simulated data. (a) time series of a dipole mesosource **P**(**r**, *t*) composed of a 15 µV sine wave added to Gaussian random noise with standard deviation 150 µV. The Gaussian random noise was low-pass filtered at 100 Hz. The sine wave has variance (power) equal 1% of the noise. (b) Power spectrum of the time series shown in (a). The power spectrum has substantial power at frequencies other than 6 Hz. (c) Time series recorded by an electrode on the outer sphere (scalp) of a 4-sphere model above the center of a dipole layer of diameter 3 cm. The dipole layer is composed of 32 dipole sources **P**(**r**, *t*) with time series constructed similar to (a) with independent Gaussian noise (uncorrelated) at each dipole source. Scalp potential was calculated for a dipole layer at a radius $r_z = 7.8$ cm in a

determined not only by the source strength but also by spatial properties of the source such as its size and synchrony. Thus, we anticipate that EEG recorded within the brain can have quite different spectra than EEG recorded on the scalp, a prediction well supported by experimental studies. *EEG dynamic behavior is generally expected to be a sensitive function of the spatial scale of the recording.*

Figure 9-7 summarizes this idea for dipole layer sources of different strength and size. Each set of symbols represents a different mesosource strength of the 6 Hz oscillation as a percentage of the total generated mesosource strength (variance). The choice of 6 Hz is only for ease of description; any other oscillation that is phase locked over the dipole layer will do just as well. For purposes of comparison we have normalized power with respect to power generated by a dipole layer of diameter 1.5 cm with very weak 6 Hz relative mesosource strength (0.5%). One strong dipole layer source (20%) with 1.5 cm diameter underneath the recording electrode produces the same scalp power at 6 Hz as a weak source (1%) of larger diameter (4.2 cm). It is evident from the parallel curves in fig. 9-7 that changes in dipole layer source size and strength can independently change scalp potential power. An increase in source diameter from 2.5 to 7 cm results in an order of magnitude increase in power. A similar increase would be observed if the relative 6 Hz source strength increases from 1 to 10% of the source variance.

Another factor that potentially influences the power spectrum is the relative phases of the 6 Hz sources within the dipole layer. Figure 9-6f shows the power spectrum at a scalp electrode generated by a dipole layer of radius 4 cm, with 6 Hz source strength equal to 1% of the total source variance. In this simulation the 6 Hz source activity was added with the same phase at each source. Figure 9-8 considers the effect of variability of phase across the sources in the dipole layer, with identical source strengths. In each plot a source distribution is shown, with the phase of the 6 Hz component of each source indicated by the gray scale. Figure 9-8a shows an example with the phase of each source randomly selected between $\pm 45°$. Source activity at 6 Hz is still synchronized across the sources but with nonzero phase difference. The introduction of phase differences reduces power at the scalp since scalp potential represents a space average of source activity, leading to partial cancellation of individual contributions to

---

4-sphere model. The model parameters were radii $(r_1, r_2, r_3, r_4) = (8, 8.1, 8.6, 9.2)$ and conductivity ratios $(\sigma_1/\sigma_2, \sigma_1/\sigma_3, \sigma_1/\sigma_4) = (0.2, 40, 1)$. Notice the time series is smoother than in the case of the individual dipole source. (d) Power spectrum of the time series shown in (c). Note the peak at 6 Hz. (e) Time series similar to (c), but due to a dipole layer of diameter of 4 cm composed of 68 dipole sources. (f) Power spectrum of the time series shown in (e). (g) Similar time series to (c), but with a dipole layer of diameter 5 cm composed of 112 dipole sources. The presence of the 6 Hz sinusoid is obvious from the time series. (h) Power spectrum of the time series shown in (g). A large spectral peak at 6 Hz is evident.

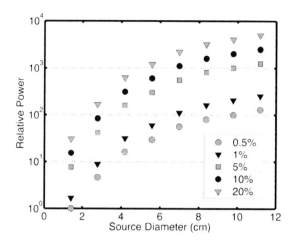

Figure 9-7 A simulated summary of the dependence of scalp power on the size and strength of a synchronous dipole layer, based on the simulation of fig. 9-6. Both source strength and source size independently contribute to the power at a scalp electrode. Source strength is expressed as the ratio of the power of sinusoid to the power of noise in the source activity and labeled with different symbols as indicated by the legend. Source diameter varies from 1.5 to 11.4 cm. Power is expressed relative to the power of the smallest dipole layer with weakest strength.

potential. In fig. 9-8b, source phases are randomly selected between $\pm 90°$ (white and black circles are $180°$ out of phase), resulting in more cancellation of scalp potentials. This results in a substantial reduction in the power at 6 Hz.

In summary, these simulations demonstrate that relative EEG power in different frequency bands and power changes between brain states can easily result from changes in source synchrony (with zero phase lag), source region size, and mesosource strength. Furthermore, mesosource strength $\mathbf{P}(\mathbf{r}, t)$, measured as dipole moment per unit volume, is itself a measure of source synchrony at smaller scales because synaptic (microsource) synchrony influences effective pole separation as shown in chapter 4. Thus, the relative power level measured by an EEG electrode at any one frequency is closely related to the degree of synchronization of synaptic currents at that frequency (with no phase lag) over tangential cortical distances up to roughly 10 cm.

6 Coherence and Phase Synchronization

In this section we introduce *spatial analysis* of the EEG by means of the analysis of a joint observation of time series $\{V_{mk}(t)\}$ consisting of $k = 1, K$ observations in $m = 1, M$ data channels. These joint observations of time series are the realization of a stochastic process distributed in space and time over the cortical surface and recorded on the scalp with EEG

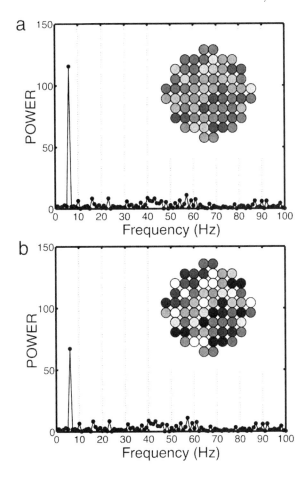

Figure 9-8 Simulation similar to fig. 9-6, but considering the phases of the sources $\mathbf{P}(\mathbf{r}, t)$. Dipole layer of diameter 4 cm with sinusoid power equal to 1% of noise power for each dipole source. The phase of the sinusoid varies within the dipole layer. (a) Source phase varies randomly by $\pm 45°$. The phase of each dipole source is indicated by the color of the dipole on the inset. Grey circles (sources) have phase zero, lighter shades are leading and darker shades are lagging. Note the loss of power at 6 Hz compared to fig. 9-6f, which plots the power spectrum with no phase differences between the dipoles. (b) Phase varies randomly by $\pm 90°$. White and black circles (sources) are 180° out of phase and generate potentials that mostly cancel at the scalp electrode. Power is lower than the examples in fig. 9-6f and (a).

electrodes. The *coherence* between pairs of EEG channels provides an entry point to examine the spatial properties of the stochastic source activity. As in the case of other statistical measures, we can never know the coherence of a stochastic process, we can only obtain estimates. In this section we define *coherence as a linear correlation coefficient* that primarily estimates the amount of phase synchronization between any two data channels. The idea of phase synchronization between two sinusoids is illustrated in fig. 9-9 where three types of phase relationships between two oscillatory

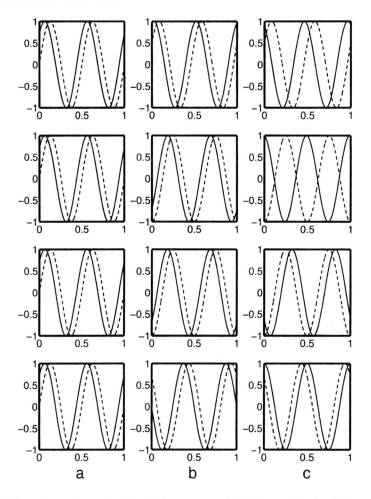

Figure 9-9 Examples of two simulated sine waves with different kinds of phase relationships, shown for four epochs. (a) The two sine waves have the same phase on every trial. (b) The two sine waves have random phase across the trials, but the phase difference is fixed at 45°. (c) The two sine waves have random phase and random phase difference across the trials.

waveforms (solid and dashed lines) are presented using four observations (epochs) of a 2 Hz sinusoid. In the first example (fig. 9-9a), the sinusoids have equal amplitudes and phases across epochs, but there is a constant phase difference of 45° between the two waveforms. This example does not represent a stationary stochastic process but rather a deterministic signal with fixed amplitude and phase at each channel on every observation, yielding a coherence of one.

In the second example (fig. 9-9b) the two signals represent a *coherent stochastic process*. At each observation, the phases of the sinusoids vary randomly, but the *relative phase* or phase difference between sinusoids is fixed at 45° and the amplitudes are equal; again the coherence is one. The third example (fig. 9-9c) represents two sinusoids from *incoherent stochastic processes.* For each realization, the absolute phases are random and the relative phases are also random. The main point of this example is that the coherence of a random process is a statistical measure of the relationship between two time series (or data channels) *across observations.* As we shall see, coherence is a measure very similar to a squared correlation coefficient, which measures the proportion of variance in one data channel that can be explained by a linear transformation of another data channel.

To calculate coherence we first define a *cross spectrum* (Bendat and Piersol 2001), which is a measure of the joint spectral properties of two data channels. The cross spectrum $C_{uv}(f_n)$ of two channels u and v at frequency f_n can be estimated from pairs of Fourier coefficients as an average over K epochs, that is

$$C_{uv}(f_n) = A_{uv}e^{j\phi_{uv}} = \frac{2}{K}\sum_{k=1}^{K} F_{uk}(f_n)F_{vk}^*(f_n) \quad n = 1, 2, N/2 - 1 \quad (9.10)$$

When $u = v$ the cross spectrum reduces to the power spectrum (9.9), and the factor of two again reflects the fact that our spectra are restricted to positive frequencies. The cross spectrum (9.10) is a measure of the *covariance* between two signals at one frequency across observations analogous to the ordinary covariance between two time series. Unlike the power spectrum, which is real valued, the cross spectrum is complex valued, and can be expressed as magnitude (or cross power) A_{uv} and phase ϕ_{uv}. The phase of the cross spectrum is the average phase difference between the two channels which we also label the *relative phase.*

If we normalize the squared magnitude of the cross spectrum by the power spectrum of each channel we obtain the coherence $\gamma_{uv}^2(f_n)$ between the two data channels:

$$\gamma_{uv}^2(f_n) = \frac{|C_{uv}(f_n)|^2}{P_u(f_n)P_v(f_n)} \quad n = 0, 1, 2, (N-1)/2 \quad (9.11)$$

This quantity is sometimes labeled "coherency" or "squared coherency" in EEG studies. We will use only "coherence" in this text. The form of (9.11) follows closely from the equation for a Pearson correlation coefficient (squared). The numerator is the squared magnitude of the cross spectrum (or squared cross power), analogous to squared covariance. The power spectrum is analogous to the variance of the signal. Thus (9.11) is analogous to dividing squared covariance by the variance of each channel, which is a squared correlation coefficient. Like the usual r^2 statistic, coherence $\gamma_{uv}^2(f_n)$ measures the fraction of variance of channel u at frequency f_n that can be explained by a constant linear transformation of the Fourier coefficients obtained at channel v. *In the frequency domain, a constant linear transformation means both constant relative amplitude and constant relative phase.*

The form of (9.10) indicates that the coherence measure is quite sensitive to the relative phase between two channels. If the relative phase is constant over epochs, the average of the product on the right-hand side of (9.10) is equal to the average product of the magnitude of the Fourier coefficients and coherence is equal to one. If the relative phase varies across the K epochs, then some cancellation will take place and coherence (9.11) will be less than one. If the phase difference is purely random from epoch to epoch, the coherence estimate will approach zero as the number of epochs K is increased.

Figure 9-10 shows power and coherence spectra obtained from a pair of simulated channels each containing a sinusoidal oscillation of 6 Hz added to independent Gaussian random noise with 100 times the variance of the sinusoid. For each epoch, the phase of the sinusoid at one channel is random, but the phase of the sinusoid at the other channel is shifted by a random phase less than $\pm45°$. The examples in fig. 9-10 show the estimated power spectrum of each channel (left column) and estimated coherence spectra between channels (right column) obtained by averaging over a different number of epochs K. With only 5 epoch averages (fig. 9-10a), the power spectrum of each channel clearly shows the peak at 6 Hz while other frequency peaks are reduced. The coherence spectrum show multiple peaks but none at 6 Hz. As the number of epochs is increased to 10 (fig. 9-10b), the power peak is reduced and a small peak becomes evident in the coherence spectrum at 6 Hz, although spurious peaks are also apparent at 3 and 16 Hz. As the number of epochs is increased to 20 (fig. 9-10c) and 40 (fig. 9-10d), coherence estimates at frequencies other than 6 Hz become negligible. With a 40 epoch average the coherence estimate is near 0.5.

A coherence of 0.5 in one frequency band indicates that at this frequency 50% of the variance in one channel can be explained by a linear transformation of the other channel. *This interpretation does not imply that there is a linear relationship between possible dynamic processes linking the data channels.* A coherence of 0.5 only indicates that we can partly account for the data by a linear model. If the relationship were purely linear, the coherence estimate would be close to one if enough epochs were averaged to remove noise effects. In the example of fig. 9-10 coherence is less than one because the linear relationship between channels is *stochastic* as the signal was constructed using random phase differences between channels restricted to a narrow range. In the case of genuine EEG data, another possibility is that the relationship between the channels is deterministic but nonlinear, in which case coherence provides a measure of the degree of linearity.

How many epochs must we average to obtain satisfactory coherence estimates? There is no easy answer since robust coherence estimates require averaging to remove noise and uncorrelated source activity whose

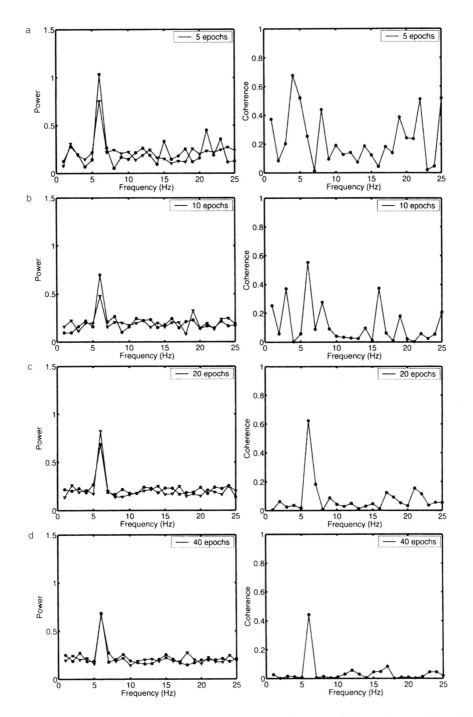

Figure 9-10 Simulated power and coherence spectra for a simulation with two channels with a 6 Hz sine wave added to Gaussian random noise with 100 times the variance of the sinusoid. In each epoch, the phase of the oscillators is random but the phase difference is less than 45°. (a) Power spectra of the channels indicated by circles and triangles, using only a 5 epoch average is shown on the left. Coherence spectrum estimate for the two channels based on the same 5 epoch average shown on the right. Same as (a) using (b) 10 epochs, (c) 20 epochs, (d) 40 epochs.

statistical properties are generally unknown in EEG. The examples in fig. 9-10 indicate that even in a relatively simple case, 40 epochs are required to obtain a reasonable coherence estimate. Somewhat fewer averages are required to estimate power spectra. In a manner similar to the usual estimates of correlation coefficients, uncertainty of coherence estimates increases as the coherence estimate becomes smaller when the number of epochs is fixed (Bendat and Piersol 2001). As a practical matter, coherence estimates should be obtained by averaging as many epochs as possible, balancing the competing goals of obtaining good frequency resolution and robust estimates, subject to the usual issue of signal stationarity. One obvious test is to determine if adding additional epochs results in negligible changes in coherence estimates.

The statistical error in coherence estimates depends on both the actual coherence of the stochastic process (which we can never know) and the number of epochs used in the coherence estimate. An approximate relation for the 95% confidence interval for the actual coherence ($\bar{\gamma}^2$) is given in terms of the standard error in the coherence estimate $\varepsilon_{\bar{\gamma}^2}$ (Bendat and Piersol 2001):

$$\frac{\gamma^2}{1 + 2\varepsilon_{\bar{\gamma}^2}} \leq \bar{\gamma}^2 \leq \frac{\gamma^2}{1 - 2\varepsilon_{\bar{\gamma}^2}} \tag{9.12}$$

where

$$\varepsilon_{\bar{\gamma}^2} = \sqrt{\frac{2}{K}} \frac{1 - \bar{\gamma}^2}{|\bar{\gamma}|} \tag{9.13}$$

In (9.13) we approximate the actual coherence (which we cannot know) with the estimated coherence, which is reasonable for $\varepsilon_{\gamma^2} < 0.2$ (Bendat and Piersol 2001). The implication of (9.12) and (9.13) is that larger coherence values have narrower confidence intervals. For instance, with $K = 100$ epochs:

$$\gamma^2 = 0.2 \Rightarrow 0.13 \leq \bar{\gamma}^2 \leq 0.40$$

$$\gamma^2 = 0.5 \Rightarrow 0.41 \leq \bar{\gamma}^2 \leq 0.63$$

$$\gamma^2 = 0.8 \Rightarrow 0.75 \leq \bar{\gamma}^2 \leq 0.85 \tag{9.14}$$

This suggests that with $K = 100$ epochs, a coherence of 0.2 can be distinguished from a coherence of 0.5, as their confidence intervals do not overlap. However, we have more confidence in the difference between stochastic processes with estimated coherences of 0.5 and 0.8, as they have narrower confidence intervals.

In describing coherence effects in EEG, we emphasize that coherence is a measure of phase synchronization. However, as defined by (9.10) and (9.11) coherence depends both on relative amplitude and on relative phase between the two channels. If the phases at two channels are identical (phase difference = 0) coherence is still less than one if the amplitudes fluctuate independently at each channel. If our main goal is to estimate phase synchronization independent of amplitude fluctuations, we can measure coherence by normalizing each Fourier coefficient by its amplitude (*phase-only coherence*) or use entropy measures on the relative phase distribution across epochs to measure synchronization (Tass et al. 1998). One reason to use coherence measures rather than directly measuring phase correlation is that coherence measures are weighted in favor of epochs with large amplitudes. This makes good practical sense because phase estimates are likely to be more reliable when amplitudes are large if large amplitudes indicate large signal-to-noise ratio as is usually the case in EEG, assuming obvious artifacts have been excluded. If only epoch phase information is used (independent of epoch amplitudes), equal emphasis is placed on low and high amplitude epochs in estimates of phase synchronization.

This point is illustrated by fig. 9-11, where two simulated waveforms each contain 6 Hz sinusoids with relative phase varying randomly (epoch to epoch) by angles less than 45° and amplitude varying randomly across 40 epochs. In these simulations, the *standard coherence estimate* (fig. 9-11, left column) is compared to a *phase-only coherence estimate* (fig. 9-11, right column) with different levels of added noise. The first row shows the estimated coherence with minimal added Gaussian random noise (variance equal to 1% of the power of the 6 Hz sinusoid). Figure 9-11a shows the usual measure of coherence with amplitude treated in the usual way (9.11) indicating a coherence of about 0.55 at 6 Hz. Figure 9-11b shows the phase-only coherence estimate obtained by normalizing the Fourier coefficients from individual epochs to equal amplitudes. In the latter case estimated coherence is about 0.8 and reflecting the strong phase synchronization. However, if signals are noisy, the advantage of removing amplitude variations is lost. Figure 9.11c and d show the standard and phase-only coherence estimates when the noise variance is twice the average power of the 6 Hz sinusoid. The standard coherence estimate with large noise (fig. 9-11c) is similar to the estimate obtained with minimal noise (fig. 9-11a). By contrast, the phase-only coherence estimate (fig. 9-11d) is reduced from about 0.8 to about 0.6. If the noise variance is increased to 4 times the sinusoid variance, both the standard coherence estimate (fig. 9-11e) and phase-only coherence estimate (fig. 9-11f) are reduced, but a greater reduction occurs in the phase-only coherence estimate (~0.2) than the reduction in standard coherence estimate (~0.4). Apparently, phase-only coherence estimates increase sensitivity to noise. In the examples here standard coherence estimates are reduced from about 0.55 to about 0.4 by adding additional noise to the data. By contrast, the

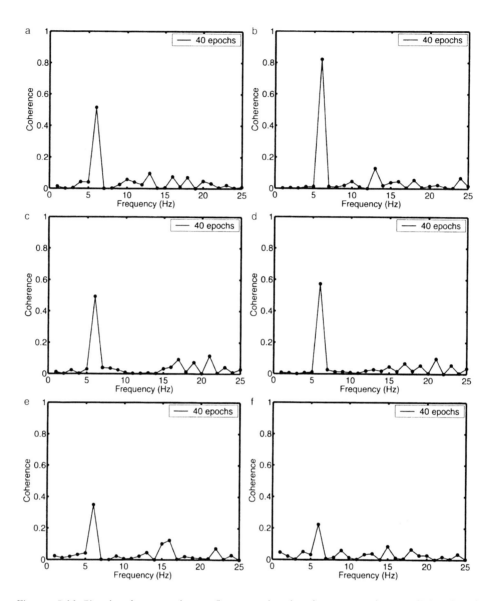

Figure 9-11 Simulated comparison of conventional coherence estimates (*left column*) calculated with (9.11) to coherence estimates obtained by first normalizing each Fourier coefficient from each epoch by its magnitude (*right column*). (a) Coherence between two channels with small variability in the phase difference between channels (less than ±45°) and random amplitudes between 0 and 100 μV for each channel and each epoch. Minimal noise is added (1% of the sinusoid power). (b) Coherence of the same channel pair in (a) calculated by first normalizing each Fourier coefficient from each epoch by its magnitude. This phase-only coherence is higher reflecting only the phase variability. (c) Same as in (a) with noise power increased to 2 times the average power of the sinusoids. (d) Same as (b) with noise power increased to 2 times the average power of the sinusoid. (e) Same as (a) with noise power increased to 4 times the average power of the sinusoid. (f) Same as (b) with noise power increased to 4 times the average power of the sinusoid. Removing amplitude information makes coherence estimates more sensitive to noise. Note that in fig. 9-10 conventional coherence estimates are robust even when noise power is 100 times the sinusoid power.

phase-only coherence estimates fall from 0.8 to 0.2 with added noise. Additionally, note that the noise used here is very small compared to the noise used to obtain fig. 9-10 where the noise variance was 100 times the power of the 6 Hz sinusoid. These simulations suggest that *ignoring amplitude information in estimates of coherence dramatically increases sensitivity to noise.*

To summarize, coherence estimates provide a measure of phase synchronization between EEG channel pairs. Fluctuations in EEG amplitude are expected to produce relatively small changes in coherence, when used with epochs containing minimal artifact. Coherence can be greater than zero or less than one for several reasons. (i) The presence of additive noise at each channel—the effects of additive noise can be minimized by averaging over a larger number of epochs. (ii) The system that gives rise to the amplitude and phase relationship between the two channels is stochastic and fluctuates across the observations. In the simulations of fig. 9-11, we have constructed signals with coherence estimates between zero and one by introducing random phase differences that were limited to less than $45°$. (iii) The system that gives rise to the relationship between the two channels is nonlinear. (iv) A mutual influence between the two systems is present in the same frequency band.

7 Effects of Spatial Filtering by Volume Conduction on Coherence Estimates

In EEG applications two other important factors determine the estimated coherence between pairs of data channels (scalp electrodes): spatial filtering by volume conduction and choice of reference electrode location. In this section we consider the effects of these factors using theoretical calculations, simulations, and examples of EEG data. In the next section this discussion is extended to consider the effects of high-resolution EEG methods on coherence estimates.

Our goal in obtaining coherence estimates is to estimate statistical properties of stochastic source processes distributed in space and time over the cortical surface. In order to develop a theoretical model relating scalp potential statistics to source statistics, it is useful to think of source statistics in terms of continuous variables of time and space rather than discrete sets of sources. EEG sources are most likely dipole layers of varying size and shape which are described in terms of continuous functions of cortical location; discrete sources are simply special cases of this picture. The so-called "EEG generators" can be expressed generally in terms of the mesosource field $\mathbf{P}(\mathbf{r}, t)$ defined over the three-dimensional volume of the brain, which generates a scalp potential field $V(\mathbf{r}, t)$. If the mesosource field $\mathbf{P}(\mathbf{r}, t)$ represents a stochastic process, we can characterize it by its mean $\mu_P(\mathbf{r}, t)$ and cross-spectral density function

$C_P(\mathbf{r}_1, \mathbf{r}_2, f)$. The cross-spectral density function is a spatial correlation function that depends on temporal frequency. The mean depends on brain location $\mathbf{r}$, and the cross-spectral density function depends on pairs of locations $(\mathbf{r}_1, \mathbf{r}_2)$. The mean $\mu_V(\mathbf{r}, t)$ and cross-spectral density function $C_V(\mathbf{r}_1, \mathbf{r}_2, f)$ of the scalp potential field $V(\mathbf{r}, t)$ are similarly defined, but are now considered continuous functions of position rather than being defined only at discrete locations by (9.8) and (9.10) for EEG channels.

For the purpose of this discussion we assume the stochastic process is weakly stationary, so that we can assume zero mean without loss of generality. The cross-spectral density function of the scalp potential is related to the cross-spectral density function of the source distribution by

$$C_V(\mathbf{r}_1, \mathbf{r}_2, f) = \int\limits_{S_1'} \int\limits_{S_2'} G_V^*(\mathbf{r}_1, \mathbf{r}_1') C_P(\mathbf{r}_1', \mathbf{r}_2', f) G_V(\mathbf{r}_2, \mathbf{r}_2') dS_1' dS_2' \qquad (9.15)$$

where $G_V(\mathbf{r}, \mathbf{r}')$ is the Green's function that gives the potential at location $\mathbf{r}$ due to a dipole source of unit strength located at $\mathbf{r}'$ and the integration is over the entire source distribution. The general form of (9.15) was initially developed in the theory of random vibrations in structural dynamics and was introduced to EEG by Katznelson (1982). In general, (9.15) is an integral over the volume of the brain, but practically this volume is constrained to conform to the geometry of the cortical surface (S). The Green's function depends on the volume conduction properties of the head, source locations, and measurement locations. For example, if all sources are radial dipoles at fixed radial location inside the brain sphere of the 4-sphere model and potentials are measured on the outer scalp sphere, $G_V(\mathbf{r}, \mathbf{r}')$ is given in spherical coordinates by (6.10).

Equation (9.15) defines a spatial filtering of the mesosource cross-spectral density function to obtain the scalp cross-spectral density function. The details depend on the volume conduction model. In chapter 6 we characterized the Green's function for scalp potentials due to a spherical surface of radial dipoles as a low-pass spatial filter, with examples shown in fig. 6-12. To examine the effects of spatial filtering on the cross spectrum or coherence estimates, we consider a simple case where the source activity is a spatially uncorrelated stationary stochastic process defined on a sphere of radius r_z in a spherical model of the head:

$$C_P(\theta_1, \phi_1, \theta_2, \phi_2, f) = p^2(f)\delta(\cos\theta_1 - \cos\theta_2)\delta(\phi_1 - \phi_2) \qquad (9.16)$$

Here ϕ and θ are the azimuth and elevation coordinates (essentially longitude and latitude) on a spherical surface, and $p^2(f)$ is the source variance as a function of frequency, in other words the power spectrum of the sources. If we place the sources in a 4-sphere model of the head, the cross-spectral density function of the scalp potentials can be calculated by substituting the Green's function (6.10) and (9.16) into (9.15) to obtain (Srinivasan et al. 1998)

$$C_V(\theta_1, \phi_1, \theta_2, \phi_2, f) = p^2(f) \sum_{n=1}^{\infty} \frac{4\pi H_n(r_z)}{2n+1} P_n(\cos \chi_{12}) \qquad (9.17)$$

where χ_{12} is the angle between two electrodes positioned at (θ_1, ϕ_1) and (θ_2, ϕ_2), the $P_n(x)$ are the Legendre polynomials (Morse and Feshbach 1953), and the H_n depend on the source radial position (r_z) and the thicknesses and conductivities of the spherical model, as discussed in appendix G. The power spectral density function can be obtained from (9.17) for the case of identical electrode positions, that is, $\chi_{12} = 0$. The coherence function γ_V^2 for the scalp potential can then be derived by substituting the cross-spectral density function given in (9.17) and the corresponding power spectral density function into (9.11) to obtain

$$\gamma_V^2(\chi_{12}) = \left[\frac{\sum\limits_{n=1}^{\infty} \frac{H_n(r_z)}{2n+1} P_n(\cos \chi_{12})}{\sum\limits_{n=1}^{\infty} \frac{H_n(r_z)}{2n+1}} \right]^2 \qquad (9.18)$$

The coherence function given by (9.18) is the scalp potential coherence predicted by the 4-sphere model if the source distribution is a spatially uncorrelated Gaussian random process. Thus, when coherence in the brain sphere between all possible source locations is zero, we can predict the scalp potential coherence that is due only to volume conduction.

We note immediately that the coherence function (9.18) is independent of frequency, which does not appear as a parameter on the right-hand side of the equation; *the effects of volume conduction on EEG coherence are independent of temporal frequency.* Second, we note that in a 4-sphere model this theoretical coherence does not depend on the position of the electrodes but only on the angular distance between electrodes χ_{12}. Figure 9-12a shows the coherence function plotted as a function of the separation distance between electrodes measured in centimeters along the spherical scalp surface. The sources consist of a superficial spherical dipole layer placed in 4-sphere models with different ratios of brain-to-skull conductivity. Coherence introduced by volume conduction falls off with distance, reaching a minimum at a surface distance of about 10 cm. At very large distances there is a small rise in the coherence as each source contributes a small negative potential at long distances due to the curvature of the closed head surface. The implication is that over

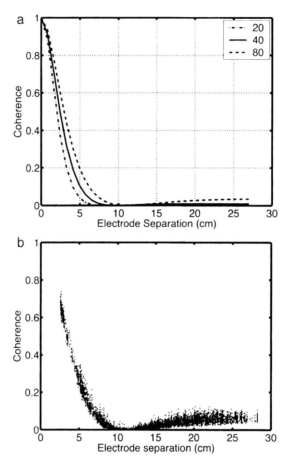

Figure 9-12 (a) Theoretical predictions of coherence between scalp potentials due to volume conduction alone, with an assumed spatial white-noise source distribution in the 4-sphere model of volume conduction in the head given by (9.15). The source is a spherical dipole layer at a radial location $r_z = 7.8$ cm. The model parameters are radii $(r_1, r_2, r_3, r_4) = (8, 8.1, 8.6, 9.2)$ and conductivity ratios $(\sigma_1/\sigma_2, \sigma_1/\sigma_3, \sigma_1/\sigma_4) = (0.2, 40, 1)$. Source coherence is zero and scalp potential coherence depends only on distance. (b) A numerical simulation in the 4-sphere model using ~3600 dipole sources distributed under an electrode array of 111 electrodes, with average electrode separation of 2.7 cm (matching the geodesic net shown in fig. 7-1). Dipole sources are independent Gaussian random processes. Again scalp potential falls off with electrode separation similar to the theoretical fall-off shown in (a).

short to moderate interelectrode distances ($<8-10$ cm in the spherical model) we may expect a significant contribution of volume conduction to coherence. This effect is similar at the three values of brain-to-skull conductivity ratio that span the range of most estimates as discussed in chapter 4. The same picture emerges from a numerical simulation (fig. 9-12b) in which roughly 3600 dipole sources were placed in the upper surface of the 4-sphere model distributed in a layer covering the extent of a 111-channel recording array ($109°$ of elevation from the vertex).

At each source location in the spherical cortical layer the source activity was treated as an independent Gaussian random process and coherences were calculated between predicted scalp potentials from the 4-sphere model using 100 epochs and 111 electrodes, thereby obtaining a similar curve to the analytic solution (fig. 9-12a). The analytic solution shows slightly lower coherence than the numerical solution, reflecting the accuracy of using an (essentially) infinite number of samples and sources versus the 100 samples and 3600 dipole sources used to generate fig. 9-12b.

This theoretical prediction of coherence due to volume conduction suggests that the main effect of volume conduction is to artificially inflate coherences at short to moderate distances, and that this effect is independent of frequency. This prediction may be evaluated with genuine EEG data. Figure 9-13 shows the coherences between an electrode labeled X and a ring of electrodes at progressively greater distances from X labeled

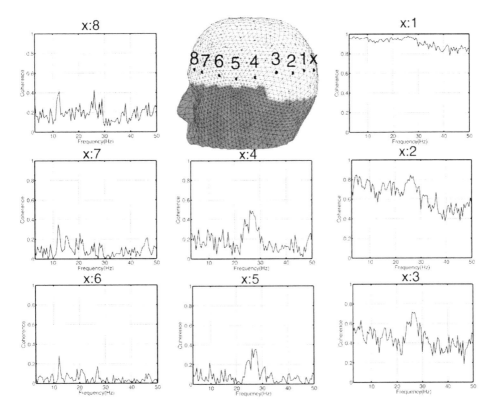

Figure 9-13   EEG coherence spectra estimates based on 100 s averages. The subject is a 36-year-old male (with *eyes open* to minimize alpha band coherence). Coherence was estimated with $T = 2$ s epoch lengths ($\Delta f = 0.5$ Hz). The head plot shows the location of nine electrodes, labeled X and 1 through 8. Coherence spectra estimates are shown between electrode X and each of the electrodes 1–8, at increasing distances along the scalp. Very close electrodes have high coherence independent of frequency as expected from the theoretical model.

1–9. The subject is at rest with eyes open, a state in which coherence is usually lower than in the eyes closed resting state or while performing a mental task (Nunez 1995). The estimated coherence between electrode X and electrode n is labeled X : n. The electrode positions are indicated and the typical distance between adjacent electrodes is 2.7 cm. At the closest electrode pair X : 1, coherence is very high (above 0.8) at all frequencies, and except for a slight decline at higher frequencies (perhaps due to artifact); coherence between these neighboring electrodes is generally independent of temporal frequency. As the electrode separation is increased, the pair X : 2 shows lower coherences, but at most frequencies coherence is still above 0.5 suggesting a strong contribution to coherence that is independent of frequency. As the sensor separation is further increased (X : 3) the floor of the coherence spectrum is reduced to about 0.2, and a peak becomes more evident in the 24–28 Hz range. For pairs of electrodes involving temporal electrodes (X : 4, and X : 5) the floor of the coherence spectrum approaches zero at most frequencies and a peak is evident in the beta band (24–28 Hz). At the still longer distances of electrodes over frontal areas (X : 6 and X : 7) the 24–28 Hz coherence peak disappears, and coherence is quite low at most frequencies. At a very long separation distance, a pair with a prefrontal electrode (X : 8), the coherences are slightly elevated across all frequencies, suggesting a very small volume conduction effect at long distances consistent with the theoretical model demonstrated in fig. 9-12.

The coherence spectra shown in fig. 9-13 have strong qualitative similarity to the coherence effects predicted by volume conduction of uncorrelated source activity. At short distances coherence is high across all frequencies. The level of coherence that is independent of frequency systematically decreases as distance increases. This suggests that it is very difficult to interpret coherence between closely spaced electrodes. The electrode pair X : 4 and X : 5 show a clear coherence peak of about 0.4 at 28 Hz, while the pair X : 3 shows a peak of about 0.7, but with elevated coherences at all frequencies. Clearly we cannot easily determine if the mesosource coherence of the pair X : 3 is genuinely higher than X : 4 or X : 5, since we observe a strong contribution by volume conduction that is independent of frequency. In addition, there is even a small rise in coherence at very large distances as predicted by the theoretical model (due to the head's closed surface). Many experimental papers on EEG coherence have ignored volume conduction effects by reasoning (incorrectly) that volume conduction effects are *additive* and can be ignored in the comparison of two or more conditions in the same subject or between groups of subjects. It is important to appreciate the underlying process is spatial filtering as expressed by (9.15). *The implication of the curves shown in fig. 9-12 is that EEG electrodes separated by less than about 10 cm are averaging over many of the same sources.* If two closely spaced electrodes record from the same source region and the power of the source region increases, coherence between these electrodes will also increase. If there are two source regions, one close to each electrode, changes in source power and changes in source coherence will both cause increases in scalp coherence when the distance between electrode pairs is small to moderate.

In fig. 9-13, potentials were expressed with respect to the (common) average reference before calculating coherence estimates. As discussed in chapter 7, any choice of reference strategy (including the average reference) introduces biases into the measured potential, although the average reference appears to be the best strategy if a sufficient number of electrode sites is used to obtain the space-averaged potential. In fig. 9-14 we consider some effects of reference electrode choice by extending the simulation of fig. 9-12b. In fig. 9-14a coherence between all pairs of (110)

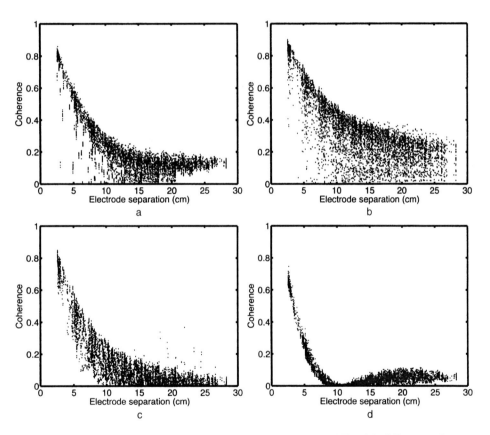

Figure 9-14   Simulations following the procedure used in fig. 9-12b with different reference electrodes. Simulated coherence between 111 electrodes using 3600 dipoles sources distributed under an array of 111 electrodes in the 4-sphere model. Dipole sources were independent Gaussian random processes. Coherence plotted as function of electrode separation excluding reference electrode. (a) Vertex reference using 110 electrodes. (b) Left mastoid reference. (c) Digitally averaged mastoids reference. (d) Coherence calculated by first referencing the potentials to the vertex and then calculating the average reference potential at 111 electrode sites. Note the average reference coherence curve closely follows reference-independent potentials.

electrodes is shown as a function of electrode separation when the potentials are referenced to the vertex electrode. For most electrode pairs coherence is elevated by more than 0.1 in comparison to reference-independent potentials shown in 9-12b. The few exceptions are sensor pairs involving electrodes very near the vertex where most of the signal cancels leaving mainly noise that yields very low coherences. Figure 9-14b shows coherences between all pairs with the reference at the left mastoid. Coherences are greatly elevated by this choice of reference. The use of a single reference site increases coherence since a common signal is being added to each channel. Figure 9-14c shows the case where all coherences are calculated based on using the average potential of the two mastoids as the reference potential. Coherences are reduced in comparison to the left mastoid reference, except for a few pairs involving one electrode over each hemisphere. Coherences are still elevated in comparison to reference-independent potentials shown in fig. 9-12. Figure 9-14d shows the coherences from potentials that were first referenced to the vertex and then the average reference was calculated before coherence estimates were obtained. With the choice of average reference, coherences are almost identical to the reference-independent coherences showing both the highly elevated coherences at short distances and a somewhat larger rise at long distances. All of the average-reference coherence estimates are within 0.1 of the reference-independent coherence estimates. These simulations and data suggest that *averaged reference coherence estimates obtained from dense electrode arrays accurately mimic theoretical reference-free coherence estimates but remain elevated by volume conduction for electrode pairs closer than about 8–10 cm.*

In this theoretical example the effect of reference electrode was to add the identical signal to all the channels, thereby artificially inflating coherences. In all cases, mesosources at the reference location were incoherent with the mesosources at each recording location. In genuine EEG data, the potential at the reference site may be partly coherent with the potential at the recording site. In this case more complicated effects can occur depending on the level of coherence and phase difference between recording and reference electrodes. For example, mesosource activity that is coherent with zero phase lag between recording and reference location will simply cancel. This can lead to changes in the pattern of coherence between the recording electrode and other recording electrodes by emphasizing the contributions from other sources. By contrast, our simulations with 111 electrodes suggest that the use of the average reference yields coherence estimates that closely approximate reference-independent potentials.

The use of average-reference potentials substantially reduces reference electrode problems associated with scalp coherence estimates, provided a large number of electrodes are available to estimate the space-averaged potential over the upper surface of the head. However, the serious problem of volume conduction "smearing" of scalp potentials remains.

Scalp potentials can be used primarily only to investigate source coherence between widely-separated electrodes over large-scale source regions. To illustrate this point, coherence between all pairs of 111 electrodes estimated from 100 seconds of *eyes-open EEG* are plotted against electrode separation in fig. 9-15 for six different frequency bands. Each of the plots has the distinguishing feature of elevated coherences at very short distances that fall off as electrode separation increases. In all cases, coherences appear to reach a minimum at about 12 cm and rise again at greater distances. Elevated long-range (>12 cm) coherences are stronger in the alpha band (9.5–12.5 Hz) than low- (<7.5 Hz) or high-frequency (>14.5 Hz) coherencies. At these frequencies power is relatively low, and the shape of the coherence versus distance is qualitatively similar to the effects of volume conduction alone. The long-range coherences in the alpha band appear to reflect large-scale coherence between electrodes that record potentials generated by large but distant source regions. These alpha coherence patterns are relatively weak compared to the coherence usually observed in *eyes-closed resting conditions* (Nunez 1995). There are also differences in short-range (<12 cm) coherences between frequency bands, but these are difficult to interpret because of the strong effects of volume conduction.

8 Effects of Surface Laplacians on Coherence Estimates

In chapter 8, we introduced high-resolution EEG methods with emphasis on the surface Laplacian method, which provides a reference-independent estimate of dura (inner skull surface) potential. *The surface Laplacian entirely eliminates the reference electrode distortion of coherence estimates.* For this reason alone, surface Laplacian coherence estimates appear to be a substantial improvement over conventional referenced EEG coherences. In addition, the improved spatial resolution of the surface Laplacian eliminates much of the volume conduction distortion of coherence estimates.

The theory and simulations discussed in chapter 8 indicate that the surface Laplacian improves the spatial resolution of EEG. The simplest summary of this effect is provided by fig. 8-7, which shows the scalp potential and surface Laplacian magnitude directly above a superficial radial dipole layer in a 4-sphere model. Scalp potentials are maximum when generated in a dipole layer (spherical cap) of about 7–8 cm (surface) radius. By contrast, the surface Laplacian is maximally sensitive to a dipole layer of radius equal to about 2 cm. The effect of the surface Laplacian estimate is to limit the sensitivity of each electrode to superficial sources within a radius of about 2–3 cm of the scalp electrode. Moreover, the surface Laplacian is much less sensitive to the dipole layer of radius 7–8 cm which contributes maximally to the scalp potential. Thus, the surface Laplacian is sensitive to a different spatial scale of mesosource activity

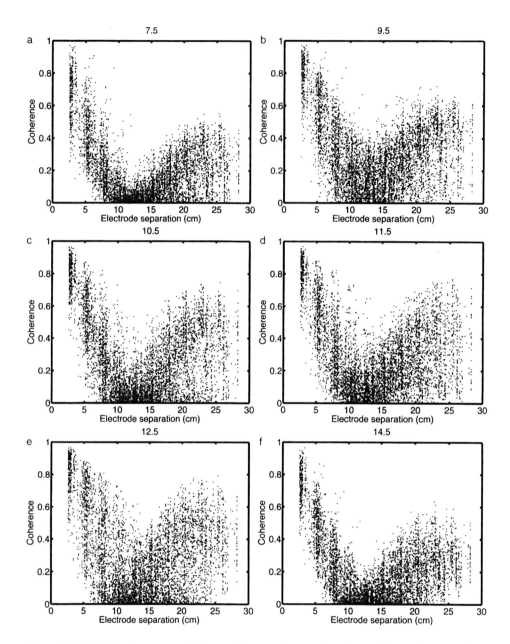

Figure 9-15 EEG coherence at different frequencies as a function of electrode separation for a 36-year-old male subject at rest with *eyes open* (chosen to minimize alpha band coherence), based on 111 electrode sites and the average reference potential. Detailed coherence spectra for this subject are shown in fig. 9-13. (a) 7.5 Hz coherence, (b) 9.5 Hz coherence, (c) 10.5 Hz coherence, (d) 11.5 Hz coherence, (e) 12.5 Hz coherence, (f) 14.5 Hz coherence. In (a) and (f) power is low and the coherence follows electrode separation consistent with the effects of volume conduction. At the other frequencies, coherence is elevated at large electrode separations.

than scalp potentials. In comparison to the low-pass spatial filtering of scalp potentials, surface Laplacians are band-pass spatial filtered as shown in fig. 8-6.

After applying the surface Laplacian to each time slice in an EEG time series recorded at many (>64) electrodes, we obtain the surface Laplacian (transformed) time series, which is then Fourier transformed using the standard FFT algorithm. In practice, these two operations can be carried out in either order since both are linear transformations. When applying the surface Laplacian to a Fourier coefficient, the real and imaginary parts are passed through the surface Laplacian separately. Given an ensemble of surface Laplacian Fourier coefficients we can calculate the power at each channel and coherence between channels following (9.9) and (9.11). Appendix J provides algorithmic details for the New Orleans spline Laplacian including Matlab code allowing easy implementation in any laboratory. Issues related to calculating power and coherence are identical to the discussion of section 3. As a practical matter, surface Laplacian time series are generally noisier than potential time series since the second spatial derivative tends to enhance noise effects at each electrode site. Thus, the use of surface Laplacians for coherence estimates generally requires averaging over many epochs.

Although in practice we estimate the surface Laplacian at a set of discrete electrode sites, the surface Laplacian may be generally considered as a stochastic field $L(\mathbf{r}, t)$ over the scalp surface. The statistics of this field can be characterized by the mean $\mu_L(\mathbf{r}, t)$ and cross-spectral density function $C_L(\mathbf{r}_1, \mathbf{r}_2, f)$. For the purpose of this discussion we assume the stochastic process is weakly stationary, so that we can assume zero mean without loss of generality. The cross-spectral density function of the surface Laplacian is related to the cross-spectral density function of the source distribution by

$$C_L(\mathbf{r}_1, \mathbf{r}_2, f) = \iint_{S_1' S_2'} G_L^*(\mathbf{r}_1, \mathbf{r}_1') C_P(\mathbf{r}_1', \mathbf{r}_2', f) G_L(\mathbf{r}_2, \mathbf{r}_2') dS_1' dS_2' \qquad (9.19)$$

where $G_L(\mathbf{r}, \mathbf{r}')$ is the Green's function that gives the surface Laplacian at location $\mathbf{r}$ on the scalp surface due to a dipole source of unit strength located at $\mathbf{r}'$ and the integrals are taken over the entire source distribution. The surface Laplacian Green's function can be obtained for the 4-sphere model by applying the definition of the surface Laplacian on a spherical surface given in (8.10) to the Green's function for scalp potentials given by (6.10).

Following the analysis of scalp potential coherence we consider the simple case where the source activity is a spatially uncorrelated stationary stochastic process defined on a sphere of radius r_z in a spherical model of the head with cross-spectral density function C_P given by (9.16). By substituting into (9.19) to obtain the cross-spectral density function of the surface Laplacian $C_{\rm L}$, and applying the definition of coherence (9.11) we obtain the coherence of the surface Laplacian:

$$\gamma_{\rm L}^2(\chi_{12}) = \left[\frac{\sum\limits_{n=1}^{\infty} \frac{n(n+1)H_n(r_z)}{2n+1} P_n(\cos\chi_{12})}{\sum\limits_{n=1}^{\infty} \frac{n(n+1)H_n(r_z)}{2n+1}} \right]^2 \tag{9.20}$$

Here the coefficients H_n depend on the radial position of the source sphere r_z and the conductivities and thicknesses of the tissue layers as given in appendix G.

The coherence function given by (9.20) is the coherence predicted for the surface Laplacian in the 4-sphere model if the source distribution is a spatially uncorrelated Gaussian random process. Similar to the coherence function for the scalp potentials (9.18), this theoretical surface Laplacian coherence is independent of frequency and depends only on the angular distance χ_{12} between electrodes. Figure 9-16a shows this coherence function for different values of the brain-to-skull conductivity ratio. In each case coherence falls off very rapidly with electrode separation, reaching zero at a distance of 3 cm as compared to 10 cm for the potentials shown in fig. 9-12a. The brain-to-skull conductivity ratio has negligible effect in this model (provided the ratio is large, greater than roughly 5 or 10). Figure 9.16b shows a numerical simulation in which roughly 3600 dipole sources were placed in the upper surface of the 4-sphere model distributed in a layer covering the extent of a 111-channel recording array (109° of elevation from the vertex) identical to the simulation of scalp potential coherence shown in fig. 9-12b. At each mesosource location in the spherical layer in the brain, the mesosource activity is an independent Gaussian random process, and coherences were estimated between surface Laplacians, that is, calculated with the 4-sphere model using 100 epochs at 111 electrode positions. *Remarkably, the surface Laplacian shows essentially zero coherence even at the closest electrode separation of 2.7 cm, accurately reflecting the spatially uncorrelated source activity.* In simulations, we have found that calculating Laplacian coherences using 111 electrodes and the New Orleans spline algorithm (appendix J) retains a small amount of inflated coherences but only between nearest-neighbor electrodes at the edge of the array (Srinivasan et al. 1998). These errors can be avoided by removing the edge electrodes from the coherence analysis (although continuing to use them to constrain the Laplacian estimate).

This result seems to suggest that the surface Laplacian solves once and for all the problem of volume conduction in EEG coherence estimates by entirely removing artificial coherence. However, life is not so simple! It is important to remember that the contribution of volume conduction to potential or Laplacian coherence is not simply additive. The underlying process is spatial filtering, expressed mathematically as the Green's functions for the potential G_V and surface Laplacian G_L and as summarized graphically in figs. 8-7 and 8-8. The potential and surface Laplacian are sensitive to different spatial scales of sources, a physical property that is reflected in coherence estimates. Large correlated dipole layers (mostly low spatial frequency components) will make large relative contributions to coherence estimates based on scalp potentials, while smaller dipole layers (composed of higher spatial frequency components) will make larger relative contributions to Laplacian coherence estimates. *This implies that*

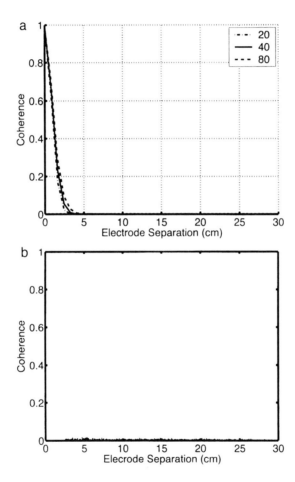

Figure 9-16 (a) Theoretical predictions of coherence between surface Laplacians due to volume conduction alone with an assumed spatial white-noise source distribution in the 4-sphere model given by (9.15). The source is a spherical dipole layer at a radial position of $r_z = 7.8$ cm. The model parameters were radii $(r_1, r_2, r_3, r_4) = (8, 8.1, 8.6, 9.2)$ and conductivity ratios $(\sigma_1/\sigma_2, \sigma_1/\sigma_3, \sigma_1/\sigma_4) = (0.2, 20\text{--}80, 1)$. Source coherence is zero. (b) A numerical simulation of Laplacian coherence using 3600 dipole sources distributed in the 4-sphere model under an electrode array of 111 electrodes with average electrode separation of 2.7 cm. Dipole sources were independent Gaussian random processes. Simulated coherence is essentially zero between all possible electrode pairs at this minimum separation distance.

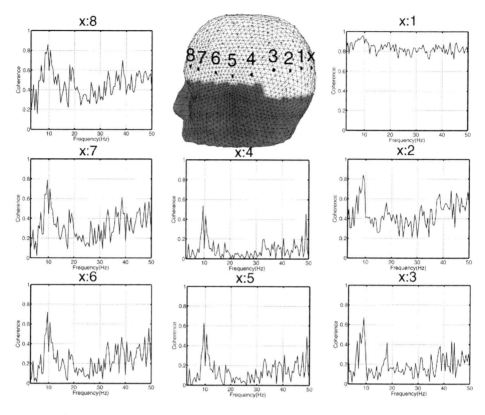

Figure 9-17   EEG (scalp potential) ordinary coherence spectra from a 22-year-old female subject at rest with eyes closed (to maximize alpha coherence). Coherence was estimated with $T = 2$ s $(\Delta f = 0.5$ Hz) in a 60 s record. The head plot shows the location of 9 electrodes, labeled x and 1 through 8. Coherence spectra between electrode X and each of the other electrodes 1–8 are shown, with increasing separations along the scalp. Note that very close electrodes have higher coherence independent of frequency as predicted by the theoretical model. Alpha band coherence is high for large electrode separations, apparently reflecting the large cortical source coherence. Power spectra for this subject are shown in fig. 9-4.

higher coherence can be observed in either potentials or Laplacians depending on the spatial bandwidth of coherent source activity.

Coherence between one electrode (labeled X) and set of electrodes (1–8) at progressively larger distances from posterior to anterior locations of the left hemisphere is shown in fig. 9-17 based on average-reference potentials and in fig. 9-18 for Laplacian-based estimates of the same data sets (spline Laplacians are estimated using the entire 111-channel data sets). The subject was at rest with eyes closed to facilitate a robust alpha rhythm. Power spectra for two midline channels of this subject are shown in fig. 9-2, demonstrating two peaks in the alpha band (9.5 and 10.5 Hz). The potential-based coherence estimates show the characteristic volume conduction effect of very high coherences at all frequencies between neighboring electrodes (X : 1). As the electrode separation increases this

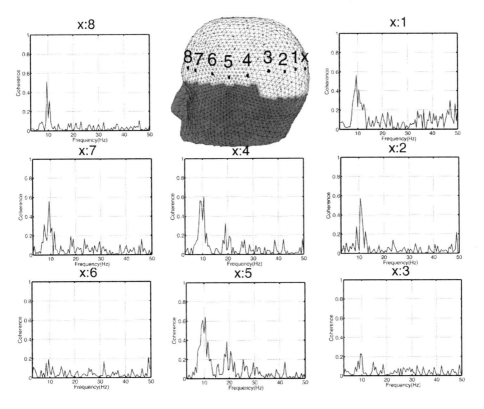

Figure 9-18 EEG (spline Laplacian) coherence spectra using the same data in fig. 9-17: the female subject at rest with eyes closed for 60 s. All 111 channels of data were submitted to the New Orleans spline Laplacian to estimate coherence spectra for these few channel pairs. The spline Laplacian coherence spectra show distinct coherence spectra between electrode X and even very closely spaced electrodes as the result of filtering out volume conduction effects.

volume conduction effect disappears. Inflated coherences at all frequencies are again apparent (more clearly than in the subject in fig. 9-13) at very large electrode separations (X:7 and X:8). The potential-based coherences show distinct peaks at 9.5 Hz and 10.5 Hz with much lower coherences at 10 Hz. For closely spaced pairs there is evidence of the 9.5 Hz coherence peak but almost no evidence of the peak at 10.5 Hz. Electrode pairs including temporal and frontal channels (X with 4–8) show two distinct coherence peaks.

Figure 9.18 shows the spline Laplacian-based coherence for the same electrode pairs. There is little evidence of elevated coherence due to volume conduction in any electrode pair. Even the closest neighbors (X:1) indicate very low coherence except at the coherence peaks at 9.5 and 10.5 Hz. At the next closest pair (X:2) a different pattern is seen with larger coherence at 10.5 Hz. For two pairs (X:3 and X:6) coherence is very low over the entire frequency range. This suggests that the source activity generating signals at these electrodes in the potentials was not local activity (small dipole layer) but rather activity generated by a larger (or deeper) dipole layer. The electrode pairs involving prefrontal electrodes (X : 7 and X : 8) show higher coherence at 9.5 Hz than 10.5 Hz. Coherences at these locations in the potential data are similar, although elevated over the entire spectrum by apparent volume conduction effects. The highest coherences at 9.5 Hz and 10.5 Hz involve temporal electrodes (X : 4 and X : 5). For these pairs additional peaks can be seen at the harmonics (19 Hz and 21 Hz). In summary, unlike the nearly homogeneous pattern of coherence seen in the potential-based coherence estimates *the Laplacian-based coherence estimates show significant spatial specificity and reveal much more detailed coherence patterns.*

Average-reference potential-based coherence between all pairs of 111 electrodes from 60 seconds of *eyes closed* EEG are plotted against electrode separation in fig. 9-19 for six different frequencies. Not surprisingly, at frequencies in the alpha band (9.5–12.5 Hz), coherences are very high at both short and long distances, and theta coherence (7.5 Hz) is lower than alpha coherence but still higher at large distances than the coherence expected due only to volume conduction. At 14.5 Hz coherences are reduced and more closely resemble the characteristics of coherence due only to volume conduction, that is, due to uncorrelated sources. Figure 9-20 shows surface Laplacian coherences at the same frequencies. At 14.5 Hz only a few coherences are greater than 0.2, and many of these involve nearest-neighbor pairs, again suggesting that potential coherence at 14.5 Hz is mostly due to volume conduction. The largest coherences occur at 9.5 and 10.5 Hz in both the potential and Laplacian-based estimates. *These data provide evidence for both a very large-scale dipole layer and smaller dipole layers that are coherent across long distances.* Many pairs of electrodes over the entire range of separation distances have high Laplacian coherences at these frequency peaks. Outside of these bands (at 7.5, 11.5, and 12.5 Hz), mainly short-range coherences remain elevated. This outcome strongly suggests that the long-range coherences observed at these frequencies are mainly due to correlated source activity in a very large-scale dipole layer.

The important point emphasized with these simulations is that more information is gained by comparing potential and Laplacian-based coherences than is obtained by considering either in isolation. *The potential and Laplacian-based coherence estimates provide complementary views of mesosource dynamics by emphasizing different spatial scales (or spatial bandwidths) of correlated source activity.*

9 Are EEG Power and Coherence Independent Measures?

The coherence estimate (9.11) normalizes the cross spectrum of two channels by the power spectrum of each channel. This suggests that if we increase power at both channels but keep relative power and relative phase constant across observations coherence should be unchanged. In practice,

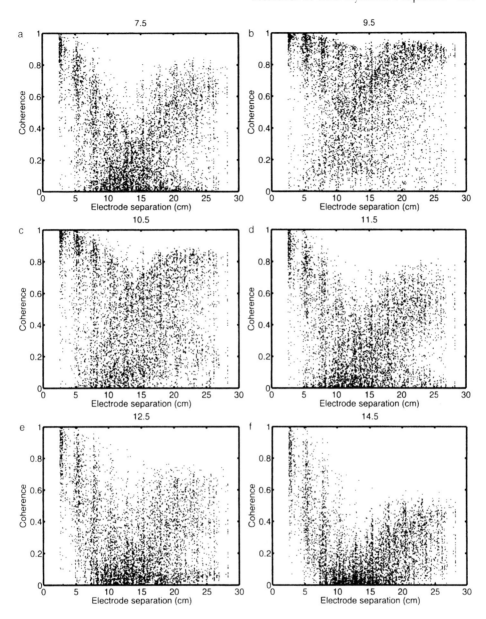

Figure 9-19   EEG (scalp potential) coherence at different frequencies as a function of electrode separation for the female subject of figs. 9-17 and 9-18 at rest with *eyes closed*. Detailed coherence spectra for this subject are shown in fig. 9-13. (a) 7.5 Hz coherence, (b) 9.5 Hz coherence, (c) 10.5 Hz coherence, (d) 11.5 Hz coherence, (e) 12.5 Hz coherence, (f) 14.5 Hz coherence. In (f) power is low and coherence follows electrode separation consistent with the effects of volume conduction. At the other frequencies, coherence is elevated at long distances.

this is not true because changes in power are usually correlated to changes in signal-to-noise ratio (SNR). Consider an ensemble of records each containing a sinusoid with random phase at one channel and the same sinusoid with a fixed phase difference at the other channel. Random noise

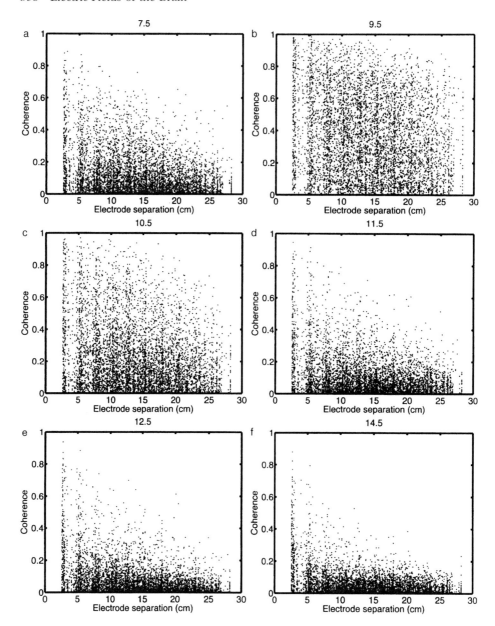

Figure 9-20   EEG (spline Laplacian) coherence at different frequencies as a function of electrode separation using the same data used in fig. 9-19. (a) 7.5 Hz coherence, (b) 9.5 Hz coherence, (c) 10.5 Hz coherence, (d) 11.5 Hz coherence, (e) 12.5 Hz coherence, (f) 14.5 Hz coherence. In (f) coherence is small for most electrode pairs. At the alpha frequencies 9.5 Hz and 10.5 Hz, a broad range of high and low Laplacian coherences are found at all distances.

at the same frequency is added to both channels. The signal-to-noise ratio (SNR) is the ratio of the sinusoid power to the noise power (or variance) at the sinusoid frequency. If sinusoid power goes up at both channels in each epoch, SNR increases. Since the sinusoids have fixed relative phase and amplitude, coherence is directly related to SNR by (Bendat and Piersol 2001)

$$\gamma_{mn}^2 = \frac{1}{\left(1 + \frac{1}{\text{SNR}_n}\right)\left(1 + \frac{1}{\text{SNR}_m}\right)} \qquad (9.21)$$

The relationships between amplitude measures (power) and coherence measures in applications to EEG are more complex, since each electrode site reflects the response to a mixture of different sources and only some of these sources are coherent. Thus, when increased power in one mesosource region causes an increase in SNR, coherence goes up only for electrode sites that are recording from other coherent source regions. Furthermore, SNR is not easily measured in EEG, so it is not clear how we can make use of (9.21) to investigate the relationship between power and coherence in genuine EEG data.

Because of the effects of volume conduction, changes in power of a source region can have strong effects on the coherence obtained from closely spaced electrodes. This follows from (9.21), with signal power reflecting the power of one source and noise power reflecting the power of all other sources (including added noise). Closely spaced electrodes may record from overlapping source regions located in an area larger than the separation distance between electrodes. This is reflected in figs. 9-12, 9-13, and 9-17 as high coherence between neighboring electrodes even when the underlying sources are completely uncorrelated. If one source becomes stronger, its SNR (relative to all other possible sources) increases at both channels. This leads to an increase in coherence between channels. Power and coherence between closely spaced electrodes are expected to be correlated due to the effect of volume conduction. At longer separation distances the effect of power on coherence is related mainly to increased SNR of distinct coherent sources that contribute signal to each electrode.

EEG power changes cannot always be predicted by changes in coherence or other measures of phase synchrony. Imagine a hypothetical cortex where phase synchrony is initially large only in some local cortical region, as indicated by the small mesosource region $\mathbf{P}(\mathbf{r}, t)$ in fig. 9-21. Suppose the synchronous region enlarges over time, starting with a synchrony scale (diameter) in the submillmeter range and spreading out to several centimeters or more as indicated in fig. 9-21b. As in the simulation shown in fig. 1-20, the synchronous region may be modeled by a dipole layer of increasing diameter. Scalp potential magnitudes depend on the (short) time averaged mesosource strength $\mathbf{P}(\mathbf{r}, t)$, here assumed be constant across the dipole layer and have constant amplitude over time. As the dipole layer enlarges with diameters in the approximate range 1 to 3 cm, large increases in scalp potential magnitudes are expected based on the exponential parts of the curves in fig. 1-20. Finally, even larger increases in dipole layer diameter (from about 3 cm to more than 10 cm), corresponding to the flatter parts of the curves in fig. 1-20, result in only modest increases in scalp potential magnitudes.

Suppose we place an electrode pair on the scalp in order to estimate coherence between two remote cortical regions as shown in fig. 9-21. Suppose further that the estimated coherence (after accounting for volume conduction) is small to moderate, but statistically significant. We can picture the underlying source distribution as composed of a large (correlated) dipole layer underneath both electrodes, plus other (uncorrelated) sources that cause scalp coherence to be less than one. In this example, the smaller scale coherence near each electrode (small dipole layer in fig. 9-21a) strongly influences scalp potential magnitudes, whereas the long-range coherence generated by the large dipole layer (fig. 9-21b) has minimal influence on magnitudes. In summary, we might anticipate that long-range coherence (in some frequency band) can either increase or decrease in different brain states independent of scalp amplitude, an effect reported for a variety of mental tasks (Petsche and Etlinger 1999). By contrast, we expect small and intermediate-range synchrony changes to result in large changes in scalp potential magnitudes, as shown in simulations (Nunez 1995).

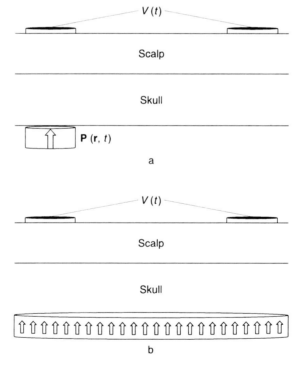

Figure 9-21 (a) A small source region modeled as a single dipole $\mathbf{P}(\mathbf{r}, t)$. (b) Large source region modeled as a dipole layer. As the dipole layer enlarges, power at the scalp electrodes depends on the synchronization of sources in the dipole layer.

Changes in synchrony as indicated in fig. 9-21 can be expected to have more complex effects on the surface Laplacian. Similar to the case of potentials, short-range synchrony increases should cause surface Laplacian magnitudes to increase up to about the 3 cm scale. For still larger dipole layers (larger correlated mesosource regions), the surface Laplacian magnitude should decrease even though the potential magnitude continues to increase (albeit slowly). At the same time, Laplacian coherence between two remote locations may increase; however, as Laplacian magnitude decreases coherence estimates become more limited by external noise.

10 Spatial Filtering Implies Temporal Filtering

Suppose some genuine dynamic system produces a signal (the *dependent field variable* $\Psi(x,t)$) that varies in time t and space x (the *independent variables*). Any such field variable (no matter how complicated) can be Fourier transformed so as to characterize the system dynamics in terms of its temporal and spatial frequency components; that is, the field may be expressed in the double Fourier series:

$$\Psi(x,t) = \sum_{n=-\infty}^{\infty} \sum_{m=-\infty}^{\infty} Z_{nm} e^{[j(\omega_m t - k_n x)]} \qquad (9.22)$$

Physical signals are measured over some finite time interval T and finite spatial extent L. In this case, the discrete frequencies and wavenumbers (spatial frequencies) are given by

$$\omega_m = \frac{2\pi m}{T} \quad k_n = \frac{2\pi n}{L} \qquad (9.23)$$

Longer epochs T and sensor array lengths L result in better temporal and spatial frequency resolutions, respectively. The square of the coefficients $|Z_{nm}|^2$ is called the *spectral density function* and may be expressed as a contour plot with m (or temporal frequency) plotted along the horizontal axis and n (or wavenumber or spatial frequency) plotted vertically. This picture requires modification in the case of data recorded on a two-dimensional surface such as a sphere or cortical surface. However, as a convenient approximation for recordings on a spherical surface of radius R, we adopt the rough correspondence

$$k_n \approx \frac{n}{R} \qquad (9.24)$$

For the remainder of this chapter, the index n is used to indicate both the one-dimensional wavenumber for waves traveling in a closed loop and the degree of the spherical harmonic function $Y_{nm}(\theta, \phi)$ for two-dimensional waves on a spherical surface. Given that genuine brains are neither one-dimensional nor spherical, corticocortical fibers are apparently anisotropic, cortical tissue may be inhomogeneous, and many other anatomical and physiological complications, this crude approximation is appropriate for our purposes.

For example, suppose we imagine a long narrow brain hemisphere (approximately one-dimensional) with multiple imbedded networks operating in different frequency ranges. Suppose further that widely distributed networks tend to operate at low temporal frequencies, but more localized networks tend to operate at higher temporal frequencies as is often the case in physical systems. If we compute the spectral density function of the source activity $P(x, t)$ using (9.22), we would find this relationship between network size and frequency expressed as a relationship between frequency and wavenumber. The spectral density function representing this stochastic process would exhibit more relative power at low wavenumbers for low temporal frequencies and high wavenumbers for high temporal frequencies. While such simple relationships may never occur in genuine brains, a plausible conjecture is that cortical source activities generally exhibit spatiotemporal organization of some kind, giving rise to some (probably complicated) relationships between frequency and wavenumber, which may be expected to change with brain state.

The scalp EEG potential field $V(x, t)$, perhaps recorded from an anterior–posterior line of scalp electrodes, can also be expanded in a spectral density function following (9.22) as in Nunez (1974). The scalp potential spectral density function is a low-pass spatial filtered version of the cortical spectral density function. The low-pass spatial filtering is given for a spherical model as a function of index n in fig. 8-8a. Since we anticipate that lower spatial frequencies k_n have spectral power at some preferred temporal frequencies ω_m, scalp EEG emphasizes these temporal frequencies. Thus, we anticipate that EEG will exhibit a different power spectrum than ECoG (or cortical source activity). The band-pass filtering of the surface Laplacian (fig. 8-8b) selects for intermediate spatial frequencies, which may then emphasize a third set of temporal frequencies. *Thus, the spatial filtering of EEG and surface Laplacians can be expected to lead to temporal filtering.* Well-known changes in temporal frequency content with brain state change might also occur with characteristic changes in spatial frequency content as suggested by Wingeier (2004) and summarized in chapter 10.

11 Steady-State Visually Evoked Potentials

In this section, signal processing approaches are introduced for experimental paradigms that (apparently) impose synchrony on populations of cortical neurons with a periodic external stimulus. This approach, pioneered by Regan (1989) and others in the 1960s, makes use of Fourier analysis to isolate the steady-state visual evoked potential (SSVEP). Recent studies have made use of periodic contrast or luminance modulation of fixed frequency, which is usually superimposed on cognitive task-related images. Steady-state evoked potentials or magnetic fields can be easily detected by Fourier analysis of EEG or MEG signals (Regan 1989; Srinivasan et al. 1999; Srinivasan 2004; Silberstein 1995; Silberstein et al. 2001; Chen et al. 2003). Steady-state responses are measured in the narrow (usually <0.1 Hz) frequency band centered on the stimulus frequency. Figure 9-22a shows the power spectrum at a channel over right occipital cortex, while the subject was presented a stimulus flickering at $f_s = 5$ Hz for 50 seconds. The power spectrum was obtained by applying the FFT to a record of length $T \sim 50$ seconds corresponding to an integer number of cycles of the flicker frequency yielding a frequency resolution $\Delta f \sim 0.02$ Hz, with only $K = 1$ epoch. The exact interval used varies with stimulus frequency in order to center one of the FFT frequency bins on the stimulus frequency. This is accomplished by choosing an epoch length T that exactly fits a sine wave of the stimulus frequency; that is, an integer number of samples per cycle. Any other choice will split the power at the stimulus frequency into multiple bands, as shown by the example in fig. 9-3. The power spectrum shows a very large peak at 5 Hz. There is also a clear peak at 15 Hz, the third harmonic of the flicker frequency. Some alpha rhythm near 10 Hz is observed but is broadband compared to the narrow response at 5 Hz. Figure 9-22b shows the response to the same stimulus flickering at $f_s = 8.14$ Hz. Again, there is a clear peak at the stimulation frequency, but in this case no harmonic response is evident in this channel. The steady-state evoked potential method concentrates stimulus responses into a narrow frequency band surrounding the stimulus frequency, resulting in a very large response in this narrow band.

Since typical EEG/MEG artifacts (such as muscle potentials) have broadband spectra, the narrow-band signal-to-noise ratio of the steady-state response can be made arbitrarily large by increasing the duration of stimulation. This approach has substantial practical value in segregating stimulus-related brain activity from both artifacts and spontaneous brain activity. This feature is illustrated in fig. 9-22c and d where Gaussian random noise (standard deviations of 50 and 100 μV, respectively) is added to the EEG data from the experiment with stimulation at $f_s = 5$ Hz (fig. 9-22a). In both cases the SSVEP peak at 5 Hz is visible despite the presence of large-amplitude noise. In fig. 9-22d we see that 100 μV noise is sufficient to obscure both the alpha rhythm and harmonic power at 15 Hz, but not the 1.3 μV rms amplitude (square root of power) SSVEP. Such broadband noise is much larger than typical EEG artifact. It has been demonstrated that adding large EEG artifact such as eye blinks and eye movements to the SSVEP data typically produces minor effects on SSVEP amplitude (Silberstein 1995). Of course, if the subject is continuously moving the eyes or blinking, the SSVEP may become contaminated.

A common misconception is that the characteristic narrow band response of the SSVEP indicates that the SSVEP is a deterministic signal rather than a stochastic process (Regan 1989). At first glance such determinism seems intuitive, since in both fig. 9-22a and b the SSVEP appears to occupy a single frequency bin with no obvious sidebands, as compared to the alpha rhythm which is distributed over 50 bins (9.5–10.5 Hz). Consider the example simulations (fig. 9-23) of amplitude modulated

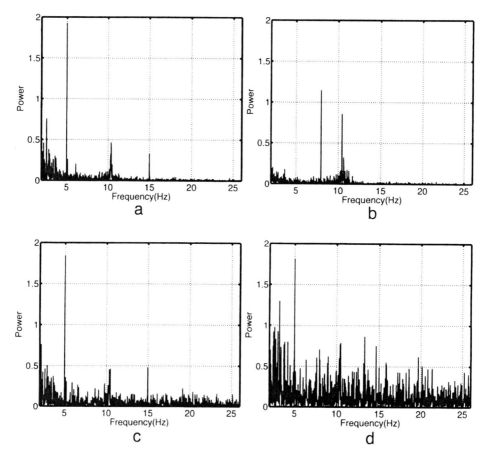

Figure 9-22 SSVEP spectra. (a) Spectrum of steady-state visually evoked potential in the female subject recorded from a channel over the right occipital lobe. The stimulus is a 5 Hz square wave flicker (20% duty cycle), in the shape of an annulus at 6° of visual angle presented for ~50 s. The exact duration was always an integer number of stimulus presentations. The spectrum shown is calculated with $T \sim 50$ s and $\Delta f \sim 0.02$ Hz. These exact parameters were selected so that Fourier transforms were calculated over an integer number of cycles of the stimulus frequency. A clear peak can be seen in the spectrum at 5 Hz with a third harmonic at 15 Hz. An alpha peak near 10 Hz is also visible. (b) Same experiment as in (a) with the stimulus frequency equal to 8.1 Hz. (c) Same as (a) with Gaussian random noise with $\sigma = 50$ mV added to EEG data. (d) Same as (a) with Gaussian random noise with $\sigma = 100$ mV added to the EEG data.

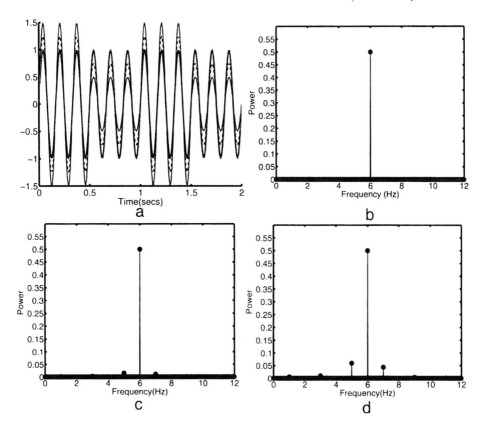

Figure 9-23 (a) Simulation of an amplitude-modulated sine wave obtained by multiplying a 6 Hz sinusoid with a 1 Hz square wave. The gray line is the 6 Hz sinusoid with 0% modulation depth, the solid line indicates 50% modulation depth, and the dashed line indicates 25% modulation depth. Only 2 s are shown of the 50 s simulation. (b) Power spectrum of the sine wave with 0% amplitude modulation. (c) Power spectrum of the sine wave with 25% amplitude modulation. (d) Power spectrum of the sine wave with 50% amplitude modulation. Even with 50% amplitude modulation, the largest sidebands at 5 and 7 Hz are only 10% of the power at 6 Hz.

6 Hz sinusoids in a 50 s record. The amplitude modulation is a 1 Hz square wave. Two seconds of the waveforms are shown in fig. 9-23a corresponding to no amplitude modulation (gray line), 25% amplitude modulation (solid line), and 50% amplitude modulation (dashed line). The corresponding power spectra are shown in fig. 9-23b–d. We see that the amplitude-modulated sine waves produce a power peak at the sinusoid frequency plus sideband power spaced by 1 Hz due to the 1 Hz square wave amplitude modulation. However, these sideband peaks are very small; even at 50% modulation the power at the sinusoid frequency is about 10 times the largest sideband peak. In the case of 25% amplitude modulation, the corresponding ratio is about 50.

In SSVEP studies signal-to-noise ratio (SNR) estimates have been obtained by comparing power in stimulation bands to power in surrounding bands yielding SNR of 3–50 (Srinivasan 2004; Srinivasan et al. 1999).

In the example SSVEPs of fig. 9-22 a and b the SNR obtained by comparing the power at the stimulus frequency to the average power in a 1 Hz band surrounding the stimulus frequency is about 15–20. We might expect that the amplitude modulation of the SSVEP is a stochastic process, and as a consequence sideband energy is unlikely to be concentrated into a single frequency band. *Thus, given the typical ratio of SSVEP power to spontaneous EEG power and other sources of noise, we cannot distinguish between sidebands and spontaneous EEG activity at these frequencies.* Thus the SSVEP response can modulate in amplitude over the interval, perhaps by up to 50%. Similarly the SSVEP can be partly phase modulated (up to $\pm 90°$) over the recording interval and the sidebands produced cannot be distinguished from background EEG activity (Srinivasan et al. 1999).

The implication of these simulations and SSVEP data is that we cannot conclude that the SSVEP is a deterministic signal embedded in background noise based only on properties of the power spectrum. SSVEP power is a *statistical measure* of average amplitude and phase consistency over a large number of cycles of the flicker. Both amplitude and phase modulation can take place during the recording interval up to a modulation depth of about 50% and still be consistent with experimental observations. Of course, as amplitude modulation approaches 100% and phase modulation approaches $\pm 180°$, sideband power becomes larger than the power at the sinusoid frequency.

In order examine the time course of amplitude and phase in more detail during the recording, the method of *complex demodulation* (also called single-cycle Fourier coefficients) is used. This method estimates single-cycle Fourier coefficients by directly applying (9.7) to epochs of duration

$$T = n\Delta t = \frac{1}{f_s} \tag{9.25}$$

which corresponds exactly to the period of a single cycle of the stimulus frequency. These single-cycle coefficients are of course broadband estimates of Fourier coefficients, since with a stimulus frequency of 10 Hz, $T = 100$ ms and $\Delta f = 10$ Hz. To improve frequency resolution, the single-cycle Fourier coefficients can be averaged (as complex numbers) over cycles. If all single-cycle coefficients are averaged the result is identical to the FFT estimate of the Fourier coefficient at f_s using the same epoch of data. In typical applications, a running average of the single-cycle Fourier coefficients may be used to obtain a compromise between frequency resolution and information about the fluctuation of the SSVEP response using coherence measures. In applications to cognitive tasks, the single-cycle Fourier coefficients can be averaged separately in different experimental conditions.

Coherence estimates can be obtained from the single-cycle Fourier coefficients following the usual formula (9.11). However, interpretation of these results is more complicated because the recording apparently does not meet the condition of stationarity (since the mean of the signal defined by (9.11) is not constant). The mean signal $\mu(t)$ over K epochs (each the length of one stimulus cycle) is a waveform consisting of oscillations at the stimulus frequency and any harmonics that are present with consistent amplitude and phase across the cycles. This signal is represented by the FFT estimate using the entire record or equivalently the average of all the single-cycle Fourier coefficients.

The presence of time-varying mean signals (nonstationarity) implies that there are two independent mechanisms that can lead to increased coherence computed by (9.11) between the SSVEP (single-cycle Fourier coefficients) recorded at a pair of channels. (i) Each channel can become better synchronized to the stimulus resulting in the amplitude and phase becoming less variable across cycles. If there is no such variability, coherence is close to 1 (limited only by noise) and the signal is deterministic. This condition should cause an increase in SSVEP power and coherence due to improved signal-to-noise ratio. (ii) Alternatively, channel pairs can become better synchronized, that is, the *phase difference* between channels may become less variable even though the phase with respect to the stimulus remains variable. In this condition, coherence is expected to increase while SSVEP power is expected to remain constant at both channels. Of course, in most instances, both effects can occur simultaneously (and in opposite directions) leading to a more complicated relationship between SSVEP power and coherence.

Partial coherence measures are useful to elucidate the difference between synchronization to the stimulus (external synchrony) and synchronization between channels (internal synchrony) as discussed with experimental data in chapter 10. Partial coherence $\gamma^2_{uv|w}(f)$ between two channels (u and v) is a frequency-dependent measure of the proportion of variance at channel u that can be explained by a linear transformation of v after removing the influence of another channel w on both u and v (Bendat and Piersol 2001):

$$\gamma^2_{uv|w}(f) = \frac{|C_{uv|w}(f)|^2}{C_{uu|w}(f)C_{vv|w}(f)} \qquad (9.26)$$

The form of this equation is identical to the usual coherence (9.11) except that the cross spectrum has been replaced by the conditioned cross spectrum. Here $C_{uv|w}(f)$ is the conditioned cross spectrum:

$$C_{uv|w}(f) = C_{uv}(f) - \left[\frac{C_{uw}(f)}{C_{ww}(f)}\right]C_{wv}(f) \qquad (9.27)$$

where $C_{uv}(f)$ and the similar terms are the usual cross spectrum estimates given by (9.10). For this purpose, the factor of 2 introduced in (9.10) accounts for negative frequencies not used. If necessary, the conditioned estimates can be doubled to account for negative frequencies but for the purpose of coherence estimates the factor of 2 is irrelevant as coherence is identical at positive and negative frequencies.

If $u = v$ the conditioned cross spectrum reduces to the conditioned or partial power spectrum (Bendat and Piersol 2001):

$$C_{uu|w}(f) = P_{u|w}(f) = \left[1 - \gamma_{wu}^2(f)\right]P_u(f) \tag{9.28}$$

The conditioned power spectrum $P_{u|w}(f)$ is the power spectrum of channel u after removing the portion of variance that is coherent with w. Similarly, conditioned cross spectrum defined in (9.27) conditions the cross spectrum of u and v by removing signals that are coherent with w. Partial coherence is closely analogous to the usual partial correlation coefficients of ordinary statistics.

In the application of partial coherence analysis to SSVEP data, we are interested in studying dynamic properties of the amplitude and phase changes at the stimulating frequency (f_s). We want to separate coherence reflecting the synchronization of two channels from the synchronization of each channel to the stimulus. *In SSVEP analysis partial coherence is used to condition coherence estimates by removing the effect of signals that are coherent with stimulus.* Thus, w in (9.27) is the stimulus record s which maintains constant amplitude and phase throughout the recording. Without loss of generality, we assume that the stimulus amplitude is one and phase is zero. In other words, the Fourier coefficient at the stimulus frequency f_s of the stimulus signal from each cycle k, F_{sk} is always one. Then the cross spectrum $C_{us}(f)$ estimated with K epochs (or cycles) reduces to

$$C_{us}(f_s) = \frac{1}{K}\sum_{k=1}^{K} F_{uk}(f_s)F_{sk}^*(f_s) = \frac{1}{K}\sum_{k=1}^{K} F_{uk}(f_s) \tag{9.29}$$

Thus, the cross spectrum of each channel u with the stimulus s reduces to the average of the single-cycle Fourier coefficients $F_{uk}(f_s)$ or equivalently the FFT estimate of the Fourier coefficient from the entire record. Note that in (9.29) we do not double the estimate of cross spectrum to account for negative frequencies. The conditioned cross spectrum (9.27) then reduces to

$$C_{uv|s}(f_s) = C_{uv}(f_s) - C_{us}(f_s)C_{sv}(f_s) \tag{9.30}$$

The conditioning given by (9.30) reduces the cross spectrum by subtracting the product of the averaged single-cycle Fourier coefficients. If $u = v$, (9.30) reduces to the partial power spectrum

$$C_{uu|s}(f_s) = P_{u|s}(f_s) = P_u(f_s) - \left| \frac{1}{K} \sum_{k=1}^{K} F_{uk}(f_s) \right|^2 \qquad (9.31)$$

The relations (9.30) and (9.31) can be used with (9.26) to calculate the partial coherence.

The application of partial coherence to remove SSVEP responses that maintain constant amplitude and phase provides a means to measure phase locking between channels independent of the phase locking between each channel and the stimulus flicker. In SSVEP experiments, the phase of the steady-state response at each stimulus frequency can vary either because of genuine fluctuations in the phase of the response or simply because of additive noise. Furthermore, coherence between channels will appear to increase as a consequence of phase locking (decreased phase variability) of the response of each channel to the stimulus flicker. Coherence may also reflect genuine consistency in the variation of phase across trials at the two channels. This contribution to coherence reflects consistency in the relative phase of the response at two channels, in the presence of cycle-to-cycle variability in the steady-state response at the stimulus frequency (Srinivasan, 2004). In order to separate these two effects in coherence data, we introduce a partial coherence estimate to remove explicitly the contributions to observed coherence of phase locking to the stimulus. If partial coherence is high it indicates that the measured coherence is not simply a consequence of each location phase locking to the stimulus. In chapter 10 we examine the behavior of ordinary and partial coherence measures in an SSVEP experiment on binocular rivalry.

12   Spectra and Coherence in Coupled Oscillators

In order to demonstrate applications of spectral analysis, ordinary coherence, and partial coherence in a genuine physical system, these three measures are calculated here for a pair of coupled oscillators, which are driven (forced) by a common sinusoidal input as indicated in fig. 9-24 (Winter 2004). A van der Pol circuit was selected for each oscillator for several reasons. The unforced van der Pol circuit may be fully characterized by only two parameters: a characteristic frequency f_0 and a nondimensional nonlinear parameter A. The unforced system exhibits well-known *limit cycle oscillations*, with frequencies close to f_0 when A is small (Nunez 1995). Limit cycles differ from oscillations of damped linear systems in being self-sustaining: no external periodic input is required to keep the oscillations going. The forced system is known to exhibit a wide range of

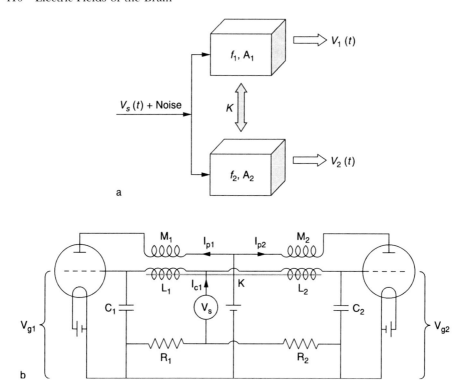

Figure 9-24 (a) A pair of coupled oscillators, which are driven (forced) by a common sinusoidal input voltage $V_S(t) = \cos(2\pi f_0 t) +$ noise. The output voltages from each oscillator are $V_1(t)$ and $V_2(t)$. Coupled van der Pol circuits were selected for simulations. Each oscillator is characterized by two dimensionless parameters: the resonance frequencies (f_1 and f_2 held fixed) and nonlinearity parameters (A_1 and A_2, varied with $A_2 = 1.2A_1$) (see Nunez 1995 for derivation of differential equation for single oscillator). The strength of inductive interaction between oscillators is given by K. (b) The van der Pol circuits are shown coupled by the pair of inductors indicated by the gray (metal) bar. The vacuum tubes (circles) provide the nonlinearity; $V_{g1} \equiv V_1(t)$ and $V_{g2} \equiv V_2(t)$ are their nondimensional grid voltages (system outputs). The common input voltage is V_S. Reproduced with permission from Winter (2004).

behavior, including simple oscillations at the driving frequency, oscillations containing multiple harmonics of the driving frequency, and chaotic oscillations.

These properties of the van der Pol system make it a useful (but, of course, vastly oversimplified) analog for the SSVEP studies described in chapter 10. The driving AC voltage of the two oscillators is then analogous to steady-state visual input to two brain hemispheres. The internal characteristic (resonant) frequencies f_1 and f_2 provide an analog to spontaneous EEG. The two oscillator outputs $V_1(t)$ and $V_2(t)$ may be considered crudely analogous to SSVEP signals recorded from the right and left hemispheres. We can vary the strengths of just two nondimensional parameters—the nonlinearity (A) and coupling between oscillators (K)—to see the effects on the two spectral outputs, as well as

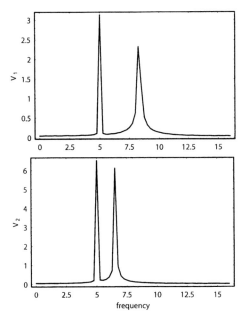

Figure 9-25 Amplitude spectra of the two outputs $V_1(t)$ and $V_2(t)$ for the linear $(A_1 = A_2 = 0)$ uncoupled $(K = 0)$ case. Both oscillators produce peaks at the driving frequency $(f_0$ in arbitrary units). The higher frequency peak in each output is the resonant frequency of the corresponding oscillator $(f_1 = 8.33$ and $f_2 = 6.53)$. Reproduced with permission from Winter (2004).

the coherence and partial coherence between the two outputs. This is accomplished by numerically solving the appropriate set of four first-order differential equations governing the behavior of the coupled oscillators and adding a small amount of white noise to the outputs. In the following simulations, the ratio of nonlinear parameters is held fixed, that is, $A_2/A_1 = 1.2$.

Figure 9-25 shows the amplitude spectra of the two outputs for the linear, uncoupled case. Both oscillators produce peaks at the driving frequency $(f_0 = 5)$. The higher frequency peak in each output spectrum is the (uncoupled) resonant frequency of the corresponding oscillator $(f_1 = 8.33$ and $f_2 = 6.53)$. Figure 9-26 shows the two amplitude spectra for uncoupled oscillators when nonlinear effects are small $(A_2 = 0.3)$. Interestingly, the addition of nonlinear interactions makes the outputs simpler in this example. Stronger nonlinearity does not alter this general result; that is, oscillations occur mainly at the driving frequency in the examples studied here.

Figure 9-27 shows the amplitude spectra for linear coupled oscillators $(K = 0.1)$. Each oscillator produces three frequency peaks: one peak at the driving frequency f_0 and two additional peaks occurring as a result of the interaction between the two systems. These new peak frequencies $(f_3$ and $f_4)$ are functions of the individual resonant frequencies and coupling

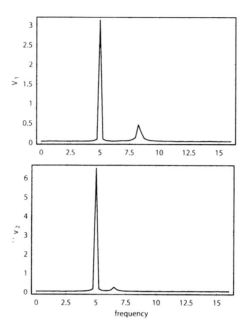

Figure 9-26 Amplitude spectra for uncoupled oscillators ($K = 0$) when nonlinear effects are small ($A_2 = 0.3$). The inclusion of non-linear dynamic behavior makes the outputs simpler in this example. Stronger nonlinearity does not alter this general result; oscillations occur mainly at the driving frequency as in the examples shown here. Reproduced with permission from Winter (2004).

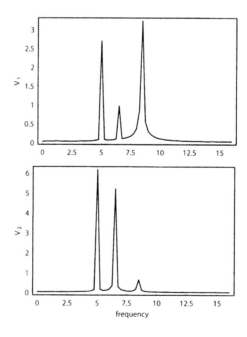

Figure 9-27 Amplitude spectra for linear coupled oscillators ($A_2 = 0$, $K = 0.1$). Each oscillator produces three frequency peaks: one peak at the driving frequency f_0 and two additional peaks f_3 and f_4 that differ from f_1 and f_2 as a result of the interaction between the two systems. Reproduced with permission from Winter (2004).

strength (f_1, f_2, and K) as illustrated in many similar systems, for example, coupled mechanical oscillators (Nunez 1995). The joint characteristic frequencies (f_3 and f_4) are approximately independent of the nonlinear parameters (A_1 and A_2) when these parameters are small. Figure 9-28 shows the nonlinear, coupled case ($A_1 = 0.3$, $K = 0.1$). Again, the addition of nonlinearity largely eliminates all but the driving frequency from the output signals.

The effects of coupling and nonlinearity on the ordinary and partial coherence between the two output signals $V_1(t)$ and $V_2(t)$ are illustrated in the following examples. The partial coherence estimate attempts to remove the common influence of the driving signal on the two outputs. Figure 9-29 shows the ordinary (top) and partial (bottom) coherence spectrum of $V_1(t)$ and $V_2(t)$ for linear, uncoupled oscillators. As expected, the ordinary coherence exhibits a sharp peak at the common driving frequency, whereas the partial coherence is essentially zero at all frequencies, accurately reflecting the fact that the oscillators are uncoupled.

The uncoupled, nonlinear example in fig. 9-30 is similar to the linear case; however, the effect of nonlinearity is to broaden the coherent band near the driving frequency and to introduce some nonzero ordinary and partial coherence outside the coherent band. Very strong nonlinearity ($A_2 = 6.0$, not shown) enhances this effect, notably by producing substantial peaks in both ordinary and partial coherence spectra at the third harmonic of the driving frequency $3f_0$.

The ordinary and partial coherence for the coupled, nonlinear case ($A_2 = 0.3$, $K = 0.3$) is shown in fig. 9-31. The three broad peaks in the ordinary coherence spectrum occur at f_0, f_3, and f_4. Note the contrast between the coherence spectra for this case and its amplitude spectra; the latter contain only a single dominant peak at f_0. That is, the coherence function is normalized to be mostly independent of amplitude differences so that small signals can produce large coherence. The partial coherence spectrum shown here is similar to the ordinary coherence spectrum except for the absence of coherence at the driving frequency f_0. Strong nonlinearity ($A_2 = 6.0$, not shown) tends to reduce both the ordinary and partial coherence at f_3 and f_4 and increase both coherence measures at the harmonic $3f_0$, as well as higher odd harmonics.

What have these simulations of coupled oscillators to do with real brains? First, we have presented these simulations primarily as a way to demonstrate the behaviors of coherence and partial coherence measures on an actual physical system. Second, these simulation results may stimulate our thinking about the origins of SSVEP power and coherence, and the ample evidence of harmonic responses, thereby helping us to interpret existing SSVEP data as well as to suggest experimental modifications or entirely new experiments. We must, of course, be quite cautious about extrapolating ideas about dynamic behaviors of driven physical systems to genuine brain science.

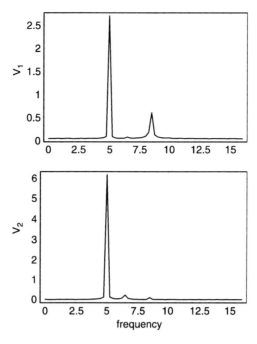

Figure 9-28 Amplitude spectra for the nonlinear, coupled case ($A_2 = 0.3$, $K = 0.1$). Again, the addition of nonlinearity largely eliminates all but the driving frequency from the output signals. Reproduced with permission from Winter (2004).

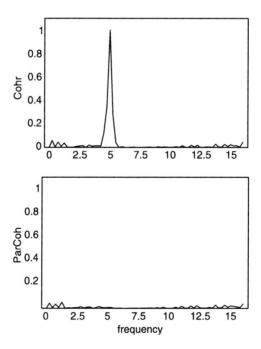

Figure 9-29 Coherence spectra. The ordinary (top) and partial (bottom) coherence spectrum of $V_1(t)$ with $V_2(t)$ for linear, uncoupled ($A_2 = 0$, $K = 0$) oscillators. As expected, the ordinary coherence exhibits a sharp peak at the common driving frequency, whereas the partial coherence is essentially zero at all frequencies, accurately reflecting the fact that the oscillators are uncoupled. Reproduced with permission from Winter (2004).

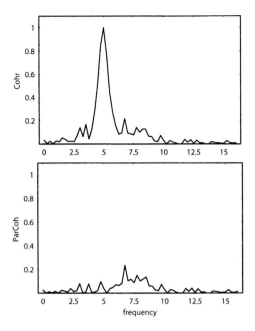

Figure 9-30 Coherence spectra. The uncoupled, nonlinear $(A_2 = 0.3, K = 0)$ example is similar to the linear case shown in fig. 9-29; however, the effect of nonlinearity is to broaden the coherent band near the driving frequency and to introduce some nonzero ordinary and partial coherence outside the coherent band.

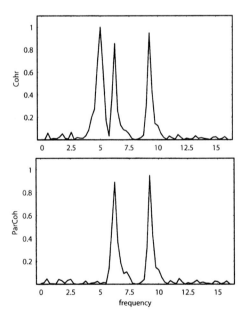

Figure 9-31 Coherence spectra. The ordinary and partial coherence for the coupled, nonlinear case $(A_2 = 0.3, K = 0.3)$. The three broad peaks in the ordinary coherence spectrum occur at f_0, f_3, and f_4. Note the contrast between the coherence spectrum for this case and its amplitude spectra (fig. 9-28); the latter contain only a single dominant peak at f_0. That is, the resonant frequencies of the coupled system show up clearly in the coherence spectra, but are largely absent from the amplitude spectra.

13 Spatial-Temporal Spectral Density Functions and Wave Propagation

Scientists who typically think of brains in terms of isolated sources or networks may find these sections on wave phenomena unnecessary or even rather tedious. They may ask what these physical waves have to do with real brains (Tucker 2000). One answer is that brain networks and waves can coexist, as in the case of networks immersed in a global environment of standing waves. Or, perhaps in some brain states, waves and networks can be complementary descriptions of the similar brain phenomena. To cite an example from another field, descriptions of traveling waves in automobile traffic are *sometimes useful*, but this does not mean that traffic patterns are generally waves, or that individual automobiles are unimportant, or wave descriptions are useful most of the time. Thus, the question *Are brain waves really waves?* is not the right question for this chapter. A better question is whether the temporary adoption of a wave-like picture of EEG recorded in some brain states may facilitate experimental designs that reveal new information about neocortical dynamics and cognition. The question of whether we are measuring genuine EEG waves is addressed in chapters 10 and 11.

The spectral density function of a field $\Psi(x, t)$ given by (9.22) can generally be applied to any physical phenomenon. A special category of fields is given the label *waves* in the physical sciences. Waves normally have the property that higher temporal frequencies occur with higher spatial frequencies as described by a relationship between spatial and temporal frequencies, the so-called *dispersion relation*:

$$\omega = \omega(k) \tag{3.29}$$

In this case, most of the coefficients Z_{nm} in the sum (9.22) are small (ideally zero). For example, consider the instantaneous potential $\Psi(x, t)$ in a transmission line forming a closed loop of length $L = 100$ m. The transmission line's physical properties include a characteristic velocity v (somewhat less than light velocity in a vacuum) and electromagnetic theory yields the dispersion relation:

$$\omega_n^2 = \omega_0^2 + v^2 k_n^2 \tag{3.33}$$

The oscillation frequency ω_n has two parts, a *local part* given by ω_0 and a *global part* $v^2 k_n^2$.

The transmission line potential $\Psi(x, t)$ is the sum of all modes as given by (9.22); however, each spatial mode n oscillates at a single frequency given by (3.33) so that the double sum over (n, m) in (9.22) may be replaced by a single sum over n. For example, the second spatial mode $(n = 2)$ has a wavenumber (spatial frequency) $k_2 = 0.1257$ m^{-1} or a spatial wavelength of 50 m. Suppose $v = 10^7$ m/s and $\omega_0 = 10^5$/s, then the oscillation frequency of the $n = 2$ mode (*second harmonic* or *first overtone*) is $\omega = 1.26 \times 10^6/\text{s}$ or $f = 200$ kHz. In chapters 10 and 11, we discuss reasons why our putative brain waves may be expected to show some rough correspondence between frequency and wavenumber. Generally, however, each temporal frequency is likely to be associated with a range of wavenumbers because of medium inhomogeneity, nonlinearity, and other factors.

The *Schumann resonances* discussed in chapter 3 provide an example of wave phenomena in two spatial dimensions; in this case wave propagation takes place in a thin spherical shell (topologically similar to one hemisphere of neocortex and its white matter layer). Like the closed loop of transmission line, the spherical shell dictates periodic boundary conditions to any continuous field variable. As a result, only waves with wavelengths dictated by the shell geometry can persist. For a linear, homogeneous medium with characteristic speed v and no local frequency contributions, the resonant frequencies in a thin spherical shell are given by

$$\omega_n = \frac{v\sqrt{n(n+1)}}{R} \quad n = 1, 2, 3 \ldots \tag{3.40}$$

As in the transmission line, the resonant frequencies consist of the fundamental mode ($n = 1$) and overtones ($n = 2, 3, 4, \ldots$). Also, as in the example of the transmission line, the overtones are not harmonics. However, in this case lack of harmonic overtones is due to the two dimensional geometry, rather than local properties in the transmission line. A theoretical dispersion relation for *quasi-linear brain waves* is discussed in chapter 11.

Figure 9-32 provides a simple example of undamped waves (that propagate without loss of energy) passing under a line of simulated "electrodes" spaced by 2.7 cm starting at electrode 1 ($x = 0$). In all the examples, the waves have a characteristic temporal frequency $f_n = 3$ Hz and spatial frequency with magnitude $|k_n| = 0.028$ cycles/cm. The first example (fig. 9-32a) shows a wave traveling from the bottom of the electrode array (13) to the top (1). The second example (fig. 9-32b) shows a wave traveling from the top (1) to the bottom of the electrode array (13). These two waves have different spectral density function with one peaked at $k = -0.028$ cycles/cm and the other peaked at $k = +0.028$ cycles/cm. The third example (fig. 9-32c) shows a case where both waves are present. In this case the two waves interfere constructively at some locations (electrodes 1, 7, and 13, doubling local amplitude) and interfere destructively at other locations (electrodes 4 and 10, canceling the signal). Perfect interference (in this idealized case) results in a standing wave. The spectral density function of this process exhibits two peaks: one at positive k and one at negative k.

Figure 9-33 shows the wavenumber spectra obtained from a linear array of 13 electrodes on the midline in an SSVEP experiment with different

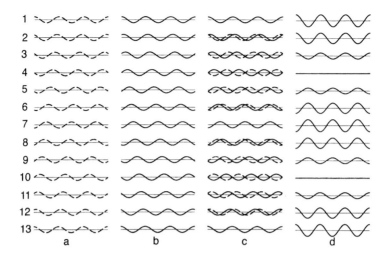

Figure 9-32   Simulation of a 3 Hz traveling under an array of 13 electrodes with zero damping. A 1 s window is displayed. (a) Wave traveling from the bottom to the top of the array, with $k = -0.028$ cycles/cm. A progressive phase shift in the sine waves is evident. (b) Wave traveling from the top to the bottom of the array with $k = +0.028$ cycles/cm. The phase shift occurs in the opposite direction. (c) The two waves shown in (a) and (b) are plotted on the same axes to illustrate the origins of interference. (d) Sum of the two waves shown in (a) and (b) showing the end result of wave interference: a standing wave.

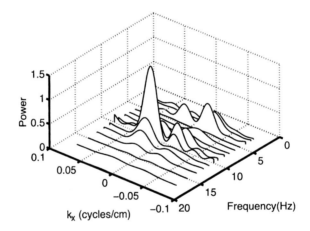

Figure 9-33   Wavenumber spectra of the SSVEP calculated with an array of 13 electrodes along the midline. The frequency label for each curve indicates the stimulating (driving) frequency. The wavenumber spectra were calculated using only the Fourier coefficient at the stimulating frequency at each electrode. Positive k indicates waves traveling from the back to the front (away from visual cortex). Negative k indicates waves traveling from front to back. Equal power at positive and negative k indicates a standing wave. The large peak $[f, k] \approx \{10 \text{ Hz}, 0.025 \text{ cycles/cm}\}$ or $[\omega, k] \approx \{63/\text{s}, 0.16 \text{ cm}^{-1}\}$ indicates a back-to-front traveling wave with phase velocity ≈ 400 cm/s along the scalp or about 800 cm/s along the folded cortical surface, consistent with corticocortical propagation speeds.

stimulation frequencies. Example power spectra at one channel from this experiment are shown in fig. 9-22. The wavenumber spectra in fig. 9-33 were obtained using (Nunez 1981)

$$P(f_s, k_x) = \frac{1}{K^2} \sum_{i=1}^{N} \sum_{j=1}^{N} C_{ij}(f_s)e^{j2\pi k_x(x_i - x_j)} \tag{9.32}$$

where C_{ij} is the cross spectrum between channels i and j located at x_i and x_j.

The wavenumber spectra were calculated at the stimulus frequency along one spatial dimension using $N = 13$ channels located on the midline. The coordinate system was selected so that positive k corresponds to waves traveling from the back to the front of the head, and negative k to waves traveling from the front to the back. The wavenumber spectra shown depend strongly on the stimulus frequency with a strong peak when $f_s = 10.0$ Hz. The wavenumber spectrum at 10.0 Hz is peaked sharply at $k \sim 0.025$ cycles/cm (~ 0.16 cm^{-1}) indicating that the spatial structure of the signal resembles a wave traveling from the back to the front on the scalp (away from visual cortex), approximately resembling fig. 9-32a. The phase velocity of this (apparent) wave packet is about 400 cm/s along the scalp or about 800 cm/s along the folded cortical surface as discussed in section 13. When the stimulus frequency is 9 Hz, power is comparable at $k \sim +0.025$ and $k \sim -0.025$ cycles/cm, more resembling a standing wave pattern, approximately like the simulation in fig. 9-32d. When the stimulus frequency is 4 Hz, waves are detected in both directions but slightly stronger in front to back directions. At least over this limited set of electrodes, it appears that different input frequencies can elicit different wave patterns in SSVEP experiments, although we have only examined a small number of electrodes on the midline in this example.

We presented this example in order to illustrate wavenumber spectra in a simple one-dimensional case where the waves can be easily visualized. In EEG, we are often more interested in spatial spectra on a two-dimensional surface. In order to prepare our readers for the experimental EEG spatial spectra discussed in chapter 10, we show the frequency response function for waves in a spherical shell in fig. 9-34A. These are the Schumann resonances (driven by white noise), but with spatial filtering to simulate the effects of volume conduction on EEG. Figure 9-34B shows the spatial-temporal spectral density function for the same simulated data shown in fig. 9-34A, but normalized so that each temporal frequency band has equal total power when summed over the five spatial modes (without this normalization nearly all power would be shown near 10 Hz). The horizontal axis is frequency (Hz) and the vertical axis is spatial mode n (the degree of the corresponding spherical harmonic function). Figure 9-34B

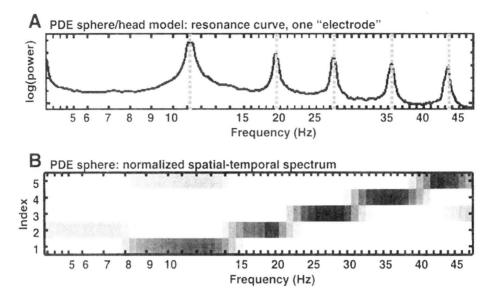

Figure 9-34 (A) The frequency response of a Schumann-like system when driven by white noise. Numerical solutions to the appropriate wave equation were obtained in a spherical shell and then passed through a volume conductor model to simulate spatial filtering. The two plots are based on 5 minutes of simulated data. In (A) the location (electrode) of the surface samples was chosen to avoid nodal lines. The numerical method was chosen over the usual analytic solution to allow for later inclusion of inhomogeneous and nonlinear effects (not shown). The dashed vertical lines are the frequencies given by (3.40) with characteristic medium velocity $v = 750$ cm/s and effective sphere radius $R = 15$ cm (after inflation to create a smooth cortical surface as discussed in chapter 11). (B) Spatial-temporal spectral density function for the same simulated data shown in (A), but normalized so that each temporal frequency band has equal total power when summed over the five spatial modes (without this normalization nearly all power would be shown near 10 Hz). The horizontal axis is frequency (Hz) and the vertical axis is spatial mode n (the degree of the corresponding spherical harmonic function, that is spatial frequency labeled "index"). The plot was obtained by sampling the upper half of the outer spherical surface (scalp) at 131 locations and applying the methods of spherical harmonic decomposition described in Wingeier et al. (2001). Identical methods were applied to EEG data as discussed in chapter 10. Reproduced with permission from Wingeier (2004).

was obtained by sampling the upper half of the outer spherical surface (scalp) at 131 locations and applying the methods of spherical harmonic decomposition described by Wingeier et al. (2001). Identical methods were used to estimate the spatial-temporal spectral density function for EEG data as discussed in chapter 10.

14 Measuring Wave Phase Velocity

Two generally distinct velocity measures are needed to describe wave propagation in complex media since such media are likely to be *dispersive*.

In such media, waves generally distort as they propagate. The measures are *phase velocity* and *group velocity*. Generally, a wave packet is composed of many component waves with individual velocities labeled phase velocities. Group velocity refers to velocity of the entire packet. In the case of nondispersive waves, phase and group velocities are equal. In this section we focus on phase velocity estimates. Group velocity estimates for EEG data are obtained in chapter 10.

Consider a field $\Psi(x, t)$ in a one-dimensional medium like a transmission line loop. For simplicity, we first focus on a single spatial mode n. From (9.22) the sum of two wave components traveling in opposite directions is given by

$$\Psi_n(x, t) = A\cos[\omega(k_n)t - k_n x] + B\cos[\omega(k_n)t + k_n x] \quad (9.33)$$

When the constant $B = 0$, the wave travels in the positive x direction. Similarly, when $A = 0$, the wave travels in the negative x direction. When $A = B$, the two traveling waves perfectly interfere and form a standing wave. However, the most general case $A \neq B$, A and $B \neq 0$ results in a mixture of traveling and standing waves.

How can we apply these ideas to EEG? Suppose we obtain bipolar recordings from an array of closely placed electrodes along the midline. The potential difference between adjacent electrode sites then yields an approximation to the scalp tangential electric field (halfway between adjacent electrodes). This measured field $\Psi(x, t)$ is independent of the reference electrode and is generally a more local measure than referenced potentials. The next step is to estimate the relative phase angle associated with the frequency $\omega(k_n)$ at each location of electric field estimate. For example, 12 midline electrodes yield 11 bipolar phase estimates. Phase estimates may be obtained several ways. Fourier transform methods are appropriate if (i) long records are used so that estimated phases correspond to narrow temporal frequency bands and (ii) most of the raw EEG signal is contained in a relatively narrow frequency band.

To connect the following examples more closely to EEG, we imagine a model cortical hemisphere with an anterior–posterior circumference (in and out of cortical folds) of about 80 cm (about 40 cm along the smooth dura). Our first imagined electrode array spans 20 cm of cortex (10 cm along the scalp). Electrode spacing is 2 cm (cortex) or about 1 cm on the scalp.

The phase function for (9.33) at frequency $\omega(k_n)$ obtained by Fourier transform is

$$\theta_n(x) = \arctan\left[\frac{A - B}{A + B}\tan(k_n x)\right] \quad (9.34)$$

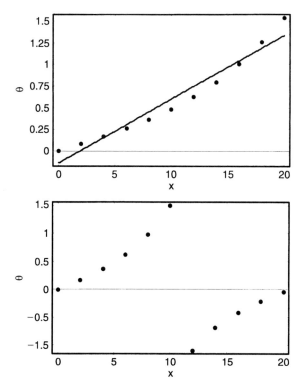

Figure 9-35 (*Upper*) The simulated phase is obtained from a mixture of traveling and standing waves, that is (9.34) with $B/A = 0.3$ (traveling wave mostly in the positive x direction), wave of cortical wavelength 81 cm (spatial frequency $k_1 = 2\pi/81 = 0.0776$ cm^{-1}), and sampling at 11 locations (2 cm spacing) over a little less than $1/4$ of this spatial wavelength, that is, $0 < x < 20$ cm on the cortex or $0 < x < 10$ cm at the scalp. Linear regression indicates excellent agreement with the traveling wave hypothesis. The correlation coefficient is 0.977 and the slope of the linear regression line is 0.0735 cm^{-1} in close agreement with the actual spatial frequency k_n. (*Lower*) The spatial mode is chosen to have a 41 cm wavelength ($k_2 = 2\pi/41 = 0.0153$ cm^{-1}). Linear increase of phase angle with x only occurs up to the location $k_2 x = \pi/2$, at which point the estimated angle abruptly changes sign due to the ambiguity associated with the arctan operation.

The spatial derivative of this phase angle is

$$\frac{\partial \theta_n}{\partial x} = \frac{(A^2 - B^2)k_n}{A^2 + B^2 + 2AB\cos(2k_n x)} \tag{9.35}$$

which reduces to $\pm k_n$ if B or A equals zero. Figure 9-35 (upper) demonstrates the results of a study for which the simulated phase is obtained from (9.34) with $B/A = 0.3$ (traveling wave mostly in the positive x direction with partial interference), cortical mode spatial frequency $k_1 = 2\pi/81 = 0.0776$ cm^{-1}, and sampling at 11 locations (2 cm spacing) over a little less than $1/4$ of this spatial wavelength, that is, $0 < x < 20$ cm on the cortex. The linear regression indicates excellent agreement with the traveling wave hypothesis. The correlation coefficient is 0.977 and the slope of the linear regression line is 0.0735 cm^{-1} in close agreement with the actual spatial frequency k_n.

The second simulation, illustrated in fig. 9-35 (lower), is identical to the first, except that the spatial mode is chosen to have a 41 cm wavelength, that is, $k_2 = 2\pi/41 = 0.0153$ cm^{-1}. A near linear increase of phase angle with x is again obtained, but only up to the location $k_2x = \pi/2$ at which point the estimated angle abruptly changes sign due to the ambiguity associated with the arctan operation. We could try to avoid this by basing phase velocity estimates on progressively shorter parts of the sensor array, but this procedure is severely limited by the poor spatial resolution available at the scalp.

In order to overcome the difficulty of phase angle flip when the EEG contains substantial power at wavelengths shorter than four times the length of the electrode array, the following procedure may be adopted.

(i) Use a Fourier transform to estimate the phase angle $\theta_n(x)$ at each location x along the array for some segment of data, defining zero phase at $x = 0$. For example, suppose SSVEP power is confined to a narrow band centered at the driving frequency. Accurate phase angle estimates for single cycles may be obtained if data are digitized with an integer number of points per cycle as discussed in section 10.

(ii) Calculate the phases associated with a range of wavenumbers k_q ($q = 1, Q$) from the expression

$$\theta_q(x) = \arctan[\tan(k_qx)] \tag{9.36}$$

(iii) Calculate the root mean square error associated with each trial wavenumber k_q using

$$\text{Error} = \sqrt{\frac{1}{Q}\sum_{q=1}^{Q}[\theta_n(x) - \theta_q(x)]^2} \tag{9.37}$$

The best estimate of k_n is expected for the choice of k_q that results in the minimum error.

Simulations of the above procedure are demonstrated in fig. 9-36. In each of these examples, the (simulated) experimental phase was calculated from (9.34) with $B = 0.1$ (minimal wave interference) and a $\pm 15\%$ random noise term (uniform distribution) added to each experimental phase calculation. The algorithm found rms errors from (9.37) by stepping

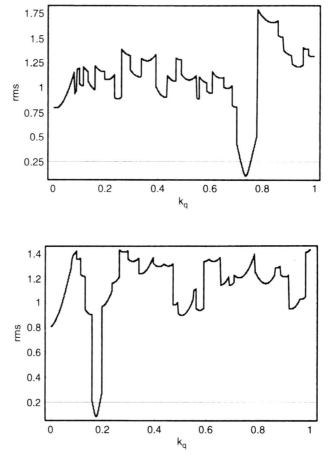

Figure 9-36 The wavenumber estimates k_n are based on trial values of k_q that minimize the error function (9.34) in several simulations. In each of these examples, the (simulated) experimental phase was calculated from (9.34) with $B = 0.1$ (minimal wave interference) and a uniformly distributed $\pm 15\%$ random noise term added to each experimental phase calculation. RMS errors are plotted versus k_q using (9.34) by stepping through trial values of k_q in increments of 0.001 cm^{-1}. This error function is shown in the upper plot for a traveling wave of length 8.45 cm or wavenumber $k_n = 0.744$ cm^{-1}. The sharp minimum in the upper plot occurs for a trial k_q close to the actual wavenumber. The traveling wave used to obtain the lower plot has a length of 36.27 cm or wavenumber of 0.173 cm^{-1}, also correctly identified by the error function (9.34).

through trial values of $k_q = [0, 1]$ cm^{-1} in increments of 0.001 cm^{-1}. This error function is shown in the upper plot of fig. 9-36 for a traveling wave of length 8.45 cm or wavenumber $k_n = 0.744$ cm^{-1}. The sharp minimum in the upper plot occurs for a trial k_q close to the actual wavenumber. The traveling wave used to obtain the lower plot of fig. 9-36 has a wavelength of 36.27 cm. Overall, the wavenumber estimates are quite accurate, although shorter waves result in broader minima in the error function. The error minima are quite robust even with much larger noise levels. For example, an error minima for the 8.45 cm wave was found at approximately the correct k_q with $\pm100\%$ noise added to calculated phase in the simulated data. The statistical significance of these error minima can be tested in separate simulations by using identical phase sets, but associated with random locations x along the array. A similar statistical test is to replace the simulated experimental data with random numbers and determine the magnitudes of false minima in the error function. When applied with these conditions, such false minima are typically in the 0.6 to 0.8 range as compared to the 0.2 range shown in fig. 9-36.

15 Empirical Orthogonal Functions and PCA

The spectral density function (9.22) requires the choice of a basis functions (a set of orthogonal functions) for the time and space variables. The time variables are naturally decomposed in Fourier series. If there is one spatial dimensional as in (9.22) Fourier series can also be applied to model the spatial dimension. If there are two spatial dimensions, as in a plane medium, a double Fourier series, one over each spatial dimension, is the natural choice. On a spherical surface, spherical harmonics are a useful set of basis functions. Spherical harmonic decompositions are used in chapter 10 to examine the spatial spectra of EEG data.

An alternative approach is to make no assumptions about the appropriate spatial basis functions, but rather to obtain the basis functions directly from the data itself (Nunez 1981). At any frequency, these *empirical orthogonal functions* can be estimated by *principal components analysis* (PCA) (Johnson and Wichern 1998). New developments in these techniques such as *independent component analysis* (ICA) (Bell and Sejnowski 1995) and *second-order blind identification* (Belouchrani et al. 1997) improve the statistical properties of this estimate by taking into consideration higher-order moments and correlation at different lags, respectively. Since these methods are relatively new, we do not attempt to evaluate them here, rather we consider some general spatial properties of the EEG covariance matrix that will influence estimates obtained with any of these techniques. As discussed throughout this chapter, volume conduction significantly influences the structure of EEG covariance as defined by the spatial filtering of cross-spectral density function (9.15).

In principal components analysis the eigenvalues and eigenvectors of the covariance matrix are evaluated to estimate the spatial basis functions. Although often applied to time series data, this method can also be applied to the cross-spectral density matrix $\mathbf{C}(f)$ with each row containing the cross spectrum of one channel with every other channel at a single frequency. This matrix is Hermitian, a mathematical label meaning here that the cross spectrum between channels u and v is the complex conjugate of the cross spectrum between channels v and u, a result following directly from the definition of the cross spectrum (9.10). As a consequence the eigenvalues

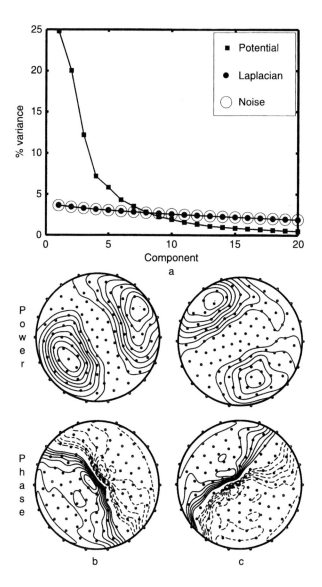

Figure 9-37 The effect of volume conduction on principal components analysis (PCA) methods to estimate empirical orthogonal functions. In this simulation, 3600 Gaussian random noise mesosources were used to simulate scalp potentials in the 4-sphere model of volume conduction in the head. Each simulation consisted of 1000 epochs, and was repeated 100 times. Scalp potential and surface Laplacians were calculated at 111 electrode locations for a dipole layer at a radius $r_z = 7.8$ cm in the 4-sphere model. Model parameters are: shell radii $(r_1, r_2, r_3, r_4) = (8, 8.1, 8.6, 9.2)$ and conductivity ratios $(\sigma_1/\sigma_2, \sigma_1/\sigma_3, \sigma_1/\sigma_4)$ $= (0.2, 40, 1)$. (a) Horizontal axis is the eigenvalue component; vertical axis is the percentage of variance accounted for by each eigenvalue. Eigenvalues of the cross spectral density matrix are obtained at one arbitrary frequency with the potentials, surface Laplacians, and random noise at 111 electrodes. Eigenvalues are expressed as a percentage of the total power (or variance) of the signals. The estimates were averaged over 100 simulations. In the case of random noise, each (mesosource) eigenvalue (large empty circles) is a small percentage of the total variance. By contrast, the first two simulated scalp potential eigenvalues (black squares) reflect 45% of the variance in the signal. The surface Laplacian eigenvalues (small black circles) are nearly identical to the random noise case.

are real and positive and reflect the variance (or power) associated with the spatial pattern given by the eigenvectors. The eigenvectors are complex valued and represent the normalized amplitude and phase at each electrode. Each set of eigenvectors represents uncorrelated modes of variability of the oscillations in one frequency band.

Estimating empirical orthogonal functions can be a useful means of data compression, perhaps as an aid to statistical analysis in cognitive tasks. However, the orthogonal functions based on scalp potentials are not connected to the underlying physiology in any obvious way. One important reason is that *volume conduction imposes spatial structure on the covariance matrix, so that estimated spatial structure is caused by both volume conduction plus any genuine mesosource spatial structure* (Silberstein and Cadusch 1992). Figure 9-37 illustrates this idea using a simple simulation of 3600 Gaussian random noise sources in a 4-sphere model of the head. Scalp potentials and surface Laplacians were calculated at 111 scalp electrodes for 100 different simulations, each consisting of 1000 epochs. For comparison purposes, we also made use of 111 uncorrelated Gaussian random noise signals with the same number of epochs. The eigenvalues of the cross spectrum matrix at one frequency obtained in each case were averaged over the 100 simulations and are expressed as a percentage of total variance (the sum of the eigenvalues) in fig. 9-37a. As expected in the simulations using Gaussian random-noise signals, the eigenvalues have similar magnitudes so that the largest eigenvalue represents less than 5% of the total variance. In the ideal case of perfectly uncorrelated signals generating an infinite data set, all eigenvalues should be equal, and each eigenvector should be sharply peaked at one electrode.

In order to simulate scalp potentials, the Gaussian random-noise sources were first passed through the 4-sphere head model. Simulated scalp potentials were then used to form the cross-spectral density matrix. In this case, the largest eigenvalue accounts for 25% of the variance and the second largest eigenvalue accounts for another 20% of the variance, even though none of the underlying sources are correlated. Figure 9-37b and c show the power (squared magnitude) and phase distribution for the first two eigenvectors (corresponding to the two largest eigenvalues). These eigenvectors show remarkably simple spatial structure, reminiscent of the potential distribution due to a tangential dipole. These patterns are also qualitatively similar to spherical harmonics of degree 1.

Volume conduction effects cause substantial spatial structure in scalp potentials even though the underlying sources have no such structure. The Laplacian removes this erroneous structure. (b) The eigenvector corresponding to largest eigenvalue for scalp potentials from one simulation. The eigenvector is complex valued, and represented here as power (squared amplitude) and phase. Note that the pattern resembles the field of a tangential dipole or a spherical harmonic of degree $n = 1$. (c) Same as (b), but showing the eigenvector corresponding to the second largest eigenvalue.

The implication of this simulation is that simple spatial structure can be found in volume-conducted EEG signals, even when there is no spatial structure in the underlying mesosource dynamics. Of course, in applications to real EEG data, genuine source coherence will also give rise to spatial structure but these two origins of spatial structure are not easily distinguished and may in fact interact with each other. By comparison to the results based on simulated scalp potentials, the surface Laplacian estimate (obtained by sampling the surface potentials) removes the artificial spatial structure due to volume conduction so that the Laplacian-based eigenvalues are nearly identical to the noise-based eigenvalues (fig. 9-37a). In this example, the Laplacian-based PCA provides a much more realistic representation of the underlying dynamics than is obtained from the potential-based PCA.

Potential-based (Nunez 1981) and Laplacian-based (Nunez 1995) eigenvalues for resting alpha rhythm suggest much more spatial structure than can be accounted for by volume conduction alone, but the relative contributions of mesosource structure and volume conduction to the eigenvectors remains unclear.

16 Summary

A general working framework for the experimental study of the large-scale dynamics of EEG is suggested here, including interpretation of data recorded at different spatial and temporal scales. This *stochastic field* framework is neutral with respect to local, regional, and global mechanisms generating EEG. We suggest that the relative importance of these contributions to EEG dynamics can vary substantially with animal species, brain state, frequency band, and measurement scale. We view source dynamics as a stochastic ("random") process having statistical properties that change with changes in behavior and cognition. This general framework has an important advantage over viewpoints that may prejudge the nature of EEG dynamics, thereby biasing experimental design. For example, dipole localization studies can only provide accurate pictures of underlying dynamics when applied to EEG phenomena that are genuinely generated by a few isolated sources. We recognize that the physiological bases for EEG are controversial and that several competing models have been widely published. The general dynamic framework advocated here for EEG analysis encompasses each of these models as a special case. As such it should be relatively noncontroversial.

We explicitly acknowledge here that brains are complex systems that can be studied with a wide range of experimental and data analysis methods. We avoid any attempts to choose the "best" methods of EEG or SSVEP data analysis because any such optimization procedure requires prior knowledge of the underlying source dynamics. Given this limitation, we have emphasized Fourier-based methods to estimate power, phase, coherence, and closely related dynamic measures in distinct frequency bands. Our stochastic field framework does not limit our methods in any obvious way. We retain complete freedom to measure important dynamic properties without prejudging the underlying nature of the source dynamics. This freedom is demonstrated with genuine EEG and SSVEP data in chapter 10.

References

Bell AJ and Sejnowski TJ, 1995, An information-maximation approach to blind separation and blind deconvolution. *Neural Computation* 7: 1129–1159.

Belouchrani A, Abed-Meriam K, Cardoso JF, and Moulines E, 1997, A blind source separation technique using second-order statistics. *IEEE Transactions on Signal Processing* 45: 434–444.

Bendat JS and Piersol AG, 2001, *Random Data. Analysis and Measurement Procedures*, 3rd Edition, New York: Wiley.

Chen Y, Seth AK, Gally JA, and Edelman GM, 2003, The power of human brain magnetoencephalographic signals can be modulated up or down by changes in an attentive visual task. *Proceedings of the National Academy of Sciences USA* 100: 3501–3506.

Cooper R, Winter AL, Crow HJ, and Walter WG, 1965, Comparison of subcortical, cortical, and scalp activity using chronically indwelling electrodes in man. *Electroencephalography and Clinical Neurophysiology* 18: 217–228.

Delucchi MR, Garoutte B, and Aird RB, 1975, The scalp as an electroencephalographic averager. *Electroencephalography and Clinical Neurophysiology* 38: 191–196.

Ding M, Bressler SL, Yang W, and Liang H, 2000, Short-window spectral analysis of cortical event-related potentials by adaptive multivariate autoregressive (AMVAR) modeling: data preprocessing, model validation, and variability assessment, *Biological Cybernetics*, 83:35–45.

Ebersole JS, 1997, Defining epileptogenic foci: past, present, future. *Journal of Clinical Neurophysiology* 14: 470–483.

Habeck CG and Srinivasan R, 2000, Natural solutions to the problem of functional integration. *Behavioral and Brain Sciences* 23:402–403.

Johnson RA and Wichern DW, 1998, *Applied Multivariate Statistical Analysis*, 4th Edition, New Jersey: Prentice Hall, pp. 458–513.

Katznelson RD, 1982, *Deterministic and Stochastic Field Theoretic Models in the Neurophysics of EEG*, Ph.D. Dissertation, La Jolla: University of California at San Diego.

Lachaux JP, Lutz A, Rudrauf D, Cosmelli D, Le Van Quyen M, Martinerie J, and Varela F, 2002, Estimating the time-course of coherence between single-trial brain signals: an introduction to wavelet coherence. *Electroencephalography and Clinical Neurophysiology* 32: 157–174.

Le Van Quyen M, Foucher J, Lachaux J, Rodriguez E, Lutz A, Martinerie J, and Varela FJ, 2001, Comparison of Hilbert transform and wavelet methods for the analysis of neuronal synchrony. *Journal of Neuroscience Methods* 111: 83–98.

Lopes da Silva FH, 1999, Dynamics of EEGs as signals of neuronal populations: models and theoretical considerations. In: E Niedermeyer and FH Lopes da Silva (Eds.), *Electroencephalography. Basic Principals, Clinical Applications, and Related Fields*, 4th Edition, London: Williams and Wilkins, pp. 76–92.

Lopes da Silva FH and Storm van Leeuwen W, 1978, The cortical alpha rhythm in dog: the depth and surface profile of phase. In: MAB Brazier and H Petsche (Eds.), *Architectonics of the Cerebral Cortex*, New York: Raven Press, pp. 319–333.

Morse PM and Feshbach H, 1953, *Methods of Theoretical Physics*, New York: McGraw Hill.

Nunez PL, 1974, Wave-like properties of the alpha rhythm. *IEEE Transactions on Biomedical Engineering* 21: 473–482.

Nunez PL, 1981, *Electric Fields of the Brain: The Neurophysics of EEG*, 1st Edition, New York: Oxford University Press.

Nunez PL, 1995, *Neocortical Dynamics and Human EEG Rhythms*, New York: Oxford University Press.

Nunez PL, 2000a, Toward a quantitative description of large scale neocortical dynamic function and EEG. *Behavioral and Brain Sciences* 23: 371–398 (target article).

Nunez PL, 2000b, Neocortical dynamic theory should be as simple as possible, but not simpler. *Behavioral and Brain Sciences* 23: 415–437 (response to commentary by 18 neuroscientists).

Percival DB and Walden AT, 1993, *Spectral Analysis for Physical Applications: Multitaper and Conventional Univariate Techniques*, Cambridge, UK: Cambridge University Press.

Petsche H and Etlinger SC, 1998, *EEG and Thinking. Power and Coherence Analysis of Cognitive Processes*, Vienna: Austrian Academy of Sciences.

Petsche H, Kaplan S, von Stein A, and Filz O, The possible meaning of the upper and lower alpha frequency ranges for cognitive and creative tasks. *International Journal of Psychophysiology* 26: 77–97.

Petsche H, Pockberger H, and Rappelsberger P, 1984, On the search for sources of the electroencephalogram. *Neuroscience* 11: 1–27.

Pfurtscheller G and Lopes da Silva FH, 1999, Event-related EEG/MEG synchronization and desynchronization: basic principles. *Electroencephalography and Clinical Neurophysiology* 110: 1842–1857.

Regan D, 1989, *Human Brain Electrophysiology*, New York: Elsevier.

Silberstein RB, 1995, Steady state visually evoked potentials, brain resonances and cognitive processes. In PL Nunez (Ed.), *Neocortical Dynamics and Human EEG Rhythms*, New York: Oxford University Press.

Silberstein RB and Cadusch PJ, 1992, Measurement processes and spatial principal components analysis. *Brain Topography* 4: 267–276.

Silberstein RB, Nunez PL, Pipingas A, Harris P, and Danieli F, 2001, Steady state visually evoked potential (SSVEP) topography in a graded working memory task. *International Journal of Psychophysiology* 42: 219–232.

Srinivasan R, 2004, Internal and external neural synchronization during conscious perception. *International Journal of Bifurcation and Chaos*, 14: 825–842.

Srinivasan R, Russell DP, Edelman GM, and Tononi G, 1999, Increased synchronization of neuromagnetic responses during conscious perception. *Journal of Neuroscience* 19: 5435–5448.

Tass P, Rosenblum M, Weule J, Kurths J, Pikovsky A, Volkmann J, Schnitzler A, and Freund H-J, 1998, Detection of n:m phase locking from noisy data: application to magnetoencephalography. *Physical Review Letters* 81: 3291–3294.

Tucker DM, 2000, Real brain waves. *Behavioral and Brain Sciences* 23: 412–413.

Wingeier BM, 2004, *A High Resolution Study of Coherence and Spatial Spectral in Human EEG*, Ph.D. Dissertation, New Orleans: Tulane University.

Wingeier BM, Nunez PL, and Silberstein RB, 2001, Spherical harmonic decomposition applied to spatial-temporal analysis of human high-density electroencephalogram. *Physical Review E* 64: 051916-1–9.

Winter W, 2005, *A Study of the Interaction Between Coupled Nonlinear Oscillators: A Metaphor for Brain Wave Dynamics*, Honors Thesis, New Orleans: Tulane University.

10

Spatial-Temporal Properties of EEG

1 Complementary Measures of EEG Dynamics

The motivations for this chapter are twofold: (i) to provide example applications of time series analysis and high-resolution methods to genuine EEG and steady-state visually evoked potential (SSVEP) data and (ii) to provide an overview of scalp EEG's most salient dynamic properties. Such efforts to pin down robust dynamic properties should require no justification for physical scientists. In contrast, animal physiologists, cognitive scientists, and medical scientists often think in terms of cortical or thalamocortical networks with emphasis on localized cell groups. Coherence and other measures of phase locking between tissue masses appear to fit naturally into this network picture. However, other dynamic measures like phase and group velocity, dispersion relations, phase transitions, and so forth, which are normally associated with physical phenomena, may seem less interesting to neuroscientists (Tucker 2000).

The short answer to this implied criticism is that complex systems, including brains, may be studied with many seemingly disparate dynamic measures. The conceptual framework outlined in chapter 1 and summarized in fig. 1-8 is based on this general idea. We conjecture cell assemblies (or networks) embedded within global cortical fields of synaptic activity. Why introduce these synaptic fields in the first place? Because they appear to be much more closely related to scalp recorded EEG than network activity. That is, in any particular cognitive experiment, a scalp electrode measures some (unknown) combination of network and global field activity. However, even if the cognitive network makes no direct contribution to measured scalp potential, it may still make an indirect contribution by altering the global field as suggested in fig. 1-8. In either case, a robust relationship between cognitive processing and EEG dynamics may be established.

Throughout this book, we use the labels *local* and *global* in two distinct but closely related contexts. When discussing experimental EEG data, our labels "local" and "global" refer to more dominant high and low spatial frequencies, respectively, somewhat analogous to the time-domain labels "fast" and "slow" oscillations. When discussing physical theory (chapter 3) or neocortical dynamic theory (chapter 11), the labels "local" and "global" refer to the basic mechanisms underlying the field oscillations. Local and global physiological mechanisms may tend to facilitate more local and global dynamic EEG behaviors, respectively. However, substantial two-way interactions between local networks and global fields are expected to cloud distinctions between "local" and "global" in both theory and experiment.

We here adopt the working hypothesis that local network dynamics, interactions between networks, and network–global field interactions (both bottom-up and top-down) are all potentially important. However, one of the central messages of this book is that different experimental designs and data analysis methods can bias EEG toward either local or global physiological interpretations. For example, a number of excellent studies have examined oscillatory activity at cellular and local network scales (Freeman 1975, 1992; Lopes da Silva 1991, 1995, 1999; Singer 1993; Steriade 1999). But millimeter-scale dynamic properties are not generally observed on the scalp because of spatial filtering by the volume conductor. That is, scalp EEG is strongly biased towards the more globally coherent dynamics that occupies the very low end of the spatial frequency spectrum. By contrast, we expect intracranial electrodes to record much larger potentials just because of their close proximity to local sources. Furthermore, *smaller intracranial electrodes often record larger potentials because of less cancellation of positive and negative source contributions* (review in Nunez 1995). Thus, in distinct contrast to scalp recordings, intracranial recordings are generally biased toward more locally dominated dynamic properties.

Given this picture, one can easily see why an animal physiologist or clinician recording from human cortex might observe quite different dynamic properties than those reported for scalp EEG, even when both groups focus on the same frequency band. *One scientist sees only the trees; the other sees only the forest.* One example is that reported ECoG propagation velocities across the cortex are typically in the millimeter/second range, consistent with intracortical propagation. By contrast, in states for which robust propagation can be identified at the human scalp, measured velocities are roughly 100 times faster, in the 5 to 10 cm/s range. Such velocities are consistent with propagation in corticocortical fibers as discussed in sections 10 and 11 of this chapter and again in chapter 11. One of the central challenges in EEG is to forge the appropriate cross-scale connections between intra- and extracranial data. By studying this issue of distinct scales with both experiments and theory, EEG scientists can design more thoughtful experiments to interpret global dynamic properties like long-range phase locking as well as locally dominated dynamics.

To illuminate the differing viewpoints of scientists recording scalp EEG and those recording from inside the cranium, consider the following musical metaphor. Imagine an orchestra playing Tchiakovsky's Piano Concerto No. 1 in New York's Central Park. Consider the different sounds heard or recorded by (i) an audience at substantial distance from the stage and (ii) a microphone attached to one of the flutes. The former group observes the (large-scale) coordinated activity of the entire orchestra, reflecting the vision of the composer. By contrast, local microphones mainly record the local instruments. Two "musical scientists" observing the same orchestra may come to quite different conclusions about the observed musical dynamics. The scientist recording more distant (global) musical data appreciates the vision of the composer and the coordination of multiple instruments to create a rewarding experience. By contrast, the scientist monitoring local flute sounds may hear only the local music, although with increased clarity. This local scientist, along with colleagues monitoring the clarinets, strings, and so forth will have valuable information to pass on to any global scientist attempting to understand the underlying bases for the concerto. At the same time, the global scientist has important large-scale information unavailable to the local scientist. Of course, if every instrument in the orchestra had an attached microphone, the concerto could perhaps be constructed by suitable integration of the local sounds.

In the brain context, genuine intracranial recordings have enormous practical limitations: severe under-sampling, uncertain cross-species extrapolations, and the apparent fractal-like dependence of measured dynamics on electrode size. For these reasons the lesson of our musical metaphor is substantially understated. In summary, *while intracranial data provide critical information, they fall short of providing the gold standard for characterizing large-scale neocortical dynamic behavior*. We have to be very clever to relate successfully the multiple data scales of electrophysiology.

2 An Overview of Human Alpha Rhythms

Discussion of human spontaneous EEG begins appropriately with alpha rhythms for both historical and clinical reasons (Kellaway 1979; Niedermeyer 1999a). Scalp alpha rhythms provide the appropriate starting point for clinical EEG exams. Initial clinical questions ask whether the patient exhibits an alpha rhythm with spatial-temporal characteristics that are age appropriate. In most adults, alpha rhythms consist of frequencies in the 9–11 Hz range when recorded from the scalp with eyes closed.

Classic alpha rhythms may be recorded in roughly 95% of healthy adults with closed eyes. By "classic" we refer to the common clinical definition of near-sinusoidal oscillations observed in raw paper or computer traces; however, "nonalpha" EEG classified this way may actually exhibit substantial spectral power in the alpha band as suggested by the simulations of chapter 9. In fact, clinicians may label rhythms with dominant 10 Hz components as nonalpha if they are not sufficiently "clean"; that is, containing a broad range of frequency components superimposed on the alpha rhythm. Normal waking alpha rhythms usually have larger amplitudes over posterior regions, but are typically recorded over widespread scalp regions. Alpha amplitude in 75% of normal adults lies in the range 15 to 45 μV when recorded from the posterior bipolar electrodes P4-O2 (6.5 cm spacing); amplitudes recorded from frontal electrodes are lower (Kellaway 1979). Tangential electric fields in the scalp are in the range of approximately 5 to 20 μV/cm for a variety of EEG phenomena.

A posterior rhythm of approximately 4 Hz develops in babies in the first three months after birth. It increases in amplitude with eye closure and is believed to be the precursor of mature alpha rhythm (Niedermeyer 1999b; Fisch 1999). Posterior scalp alpha amplitudes in children older than about three years are substantially larger than adult amplitudes, perhaps due partly to volume conduction effects, for example, incomplete skull "closure" (in the electrical if not physical sense). By contrast, anterior amplitudes and anterior–posterior coherence is substantially lower in children than in adults (Srinivasan 1999). Maturation of the alpha rhythm is characterized by increased alpha frequency and coherence between ages of about three and ten (Thatcher 1996). A corresponding reduction in delta activity (0 to 4 Hz) is also common. Such delta reductions may continue through age 25 to 30 (Pilgreen 1995; Niedermeyer 1999b), a time when myelination of corticocortical fibers is nearly complete (Yakovlev and Lecours 1967; Courchesne 1990).

Normal awake alpha rhythms may be "blocked" (substantially reduced in amplitude) by eye opening, drowsiness, and by moderate to difficult mental tasks. EEG phenomena typically exhibit an inverse relationship between amplitude and frequency (Barlow 1993). Hyperventilation and some drugs often cause reduction of alpha frequencies together with increased amplitudes (Bickford 1979). This effect may occur with alcohol, for example (Shichijo et al. 1999). Other drugs, notably barbiturates, are associated with increased amplitude of the small amount of beta activity often superimposed on scalp alpha rhythms (Niedermeyer and Lopes da Silva 1999). The physiological bases for inverse relations between amplitude and frequency and most other salient characteristics of EEG are unknown, although several physiologically based theories have been advanced to account for such properties, as outlined in chapter 11. For example, limit cycle oscillations typically occur at larger amplitudes with lower frequencies. The most obvious influence on scalp amplitudes is the spatial scale of the synchronous sources forming the underlying cortical dipole layer (the *effective correlation length*) as indicated in figs. 1-20, 9-7, and 9-8. To the extent that higher temporal frequencies are generated by smaller dipole layers (more relative power at higher spatial frequencies), we expect lower scalp amplitudes to be associated with higher frequencies.

The EEG literature sometimes treats alpha primarily as a unitary occipital-parietal rhythm. In extreme cases, a few "equivalent alpha dipoles" have been proposed to account for observed data. Yet in the classic studies by Jasper and Penfield (1949), alpha rhythms were recorded from nearly the entire upper cortical surface (including frontal and prefrontal areas) in a large population of patients awake prior to surgery as indicated in fig. 1-5. The exceptions involved regions close to the central motor strip where dominant beta activity (>13 Hz) was reported. These classic studies were published without using spectral analysis so the magnitude of alpha contribution to rhythms reported as "nonalpha" is unknown.

Some discrepancy of views about the spatial distribution of alpha can be explained as follows. First, EEG clinical populations are biased toward patients who are older, have neurological problems, and may be anxious during the recording. These factors tend to work against production of robust, widespread alpha rhythms. Second, the clinical definition of alpha is based on raw waveforms rather than spectra. With this view, "alpha rhythms" have quasi-sinusoidal waveforms, that is, a distinct spectral peak (or peaks) between 8 and 13 Hz. Often alpha is identified clinically by simply counting zero crossings. While this definition of alpha is apparently appropriate clinically, it can provide misleading views of possible physiological bases. The reason is that raw EEG composed of broad frequency bands can appear very "nonalpha" to visual inspection, even though amplitude spectra show a substantial (or even maximum) contribution from the alpha frequency band as in the simulations of chapter 9. This potential misconception can be especially pronounced when the raw record contains substantial beta activity (>13 Hz), which tends to attract the eye and increase number of zero crossings, perhaps leading to overemphasis in qualitative descriptions. A third reason for differing views about spatial properties of alpha is that the human alpha band contains multiple rhythms and origins that potentially interact to varying degrees in different brain states. Some alpha phenomena are widely distributed and some are more localized. In this context, we repeat the following description by EEG pioneer Grey Walter (quoted in Basar et al. 1997) based on extensive intracranial recordings

> We have managed to check the alpha band rhythm with intra cerebral electrodes in the occipital-parietal cortex; in regions which are practically adjacent and almost congruent one finds a variety of alpha rhythms, some are blocked by opening and closing the eyes, some are not, some respond in some way to mental activity, some do not. What one can see on the scalp is a spatial average of a large number of components, and whether you see an alpha rhythm of a particular type or not depends on which component happens to be the most highly synchronized processes over the largest superficial area; there are complex rhythms in everybody.

In scalp recordings, larger frontal alpha is often observed as subjects become more relaxed, for example, while slowly counting breaths or with other relaxation techniques. Alpha rhythm of unusually large amplitude, occurring over the entire scalp, and sometimes exhibiting frontal dominance, may be associated with mental retardation in children (Bickford 1973) or some types of epilepsy (Kellaway 1979). Large amplitude frontal alpha rhythms may also be recorded in coma and anesthesia states (Nunez 1981, 1995; Niedermeyer and Lopes da Silva 1999; Fisch 1999). In summary, frontal alpha rhythms of moderate amplitude are common in healthy relaxed subjects with closed eyes as shown in figs. 1-4 and 10-5. Widespread alpha of large amplitude (often larger in frontal regions) may occur with trauma, disease, or anesthesia. The physiological relationships between these disparate alpha phenomena are unknown. Nevertheless, because they have similar frequencies (similar time constants), one may conjecture that they share some underlying physiology.

3 A High-Resolution Experimental Study of Human Rhythms

Sections 3 through 9 of this chapter outline an experimental study of relationships between spontaneous EEG and cognition carried out at the Brain Sciences Institute in Melbourne, Australia, over the period 1999–2001 (Nunez et al. 2001; Wingeier et al. 2001; Wingeier 2004). Our motivation for presenting these data and analyses methods is to demonstrate: (i) high-resolution EEG, (ii) quantitative measures emphasizing both local and global dynamic behavior, (iii) the quasi-stable global phase structure of alpha rhythm, (iv) the sensitivity of EEG dynamic properties to measurement scale, and (v) upper alpha and theta phase locking during mental calculations. The cognitive task was chosen mainly as a convenient means to manipulate EEG properties, rather than to study specific cognitive functions. Our experimental measures directly address theoretical dynamic models, brain binding, and the functional significance of EEG. We show that different measures of EEG dynamics can substantially bias physiological interpretations toward either extreme local or extreme global physiological interpretations.

Spontaneous EEG was recorded from five healthy subjects with eyes closed. One subject (BMW) was studied a second time on another day. The general dynamic behavior of his EEG was found to be reproducible (unless otherwise noted below). The resting state was alternated each minute with a mental calculation task (the "cognitive period," also eyes closed). Resting and cognitive periods were each repeated four to six times (depending on subject) to obtain a series of one-minute alternating periods with 7 to 11 transitions between distinct brain states. Three subjects were chosen for detailed analyses based on data being nearly free of obvious artifact in all channels.

A commercial electrode cap with 131 embedded electrodes (diameter = 0.5 cm) was used to record EEG. Electrode placement and impedance checks required approximately one hour. Average center-to-center and edge-to-edge electrode spacing were 2.2 and 1.2 cm, respectively. Because of gel spreading beyond electrodes, the effective edge-to-edge separation was somewhat less than 1 cm. Each data channel was tested individually to ensure that no salt bridges between electrode pairs occurred due to excessive gel spreading. In order to maintain good electrode contact, reference and ground electrode impedances were checked regularly and kept below 10 kΩ by re-abrading the local scalp or shifting the electrode. In addition EEG raw waveform signal spectra were monitored visually to maintain minimal line noise (50 Hz in Australia) as suggested in chapter 7. Electrode positions are shown in fig. 10-1. Signals were band-pass filtered with cutoffs at 0.5 and 80 Hz and subsequently digitized at 500 Hz.

Data were recorded with respect to a right ear reference with amplifiers grounded to the nose using the EEG system described by Simpson (1998). A separate channel recorded left ear potential with respect to the right ear.

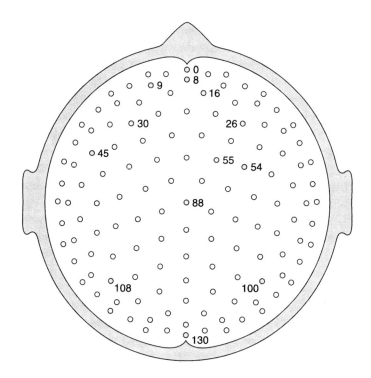

Figure 10-1 These 131 electrode positions were used in several simulations in chapters 8 and 9 and for EEG recordings in sections 3–9 of this chapter. Circles shown are smaller than effective electrode sizes (0.5 cm diameter plus gel). Average center-to-center and edge-to-edge electrode spacings are 2.2 and 1.2 cm, respectively. The electrode cap was purchased from Electro-Cap International Inc., Eaton, Ohio. Reproduced with permission from Nunez et al. (2001).

Prior to analyses, data were transformed to the instantaneous digital average potential of the two ears to provide data consistent with other laboratories; however, almost none of the results shown here are based on this mathematically linked-ears reference. Rather, data were transformed to the common average reference and then passed through the Melbourne dura imaging algorithm. Artifact rejection was by visual inspection of raw data. In several cases a few bad data channels (less than five) were replaced by nearest-neighbor interpolations because of high impedance, degraded connections, or other malfunctions. Muscle and eye blink artifact were also recorded in two subjects, mainly to facilitate interpretation of power and coherence results for the delta, beta, and gamma bands where the ratio of signal to artifact noise is typically low in EEG studies.

Recording sessions started with a five-minute period when subjects were asked to relax with eyes closed, using slow breath counting or other personal relaxation exercises. Each one-minute mental calculation period was seeded with a two digit integer X and involved summing the series $X + (X + 1) + (X + 2) + (X + 3) + \cdots$ to sums of several hundred. A break of 10 seconds between each one-minute period allowed subjects to make comfortable transitions between states, that is, to get back into relaxed states after each cognitive pressure period. This mental task had several important technical features making it easy to implement with EEG: minimal artifact because of closed eyes and lack of motor components, ease of task lengthening to improve statistics, and robust changes of amplitude and coherence with brain state changes (Nunez 1995; Nunez et al. 1997, 1999). However, the task was not "clean" from a cognitive science viewpoint. That is, the task combined a short-term memory component (holding both the last number and the partial sum of the series in short term memory) and an active component (adding the partial sum to the next largest integer). Obtaining fine distinctions between these mental processes is appropriate for separate studies, hopefully putting the methods and data reported here to efficient use. However, this project was mainly concerned with robust dynamical properties of human spontaneous EEG, which were easily and reliably manipulated with this simple mental task.

Standard (MATLAB release 11) fast Fourier analysis was applied to each data channel using a Hanning window, often with one-second epochs providing 1.0 Hz frequency resolution. Other studies involved five-second epochs to obtain 0.2 Hz frequency resolution. Real and imaginary Fourier coefficients yielded magnitude, phase, and coherence estimates based on the average potential of the two ears or common average reference. In a few cases, phase estimates were based on the Hilbert transform (MATLAB release 11) for comparative purposes. For *dura imaging* calculations, raw data were transformed to potentials referenced to the instantaneous average potential of all 131 electrode sites (the *common average reference*). With large electrode arrays, the common average reference potential normally approximates the theoretical potential at infinity (Bertrand et al.

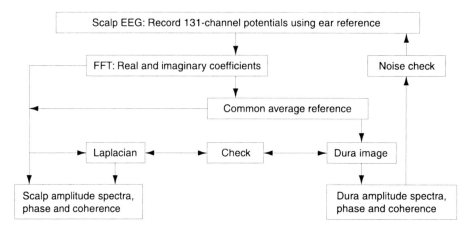

Figure 10-2 Outline of methods used in the high-resolution study of spontaneous EEG. Laplacian and dura image algorithms may be applied either before or after the fast Fourier transform (FFT), but the latter approach is computationally much faster when only very limited frequency ranges are analyzed. Periods with obvious artifact were eliminated by visual inspection (not shown). The check for agreement between Laplacian and dura imaging was applied to a subset of the data. No one-second epochs with substantial differences in spatial properties were found. (Note that such close agreement requires dense electrode arrays.) The "Noise check" box refers to the purposeful addition of noise to raw data (or Fourier coefficients) to test robustness of high-resolution estimates (especially phase). See Group 5 of table 8-1 for a noise check example.

1986; Srinivasan 1999) as discussed in chapter 7. As such, it is the appropriate reference for submission to the Melbourne dura imaging algorithm. Transformation to average reference has no effect on spline-Laplacian estimates, which are entirely reference free.

The average-referenced data were passed through the dura imaging algorithm to obtain spatially filtered (high-resolution) estimates of amplitude, phase, and coherence as indicated in fig. 10-2. Dura estimates were spot checked against the spline-Laplacian algorithm (using ear-referenced data), which also provided estimates of dura potential as shown in chapter 8. No substantive differences between Melbourne dura image (with zero smoothing parameter) and New Orleans spline-Laplacian estimates of dura potential were found (see table 8-1). Note that Laplacian and dura imaging algorithms may be applied either before or after Fourier transform. That is, the algorithms may accept either raw EEG data or real and imaginary Fourier coefficients, but not power which lacks phase information. Computation is much faster if the fast Fourier transform (FFT) is applied first because only the part of the bandwidth with relatively large signal-to-noise ratio is of interest. Dura imaging of raw data was only implemented to check software and to produce a few example dura image time series.

Peak power plots, used to supplement information obtained from average amplitude spectra, were obtained as follows. Four- to six-minute records corresponding to estimates of resting scalp potential, resting dura potential, cognitive scalp potential, and cognitive dura potential were divided into five-second epochs for each of the 131 channels. Fourier transforms then yielded estimates of amplitude (or power) versus frequency with 0.2 Hz resolution for each channel and for each epoch. The frequency component on the interval ($3 \leq f \leq 20$ Hz) with maximum power for a particular channel and epoch was stored for plotting. The lower delta range ($f \leq 2.8$ Hz) was excluded from the peak power test because delta artifact (due to subject movement, eye blinks and movement, EKG, and so forth) is very difficult to distinguish from genuine source dynamics. Power at frequencies greater than 15 or 20 Hz was generally very low. We were not confident that we could reliably distinguish beta and gamma brain rhythms from artifact in the spontaneous EEG so these frequency ranges are not emphasized here, although some of our beta band results may be brain related.

The method of peak power defines each five-second epoch at each electrode site by a single frequency that best characterizes that epoch. This procedure has several motivations. First, a better feeling for nonstationary EEG behavior is obtained than by using only average amplitude spectra. Second, it allows spectral properties over the entire scalp to be viewed in a single plot. Most importantly, the dominant frequency components in low-amplitude signals show up nicely. This feature is important for frontal regions, which often exhibit lower EEG amplitudes over most frequency bands.

Phase estimates were obtained at each electrode site for each one-second epoch by transforming real and imaginary Fourier coefficients so that a zero phase angle was obtained at Cz (site 88 in fig. 10-1). Without such transformation, "phase" would be physiologically meaningless, depending on the arbitrary separation times of records into epochs. Phase estimates are often sensitive to noise, especially at locations with low amplitude signals or when based on short time segments. In order to test this sensitivity, phase estimates presented here were spot-checked by purposely adding 15% uncorrelated noise directly to raw EEG data and, in separate tests, by first passing the noise through a forward head model to simulate intracranial biologic noise, which was spatially correlated only because of the head volume conductor (see "Noise check," fig. 10-2). Thus, our conclusions about EEG phase estimates are based on the conservative proposition that genuine noise of this magnitude might have contaminated raw data. Delta, beta, and gamma frequency ranges typically have much lower signal to (artifact) noise ratios than theta and alpha bands. Delta or beta phase appeared to be much less well defined in our data because of phase instability, low signal to noise ratio, or some combination of factors.

As discussed in chapter 9, coherence is a correlation coefficient (squared); it provides one important measure of dynamic relations between signals (scalp or dura) recorded at pairs of electrode sites. We defined phase based on records over a range of epochs, between one second and one minute with FFT methods. In addition, a 1 Hz band *instantaneous phase*, based on the Hilbert transform, was also used to check FFT-based phase estimates. Tests for consistency of such phase estimates over time and frequency band provided supplementary information about accuracy and stability of neocortical phase structures.

Our coherence estimates are based on Fourier coefficients for one-second epochs, averaged over five-minute periods. Such averages over 300 epochs provide high statistical confidence, but fail to provide information about variations in phase synchrony over time. Coherence issues relating to statistical significance, volume conduction, reference electrode, high-resolution estimates, and interpretation at multiple spatial scales are discussed in chapters 8 and 9 and in several references (Nunez 1995; Nunez et al. 1997, 1999). In the current study, each coherence estimate was associated with one minute of data (resting or cognitive periods) for each of the $131 \times 130/2 = 8515$ electrode pairs and each 1 Hz band. Many coherence changes were fully consistent with all (7 to 11) transitions between brain states, as demonstrated in an earlier study (Nunez et al. 1999).

4 Topography of Resting Alpha Rhythms

Scalp amplitude distributions of resting alpha rhythm at six successive times are displayed in fig. 10-3. Individual plots are separated by about

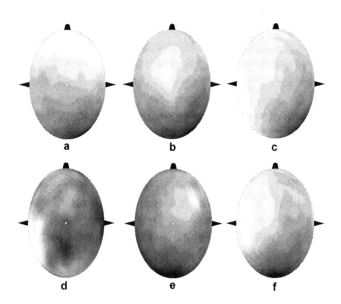

Figure 10-3 The alpha potential topography for one subject. Amplitude distributions of (average referenced) resting alpha rhythm at six successive times separated by about 90 ms are shown in (a–f). The times correspond to positive peaks in the potential recorded by posterior-midline electrode 130. Each plot was constructed by averaging over five adjacent time slices with 2 ms separation between adjacent slices. Amplitudes were normalized with respect to the maximum positive and negative potentials. Plots generated by Wingeier (2004).

100 ms and correspond to positive peaks in the average reference potential recorded by posterior-midline electrode 130. Each plot was constructed by averaging over five adjacent time slices to minimize noise effects, a 10 ms average with the 500 Hz sample rate. This step was not needed for raw potentials since single time slices (very short time averages) were very similar to the 10 ms averages. Rather the averaging was introduced to smooth the dura imaging waveforms. Generally, anterior and posterior scalp potentials oscillate out of phase, dynamics corresponding to the low end of the spatial frequency spectrum (mostly $n = 1$ or 2 of the spherical harmonics). Dura spatial patterns shown in fig. 10-4 exhibit far more complexity than the corresponding raw scalp potentials as a result of filtering out the very low spatial frequencies, which are associated with volume conduction as well as any genuine low spatial frequency dynamic source patterns that may occur (as discussed in chapter 8). *We have no way to distinguish these two contributions to the low end of the scalp spatial frequency spectrum.* The New Orleans spline-Laplacian and Melbourne dura imaging algorithms yield nearly identical patterns as expected from table 8-1.

All magnitudes in figs. 10-3 and 10-4 were normalized with respect to potential extrema observed within the 10 ms period in order to facilitate comparisons between scalp and dura estimates. This is an appropriate step because, in simulations, dura imaging and spline-Laplacian algorithms accurately estimate relative, but not absolute, potential magnitudes. The reasons are clear: absolute scalp potentials and Laplacians depend strongly

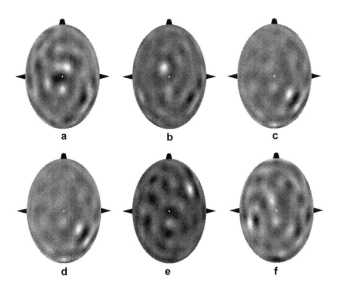

Figure 10-4 Estimates of dura potential for the same data shown in fig. 10-3, obtained by passing average referenced data through the Melbourne dura imaging algorithm (with smoothing parameter set to zero). Normalized dura potentials are plotted. The New Orleans spline-Laplacian yields very similar patterns of dura potential; correlation coefficients obtained with an electrode-by-electrode comparison are in the 0.95 range. Plots generated by Wingeier (2004).

on skull tissue resistance and Laplacians (microvolts/cm^2) do not even have electric potential units.

The plots in figs. 10-3 and 10-4 demonstrate that alpha rhythms present distinct maps when different cycles are observed or when viewed at different spatial and temporal scales. Each time slice of scalp potential (roughly the 5–10 cm spatial scale and 10 ms temporal scale) exhibits a generally different spatial distribution. The corresponding dura image estimates (roughly the 2–3 cm and 10 ms scales) show that when low spatial frequency scalp potentials (due to some unknown combination of volume conduction and genuine source dynamics) are filtered out, the remaining spatial patterns are complex and quite variable over time.

Time averaging, obtained by either averaging amplitude maps or Fourier coefficients, generally produces a potentially misleading picture of the spatial distribution of alpha sources. Time averaging over (say) one-minute records may produce topographic maps that are relatively consistent from minute to minute, that is, stable spatial structures at one-minute time scales. However, no such stability is observed at the 10 ms timescale. In summary, the better the time and spatial resolutions, the more detail is observed in amplitude maps, at least down to some limiting resolution. This fractal-like behavior of scalp EEG appears to be limited to timescales greater than about 10 ms. That is, with most phenomena we do not find more detail by increasing the sampling rate above about 100 Hz, the brainstem auditory evoked potential being an exception. We are not able to approach an equivalent limiting spatial scale with scalp recordings. No such scale is likely to be found even with intracortical electrodes where dynamic behavior is likely to be a sensitive function of electrode size and location; that is, *fractal all the way down to the molecular level and below*.

Subject BMW produced two distinct frequency peaks in the alpha band, at 8.5 and 10.0 Hz. Lower and upper alpha peaks generally have different spatial distributions over the scalp, as shown in earlier studies (Nunez 1974, 1981; Nunez et al. 2001); this dynamic property held for subject BMW. Our conceptual framework outlined in fig. 1-8 and the data shown in figs. 8-12 and 8-13 suggest that local alpha (and other) networks may be immersed in a global alpha environment as discussed in more detail in chapter 11. If these alpha networks are relatively fixed in location, this idea suggests that cross-frequency dura amplitude estimates of alpha rhythm may be more similar to each other than the corresponding cross-frequency scalp amplitudes. That is, we conjecture that if we compare amplitude (square root of power) maps across different parts of the alpha band, the dura image maps will be more similar to each other than the potential maps. This conjecture is based on the idea that smaller regions of alpha generation are more spatially stable than the global process. Fixed dipoles provide an extreme example in which the local regions are quite small. By contrast, substantial changes in global mode spatial patterns are conjectured to occur as frequency changes, as in the case of standing waves in physical systems and possibly neocortex (see chapters 3 and 11).

To investigate this idea in a subject with a double alpha peak, we computed cross-frequency (8.5 and 10.0 Hz) correlation coefficients for 300 successive one-second epochs, for both log(scalp potential amplitude) and log(dura image amplitude). Correlation coefficients were obtained from 92 electrode-by-electrode comparisons, excluding the outer ring of 39 electrodes where dura estimates are less accurate. The average (over 300 epochs) cross-frequency scalp potential correlation was 0.169, whereas the average cross-frequency dura image correlation was 0.307. That is, *the local spatial properties of low- and high-frequency alpha oscillations were more similar to each other than the corresponding global spatial properties.*

This result may, at first, appear counterintuitive: the smooth maps of potential are less stable across frequencies than the complex dura maps. *However, this outcome is consistent with the presence of relatively stable (in space) local networks operating over several frequencies within the alpha band (or the entire band), but immersed in global standing waves of synaptic action that encompasses the same range of frequencies.* This result is very tentative because it has been verified in only the one subject with a clear double alpha peak. Furthermore, we do not have a direct check of dura image accuracy, which is somewhat limited by head model accuracy. For these reasons, we do not claim verification of any theory. Rather, the methods are presented here as a suggestion for future study.

5 Spectral Properties of Resting Alpha

Amplitude spectra recorded in two subjects in the resting state are shown in figs. 1-4 and 10-5. Potentials in fig. 10-5 were recorded with respect to the digital average potential of the two ears, mainly for easier comparisons with other laboratories. The four scalp locations are channels 30 and 26 (left and right frontal, upper row) and channels 108 and 100 (left and right posterior, lower row). These electrode positions are shown in fig. 10-1. These are typical spectra for young, healthy, relaxed subjects (and many not so young). They indicate dominance of alpha rhythms over most of the scalp. In order to view changes in spectral properties over the entire scalp with changes in brain state and spatial scale, we adopted plots of peak power in five-second epochs as discussed in section 2.

The global effects of spatial filtering are illustrated by the estimates of peak power in fig. 10-6. As discussed in section 3, each five-second epoch of each data channel was Fourier transformed to find the single frequency component with the highest amplitude (0.2 Hz resolution). All smaller frequency peaks were excluded by this procedure. The scalp (left) and dura (right) peak power estimates for three subjects are shown. The smaller electrode numbers on vertical axes near the upper parts of these plots correspond to frontal scalp locations (see fig. 10-1). Each peak power plot contains (60 five-second epochs) × (131 electrodes) or 7860 plotted points. The dominance of alpha band activity over the entire scalp is evident in all

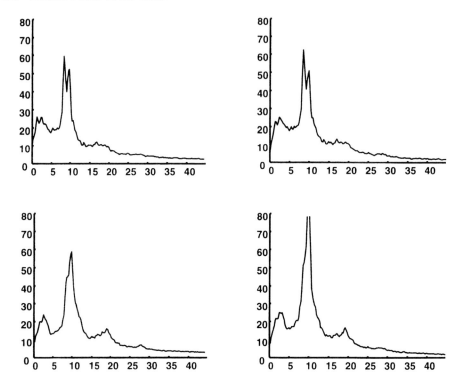

Figure 10-5 Amplitude spectra based on 5 minutes of resting EEG (0.2 Hz resolution) with eyes closed, referenced to the digitally averaged potential of the two ears. The subject is a 38-year-old female engineering graduate student. The four locations correspond to left and right frontal and left and right posterior scalp, roughly sites F3, F4, P3, and P4 in this order (nose up).

three subjects in the plots based on unprocessed scalp potential. All three subjects show two or three (apparently) distinct bands of global alpha rhythm in the scalp potential plots.

These data are consistent with multiple local alpha rhythms, multiple modes of a global standing wave field, or some combination of source activity. By contrast, the corresponding dura image plots show more sparsely patched alpha activity, perhaps highlighting local alpha networks after removal of the global alpha field by the dura image spatial filter. Other data (Nunez 1995, 2000a,b; Andrew and Pfurtscheller 1996, 1997; Nunez et al. 1997, 1999; Florian et al. 1998) also suggest that the usual eyes

---

Figure 10-6 Peak power histograms for scalp potential (*left column*) and corresponding dura image (*right column*) estimates for the three subjects (BMW, CVR, and RS). Smaller electrode numbers on vertical axes near the upper portions of the plots correspond to more frontal scalp locations (see fig. 10-1). For each five-second epoch and each electrode site, the frequency component (0.2 Hz resolution) with the largest power in the range $3.0 \leq f \leq 20.0$ Hz was selected by the FFT. Each plot contains 60 epochs $\times$ 131 electrodes = 7860 points. Other frequency components at each site are not plotted, even though they may be nearly as large as the peak components. The test was repeated with the same data

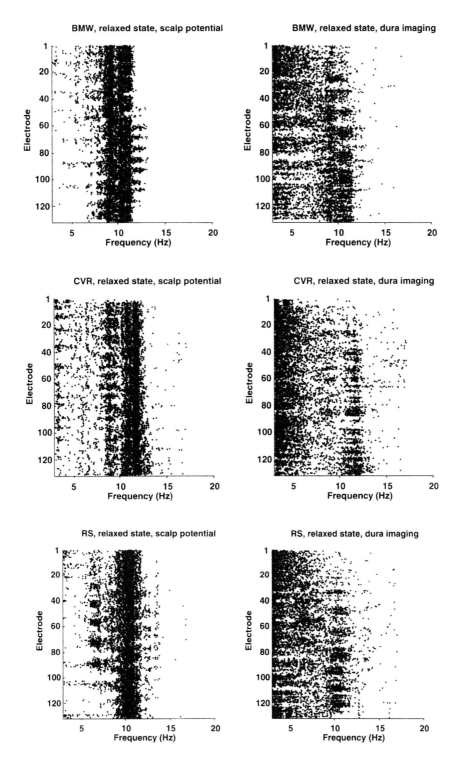

first passed through the dura imaging algorithm (*right column*). The dominance of alpha band activity over the entire scalp is evident in all three subjects in the average reference potential plots, but somewhat less evident in the dura image plots as a result of filtering out the more global activity. Reproduced with permission from Nunez et al. (2001).

closed resting EEG in humans has at least several distinct contributions: long-wavelength (low spatial frequency) activity near the alpha peak frequency that often exhibits moderate to high coherence over large scalp distances (10 to 25 cm) and more localized, incoherent delta, theta, (additional) alpha, and beta activity contributing mainly to dynamics at shorter spatial wavelengths, perhaps as part of specific networks.

These data may be interpreted naturally in the context of cortical source activity expressed in the spherical harmonic expansion (8.11) for the idealized case of spherical scalp and cortical surfaces. Cortical mesosource strength, that is, dipole moment per unit volume $P(\theta, \phi, t)$ at surface locations (θ, ϕ), may be expressed as a sum over spherical harmonic functions (a sum over characteristic spatial functions or *eigenfunctions*) with progressively higher spatial frequencies. The coefficients in this expansion $\Phi_{nm}(t)$ are generally determined by the underlying dynamics.

The combined effects of spatial filtering by the volume conductor and high-pass high-resolution estimates of source activity are illustrated by fig. 8-6. These data show the effects of filtering out the lowest spatial frequencies (mainly the $n = 0$ and 1 modes of the spherical harmonics) with Laplacian or dura imaging algorithms. That is, measured EEG on an idealized spherical head may be generally expressed as a sum over the spherical harmonic functions, but with weighting coefficients $\Phi_{nm}(t)$ depending partly on spatial filtering. By mostly removing the lowest modes ($n = 0$, $m = 0$ and $n = 1$, $m = -1, 0, 1$) with Laplacian or dura imaging methods, we shift the weighting away from the more global towards more local dynamics. Whereas globally dominated dynamics (as measured by peak power potentials) occurs mostly in the alpha band, more locally dominated dynamics (as measured by dura imaging) was more evident in delta, theta, and beta bands.

6 Spectral Power as a Function of Brain State

Figure 10-7 shows peak power estimates obtained from average reference potentials (left) and dura image estimates (right) for the cognitive periods. Comparison with the corresponding resting plots in fig. 10-6 indicates that alpha blocking of scalp potential in subjects BMW and RS was minimal. Both subjects have engineering Ph.D. degrees. Alpha blocking was more evident in subject CVR, a psychology student having less experience with computational exercises. This outcome suggests adding a verbal task to future experiments to possibly differentiate subjects with distinct educational backgrounds.

Subject RS showed a robust theta rhythm at many frontal and central sites in the resting state. His theta was enhanced, became more narrow band, and more widespread during cognition. The other two subjects produced dominant theta mainly during cognitive periods. While theta

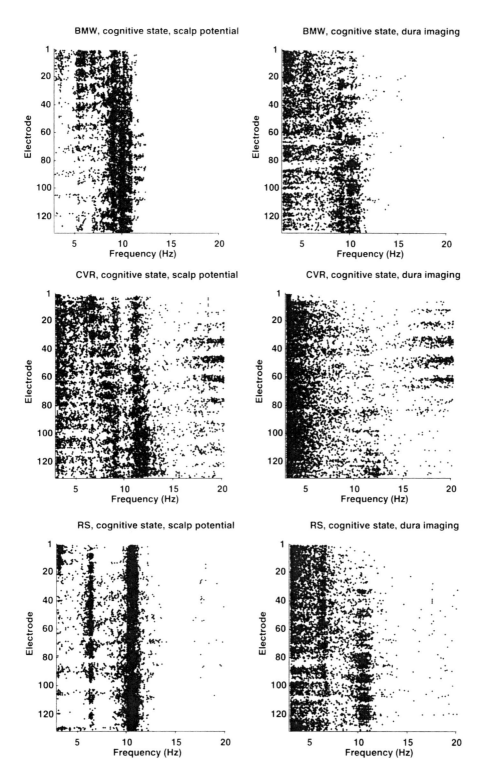

Figure 10-7 Peak power estimates obtained from average referenced potentials (*left*) and dura image estimates (*right*) for the cognitive periods. The methods are identical to those used in fig. 10-6. Reproduced with permission from Nunez et al. (2001).

activity was often evident in frontal regions, it was more widespread than implied by the usual description "frontal midline theta," reported in several working memory studies (review by Gevins et al. 1997). If theta were highly localized, locally dense clusters of points in the peak power dura image plots would be expected. Instead, upper theta (5 to 6 Hz) was actually quite evident in the peak power potential plots, indicating dynamics at relatively low spatial frequencies. Of course, theta could have multiple origins, occur in both low and high spatial frequency bands, be sensitive to task details, or some combination of all these effects.

Subject RS showed pronounced narrowing of both theta and alpha band activity (peak power points) during cognitive states. Some shifting of alpha to theta activity occurred over both anterior and posterior scalp. Subject BMW produced somewhat similar behavior, but theta production was mostly frontal. Subject CVR, female and physically smaller than the other two subjects, showed a substantial number of peak power points in the beta band, especially during the cognitive state. This could have been due to subtle muscle artifact, an indirect consequence of more alpha blocking, genuine cortical source activity in the beta band that was more evident because of a lower resistance or perhaps thinner skull (implied by her smaller size), or a combination of these factors. CVR's cognitive peak power plots (fig. 10-7) indicate a number of electrode sites with sparse points in the approximate range $13 \leq f \leq 16$ Hz, but a much higher density of peak power points in the range $17 \leq f \leq 20$ Hz. This suggests contribution from brain rather than muscle sources in the beta range since muscle spectra are normally relatively flat over $13 \leq f \leq 20$ Hz, falling off slowly with increasing frequency. On the other hand, many of these channels were located near temporal muscles. Thus, our best guess is that these beta points reflect some combination of brain activity and subtle muscle artifact.

One should keep in mind that the peak power plots present a very conservative view of dominant frequencies of cortical source activity. That is, each plotted point in the theta or beta band means for that particular electrode site and five-second epoch, a particular frequency was the *single component* (with 0.2 Hz resolution) with the largest power in the range $3 \leq f \leq 20$ Hz. Thus, absence of theta or beta points (especially in posterior regions) does not necessarily mean absence of substantial theta or beta activity. Generally, it means that whatever theta or beta power was produced, it was dominated by larger alpha or high-end (>3 Hz) delta power. Similarly, absence of alpha points in frontal regions during the cognitive task does not imply absence of alpha rhythm.

Additional observations on so-called *alpha blocking* are of interest here (Wingeier 2004). In four of the six studies (five subjects, one repeated), the following spectral changes were observed when comparing cognitive with resting states. Power in the lower part of each subject's alpha band (1 or 2 Hz below the peak) decreased at the same time that power in the upper part (1 or 2 Hz above the subject's peak) increased. However, the changes were asymmetric in at least two ways. (i) The magnitudes of lower alpha band reductions were larger than the magnitudes of upper alpha band increases. Thus, if the entire alpha band had been studied as a unitary process, traditional alpha blocking would have been observed. The subjects in this category include RS, but not CVR. Subject BMW showed this behavior in the first experiment; his behavior in the second experiment was more mixed. (ii) Alpha band power decreases with cognition were sometimes biased towards lower spatial modes, and increases with cognition were sometimes biased toward higher spatial modes. The spatial modes of the spherical harmonic functions provide an overall measure of the spatial frequencies in the scalp potential topography as discussed in section 11.

Five of the six experiments resulted in increased theta power during cognitive states; three of these showed simultaneous increases in upper alpha band power. The one subject (KR) that failed to show increases in theta power during cognitive periods had increased upper alpha power with cognition. She (and two other subjects) also exhibited scattered increased power and coherence in beta and gamma bands that were not obviously caused by muscle artifact, but we cannot be certain that this effect was brain-generated. In summary, all subjects exhibited power increases in the theta band, upper alpha band, or both during cognitive periods. *These data suggest that an updated view of traditional alpha blocking is needed. Our results are consistent with the formation of regional cognitive networks that operate in the theta, upper alpha, and (probably) higher frequency bands. Activation of these networks appears partly to disrupt lower alpha band oscillations, which have more global structure than upper alpha, theta, or higher frequency bands. Thus, the traditional term "alpha blocking" is somewhat misleading.*

7 Stability of Alpha Phase Structure

Dura image phase plots indicate many alternating regions out of phase as indicated in fig. 10-8. Regions of constant phase ("zero phase lag") were separated by several centimeters. In other words, regions 180° out of phase were typically separated by about 2 to 3 cm, or roughly the dura image spatial resolution. Many alpha phase structures based on dura imaging with epochs ranging from one second to one minute were studied. All dura phase structures obtained with zero smoothing parameter showed qualitatively similar complex structures at the same approximate scale of the EEG spatial resolution, suggesting even more complexity at scales too small to observe from the scalp. Dura image with nonzero smoothing parameters had levels of detail intermediate between those of raw scalp potential and dura image with zero smoothing parameter.

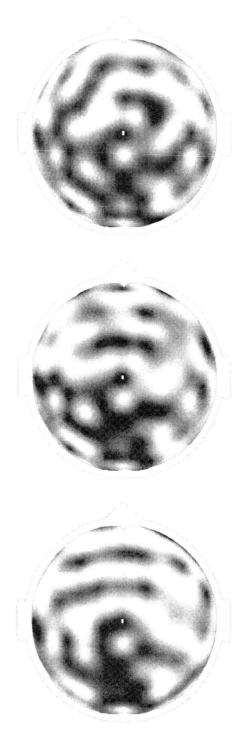

Figure 10-8 Estimated phase structures of human alpha rhythm on the dura surface based on dura imaging of 131-channel scalp data. Cosine (phase) plots are based on successive 20-second epochs with zero phase fixed at Cz (white dot). Phase is calculated at the peak alpha frequency (10 Hz) with 1 Hz bandwidth. The centers of white (-1) and black ($+1$) regions are $180°$ out of phase. Plots generated by Wingeier (2004).

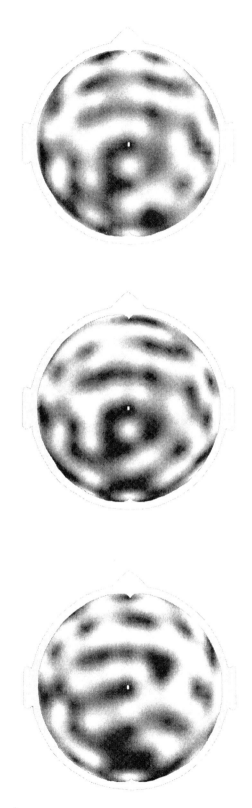

Figure 10-8 Continued.

453

In order to test whether these phase structures genuinely represented cortical source dynamics, the accuracy and stability of dura phase estimates were studied as follows:

(i) Correlation coefficients comparing successive estimates of cosine phase over the 131 electrode sites at all integer frequencies on $3 \leq f \leq 40$ Hz were calculated for 5 minutes of resting alpha using one-second epochs. That is, phase at each electrode site was determined for each one-second block of data by conventional Fourier transform methods. Each resulting phase map was then compared with the successive phase map. Correlation coefficients (obtained from electrode-by-electrode phase comparisons), averaged over all 299 successive epoch pairs, are plotted versus frequency in the upper part of fig. 10-9. The correlation coefficients were all less than 0.2, reflecting large second-to-second changes in dura phase structure. However, these correlation coefficients were substantially larger in the approximate range $6 \leq f \leq 11$ Hz, indicating much more stability of dura phase estimates in this frequency range.

(ii) Phase stability at the peak alpha frequency was also studied by using different epoch lengths in five-minute records of resting alpha. Correlation coefficients comparing successive epochs at individual alpha peaks 10 Hz (subject BMW) and 10 Hz (subject RS) are plotted versus epoch length in lower part of fig. 10-10. Correlation coefficients, averaged over all epoch pairs, increased monotonically with epoch length, ranging from about 0.1 for 1-second epochs to about $0.35-0.50$ for 20-second epochs. Adjacent frequency bins were averaged to hold frequency resolution fixed at 1 Hz. The result for the alpha and upper theta band was: *the longer the epoch used to define phase, the more stable the phase estimates.*

(iii) Uncorrelated Gaussian noise with amplitude equal to 15% of the RMS amplitude of the raw data (averaged over all electrodes) was added directly to raw scalp potential measurements. This purposely contaminated data (noise plus genuine EEG) were then passed through the dura image algorithm. All phase correlation coefficients in fig. 10-9 were re-calculated with this purposeful addition of noise. No substantial differences were obtained, as suggested by Group 5 of table 8-1.

(iv) Uncorrelated $1/f$ noise with amplitude equal to 15% of the RMS amplitude of the raw data was passed through the forward solution of the 4-sphere head model to produce simulated, spatially correlated noise. This noise was then passed to the dura image and Fourier transform algorithms to produce phase estimates for successive epochs of varying lengths. The circles in the lowest plot of fig. 10-9 (the *random simulation*) show epoch-to-epoch

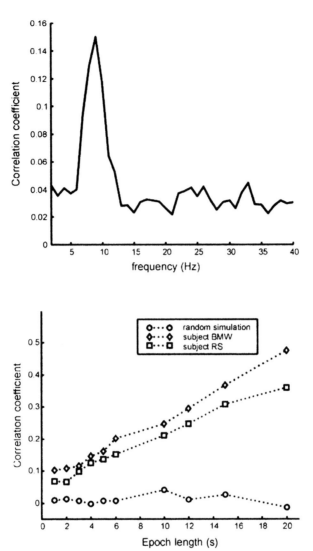

Figure 10-9 (*Upper*) Correlation coefficients comparing successive (one-second epoch) estimates of cosine dura image phase over the 131 electrode sites are plotted versus integer frequencies. Phase plots were calculated for 5 minutes of resting alpha using one-second epochs with phase at site 88 (Cz) defined as zero for each epoch. Correlation coefficients (obtained from electrode-by-electrode phase comparisons) were averaged over all 299 successive epoch pairs. Subject BMW. (*Lower*) Dura cosine phase correlation coefficients comparing successive epochs at individual alpha peaks (10 Hz for both BMW and RS) are plotted versus FFT epoch length. Correlation coefficients, averaged over all epoch pairs, increase monotonically with epoch length, ranging between about 0.1 for one-second epochs to about 0.4 to 0.5 for 20-second epochs (frequency resolution held fixed at 1 Hz by bin averaging). The lower plot ("random simulation") was generated using $1/f$ noise passed through the 4-sphere head model (forward solution) to simulate spatially correlated scalp noise, which was then passed through the dura imaging and FFT algorithms to estimate dura phase. These data suggest the existence of phase structure within the upper theta and alpha bands, which becomes progressively more stable when based on longer epochs (essentially longer time averages). No such phase structure is evident at other frequencies. Reproduced with permission from Nunez et al. (2001).

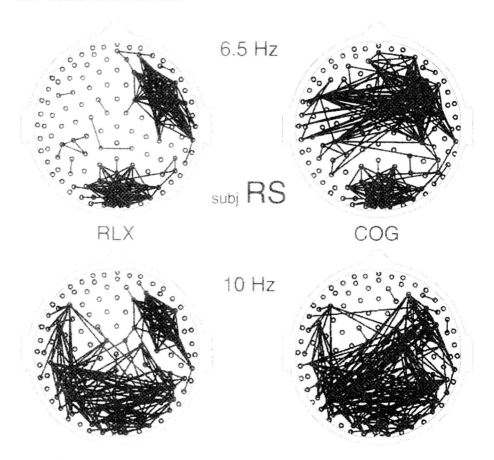

Figure 10-10 Dura image interelectrode coherence for subject RS in the relaxed state (RLX) and cognitive state (COG). Each coherence map is based on 5 minutes of data. All interelectrode coherences greater than 0.1 at the 99% confidence level are indicated by lines between the appropriate electrode pair, excluding nearest-neighbor edge electrodes. Actual coherence estimates indicated by lines vary widely. For example, all are in the range 0.33 to 0.65 for electrode separations greater than 10 cm. Both upper 6.5 Hz theta coherence (*upper row*) and 10.0 Hz upper alpha coherence (*lower row*) generally increased during the cognitive task. By contrast, 8.0 Hz alpha coherence decreased during the cognitive task (not shown). Simulations confirmed that these patterns represent genuine source coherence, rather than volume conduction or statistical artifact. Reproduced with permission from Nunez et al. (2001).

phase correlations as a function of epoch length resulting from this spatially correlated noise. All noise-simulated correlation coefficients are close to zero as expected, thereby supporting the idea that the EEG dura phase correlations in fig. 10-9 represent genuine brain dynamic processes.

These studies show that the phase structure of the alpha rhythm in these subjects is *quasi-stable*. From one viewpoint this result is perhaps expected; however, our data differ substantially from that expected in either of two distinct dynamic models. In the simplest possible model, alpha sources would have some fixed spatial distribution, due perhaps to a few fixed dipole layers. If this dynamic model were correct, the phase correlations of fig. 10-9 would be uniformly high and independent of epoch length in sharp contrast to actual observations. The other extreme model is spatial-temporal white noise in which the phase correlations should be low and independent of both frequency and epoch length, again in sharp contrast to observations. This latter model is roughly consistent with data outside the alpha band, but inconsistent with alpha band observations. Thus, *EEG dynamics within the alpha band lies between the extremes of full determinism and full randomness.*

This alpha quasi-stability depends on both the temporal and spatial scales of phase estimates. That is, phase estimated with long epochs shows much less epoch-to-epoch variation. Furthermore, phase estimated at large scales with raw potentials shows less epoch-to-epoch variation than (smaller-scale) dura image phase (not shown). We conjecture that the observed phase structures may represent interference patterns of standing waves of synaptic action. Such synaptic action may be superimposed on and interact with local networks that are embedded within the synaptic action fields as discussed in chapters 1, 8, and 11.

8 Alpha and Theta Coherence

Theta and upper alpha coherence patterns in subject RS are shown in fig. 10-10. Electrode pairs with dura coherence greater than 0.1 at the 99% confidence level (Bendat and Piersol 2001) have connecting lines drawn. The columns represent five minutes of relaxed (left, RLX) and five minutes of cognitive (right, COG) state. During states of mental calculation, coherence at both 6.5 Hz and 10.0 Hz were generally higher in subject RS (averaged over five-minute periods), whereas lower alpha band coherence was reduced (not shown). That is, widespread coherence increases were observed at integer frequencies $(6, 7, 10, 11)$ Hz simultaneously with coherence decreases at $(8, 9)$ Hz as shown in Wingeier (2004). The coherence estimates between specific electrode pairs vary widely. For example, for electrode pairs separated by 10 cm or more, coherence estimates (with lines drawn) varied from 0.33 to 0.65. The lower coherence estimate is the minimum required to satisfy the criterion for coherence greater than 0.1 at the 99% confidence level. Since coherence is a correlation coefficient squared, these data imply estimated alpha band dynamic correlations in the 0.57 to 0.81 range between remote cortical locations, providing some justification for our characterization of resting alpha rhythm as *more globally dominated dynamics.*

The general behavior of coherence patterns varied substantially between the three subjects studied, but was robust over different periods within individual subjects. It is further emphasized that dura coherence estimates are conservative in the sense that they may be artificially low because of the spatial filtering by the dura imaging algorithm. That is, *removal of erroneous high coherence due to volume conduction by dura imaging may also remove genuine source coherence associated with very low spatial frequency source activity* (Nunez et al. 1997, 1999). Finally, coherence can vary substantially over time even with our attempts to fix brain states over one-minute periods. Such time variations in phase locking are described in section 9.

The significance of these coherence estimates was first checked by passing random noise through the 4-sphere head model to simulate scalp potentials generated by uncorrelated dura sources. These simulated scalp potentials were then passed through the dura imaging and Fourier transform algorithms to obtain dura coherence estimates. The resulting coherence plots based on the same 99% confidence level used for the EEG data were empty as expected, except for adjacent electrode positions on the outer ring. These erroneous coherence estimates resulted from inaccurate dura estimates at edge electrodes. Thus, all lines connecting adjacent electrodes in the outer ring were removed from the coherence plots for the genuine data in fig. 10-10. In a second test, the coherence pattern at 37 Hz was obtained for subject RS. Only five pairs of electrodes passed the 99% test and all such sites were closer together than 5 cm. *This test shows that 37 Hz gamma activity was globally incoherent, and that neither volume conduction nor the dura imaging algorithm could substantially inflate dura coherence estimates*, a finding consistent with earlier high resolution coherence studies (Nunez et al. 1997, 1999; Srinivasan et al. 1996, 1998; Srinivasan 1999).

9 Theta Phase Synchronization During the Cognitive Task

Subjects BMW and RS displayed more coherent theta band activity at many frontal and frontal-parietal electrode pairs during mental calculations than in the resting state. Several such electrode pairs were selected for more detailed phase analyses so that changes over shorter times could be observed. Phase estimates for each signal were obtained by Fourier transforms at the (observed) maximum coherent theta frequency. A Hanning window and overlapping one-second epochs were used. The window was stepped by 0.1 second to obtain successive phase estimates. A series of relative phase offsets between pairs of recording sites was calculated for signals over the entire recording (approximately 10 minutes). In order to visualize the phase offsets, statistical distributions of phase estimates were computed in a series of 10-second sliding windows. When phase offset was near random over the immediate 10-second window, phase distributions were relatively uniform. However, when phase offset was more consistent over multiple phase measurements within the 10-second window, phase distribution was peaked at this phase offset.

In fig. 10-11, the upper rows of each plot pair display 10-second phase distributions (represented as grayscale histograms) through successive

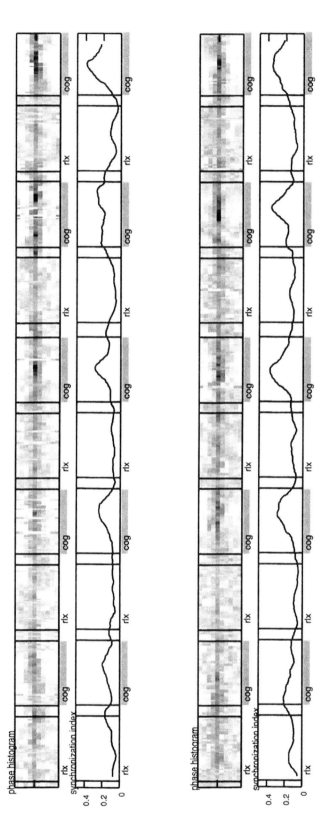

Figure 10-11 The upper rows of each plot pair display 10-second phase offset distributions (phase differences between electrode pairs) represented as grayscale histograms. Successive 1-minute periods of constant brain state are shown, alternating between resting and cognitive states (the mental summing of series). Cognitive periods are indicated by shaded bars and the word "cog." The lower row of each plot pair is the synchronization index used by Tass et al (1998). Phase offset peaks at approximately 140 to 180 degrees. (*Upper pair*) Electrode sites 9–55. (*Lower pair*) Sites 16–55 (essentially frontal midline theta), see fig. 10-1. Subject RS. Reproduced with permission from Nunez et al. (2001).

one-minute periods of constant state, alternating between resting and cognitive states, the latter indicated by the word "cog." Example plots are presented for subject RS for electrode pair 45–54 (cross hemispheric frontal-central) in the upper plot pair, and sites 9–55 (frontal-central) in the lower plot pair. In these examples, phase offset distributions peak in roughly the 140° to 180° range. Additional examples may be found in Nunez et al. (2001).

A synchronization index was adopted to quantify divergence of these phase distributions from uniformity (Tass et al. 1998; Lechaux et al. 1999). For each phase distribution, the index was calculated from $\rho = (S_{max} - S)/S_{max}$, where $S_{max} = \ln N$ and N is the number of bins in the distribution. S is the entropy, defined in the context of information theory as

$$S = \sum_{i=1}^{N} q_i \log_2 q_i \qquad (10.1)$$

where q_i is the probability that a phase estimate falls within bin i. The synchronization index ρ ranges from 0 to 1, where indices of 0 and 1 indicate no synchronization and perfect synchronization, respectively. The theta synchronization index (phase offset consistency) increased with mental calculation in these electrode pairs, as shown in the lower row plots of each pair. The synchronization effect tended to increase as the one-minute cognitive periods progressed. This was contrary to habituation often observed in extended mental tasks. Facilitation of cell assembly formation by repetition of the mental task is a possible explanation.

In order to check further the statistical significance of phase estimates, phase distribution and synchronization index were also calculated for a surrogate data set with amplitude retained and phase estimates presented in random order, independent of brain state. The residual synchronization was low (<0.2) so no task effect was found in the surrogate data as expected. Finally, instantaneous phase was estimated with the Hilbert transform after band passing (1 Hz band) raw data, as described in Rosenblum et al. (1996). Comparison of Hilbert transform and FFT methods revealed no substantial differences in several spot checks of phase estimates.

10 SSVEP Dynamics During Binocular Rivalry

The SSVEP is a method to elicit stimulus-related responses in the EEG for cognitive and clinical studies. In SSVEP studies, a stimulus is luminance or contrast modulated at a fixed frequency, and scalp potential responses are examined in a narrow frequency band surrounding the stimulus frequency. The simulations and genuine data shown in chapter 9 demonstrate that the SSVEP response is robust in the face of artifacts. This property is itself a strong motivation to choose SSVEPs in experimental studies.

The methods used to estimate SSVEPs are detailed in chapter 9. In this section some of the general properties of the SSVEP that are known at this time are examined using an example experiment on binocular rivalry (Srinivasan et al.1999; Srinivasan 2004).

Early studies of steady-state responses used electrodes positioned over occipital and parietal cortex in humans (Tyler et al. 1978; Regan 1989), and local field potentials recorded in monkey visual cortex (Nakayama and Mackeben 1982) demonstrated that steady-state responses in visual cortex are sensitive to the temporal frequency of the visual input. The dependence of the steady-state response magnitude on input frequency is characterized by at least three different "resonant" frequencies, that is, peaks in the response amplitude at the stimulation frequency. The reported resonant bands are 7–10 Hz (alpha), 15–30 Hz (beta), and 40–50 Hz (gamma) (Regan, 1989). Even at a single electrode site, individual subjects can show multiple peaks within these resonant bands. A more recent study of multiunit activity (MUA) in the cat visual cortex with periodic stimulation has also shown a similar banded structure with response peaks at multiple stimulus frequencies in the 4–8 Hz, 16–30 Hz, and 30–50 Hz ranges (Rager and Singer 1998). Steady-state responses in these different frequency bands show quite different sensitivities to physical stimulus parameters (color, spatial frequency, modulation depth, etc.) suggesting that flicker can entrain functionally distinct although spatially overlapping (at the cm scale of EEG) neocortical dynamic processes (Regan, 1989).

Because of the limited number of electrodes used in these earlier studies, only minimal information about the spatial properties of dynamics within these different frequency bands was obtained. With the advantages of modern technology, the power, phase, coherence, and partial coherence of steady-state responses have been studied more recently using large numbers of EEG electrodes and MEG sensors covering the entire scalp. These SSVEPs were recorded in subjects performing a number of cognitive tasks such as binocular rivalry (Srinivasan et al. 1999; Srinivasan 2004) selective attention (Chen et al. 2003) and higher cognitive functions such as working memory (Silberstein et al. 2001, 2003, 2004). In these studies, task-related modulations of steady-state responses to visual input were recorded at many scalp locations including temporal, frontal, and prefrontal regions far from primary visual cortex. These experiments have also shown that the amplitude and spatial distribution of the SSVEP or steady-state MEG over the scalp is a sensitive function of stimulus frequency f_s.

Figure 10-12 illustrates this exquisite sensitivity to stimulus frequency in a *binocular rivalry experiment* (Srinivasan 2004). Generally, binocular rivalry experiments involve presentation of two incongruent flickers (one to each eye), and subjects report that their percept spontaneously changes from perceiving only one flicker (red) to perceiving only the other (blue). Figure 10-12 shows the power spectrum recorded at one channel over the

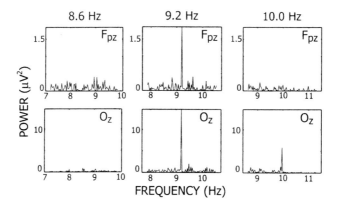

Figure 10-12 SSVEP power spectra (average referenced) at two channels calculated from individual epochs ($T \sim 20$ s, $\Delta f = 0.05$ Hz) in subject RY (22-year-old male). Each epoch corresponds to a period where a blue stimulus was flickered at 8.6, 9.2, and 10 Hz. The red stimulus was presented at another, higher frequency. The two electrodes (two rows) are located along the midline and are labeled by the closest 10/20 electrode. Power spectra were calculated using conventional FFT methods and are expressed in units of μV^2. In each case, the epoch submitted to the FFT algorithm was equal to an integer number of cycles of the stimulus frequency. Reproduced with permission from Srinivasan (2004).

occipital pole and another channel over the frontal pole with stimulus frequencies f_s equal to 8.6, 9.2, and 10 Hz. The stimulus is a blue pattern flickered into the left eye while a different red pattern is flickered into the right eye at another frequency (not shown). The magnitude of the response depends sensitively on the stimulation frequency at both scalp locations. With $f_s = 8.6$ Hz, no SSVEP response is observed at either channel. With $f_s = 9.2$ Hz, a robust response is recorded at both locations. With $f_s = 10$ Hz only the occipital channel shows a response, but it is substantially smaller than the 9.2 Hz response. Figure 10-13 indicates the SSVEP responses at all 111 channels for this subject for each of the selected stimulation frequencies. The channels have been organized into regional groups. The largest SSVEP magnitudes were recorded with $f_s = 9.2$ Hz at occipital and parietal electrodes. At 9.2 Hz a response is also apparent at central, frontal, and prefrontal channels, but the magnitudes are much smaller than responses at occipital and parietal electrodes. However, the sharp spectral peak shown at electrode Fpz in fig. 10-12 indicates that even these smaller responses are well above the noise level (in SSVEP studies, "noise" is mostly spontaneous EEG). To measure whether a stimulus frequency peak is obtained above the spontaneous EEG, a measure of signal to noise ratio may be obtained by comparing the power at the stimulus frequency f_s with power at neighboring frequencies (Srinivasan et al. 1999) or using the power measured at f_s in trials where the stimulus is flickered at a different frequency (Srinivasan 2004).

This finding suggests cortical rather than subcortical resonance since we expect small changes in input frequency (with all other stimulus

F(Hz)   F(Hz)

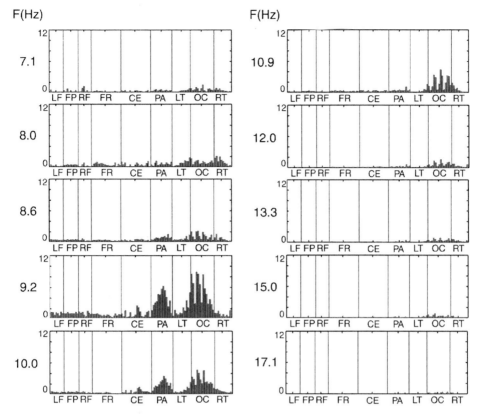

Figure 10-13 SSVEP power at the stimulus frequency at 111 channels for subject RY (22-year-old male). Each bar plot corresponds to a different stimulus frequency and is organized according to channel groups: LF, left prefrontal; FP, frontal pole; RF, right prefrontal; CF, central frontal; CE, central; PA, parietal; LT, left temporal; OC, occipital; RT, right temporal. Power values are given in μV^2. Note that the magnitude and spatial distribution of the steady-state response at the stimulus flicker frequency depend strongly on the flicker frequency. Reproduced with permission from Srinivasan (2004).

parameters held constant) not to change the spatial location of cortical inputs (Silberstein 1995). In this subject, the response at 9.2 Hz appears to cover a large number of electrode sites in a large-scale pattern over the scalp. Robust SSVEP responses can usually be detected by electrodes or sensors positioned over the frontal pole (far from primary visual areas) but only at specific frequencies, usually around 10 Hz for structured stimuli such as gratings (Narici et al. 1998; Srinivasan et al. 1999; Srinivasan 2004). The dynamics of these frontal responses appears sensitive to both the input frequency and the cognitive task (Srinivasan et al. 1999; Srinivasan 2004; Silberstein et al. 2001).

In binocular rivalry experiments, SSVEP responses recorded at frontal electrodes are sensitive to whether the subject consciously perceives the stimulus flicker. This observation applies to both SSVEP (Srinivasan 2004) and steady-state evoked magnetic field recordings

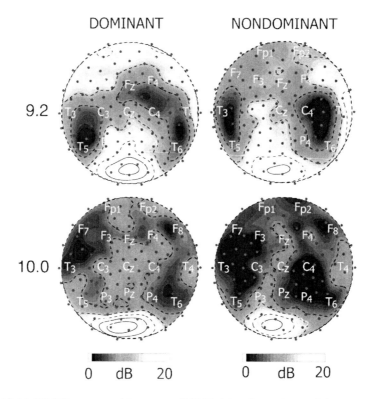

Figure 10-14 SSVEP topographic maps of SNR (signal-to-noise ratio) at two different stimulus frequencies for subject RY (22-year-old male). The rows corresponds to stimulus frequencies of 9.2 and 10.0 Hz. The column on the left shows a map of SNR during perceptual dominance (subject is perceiving the target stimulus at the given frequency). The column on the right shows maps of SNR during perceptual nondominance (the subject is perceiving a rival stimulus presented at a different frequency). Contour lines are at intervals of 3.3 dB, with solid contour lines at and above 20 dB and dashed lines below 20 dB.

(Srinivasan et al. 1999). The episodes of conscious perception of one flickering stimulus (*perceptual dominance*) typically last about 1 to 3 seconds. There are also periods when the subject does not perceive the stimulus flicker (*perceptual nondominance*) but instead perceives the rival stimulus flickering at a different frequency. By contrasting data recorded in these distinct states (while the stimuli characteristics are held fixed), we seek information about the SSVEP (and by implication, source) dynamics of consciousness. In order to distinguish SSVEP dynamic behavior between periods of perceptual dominance and nondominance, complex demodulation was used to calculate single-cycle Fourier coefficients at the stimulus frequency as discussed in chapter 9. The single-cycle Fourier coefficients were selectively averaged over episodes of dominance and nondominance. Figure 10-14 shows topographic maps of the power at the stimulus frequency f_s during periods of dominance (left column) and nondominance (right column) expressed in units of signal to noise ratio (SNR) at

9.2 and 10 Hz for the same subject indicated in figs. 10-12 and 10-13. SNR is defined by

$$\text{SNR} = 20 \log \left(\frac{P(f_s)}{N(f_s)} \right) \tag{10.2}$$

In this case the noise power $N(f_s)$ was estimated by applying the identical complex demodulation procedure at f_s and selectively averaging during dominance and nondominance periods to trials with the stimulus flickering at a different frequency from f_s. Solid lines indicate that the SNR is greater than 20 dB, in other words signal power is 10 times noise power. The response at 9.2 Hz during dominance is around 7–10 times the noise power at a large number of frontal channels. This response is significantly reduced when the subject is not aware of the stimulus flicker (and is aware of the rival stimulus flicker). Changes of power between the two states at occipital channels is somewhat smaller, and right temporal channels appear to increase power when the subject is unaware of the stimulus. At this subject's 9.2 Hz resonant frequency we note strong effects of consciousness of the stimulus across the array of electrodes. At 10 Hz, similar but weaker effects are observed. Figure 10-15 shows the SSVEP response at resonant frequencies in four other subjects, two with peak response at 9.2 Hz and two with apparent peak response at 10 Hz (technical limitations limited the spacing of possible stimulus frequencies). In each case, power is modulated by awareness of the stimulus, an effect that is largest at frontal electrodes and smaller at occipital electrodes. This basic finding is consistent with earlier MEG studies (Srinivasan et al. 1999) in which the most significant effects were found at frontal channels with weaker effects at occipital and parietal channels.

Modulation of SSVEP power has been reported in other cognitive tasks, most notably tasks involving selective attention (Chen et al. 2003; Morgan et al. 1996; Muller et al. 1998). What mechanisms can modulate SSVEP power? As discussed in chapters 4 and 9, the two ways EEG power can increase at some location are by increased mesosource strength $\mathbf{P}(\mathbf{r}, t)$ and increased size of correlated source region, both of which reflect changes in the synchronization of cortical source activity in the local region, that is, a tissue volume within roughly 5 to 10 cm of the electrode. These general physiological mechanisms of EEG power modulation discussed in chapters 4 and 8 apply also to the SSVEP. In addition to the influences on estimated SSVEP power, we note that the single-cycle Fourier coefficients obtained by complex demodulation are averaged (as complex numbers) over several cycles of the stimuli to improve SNR. In the examples shown in figs. 10-13 and 10-14 the averages were obtained over several hundred cycles. SSVEP power is sensitive to distribution of phase across these cycles. If the distribution of phase of the response over the cycles is narrow, SSVEP power is high. If the phase is highly variable across the cycles, SSVEP

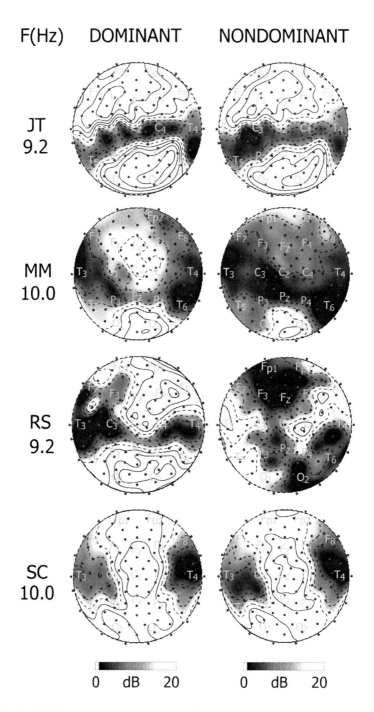

Figure 10-15 SSVEP topographic maps of SNR at the frequency that exhibited highest power over the array for four other subjects. Each row corresponds to a different subject and stimulus frequency: MM at 10 Hz, RS at 9.2 Hz, RY at 9.2 Hz, and SC at 10 Hz. The column on the left shows maps of SNR during perceptual dominance The column on the right shows maps of SNR during perceptual nondominance . Contour lines are shown at intervals of 3.3 dB, with solid contour lines plotted at and above 20 dB and dashed lines plotted below 20 dB. Reproduced with permission from Srinivasan (2001).

power is dramatically reduced. SSVEP power is a *statistical measure* of average amplitude and phase consistency over a large number of cycles of the flicker.

11 Coherence and Partial Coherence of the SSVEP in Binocular Rivalry

In SSVEP experiments, both coherence and partial coherence provide a means to study synchronization between distant brain areas due to cognitive processes (Silberstein et al. 2001). Partial coherence is a measure of coherence between two signals, after removing signals at each channel that are linearly related to a third signal, as discussed in chapter 9. In SSVEP applications, partial coherence is used to remove signals that are linearly related to the stimulus flicker. With this method, we remove any signals that maintain constant amplitude and phase with respect to the stimulus throughout the record.

Figure 10-16 summarizes the ordinary and partial SSVEP coherence obtained during periods of perceptual dominance and nondominance in the binocular rivalry experiment. Coherence and partial coherence measures are shown only at the stimulus frequency in the form of matrices containing all channel pairs. The channels are grouped into regions, as indicated by the labels, according to their proximity to 10/20 electrodes as detailed in the figure caption. Ordinary coherence is very high (>0.8) between many electrode pairs during both dominance and nondominance. Such high coherence reflects both genuine mesosource phase correlation and volume conduction effects. In chapter 9, it was shown that coherences between distant electrodes (>12 cm) are much less influenced by volume conduction (Nunez et al.1997; Srinivasan et al. 1998) and indicate genuine correlations between large-scale source regions in distant cortical areas.

In all the subjects, ordinary coherence at the stimulus frequency almost always increased during conscious perception of the stimulus; only a few channel pairs show significant decreases in coherence. Increases in coherence as large as 0.4 were observed during perceptual dominance, indicating large increases in cortical synchrony. However, specific coherence patterns varied considerably between subjects. All subjects showed increases in long-range coherence including coherences between occipital or parietal electrodes and frontal or prefrontal electrodes. By contrast, relatively few of the coherences within any local area, for example among occipital electrodes, are modulated by conscious perception. Volume conduction dominates these coherences between closely spaced electrodes (as discussed in chapter 9) making it difficult to observe changes related to cognitive or perceptual processes.

Synchronization of each electrode site to the stimulus flicker ("external" synchronization) narrows the width of the phase distribution at each channel and is associated with increases in both SSVEP power and

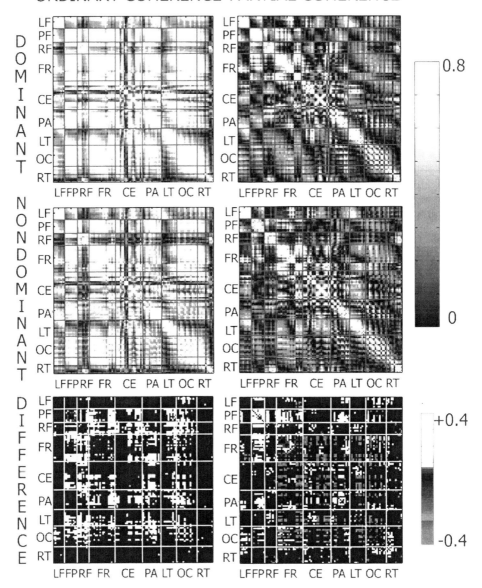

Figure 10-16 Matrix plots of SSVEP ordinary (*left column*) and partial coherence (*right column*) at 10 Hz between all possible pairs of 111 electrodes in subject MM. Each matrix has rows and columns organized according to channel groups: LF, left prefrontal; FP, frontal pole; RF- right prefrontal; CF, central frontal; CE, central; PA, parietal; LT, left temporal; OC, occipital; RT, right temporal. The top row shows ordinary and partial coherence during perceptual dominance. The middle row shows ordinary and partial coherence during perceptual nondominance. The bottom row shows the difference in ordinary and partial coherence between dominance and nondominance. Only significant differences are shown as indicated by white for positive and gray for negative. Insignificant differences are set to zero (black).

coherence. Partial coherences were also computed, thereby removing the average stimulus-locked response from each epoch at each channel. Partial coherences are substantially reduced in comparison to ordinary coherence, but still remain high between many electrode pairs. High partial coherences indicate that the residual signal, after removing responses that maintain constant amplitude and phase with respect to the stimulus across epochs, exhibits phase correlation between electrodes. This phase correlation reflects consistency in relative phase between channels within the portion of the steady-state response that varies in phase and amplitude across epochs. Ordinary coherence reflects a mixture of this "internal" synchronization and "external" synchronization imposed by the stimulus flicker. It should be noted that volume conduction influences partial and ordinary coherence in essentially the same way. Partial coherence between distant electrode pairs can be meaningfully interpreted as a measure of large-scale phase synchronization between distant cortical areas, independent of the local synchronization of each area by the stimulus flicker.

Figure 10-16 shows that partial coherences are also modulated by conscious perception of the stimulus as shown by the matrix plot of the difference between partial coherence during dominance and nondominance periods. At some electrode pairs partial coherence increases during perceptual dominance similar to ordinary coherence (indicated in white). At other channel pairs, partial coherence decreases (indicated in gray), even though ordinary coherence increases. In addition, a few electrode pairs that show no significant change in ordinary coherence modulate partial coherence during conscious perception. Figure 10-17 shows the relationship between ordinary coherence differences and partial coherence differences in each subject. Each point shown on the plots indicates a channel pair with a significant modulation of ordinary coherence. The large black dots represent channel pairs where both ordinary and partial coherence were significantly modulated. Three distinct clusters of channel pairs, occupying three quadrants of the diagram which we describe as two different patterns of ordinary and partial coherence modulation during conscious perception were observed. No electrode pairs showed significant increases of partial coherence while ordinary coherence decreased (lower left).

Two groups of electrode pairs, located in the upper right and lower left quadrants of each plot, show ordinary and partial coherence that both significantly increase or significantly decrease during dominance. Examining these pairs of electrode sites, we found that increases in both power and partial power were coupled with these increases in ordinary coherence and partial coherence. Partial power is estimated from the power spectrum by removing the portion of the power spectrum that is phase locked to the stimulus across epochs as discussed in chapter 9. A smaller group of electrodes show decreases in both ordinary and partial coherence with corresponding decreased power and partial power. These complementary patterns suggest that at these electrode sites modulation of power and coherence by conscious perception is independent of the synchronization of each channel with respect to the stimulus flicker. This result implies an "internal" synchronization that measures functional integration of (often) widely separated cortical areas. Another group of electrode pairs, in the

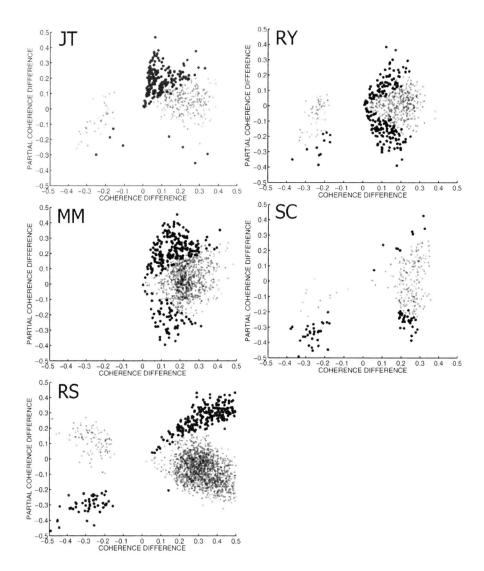

Figure 10-17 Modulation of SSVEP ordinary and partial coherence by conscious perception. The difference in ordinary coherence between perceptual dominance and nondominance is plotted against the equivalent difference in partial coherence for five subjects. Each dot in each graph represents a channel pair with significant modulation of ordinary coherence during conscious perception. Large dots indicate channel pairs that significantly modulate both ordinary coherence and partial coherence. Small dots indicate channel pairs that significantly modulate ordinary coherence but not partial coherence. Note that some channels modulate both ordinary and partial coherence in the same direction, while others increase ordinary coherence while decreasing partial coherence. Reproduced with permission from Srinivasan (2004).

lower right quadrant of each plot, shows increased ordinary coherence but decreased partial coherence during dominance versus nondominance. These channels were characterized by small increases in power and significant decreases in partial power. This pattern is consistent if the main effect at these channels is increased synchronization with respect to the stimulus flicker during conscious perception. This "external" synchronization of cortical sources in each area by the flicker gives rise to increased coherence between electrodes.

Internal and external synchronization give rise to distinct modulation patterns of the statistical structure of the steady-state response, as analyzed using the ordinary and partial coherence measures described here. One naturally asks what neural mechanisms produce these distinct patterns of coherence modulation during conscious perception of the stimulus. External synchronization is a phenomenon of reduced variability of the mesosources in a cortical area in response to the stimulus, that is, a more precise synchronization of individual cortical areas to the stimulus. Although this effect could be a consequence of feedback from other areas, strictly local models can adequately explain the observed external synchronization. As demonstrated in the cat, neurons in primary visual cortex can be precisely synchronized at the stimulus flicker frequency (Rager and Singer 1998). Internal synchronization is necessarily mediated by mechanisms involving feedback interactions between cortical areas, since internal synchronization is independent of the phase of the response with respect to the stimulus. As the phase of each channel varies with respect to the stimulus, the relative phase between channels is constrained.

We present this example experiment to illustrate ordinary and partial SSVEP coherence to study neocortical dynamics related to behavior and cognition. SSVEP is an active research area so we anticipate that much more information about SSVEP dynamic behavior will be obtained in the near future. Again, we emphasize that even if one were to calculate only SSVEP power (ignoring coherence, partial coherence, and other measures), the substantial benefit of obtaining robust estimates in the presence of (perhaps) subtle artifacts provides strong motivation for adopting SSVEPs in cognitive and clinical studies. SSVEPs are also interesting as a means to study dynamic source properties to facilitate connections to theoretical models of source dynamics and the underlying physiology as discussed in chapter 11.

12 Estimates of EEG Phase Velocity

As outlined in chapter 9, two generally distinct velocity measures are needed to describe wave propagation when the waves are *dispersive* (wave distorts as it propagates). The measures are *phase velocity* and *group velocity*. Generally, a wave packet is composed of many component waves with individual phase velocities. We may visualize the wave packet as similar to a compound action potential in a nerve with axons of different diameter (having different action potential speeds). Group velocity refers to velocity of the entire packet. In the case of nondispersive waves, phase and group velocities are equal.

One fundamental question concerning EEG dynamics is whether evidence of propagating activity can be observed in scalp data. Even if traveling waves actually occur, but they propagate in multiple directions along the scalp, can we ever observe them in scalp recordings? One indication of traveling waves is observation of continuous phase shifts along a line of electrodes as discussed in chapter 9. By estimating phase shifts in relatively narrow temporal frequency bands, we tend to pick out velocities of single components of putative wave packets, that is, phase velocities. A number of phase velocity estimates have been published for putative waves traveling in posterior-to-anterior or anterior-to-posterior directions near the midline, for example with SSVEPs (Hughes et al. 1992, 1995). However, many early studies have relied on monopolar (reference) recordings, which are distorted by volume conduction and reference electrode effects. These phenomena tend to add common signals to closely placed electrodes (volume conduction) and to all electrodes (reference). We then expect reference recordings to overestimate phase velocity because the addition of these common signals is essentially instantaneous; it occurs with infinite velocity. A more accurate approach uses bipolar recordings from closely spaced electrodes (Nunez 1974). With this experimental design, the reference effect is eliminated and volume conduction effects are substantially reduced. The bipolar pairs provide estimates of instantaneous tangential electric fields half way between each electrode pair. The propagation velocity of electric field components may then be estimated.

One comprehensive study of propagation velocity adopted a combination of MEG and bipolar EEG (Silberstein 1995; Burkitt et al. 2000). In 14 of 18 subjects, traveling waves were indicated in scalp-recorded SSVEPs (driven at peak alpha frequency) and magnetic fields (MEG). Measured phase velocities were generally in the range 3–7 m/s along the scalp or about 6–14 m/s along the folded cortical surface, as shown in fig. 10-18. As expected, propagation velocity estimates obtained with reference recordings were substantially higher. These data agree nicely with the estimated peak in the distribution of myelinated corticocortical propagation speeds of roughly 6–9 m/s (Katznelson 1981; Nunez 1995). Checkerboard patterns were more likely to produce the posterior to anterior negative phase shift associated with (back to front) traveling waves. By contrast, the unstructured stimulus had more tendency to produce an abrupt phase change in central regions of the array, more consistent with standing waves, as summarized in fig. 10-19. One possible interpretation is that standing waves occur as a result of the interference of waves traveling in opposite directions as discussed in chapters 3, 9, and 11.

In the SSVEP phase velocity studies cited above, it was conjectured that the checkerboard stimulus was more likely than the unstructured stimulus

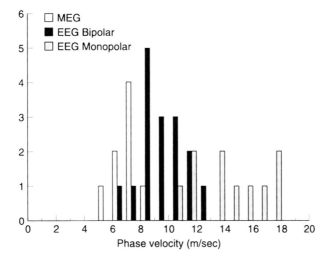

Figure 10-18 Histograms of estimated SSVEP phase velocities along the midline using three different measures are shown. These velocities are double scalp recorded velocities to estimate velocities along the folded cortical surface. Monopolar SSVEP recordings were referenced to the digital average potential of the two earlobes. Bipolar SSVEP recordings were obtained from closely placed electrode pairs, thereby obtaining estimates of tangential electric field halfway between each pair. Phase velocity estimates require a smooth phase change across the nine midline recording sites. This test was based on linear regression of phase versus distance with a correlation coefficient greater than 0.9. The SSVEP was elicited by a checkerboard 10 Hz flicker. An unstructured flicker tends to produce more abrupt phase changes more consistent with standing waves (due perhaps to the interference of waves traveling in opposite directions). Reproduced with permission from Silberstein (1995).

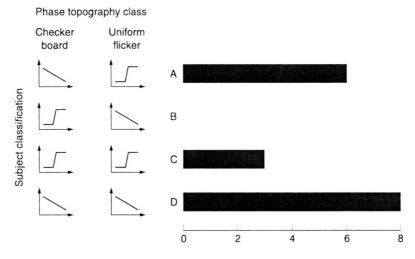

Figure 10-19 Classification of general SSVEP phase topography. The two left-hand columns depict four different combinations of progressive and discontinuous phase shifts along the midline driven by either a checkerboard pattern or full-field flicker. The histogram at right shows the number of subjects with each type of phase topography combination. For example, the six class A subjects switched their general phase topography with stimulus change. Reproduced with permission from Burkitt et al. (2000).

to produce spatially damped waves that would propagate from primary visual cortex to anterior regions. If so, the propagation direction could be expected to remain constant and long data records (several minutes) used to estimate phase velocity in a narrow frequency band centered on the driving frequency. In order to test both the robustness of these SSVEP phase velocity estimates and a modified approach more appropriate for spontaneous EEG, new data were recorded in five subjects and analyzed as follows (Silberstein et al. 1993; Nunez 1995): SSVEP data were recorded with respect to a neck reference and transformed to sets of eight bipolar signals from the nine midline electrodes (3 cm spacing). *Data were digitized at exactly 16 samples per stimulus cycle to obtain accurate estimates of single-cycle Fourier coefficients used to determine phases for each short epoch. The choice of an integer number of samples per cycle is essential to prevent power spillage into side bands by the Fourier transform* (see discussion below and chapter 9). SSVEP (integer) frequency was varied from 9 to 13 Hz so epoch lengths varied from 142 to 77 ms. Each stimulus frequency lasted approximately 3 minutes.

Two separate issues were addressed. First, we asked if the number of cycles satisfying the linear regression test (based on phase versus distance) was sufficiently large to justify the claim of posterior to anterior traveling waves. About 8% of the approximately 50,000 cycles satisfied the statistical criterion ($p = 0.01$). Alternative tests of statistical significance of traveling wave cycles were based on (i) random (simulated) data and (ii) the genuine phases at random electrode locations. Less than 0.1% of these surrogate data satisfied the statistical test, thereby providing evidence for substantial propagating activity in the genuine data. The second task was to estimate the phase velocities in these data. Phase velocity estimates along the scalp were obtained from the slope of the linear regression fit to phase versus distance. That is, the phase velocity of a wave component of frequency f traveling over a distance x and exhibiting a phase shift θ in the x-direction is given by $v_P = 2\pi f x / \theta$. (see Nunez 1995 for details). Nearly all phase velocity estimates were in the 2 to 6 m/s range along the scalp, corresponding to about 4 to 12 m/s along the cortical surface in approximate agreement with the earlier study of figs. 10-18 and 10-19.

In contrast to SSVEP, spontaneous EEG has no obvious preferred propagation direction. Even if traveling waves do occur, they might propagate in multiple directions, interfere, and generally produce very complex patterns as indicated by the topography shown in figs. 10-3 and 10-4. Thus, the identification of any kind of wave propagation at the scalp might seem unlikely. In order to investigate this idea, the SSVEP single-cycle analysis method was applied to resting alpha rhythm data (10 Hz) in one subject (Silberstein et al. 1993). This subject's alpha bandwidth was relatively narrow (1–2 Hz), but broader than the SSVEP response. Thus, we were not able to eliminate side-band spillage of the Fourier transform by choosing an integer number of samples per cycle. This suggests that our phase velocity estimates for the spontaneous EEG are less accurate than SSVEP velocities. Nevertheless, we present these tentative estimates. About 8% of the cycles were found to satisfy the statistical test for posterior-to-anterior midline traveling waves. Another 8% satisfied the same test for anterior-to-posterior midline traveling waves (Nunez 1995). Again, the expected percentage based on the (random) surrogate data tests was less than 0.1%. Propagation velocity estimates for single cycles were nearly all in the 3 to 7 m/s range along the scalp or about 6 to 14 m/s along the folded cortical surfaces. In summary, about 84% of alpha cycles could not be associated with midline propagation. We conjecture several confounding influences that might prevent such wave observation: interference of midline waves traveling in opposite directions (forming standing waves), oblique propagation, spatially damped waves, lack of good frequency resolution, waves originating under the electrode array, and nonwave phenomena. Nevertheless, 16% of the cycles showed evidence for midline traveling waves.

The search for traveling EEG waves has been extended to slow-wave sleep using a 256-electrode array (Massimini et al. 2004). Sleep data were band passed ($0.1 < f < 4.0$ Hz) and single cycles were defined by zero crossing and extrema criteria. Such cycles were identified as waves (or perhaps wave packets) originating in definite regions and traveling over the scalp. Waves originated more frequently in prefrontal regions and propagated in an anterior–posterior direction. Their rate of occurrence increased progressively, reaching almost one per second as sleep deepened. Phase velocities were estimated for a subset of waves that traveled in midline directions (55% of cycles in all subjects). Estimated scalp velocities were all in the 1 to 7 m/s range, with most scalp velocities in the 2 to 3 m/s range or 4 to 6 m/s along the folded cortex. The authors suggest that *wave propagation is probably mediated by corticocortical fibers* because slow sleep oscillations survive surgical isolation of the thalamus (Steriade et al. 1993) but are disrupted by disconnection of cortical pathways by surgical and pharmacological means (Amzica and Steriade 1995).

The following caveats are offered to facilitate interpretation of EEG phase velocity estimates.

(i) In many studies, the SSVEP frequency closely matches the driving frequency as shown in fig. 10-12. That is, the scalp signal is close to a sinusoidal oscillation of known frequency. Fourier coefficients for single cycles may then be calculated by integrating the signal with sine and cosine functions of this frequency, thereby obtaining slow Fourier transforms (*complex demodulation*) (Silberstein 1995). The usual power spillage into side bands, which occurs when Fourier transforms of unknown signals are calculated, is avoided if the signal is digitized at an integer number of samples per (known) cycle length. That is, the signal bandwidth Δf normally equals $1/T$, where T is the chosen epoch (integration period). The single cycles used in the second

SSVEP study cited above (Silberstein et al. 1993; Nunez 1995) had epochs T of 77 to 142 ms, corresponding to very poor frequency resolutions Δf in the range 7 to 13 Hz. However, if brain response is such that nearly all SSVEP is contained in a narrow band Δf_s centered on the driving frequency f_s, narrow band Fourier transforms and the corresponding phase estimates are essentially achieved with short epochs.

(ii) Application of the single-cycle methods to spontaneous EEG is more problematical because of multiple and possibly drifting frequencies in typical signals. However, when relaxed with eyes closed, many healthy subjects produce relatively narrow band (1 to 2 Hz) alpha rhythms with peak frequency variations over time less than about 0.5 Hz. The single cycle phases in the slow wave sleep study (Massimini et al. 2004) were not determined by Fourier transforms, rather data were band-pass filtered so that phase velocity estimates apply to a 4 Hz bandwidth probably centered near 1 Hz. Lack of good frequency resolution may contribute to distributing phase velocity estimates over a wider velocity range. One possible reason is that phase velocity may change with wave frequency as discussed in chapter 9 and in section 13. Also, the slow sleep wave phase velocity estimates were obtained with ear reference recordings of potential which tend to overestimate phase velocity as demonstrated in earlier studies (Silberstein 1995; Burkitt et al. 2000).

13 Dispersion Relations and Group Velocity

As discussed in chapter 9, wave phenomena constitute a special subset of spatial-temporal functions that satisfy dispersion relations, given by some relation between temporal and spatial frequencies; that is, $\omega = \omega(k)$ in one spatial dimension. In the case of waves in a spherical or prolate spheroidal shell like the Schumann resonances discussed in chapters 3 and 9, dispersion relations may take the form $\omega = \omega_{nm}$, where n and m specify the particular spherical harmonic function corresponding to different spatial frequencies in latitudinal and longitudinal directions. A plausible question to ask of EEG phenomena that appear to be globally dominant is whether we can observe a consistent increase in spatial frequency with increased temporal frequency.

An early attempt to address the issue of possible wave dispersion effects adopted a midline array of nine electrodes so that tangential electric field estimates were obtained at eight midline locations (Nunez 1974, 1981). In each subject, the peak alpha frequency f_0 was determined. One-dimensional spatial spectra for power in the low and high alpha frequency bands $(f_0 - \Delta f)$ and $(f_0 + \Delta f)$ were obtained, where $\Delta f = 1.5$ Hz. In all 13 experiments (8 subjects with repeat experiments), the spatial spectra shifted such that higher alpha frequencies were found to occur with higher spatial frequencies. Accurate estimates of phase and group velocities were not obtained due to experimental limitations: notably the small number of electrodes and limited length of the electrode array (making accurate estimates of long-wave activity impossible). Recently, this experiment was repeated on one subject with similar results (Wingeier 2004, unpublished).

A second approach to determine if alpha rhythms show evidence for a dispersion relation used an electrode array around a horizontal circumference (60 cm) of the head (Shaw 1991, reviewed in Nunez 1995). This array allowed much more accurate estimates of long-wavelength scalp potentials. Spatially aliased power was estimated as a function of frequency by comparing power obtained with 2 and 5 cm electrode spacings. In the four subjects studied, aliased power showed a minimum near the peak alpha frequency f_0 in both eyes open and eyes closed states. Aliased power increased monotonically for frequencies $f_0 < f < 40$ Hz, consistent with the existence of a dispersion relation (or multiple dispersion relations) for dynamic activity above f_0.

In a third experiment to test for an alpha wave dispersion relation(s), two-dimensional spatial spectra were obtained from the 131-channel array shown in fig. 10-1 (Wingeier et al. 2001; Wingeier 2004). The methods involve fitting spatial data to a series of spherical harmonic functions corresponding to progressively higher spatial frequencies as discussed in chapter 9. This process involves a number of technical issues discussed in the references. The most obvious limitation occurs because of sampling only part of a surface (roughly the upper half of an equivalent sphere). The $n = 0$ mode (zero spatial frequency) corresponds to a constant potential over the entire sphere, whereas the $n = 1$ mode corresponds to constant potential over each half of the sphere, but with opposite signs on the two halves. Thus, we cannot distinguish between the spatial modes $n = 0$ and 1 by sampling on only one half the surface. Of course, we do not know in advance where a nodal line separating the two halves might be located, but this does not alter the general argument.

Figure 10-20 shows spatial-temporal spectral power (*frequency–wavenumber spectra*) in five subjects recorded in the eyes closed, resting state. Power is normalized so that each temporal frequency band has the same total power in the six spatial modes shown ($n = 1, 6$). Without this normalization nearly all power would occur near $f = 10$ Hz and $n = 1$. The plots indicate greater power in lower left (low temporal and spatial frequencies) and upper right (high temporal and spatial frequencies), again consistent with the existence of a dispersion relation (or multiple dispersion relations) for dynamic activity above f_0. During the cognitive task, this general result held, but some changes occurred with apparent biases toward certain n ranges. For example, both power increases (at large values of n) and power decreases (at small values of n) can occur within a single temporal frequency band.

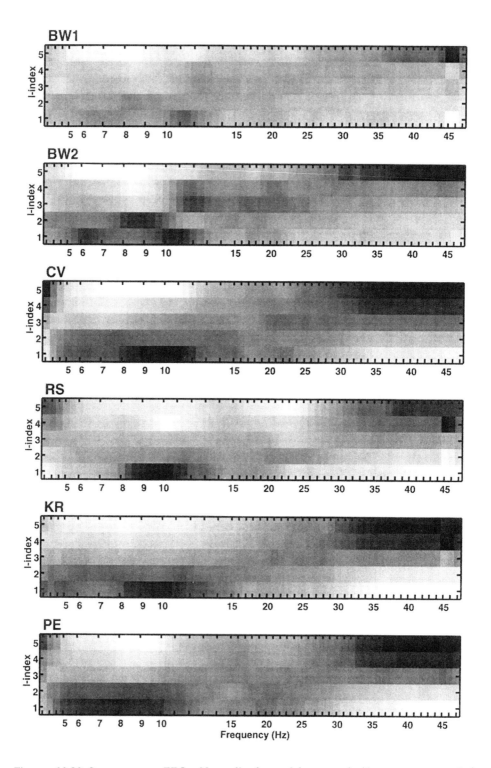

Figure 10-20 Spontaneous EEG. Normalized spatial-temporal (*frequency–wavenumber*) spectral power in five subjects (one repeat). Power is normalized so that each temporal frequency band has the same total power in the six spatial frequencies shown (spherical harmonics of degree n, plotted as l here). Without this normalization nearly all power

We must be skeptical of all scalp studies of high-frequency activity, including these involving putative EEG dispersion relations, because of likely artifact contamination. To address this question, four subjects were subjected to arduous studies using sinusoidal driving of their visual systems (SSVEP) by Wingeier (2004). Normalized spatial-temporal SSVEP spectral power in four subjects is shown in fig. 10-21. Single-cycle Fourier coefficients were decomposed into spatial power spectra for each of 60 stimulus frequencies (mostly integer frequencies, some half integer near 10 Hz). Each stimulus frequency was presented in random order for one minute. Figure 10-21 suggests again that *higher spatial frequency dynamics tends to occur with higher temporal frequencies.* Since SSVEP power occurred mainly at the driving frequency in these studies, fig. 10-21 adds additional support to validity of the spontaneous EEG spectra shown in fig. 10-20, although the problem of possible artifact contamination was not fully solved.

There were two complementary motivations for this study of spatial spectra: (i) to see if EEG and SSVEP dynamics exhibit consistent relationships between temporal and spatial frequencies and (ii) if such relationships were established with spatial frequencies increasing monotonically with temporal frequencies, an apparent group velocity may be defined. Such apparent group velocities were estimated in terms of smoothed estimates of the function $\omega = \omega(k)$, where the one-dimensional spatial frequency was identified as

$$k \approx \frac{n}{R}$$

where $R \approx 15$ cm is an effective sphere radius (for the anterior–posterior circumference) of the unfolded cortex (see chapter 11). Group velocity may then be estimated as

$$v_G \approx \frac{\Delta\omega}{\Delta k}$$

We emphasize that general dynamic patterns do not usually show evidence for wave-like behavior; no phase or group velocity estimates are possible in such dynamics. Rather statistical tests indicating monotonic increases in ω with increasing k must be passed as in these EEG data. In all, 15 estimates of group velocity in the 5 subjects were obtained for the 3 states for frequencies in the range $7.25 < f < 40$ Hz, where possible dispersion relations were conjectured. Based on an effective cortical radius of $R = 15$ cm, group velocity estimates expressed in terms of propagation along the folded cortical surface are: resting (6.9 to 8.5 m/s), cognitive

would occur near $f = 10$ Hz and $n = 1$. Each plot is based on 5 minutes of 131-channel data recorded in the eyes closed, relaxed state using a common average reference. Darker shades indicated greater power. All plots indicate greater power in lower left quadrants (low temporal and spatial frequencies) and upper right quadrants (high temporal and spatial frequencies). Methods are identical to analysis of Shumann resonances shown in fig. 9-34. Reproduced with permission from Wingeier (2004).

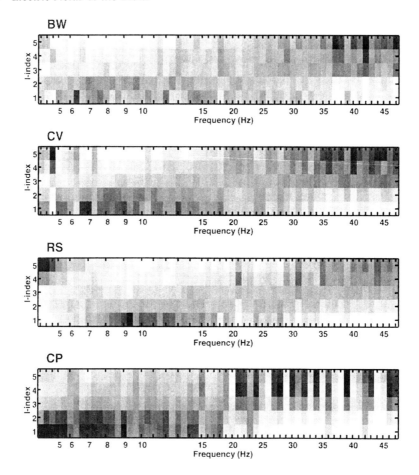

Figure 10-21 SSVEP spectra. Normalized spatial-temporal (*frequency-wavenumber*) spectral power in four subjects (relaxed state) calculated in a similar manner to the spontaneous EEG in fig. 10-20. The subjects viewed 60 flicker frequencies presented in random order. Single-cycle Fourier coefficients were decomposed into spatial power spectra for each stimulus frequency. Reproduced with permission from Wingeier (2004).

(7.1 to 9.1 m/s), and SSVEP (7.4 to 12.8 m/s). The grand mean and standard deviation are 8.4 ± 1.6 m/s. The effective cortical radius R is not well known in this study because the frequency–wavenumber spectra mix waves traveling in the long anterior–posterior direction with transverse waves. With an effective $R = 11$ cm, the grand mean of estimated group velocity is 6.2 ± 1.2 m/s. Group velocities along the scalp are about half these values.

14 Summary of the Complementary Dynamic Measures of EEG and SSVEP

Example applications of time series analysis and high-resolution methods to genuine EEG and SSVEP data are outlined. A brief overview of dynamic properties observed from the scalp is furnished. Like most neuroscientists, we view brain function in terms of *cell assemblies* (or less precisely *neural networks*). Evidence is presented that is consistent with multiple alpha and theta networks immersed within the global synaptic fields closely associated with scalp potentials. Alpha rhythms are shown to exhibit quasi-stable stable spatial structure; both networks and fields may contribute to such structure. We demonstrate here that coherence and other measures of phase locking in specific frequency bands, often between remote scalp locations, are reliably associated with behavior and cognition as in the experiment using mental calculations. Phase locking seems to fit naturally in the network picture, suggesting that different brain functions require phase synchronization between remote cell groups. In a prominent example of this general phenomenon, the conscious perception of a target stimulus was shown to occur with substantial coherence increases between remote cortical regions. These data support the idea that consciousness is associated with widespread cortical interactions required to provide some minimal level of "binding" of remote cell groups.

Other dynamic measures discussed here—phase and group velocity, dispersion relations, and standing and traveling waves—which are more closely aligned with physical phenomena, may seem less compatible with genuine neural networks. However, we argue that such measures are complementary to coherence and other synchronization measures, especially in the context of conjectured interactions between networks and global fields as suggested by fig. 1-8. One may properly question, Are brain waves really "waves"? Rather, let us pose an easier question: is the depiction of large-scale EEG dynamics in terms of traveling or standing waves useful in some experiments? Or, do such physical measures provide important information that can help in the design of better cognitive experiments? The experimental data and theoretical arguments of this book suggest affirmative answers to these questions. To cite a simple example, *no fixed dipole can account for either the progressive phase shifts or coherence patterns described here*. Such vastly oversimplified views of complex neocortical dynamics are quickly discredited when exposed to even moderately sophisticated experimental studies. By contrast, a combination of network and global field processes is tentatively proposed here, with different brain states based on different mixtures of local and global processes. The best global wave candidates appear to be associated with minimal cognition: anesthesia, deep sleep, some SSVEP, and the more global alpha rhythms. We conjecture that low levels of cognition involve cell assemblies embedded within such global environments, but higher cognitive loads may obviate such wave-like behavior. That is, if too much of the global environment is devoted to specific networks, the global wave-like picture is expected to fail. Alpha blocking when the eyes are opened may be the simplest example.

In this general context of locally versus globally dominated dynamics, Penfield and Jasper's (1954) extensive studies of cortical rhythms concluded that the normal ECoG differentiation between cortical areas is eliminated with anesthesia. This observation of transitions from a conscious to unconscious states with anesthesia may apply, at least in part, to hypoxia, coma, some epilepsies, and to a lesser extent normal deep sleep. It also appears consistent with our SSVEP binocular rivalry study. Thus, the general idea of local networks embedded in global fields provides one theoretical "entry point" to the complex world of large-scale neuroscience that can perhaps facilitate future studies of brain dynamics and cognition in a more parsimonious manner. We outline more details concerning such theoretical entry point to neocortical dynamics in chapter 11.

References

Amzica F and Steriade M, 1995, Disconnection of intracortical synaptic linkages disrupts synchronization of a slow oscillation. *Journal of Neuroscience* 15: 4658–4677.

Andrew C and Pfurtscheller G, 1997, On the existence of different alpha band rhythms in the hand area of man. *Neuroscience Letters* 222: 103–106.

Barlow JS, 1993, *The Electroencephalogram. Its Patterns and Origins*, Cambridge, MA: MIT Press.

Basar E, Schurmann M, Basar-Eroglu C, and Karakas S, 1997, *International Journal of Psychophysiology* 26: 5–29.

Bendat JS and Piersol AG, 2001, *Random Data. Analysis and Measurement Procedures*, 3rd Edition, New York: Wiley.

Bertrand O, Perrin F, and Pernier J, 1986, A theoretical justification of the average reference in topographic evoked potential studies. *Electroencephalography and Clinical Neurophysiology* 62: 464.

Bickford RG, 1973, *Clinical Electroencephalography*, New York: Medcom.

Burkitt GR, Silberstein RB, Cadusch PJ, and Wood AW, 2000, The steady-state visually evoked potential and travelling waves. *Clinical Neurophysiology*, 111: 246–258.

Chen Y, Seth AK, Gally JA, and Edelman GM, 2003, The power of human brain magnetoencephalographic signals can be modulated up or down by changes in an attentive visual task. *Proceedings of the National Academy of Sciences USA* 100: 3501–3506.

Courchesne E, 1990, Chronology of postnatal brain development: event-related potential, positron emission tomography, myelinogenesis, and synaptogenesis studies. In: JW Rohrbaugh, R Parasuraman, and R Johnson (Eds.), *Event-Related Potentials of the Brain*, New York: Oxford University Press, pp. 210–241.

Fisch BJ, 1999, *Fisch & Spehlmann's EEG Primer*, Amsterdam: Elsevier.

Florian G, Andrew C, and Pfurtscheller G, 1998, Do changes in coherence always reflect changes in functional coupling? *Electroencephalography and Clinical Neurophysiology* 106: 87–91.

Freeman WJ, 1975, *Mass Action in the Nervous System*, New York: Academic Press.

Freeman WJ, 1992, Predictions on neocortical dynamics derived from studies in paleocortex. In: E Basar and TH Bullock (Eds.), *Induced Rhythms in the Brain*, Boston: Birhauser, pp. 183–201.

Gevins AS, Smith ME, McEvoy L, and Yu D, 1997, High-resolution mapping of cortical activation related to working memory: effects of task difficulty, type of processing, and practice. *Cerebral Cortex* 7: 374–385.

Hughes JR, Ikram A, and Fino JJ, 1995, Characteristics of traveling waves under various conditions. *Electroencephalography and Clinical Neurophysiology* 26: 7–22.

Hughes JR, Kuruvilla A, and Kino JJ, 1992, Topographic analysis of visual evoked potentials from flash and pattern reversal stimuli: evidence for "traveling waves". *Brain Topography* 4: 215–228.

Jasper HD and Penfield W, 1949, Electrocorticograms in man. Effects of voluntary movement upon the electrical activity of the precentral gyrus. *Archiv. Fur Psychiatrie und Zeitschrift Neurologie* 183: 163–174.

Katznelson RD, 1981, Normal modes of the brain: neuroanatomical basis and a physiological theoretical model. In PL Nunez (Au.), *Electric Fields of the Brain: The Neurophysics of EEG*, 1st Edition, New York: Oxford University Press, pp. 401–442.

Kellaway P, 1979, An orderly approach to visual analysis: the parameters of the normal EEG in adults and children. In: DW Klass and DD Daly (Eds.), *Current Practice of Clinical Electroencephalography*, New York: Raven Press, pp. 69–147.

Lachaux JP, Rodriguez E, Martinerie J, and Varela FJ, 1999, Measuring phase synchrony in brain signals. *Human Brain Mapping* 8: 194–208.

Lopes da Silva FH, 1991, Neural mechanisms underlying brain waves: from membranes to networks. *Electroencephalography and Clinical Neurophysiology* 79: 81–93.

Lopes da Silva FH, 1995, Dynamics of electrical activity of the brain, local networks, and modulating systems. In: PL Nunez (Au.), *Neocortical Dynamics and Human EEG Rhythms*, New York: Oxford University Press, pp. 249–271.

Lopes da Silva FH, 1999, Dynamics of EEGs as signals of neuronal populations: models and theoretical considerations. In: E Niedermeyer and FH Lopes da Silva (Eds.), *Electroencephalography. Basic Principals, Clinical Applications, and Related Fields*, 4th Edition, London: Williams and Wilkins, pp. 76–92.

Massimini M, Huber R, Ferrarelli F, Hill S, and Tononi G, 2004, The sleep slow oscillation as a traveling wave. *Journal of Neuroscience* 24: 6862–6870.

Morgan ST, Hansen JC, and Hillyard SA, 1996, Selective attention to stimulus location modulates the steady-state visually evoked potential. *Proceedings of the National Academy of Sciences USA* 93: 4770–4774.

Muller MM, Picton TW, Valdes-Sosa P, Riera J, Teder-Salejarvi WA, and Hillyard SA, 1998, Effects of spatial selective attention on the steady-state visually evoked potential in the 20–28 Hz range. Brain research. *Cognitive Brain Research* 6: 249–261.

Nakayama K and Mackeben M, 1982, Steady-state visual evoked potentials in the alert primate. *Vision Research* 22: 1261–1271.

Narici L, Portin K, Salmelin R, and Hari R, 1998, Responsiveness of human cortical activity to rhythmical stimulation: a three-modality, whole cortex neuromagnetic investigation. *Neuroimage* 7: 209–223.

Niedermeyer E, 1999a, The normal EEG of the waking adult. In: E Niedermeyer and FH Lopes da Silva (Eds.), *Electroencephalography. Basic Principals, Clinical Applications, and Related Fields*, 4th Edition, London: Williams and Wilkins, pp. 149–173.

Niedermeyer E, 1999b, Maturation of the EEG: development of waking and sleep patterns. In: E Niedermeyer and FH Lopes da Silva (Eds.), *Electroencephalography. Basic Principals, Clinical Applications, and Related Fields*, 4th Edition, London: Williams and Wilkins, pp. 189–214.

Niedermeyer E and Lopes da Silva FH (Eds.), 1999, *Electroencephalography. Basic Principals, Clinical Applications, and Related Fields*, 4th Edition, London: Williams and Wilkins.

Nunez PL, 1974, Wave-like properties of the alpha rhythm. *IEEE Transactions on Biomedical Engineering* 21: 473–482.

Nunez PL, 1995, *Neocortical Dynamics and Human EEG Rhythms*, New York: Oxford University Press.

Nunez PL, 2000a, Toward a large-scale quantitative description of neocortical dynamic function and EEG (Target article), *Behavioral and Brain Sciences* 23: 371–398.

Nunez PL, 2000b, Neocortical dynamic theory should be as simple as possible, but not simpler (Response to 18 commentaries on target article). *Behavioral and Brain Sciences* 23: 415–437.

Nunez PL, Silberstein RB, Shi Z, Carpenter MR, Srinivasan R, Tucker DM, Doran SM, Cadusch PJ, and Wijesinghe RS, 1999, EEG coherence: II. Experimental measures of multiple EEG coherence measures. *Electroencephalography and Clinical Neurophysiology* 110: 469–486.

Nunez PL, Srinivasan R, Westdorp AF, Wijesinghe RS, Tucker DM, Silberstein RB, and Cadusch PJ, 1997, EEG coherency: I. Statistics, reference electrode, volume conduction, Laplacians, cortical imaging, and interpretation at multiple scales. *Electroencephalography and Clinical Neurophysiology* 103: 516–527.

Nunez PL, Wingeier BM, and Silberstein RB, 2001, Spatial-temporal structures of human alpha rhythms: theory, micro-current sources, multiscale measurements, and global binding of local networks. *Human Brain Mapping* 13: 125–164.

Penfield W and Jasper HD, 1954, *Epilepsy and the Functional Anatomy of the Human Brain*, London: Little Brown.

Pilgreen KL, 1995, Physiologic, medical and cognitive correlates of electroencephalography. In: PL Nunez (Au.), *Neocortical Dynamics and Human EEG Rhythms*, New York: Oxford University Press, pp. 195–248.

Rager G and Singer W, 1998, The response of the cat visual cortex to flicker stimuli of variable frequency. *European Journal of Neuroscience* 10: 1856–1877.

Regan D, 1989, *Human Brain Electrophysiology*, New York: Elsevier.

Rosenblum M, Pikovsky A, and Kurths J, 1996, Phase synchronization of chaotic oscillators. *Physical Review Letters* 76: 1804–1807.

Shichijo F, Nagahiro S, Kubo S, and Takimoto O, 1999, Acute effects of alcohol drinking on the EEG, International Society of Brain Electromagnetic Topography, Adelaide, Australia (Poster).

Silberstein RB, 1995, Steady-state visually evoked potentials, brain resonances, and cognitive processes. In: PL Nunez (Au.), *Neocortical Dynamics and Human EEG Rhythms*, New York: Oxford University Press, pp. 272–303.

Silberstein RB, Danieli F, and Nunez PL, 2003, Fronto-parietal evoked potential synchronization is increased during mental rotation. *NeuroReport* 14: 67–71.

Silberstein RB, Nunez PL, Pipingas A, Harris P, and Danieli F, 2001, Steady-state visually evoked potential topography in a graded working memory task. *International Journal of Psychophysiology* 42: 219–232.

Silberstein RB, Nunez PL, and Wijesinghe R, 1993, Unpublished data recorded in Melbourne and partly analyzed in New Orleans.

Silberstein RB, Song J, Nunez PL, and Park W, 2004, Dynamic sculpting of brain functional connectivity is correlated with performance measures. *Brain Topography* 16: 249–254.

Simpson DG, 1998, Instrumentation for high spatial resolution steady state visual evoked potentials. Report of the Brain Sciences Institute & Biophysical Sciences and Electrical Engineering, Swinburne University of Technology, Melbourne, Australia.

Singer W, 1993, Synchronization of cortical activity and its putative role in information processing and learning. *Annual Reviews of Physiology* 55: 349–374.

Srinivasan R, 1999, Spatial structure of the human alpha rhythm: global correlation in adults and local correlation in children. *Clinical Neurophysiology* 110: 1351–1362.

Srinivasan R, 2004, Internal and external neural synchronization during conscious perception. *International Journal of Bifurcation and Chaos* 14: 825–842.

Srinivasan R, Nunez PL, and Silberstein RB, 1998, Spatial filtering and neocortical dynamics: estimates of EEG coherence. *IEEE Transactions on Biomedical Engineering* 45: 814–826.

Srinivasan R, Russell DP, Edelman GM, and Tononi G, 1999, Frequency tagging competing stimuli in binocular rivalry reveals increased synchronization of neuromagnetic responses during conscious perception. *Journal of Neuroscience* 19: 5435–5448.

Steriade M, 1999, Cellular substrates of brain rhythms. In: E Niedermeyer and FH Lopes da Silva (Eds.), *Electroencephalography. Basic Principals, Clinical Applications, and Related Fields*, 4th Edition, London: Williams and Wilkins, pp. 28–75.

Steriade M, Contreras D, Curro Dossi R, and Nunez A, 1993, The slow (<1 Hz) oscillation in reticular thalamic and thalamocortical neurons: scenario of sleep rhythm generation in interacting thalamic and neocortical networks. *Journal of Neuroscience* 13: 3284–3299.

Tass P, Rosenblum M, Weule J, Kurths J, Pikovsky A, Volkmann J, Schnitzler A, and Freund H-J, 1998, Detection of n:m phase locking from noisy data: application to magnetoencephalography. *Physical Review Letters* 81: 3291–3294.

Thatcher RW, 1996, Neuroimaging of cyclic cortical reorganization during human development. In: RW Thatcher, LG Reid, J Rumsey, and N Krasnegor (Eds.), *Developmental Neuroimaging: Mapping and Development of Brain and Behavior*, San Diego: Academic Press.

Tucker DM, 2000, Real brain waves. *Behavioral and Brain Sciences* 23: 412–413.

Tyler CW, Apkarian P, and Nakayama K, 1978, Multiple spatial frequency tuning of electrical responses from the human visual cortex. *Experimental Brain Research* 33: 535–550.

Wingeier BM, 2004, *A High Resolution Study of Coherence and Spatial Spectral in Human EEG*, Ph.D. Dissertation, New Orleans: Tulane University.

Wingeier BM, Nunez PL, and Silberstein RB, 2001, Spherical harmonic decomposition applied to spatial-temporal analysis of human high-density electroencephalogram. *Physical Review E* 64: 051916-1-9.

Yakovlev PI and Lecours AR, 1967, The myelogenetic cycles of regional maturation of the brain. In: A Minkowski (Ed.), *Regional Development of the Brain in Early Life*, Philadelphia: FA Davis, pp. 3–70.

11

Neocortical Dynamics, EEG, and Cognition

---

1 Neocortical Dynamic Properties for the Millennium

For more than a century, neuroscientists have pursued the *Holy Grail of connecting psychology with physiology*, but such achievements have been quite difficult to accomplish. Many robust EEG links to psychology have been established over the past 80 years. General states of consciousness, brain pathology, and specific cognitive processes have been shown to be moderately to strongly correlated with EEG dynamic measures (Kellaway 1979; Gevins and Cutillo 1995; Silberstein 1995a; Uhl 1998; Klimesch 1999; Niedermeyer and Lopes da Silva 1999; Aminoff 1999). Thus, an indirect approach to establishing connections between psychology and physiology is to link EEG data to the underlying physiology as indicated in fig. 11-1; this chapter provides several views at this issue from a theoretical perspective. Several preliminary mathematical theories are proposed so that stronger links may be added to the serial chain physiology–EEG–psychology.

New relations between cognitive events and EEG measures are discovered on a regular basis. We have not described many such connections in this book. Rather, a few cognitive experiments are cited mainly as a means to demonstrate the data analyses that seem effective in revealing dynamic properties of EEG. Naturally, we would also like to focus on critical cognitive experiments that are most likely to endure, but who can say what cognitive science will look like in 50 or 100 years? By contrast to the cognitive theories that motivate many of today's experiments, EEG dynamic properties are determined by natural selection; they will be just as valid in a century or so as they are today. We guess that future cognitive experiments, whatever form they may take, will benefit from such

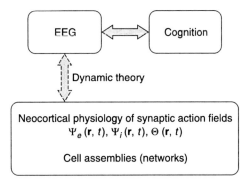

Figure 11-1   Indirect connections between cognitive science and physiology may be achieved through the established EEG–cognitive links (solid arrow) and new links between EEG and physiology (dashed arrow) facilitated by mathematical theory. In the lower box, synaptic and action potential fields are shown above networks suggesting that such fields are more directly related to EEG data than neural networks (or probably more accurately, *cell assemblies*).

dynamic knowledge. An abbreviated summary of some of today's established dynamic EEG properties is as follows.

(i) Eyes closed, resting alpha rhythms with frequencies in the 8 to 13 Hz range are easily recorded from the scalp in perhaps 95% of the adult population. Alpha rhythms have been recorded from nearly the entire upper surface of exposed neocortex (Jasper and Penfield 1949). High-density scalp EEG also reveals widespread alpha rhythms over the entire scalp as discussed in chapter 10 (Nunez et al. 2001). Cortical and scalp recordings have revealed the existence of multiple alpha rhythms in different parts of cortex (Pfurtscheller and Neuper 1992; Andrew and Pfurtscheller 1997; Florian et al. 1998; Sarnthein et al. 1998; Pfurtscheller and Lopes da Silva 1999). Some are blocked by eyes opening; some are not. Some are blocked by mental activity; some are not. Scalp recordings of alpha rhythm are space averages of apparent multiple processes. As a result of this spatial filtering, scalp potentials are biased towards cortical *global activity*; that is, activity in the low end of the spatial frequency spectrum (Nunez 1974b; Wingeier et al. 2001). Comparison of temporal frequency spectra obtained from high-resolution and conventional scalp recordings reveals that alpha rhythms show both global and local dynamic behavior (Nunez et al. 2001). That is, high-resolution EEG methods spatially filter out both the global source dynamics and volume conducted potentials leaving only mid-scale dynamics (which is still much larger scale than cortical recordings). These scalp EEG studies are fully consistent with Grey Walter's early ECoG observations.

(ii) When recorded from the scalp, the low and high frequencies of the alpha band have somewhat different spatial distributions. The high alpha band has more relative power at higher spatial frequencies (Nunez 1974b, 1995; Shaw 1991; Wingeier et al. 2001; Wingeier 2004). Furthermore, power and coherence changes with transitions between resting and cognitive states (mental tasks) can occur in opposite directions in the upper and lower alpha bands (Klimesch et al. 1999; Nunez et al. 2001; Wingeier 2004). Again, these data are consistent with Walter's ECoG observations of multiple alpha rhythms.

(iii) Scalp recordings during deep sleep and some coma and anesthesia states produce large-amplitude, widespread delta (0 to 4 Hz) activity over the scalp. With halothane anesthesia, it is possible to "tune" the brain (Stockard 1996; Nunez et al. 1976, 1977, 1995). Halothane-dominant oscillation frequency can vary from about 4 to 16 Hz depending on inspired concentration; high concentrations result in lower frequencies and larger amplitudes. Multimode oscillation frequencies go up and down together with inspired concentration as shown in the example of fig. 11-2.

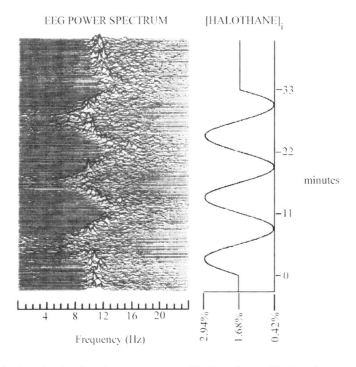

Figure 11-2 Anesthesia time-frequency plot. Multimode oscillation frequencies go up and down together with inspired concentration of halothane (sine wave modulated shown at right). EEG is large amplitude ($\approx$50–100 μV) over the entire scalp. All eight subjects in the study showed similar EEG behavior, but with differences in number and intensity of apparent modes. Reproduced with permission from Stockard (1976) and Nunez et al. (1977).

(iv) Differences in observed ECoG dynamic behavior between cortical areas disappear during anesthesia based on visual inspection of raw time series (Bickford 1950; Penfield and Jasper 1954). That is, transitions from normal waking to anesthesia states appear to correspond to transitions from more local to more global dynamic states. A large variety of EEG behavior may be observed depending on depth and type of anesthesia as well as type of coma. These include sinusoidal oscillations and complex waveforms (combinations of oscillations) in the delta, theta, alpha, and beta bands. However, as a *general rule of head*, lower temporal frequency oscillations tend to occur with larger amplitudes in a wide range of brain states (Barlow 1993).

(v) Mental activity of various sorts tends to enhance EEG power in certain frequency bands and suppress power in other bands. Many of the details are subject and task dependent, but increased frontal power in the theta band (4–7 Hz) during mental activity is a common finding (Gevins et al. 1997; Klimesch 1999). In some subjects, power increases may also occur in upper alpha (10–13 Hz) and perhaps beta bands (>13 Hz), while power in the lower alpha band (8–9 Hz) decreases (Petsche et al. 1997; Petsche and Etlinger 1998; Klimesch et al. 1999; Nunez et al. 2001). Based on evidence from intracranial studies in animals (Singer 1993; Bressler 1995) and scalp experiments in humans (Lachaux et al. 1999), there are reasons to believe that mental activity is also associated with changes in the 40 Hz range (and possibly higher); however, the high probability of muscle artifact contamination has limited interpretations of gamma recordings from the human scalp.

(vi) Changes in the long-range covariance of transient event-related potentials are associated with correct performance on various mental tasks (Gevins and Cutillo 1995). These covariance patterns are presumably due to selective source synchrony at the relatively low temporal frequencies of the theta and alpha bands. These data suggest that cognition is associated with rapidly shifting patterns of statistical interdependency between (often) remote cortical locations.

(vii) Amplitude, phase, and coherence changes of 13 Hz *steady-state visually evoked potentials* (SSVEPs) are correlated with performance on mental tasks (Silberstein 1995a; Silberstein et al. 2001, 2003, 2004). Long-range coherence between some regions increases during mental activity (suggesting formation of regional networks) while coherence between other regions decreases. The latter effect can be interpreted as indicating dissolution of irrelevant networks, reduction in global field effects (discussed in section 3) or some combination.

(viii) In studies of binocular rivalry, where two incongruent images are flickered (one to each eye) at 7–12 Hz, *steady-state evoked magnetic fields* and SSVEPs show that conscious perception of only one of the two images (a unitary consciousness) is associated with increased inter-hemispheric coherence (Srinivasan et al. 1999; Edelman and Tononi 2000).

(ix) Mental activity of various sorts tends to enhance EEG coherence in certain frequency bands and electrode pairs and suppress coherence in other bands and electrode pairs (Nunez et al. 1997, 1999). Many of the details are subject dependent, but increased coherence in frontal electrodes in the theta band (4–8 Hz) during mental activity is a common finding (Nunez et al. 2001). Coherence changes may be either coincident or occur independently of power changes (Petsche et al. 1997, 1998), apparently depending on the spatial scale of coherent source activity as discussed in chapter 9 and Nunez (2001). One study has reported coupling of theta and gamma band activity during human short-term memory processing, as measured by *bicoherence* (Schack et al. 2002). These data have direct relevance to the resonance phenomena outlined in sections 7 and 8.

2 A Tentative Framework for Brain Dynamics and Several Conjectures

The framework outlined in chapter 1 (see fig. 1-8) appears to be well supported by these general properties of EEG data together with the various theoretical considerations discussed throughout this book, including both dynamic and volume conduction theory. That is, neocortical source dynamics may be viewed in terms of rapidly changing cell assemblies (or networks) embedded within a global environment. We choose to express this global environment in terms of *synaptic and action potential fields*. Scalp potentials evidently provide signatures of some (generally unknown) combination of the synaptic action fields and network activity, but are strongly biased towards dynamics with low spatial frequencies, suggesting substantial (or perhaps dominant) contributions from globally coherent synaptic fields. We further conjecture that both bottom-up (networks to global) and top–down (global to networks) interactions provide important contributions to the neocortical dynamics of behavior and cognition. Such two-way interactions appear to substantially facilitate so-called *brain binding*, the ability to coordinate separate functions into unified behavior and consciousness. Our proposed framework is consistent with the following descriptions by other scientists.

(i) In the following quote by Mountcastle (1979) we may substitute *local networks* or *small-scale cell assemblies* for "systems":

The brain is a complex of widely and reciprocally interconnected systems and the dynamic interplay of neural activity within and between these systems is the very essence of brain function.

(ii) Based on extensive studies of evoked potential covariance associated with mental activity, Gevins and Cutillo (1995) state:

…many (cortical) areas probably are involved in a constellation of rapidly changing functional networks that provide the delicate balance between stimulus-locked behavior and purely imaginary ideation.

(iii) Based on synchronization and other studies in human and nonhuman primates, Bressler (1995) conjectures:

…elementary functions are localized in discrete cortical areas, whereas complex functions are processed in parallel in widespread cortical networks. Control processes, operating at cortical and sub-cortical levels by a variety of mechanisms, dynamically organize and regulate large-scale cortical networks.

(iv) The following view is expressed by Edelman and Tononi (2000) in the context of a quantitative complexity measure associated with consciousness and brain binding:

…high values of complexity correspond to an optimal synthesis of functional specialization and functional integration within a system. This is clearly the case for systems like the brain—different areas and different neurons do different things (they are differentiated) at the same time they interact to give rise to a unified conscious scene and to unify behaviors (they are integrated).

In this latter view complexity (and by implication, cognition) tends to maximize between the extremes of isolated networks and global coherence. We find this to be a compelling working hypothesis. It then follows that both local network dynamics and interactions between networks are important for brain function. However, one of the central messages of this book is that different experimental designs and methods of data analysis can bias EEG (or MEG or fMRI or PET) physiological interpretations in either local or global directions.

Silberstein (1995b) has taken this general local versus global dynamic picture a step further in the physiological and clinical directions by suggesting several ways in which brainstem neurotransmitter systems might act to change the coupling strength between global fields and local or regional networks. He outlines how different neurotransmitters might alter the coupling strengths by selective actions at different cortical depths, thereby changing resonance properties. He further conjectures that *several diseases (Parkinson disease, some schizophrenias) may be manifestations of hyper-coupled or hypocoupled dynamic states brought on by the faulty actions of the neurotransmitters*. With this background in mind, we examine possible properties of networks and global fields in the following sections.

3 Multiscale Dynamic Theory Illustrated with a Metaphorical Field

Throughout this book, we have emphasized the importance of spatial scale in both experimental and theoretical studies of brain dynamics. In order to facilitate better understanding of relationships between dynamic variables defined at different scales and their association with putative brain networks, a metaphorical theory is outlined here. Our general conceptual framework is expressed by fig. 1-8, in which we imagine cell assemblies (or probably less accurately neural networks) immersed in *global fields* of synaptic action. These synaptic fields are distinguished from the electric and magnetic fields that they generate. *The existence of these fields is noncontroversial.* For example, all we mean by the excitatory synaptic action field $\Psi_e(\mathbf{r}, t)$ is simply the number density of active excitatory synapses in some tissue voxel located at $\mathbf{r}$, defined over the entire cortical surface. Such definition implies a *coarse graining* over small time and space scales so that $\Psi_e(\mathbf{r}, t)$ varies relatively smoothly in time and space. The only possible controversy is whether the introduction of such field concepts is helpful to neuroscience.

Modern theories of large-scale neocortical dynamics are likely to be *field theories* (or *mean-field theories*) for both theoretical and experimental reasons. In order to facilitate better communication between biological and physical scientists and between experimentalists and theoreticians, we here consider a fanciful field theory of human alcohol consumption over the earth's surface. Suppose our first choice of dependent variable is $\Psi_a(\mathbf{r}, t)$, the volume of alcohol consumed at surface location $\mathbf{r}$ and time t. This choice causes immediate problems for theory development. The variable $\Psi_a(\mathbf{r}, t)$ can only be nonzero at the discrete locations of human drinkers, and humans are continually on the move. Also, the drinking process also tends to be discontinuous in time. Thus, our variable $\Psi_a(\mathbf{r}, t)$ must fluctuate widely in both space and time in a manner similar to very small-scale (perhaps fractal) measurements of synaptic current source activity. Such discontinuous dynamic behavior creates substantial problems, not only for theory development, but also for experimental attempts to measure alcohol consumption and check the theory. For these reasons, we may define a set of *coarse-grained variables* (*fields*) in terms of time and space averages, that is

$$\Psi(x, y, t; X, Y, T) = \frac{1}{XYT} \int\limits_{x}^{x+X} dx' \int\limits_{y}^{y+Y} dy' \int\limits_{t}^{t+T} dt' \Gamma(x', y') \Psi_a(x', y', t') \qquad (11.1)$$

Here the (x, y) are surface coordinates and $\Gamma(x, y)$ is some weighting function. The spatial and temporal scales of the theory or experiment are given by the coarse graining parameters (X, Y, T). The weighting function (or *distribution function* or *kernel*) $\Gamma(x, y)$ is constant (equal to one) if the field Ψ is a simple space-average of alcohol consumption. Alternatively, Ψ might represent another large-scale variable that depends on small-scale consumption, say alcohol-related traffic accidents, in which case the integral weighted by $\Gamma(x, y)$ would effect the transformation from small-scale variable $\Psi_a(\mathbf{r}, t)$ to the new field. Of course, finding the appropriate weighting function $\Gamma(x, y)$ typically requires a separate theory. Some poorly informed sociologist working at the small scales of individual family behaviors might display *scale chauvinism* by labeling the macroscopic field Ψ as an *epiphenomenon*, displaying an attitude found in several scientific fields. A more enlightened viewpoint would consider the large-scale variable $\Psi(\mathbf{r}, t)$ to result from a *bottom-up interaction across spatial scales*. Even this would not be fully accurate if the small-scale drinking rate $\Psi_a(\mathbf{r}, t)$ were substantially influenced by (say) global laws or police action resulting from excessive alcohol-related accidents, *a top-down interaction across spatial scales*. This system would then experience *circular causality* as discussed in section 10, or symbolically $\Psi_a(\mathbf{r}, t) \leftrightarrow \Psi(\mathbf{r}, t)$.

A theory developed for particular spatial and temporal scales, say the (1 mile, 1 day) scales might provide some prediction of the rate of alcohol consumption in neighborhoods on a day-by-day basis. Such theory might predict "fast" sinusoidal oscillations in time with a constant period of one week and "spikes" at holidays, but would be unable to predict hourly oscillations. These particular scales might be chosen in the theory with the aim of matching experimental data, perhaps obtained by contacting neighborhood merchants every morning. Alternatively, we might imagine that alcohol data are available only at quite different scales, say at city or state levels. Naturally, we want our theory to match these experimental scales. Just as in the case of synaptic fields, any global alcohol function Ψ must satisfy two fundamental mathematical conditions: Ψ must be finite at all earth surface locations, and it must be a single-valued function of surface coordinates. The latter condition requires that Ψ satisfy periodic boundary conditions. By contrast, strictly local theories do not require global boundary conditions. We might, for example, just prohibit drinking in the countryside, that is set $\Psi = 0$ at the boundaries of our cities of interest.

Several physiological examples of this kind of coarse graining are provided in this book. One such example (but in three spatial dimensions) is the definition of the mesosource function in terms of the synaptic microcurrent sources (4.26). In this case, the weighting function Γ is simply the location vector $\mathbf{w}$ of microsources within the tissue mass and no time averaging is needed. Another example, is the expression for (macroscopic) scalp potential in terms of the mesosource function given by (2.2), where the weighting function Γ is the Green's function containing all information about the head volume conductor. The standard scalp-recorded evoked or event-related potential represents an experimental coarse graining of cortical potential with space averaging forced by the head volume conductor. Finally, we note that investors in financial markets are intimately familiar with the coarse graining of experimental data. The usual running average of market indices over perhaps $T = 90$ or 200 days provides the time averaging, while the market index itself (say the S&P500) is essentially the space average, calculated with the market capitalizations of individual stocks forming the weighting function Γ.

4 A Simple Model for Global Fields

In order to distinguish the various theories of large-scale neocortical dynamics, we adopt the label *local theory* to indicate mathematical models of cortical or thalamocortical interactions (feedback loops) for which corticocortical propagation delays are assumed to be zero. The underlying timescales in these theories are typically postsynaptic potential (PSP) rise and decay times. Thalamocortical networks are also "local" from the viewpoint of a surface electrode, which cannot distinguish purely cortical from thalamocortical networks. Finally, these theories are "local" in the sense of being independent of global boundary conditions dictated by the size and shape of the cortical–white matter system.

By contrast, we adopt the label *global theory* to indicate mathematical models in which delays in the corticocortical fibers forming most of the white matter in humans provide the important underlying timescale for the large-scale EEG dynamics recorded by scalp electrodes. Periodic boundary conditions are generally essential to global theories because the cortical–white matter system of one hemisphere is topologically close to a spherical shell as indicated in figs. 11-3 and 3-12. The most recent theories of neocortical dynamics include selected aspects of both local and global theories, but typically with more emphasis on one or the other.

Figure 11-4a indicates the two halves of the cerebral cortex with several modular columns of diameter ≈ 300 μm, each containing about 1,000 to 10,000 neurons (Szentagothai 2004). Several axons are shown crossing through the corpus callosum (the total number is of the order of 10^8 in the human brain), one corticocortical axon (total number about 10^{10}) and two corticothalamic axons (total number about 10^8). Figure 11-4b shows just a few network details in a single column through the entire cortex (with transverse diameter stretched to show more detail). In this section, *we imagine a neocortex entirely devoid of networks*. That is, all preferential cell interactions are ignored and only global synaptic fields due to simple input–output relations in cortical tissue masses are considered. We do not suggest that this is a realistic picture for all (or even most) brain states. Rather, we conjecture some approximate correspondence with sleep, resting, or anesthesia states. We further suggest that global fields may play

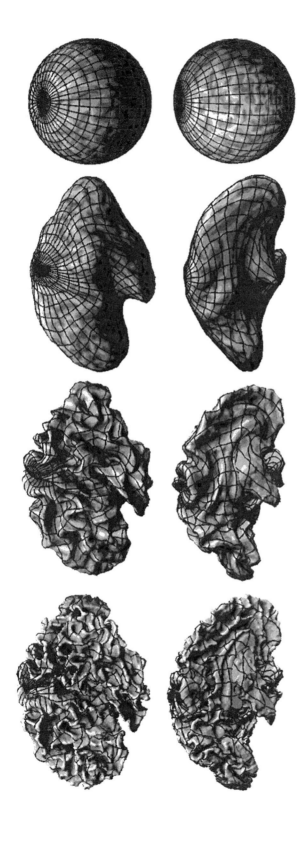

Figure 11-3 Periodic boundary conditions are generally essential to global theories because the cortical–white matter system of one hemisphere is topologically nearly identical to a spherical shell. Here a computer algorithm progressively inflates each brain hemisphere and transforms them into spheres. The figure was generated by Armin Fuchs and kindly transmitted to Nunez for this publication. The computer algorithm was developed by Dale et al. (1993, 1999) and Fischl et al. (1999).

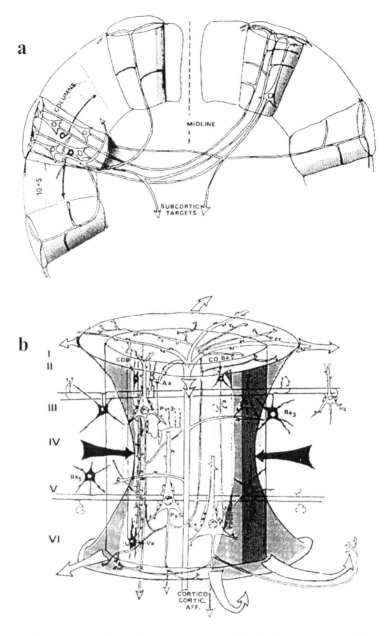

Figure 11-4 (a) Several corticocortical columns (modules) with diameters ≈200 to 300 μm through the entire cortex are shown. Column widths are greatly exaggerated to show interiors. The modules are defined as the width of aborization of corticocortical afferents, that is, the input scale for long-range cortical connections. Several callosal and one corticocortical axons are shown. The human brain has about 10^{10} corticocortical and perhaps 10^8 thalamocortical fibers (Braitenberg and Schuz 1991). (b) Some details of networks inside one column are shown. Each corticocortical column has about 1,000 to 10,000 neurons and most neurons send an axon into the white matter to connect to other cortical regions or to thalamus. The hourglass shape was chosen to suggest the dynamic distortion of a cylindrical module by the tendency for lateral (intracortical and corticocortical) excitation to spread to neighboring columns from layers I and VI (white arrows) with inhibitory interactions act mainly on middle layers III, IV, and V (black arrows). Reproduced with permission from Szentagothia (2004).

important roles in facilitating communication between separate networks. Mainly, this basic global theory should be considered a crude limiting approximation that suggests some general global properties to look for in experimental EEG data. For purposes of the simplest version of the global brain theory we assume the following:

(i) Excitatory action potentials are transmitted along intracortical and the corticocortical axons that form most of the white matter layer directly below neocortex. Since axon propagation velocities are finite, action potentials at one cortical location produce synaptic activity at distant locations after time delays that are proportional to separation distance on an inflated (idealized) smooth surface.

(ii) The intracortical and corticocortical axons are parceled into M excitatory systems. For each fiber system ($m = 1, M$), the density of connections between any two cortical regions falls off exponentially with separation distance. The characteristic lengths of the individual exponential decays are given by λ_m^{-1}. An example three-fiber system is depicted in fig. 11-5.

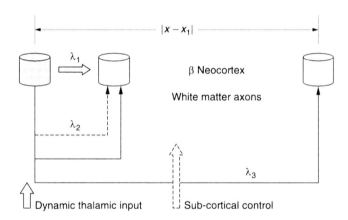

Figure 11-5 In the global theory, the assumed fall-off in excitatory fiber density between any two cortical locations separated by distance $|x-x_1|$ is given by a sum of M exponential decays corresponding to M fiber systems with characteristic lengths λ_m^{-1}. This example pictures $M = 3$ fiber systems: a short-range intracortical system (*recurrent collaterals*, $\lambda_1 > 10$ cm^{-1}) represented by the short arrow, an intermediate length system (*U fibers and somewhat longer corticocortical fibers*, $\lambda_2 < 1$ cm^{-1}) represented by the dashed line, and a long corticocortical fiber system ($\lambda_3 \approx 0.1$ to 0.2 cm^{-1}) represented by the solid line. Only efferent fibers exiting the gray column are indicated in this picture except for dynamic input from the thalamus (vertical gray arrow). All cortical tissue masses are assumed to have both afferent and efferent fibers. In the simplest version of the global theory, the influences of the shorter excitatory fibers (larger λ_m values) and all inhibitory fibers are lumped into the cortical excitability parameter β, which acts to control neocortex by means of chemical and electrical input from subcortical regions (dashed white arrow). This input is assumed to act on much longer timescales (seconds to minutes) than the millisecond-scale dynamic input from the thalamus. See appendix L and Nunez (1995) for details.

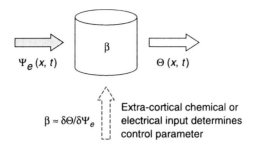

Figure 11-6 A mesoscopic cortical tissue mass (say millimeter scale) is represented with *excitatory synaptic input* $\Psi_e(x, t)$ from other cortical tissue indicated by the gray arrow (intracortical and corticocortical). As a result the tissue mass produces a certain number of action potentials (per volume or cortical surface area): the tissue mass *output* $\Theta(x, t)$. The linear approximation of the global theory postulates that small changes in this input $\delta\Psi_e(x, t)$ cause proportional changes in output $\delta\Theta(x, t)$. The text uses the simplified notation $\delta\Psi_e(x, t) \equiv \Psi(x, t)$. The proportionality constant β depends on tissue excitability as determined by chemical and electrical cortical input that occurs on timescales much longer than synaptic field cycle times. In the quasi-linear approximation proposed in this chapter, it is conjectured that large excitatory fields $|\Psi_e(x, t)|$ cause recruitment of additional inhibitory input to prevent instability (epilepsy) in healthy brains.

(iii)   An incremental change in number density of action potentials $\delta\Theta(\mathbf{r}, t)$ produced in a mesoscopic mass of cortical tissue increases roughly in proportion to small increases in number density of excitatory synaptic inputs $\delta\Psi_e(\mathbf{r}, t)$ as suggested in fig. 11-6. Similarly, action potential density tends to decrease in approximate proportion to small increases in number density inhibitory synaptic inputs $\delta\Psi_i(\mathbf{r}, t)$. This is the basic linear approximation that ignores nonlinear feedback as well as all local network effects expected in most brain states.

(iv)   The magnitudes of the action potential changes in (iii) are determined by a single control parameter β, *the background excitability of neocortex*. This excitability parameter β, which partly determines brain state, may be changed by unspecified chemical and electrical input from midbrain or neocortex. In the simplest version of the global theory, influences of the inhibitory input $\delta\Psi_i(\mathbf{r}, t)$ and shorter corticocortical fibers (excitatory) are lumped into β. Changes in β occur on much longer timescales (seconds to minutes) than EEG cycle times.

(v)   As the excitatory synaptic action density $|\Psi_e(\mathbf{r}, t)|$ in some neocortical region $\mathbf{r}$ becomes progressively larger, extra inhibitory input to the local tissue mass is recruited in healthy brains as a result of negative feedback from contiguous cortex, thalamus, or both. This is a quasi-linear approximation that may cause limit cycle-like oscillations of global modes, but still ignores the local network effects expected in most brain states.

The model cortex outlined above has been considered in a series of theoretical papers (Nunez 1972, 1974, 1989, 1995, 2000a, b; Katznelson

1981). A short summary of the one-dimensional version appears in appendix L. The general predictions of this theory are as follows.

The modulation of excitatory neocortical synaptic action may be expressed as a weighted sum of contributions of the form

$$\delta \Psi_e(\mathbf{r},t) = \sum_n \xi_n(t) \psi_n(\mathbf{r}) \qquad (11.2)$$

Here the functions $\xi_n(t)$ are called the order parameters in the field of *synergetics, the science of cooperation* (Haken 1983). The general form of the expression (11.2) applies to a large variety of complex physical systems. In some quasi-linear approximations, the order parameters $\xi_n(t)$ in the sum may be approximated by

$$\xi_n(t) \cong C_n \cos[\omega_n t - \theta_n] \qquad (11.3)$$

The spatial functions (*eigenfunctions*) $\psi_n(\mathbf{r})$ are severely restricted by cortical boundary conditions; that is, by the size and shape of the cortical surface. For example, the theory predicts standing waves in a spherical shell (Katznelson 1981; Nunez 1995), in which case the $\psi_n(\mathbf{r})$ are the spherical harmonics $Y_{nm}(\theta, \phi)$. Here we outline the simplest version of this work in which oscillation frequencies of multiple modes occur in a closed one dimensional loop representing the anterior–posterior circumference of one cortical hemisphere. As outlined in appendix L, each spatial mode oscillates with its characteristic mode frequency

$$f_n = \frac{\omega_n}{2\pi} \approx \frac{v}{L} \sqrt{n^2 - \left(\frac{\beta \lambda L}{2\pi}\right)^2} \quad n = 1, 2, 3, \dots \qquad (11.4)$$

The neocortical parameters in (11.4) and their probable ranges are as follows:

(i) *Characteristic velocity* (peak in the velocity distribution function) for propagation in corticocortical fibers (review in Nunez 1995):

$$v \approx 600\text{--}900 \text{ cm/s} \qquad (11.5)$$

(ii) Effective front-to-back circumference of one cortical hemisphere after inflation to smooth the surface as shown in fig. 11-3. For waves on a spherical surface with area equal to 1500 cm^2, the effective radius is about 11 cm, corresponding to a circumference of about 70 cm. However, each brain hemisphere is shaped more like an eccentric prolate spheroid with a long (smooth) circumference in roughly the range

$$80 < L < 90 \text{ cm} \qquad (11.6)$$

(iii) Nondimensional cortical excitability control parameter β. The excitability control parameter is roughly proportional to the incremental increase in action potential density $\delta\Theta(\mathbf{r}, t)$ produced within a cortical mass element (the output) due to an incremental increase in excitatory synaptic input, that is

$$\beta \propto \frac{\delta\Theta}{\delta\Psi_e} \tag{11.7}$$

A plot of action potential output Θ versus excitatory input Ψ_e is expected to have a sigmoid shape if there are no local circuit effects. In this case, β is proportional to the local slope of the sigmoid. In the linear limiting case, $\beta > 1$ causes all modes to become unstable. However, we assume here that *natural selection has provided for enhanced negative feedback from thalamus or contiguous cortex to prevent such instability in healthy brains.* We do not now have accurate estimates for the range of β, which is expected to vary with brain state, but a plausible guess is something like $0 < \beta < 10$ (Nunez 1995). As discussed below, ignorance of β does not prevent us from obtaining several rough theoretical predictions.

(iv) The longest corticocortical fiber system density is assumed to fall off according to

$$\exp[-\lambda_M/\mathbf{r} - \mathbf{r_1}/]$$

between any two cortical locations $\mathbf{r}$ and $\mathbf{r_1}$ (or x and x_1 in the one-dimensional version), as indicated in fig. 11-5. The effects of short excitatory fibers (larger λ_m values in both intracortical and corticocortical systems) are included (approximately) in the excitability parameter β (for details see pp. 488–490 of Nunez 1995). This assumed exponential fall off in fiber connection density is chosen for mathematical convenience rather than physiological reality in order to facilitate analytic solutions. Nevertheless, by fitting a slightly more complicated function to the measured (and scaled) fall-off of corticocortical fiber density in mouse brain, very similar theoretical results are obtained (for details see pp. 506–511 of Nunez 1995). We simplify the notation using $\lambda_M \rightarrow \lambda$. An estimated range for the average (long) fiber length λ^{-1} for an inflated cortex is 5 to 10 cm (Nunez 1995). Thus, the following nondimensional parameter range is suggested:

$$1 < \left(\frac{\lambda L}{2\pi}\right)^2 < 3 \tag{11.8}$$

By applying these estimates to the predicted angular frequencies (11.4) yields

$$7 < \frac{v}{L} < 11 \text{ Hz} \qquad (11.9)$$

In this case of one-dimensional waves around the circumference, the $n = 1$ mode appears to be nonoscillatory (imaginary frequency). Both the $n = 1$ and $n = 2$ modes appear to be roughly consistent with the average spatial distribution of scalp alpha rhythms. To consider a (partly arbitrary) numerical example, the parameter choices

$$(v, L, \lambda, \beta) = (750 \text{ cm/s}, 80 \text{ cm}, 0.1 \text{ cm}^{-1}, 1.3) \qquad (11.10)$$

yield the following predicted mode frequencies:

$$f_2 = 10.5 \text{ Hz}, \quad f_3 = 23.5 \text{ Hz}, \quad f_4 = 34.1 \text{ Hz} \qquad (11.11)$$

While the exact frequencies cannot be taken seriously, one general prediction is multiple global oscillatory modes with progressively higher frequencies. *These overtones are not harmonics, which are normally associated with nonlinear effects.* We have ignored many details; for example, the mode frequencies of standing waves in a closed surface (a prolate spheroidal shell, for example) tend to occur in clusters near the frequencies of the major modes associated with the largest circumference (Nunez 1995). Thus, we might expect to find several modes clustered near 10 Hz due only to the shape of the two-dimensional surface. The frequencies predicted by (11.4) are generally in the EEG range, suggesting that the general global picture of standing waves warrants deeper study. However, parameter uncertainty prevents quantitative verification of the theory based only on frequency estimates.

Each hemisphere of neocortex is topologically very close to a spherical shell as indicated in fig. 11-3. The choice of the *eigenfunctions* $\psi_n(\mathbf{r})$ is severely restricted in closed systems for two fundamental physical reasons. First, because they represent genuine (measurable) variables, the functions $\psi_n(\mathbf{r})$ must be finite everywhere on the closed surface. Second, they must be single-valued functions of surface coordinates. For example, suppose we choose some function to represent population density over the earth. The population of (say) New York predicted by our function cannot depend on whether the coordinate path is measured east to west or west to east. The most common eigenfunctions used on spherical surfaces are the spherical harmonics $Y_{nm}(\theta, \phi)$. These functions satisfy both physical constraints and arise naturally as a result of the spherical geometry and

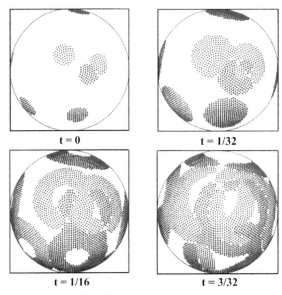

t = 0   **t = 1/32**

t = 1/16   **t = 3/32**

Traveling waves on a sphere

Figure 11-7 Traveling waves in a spherical shell. Wave packets originate at eight cortical locations perhaps as a result of subcortical input. Dark and light patches indicate regions of positive and negative variations of the excitatory synaptic action field $\delta\Psi_e(\mathbf{r}, t) \equiv \Psi(\mathbf{r}, t)$, respectively. Empty spaces show regions with excitatory synaptic action close to the background field $\Psi_e(\mathbf{r}, t)$. Constructive and destructive interference is observed in all but the first plot. These plots represent generic weakly damped *waves*; they do not depend on any specific model. Reproduced with permission from Nunez (1995).

the Laplacian operator, which occurs in the equations of physics that are most frequently applied to physical systems as well as in volume conduction in the head.

Nondispersive and weakly damped traveling waves in a thin spherical shell are illustrated in fig. 11-7. These example wave packets are generated at eight discrete locations and spread out in the shell in a manner similar to water waves due to raindrops in a pond or electromagnetic waves due to multiple lighting strikes in the atmosphere. Overlapping wave packets exhibit interference phenomena; that is, regions with negative field values tend to cancel regions of positive field values. After the external input stops, the fields settle into standing wave patterns for some additional time (depending on the magnitude of damping) as in the examples shown in fig. 11-8. A similar interference phenomenon is postulated in neocortical tissue at mesoscopic scales. That is, if a portion of a wave packet having excess excitatory synaptic action $\Psi(\mathbf{r}, t) \equiv \delta\Psi_e(\mathbf{r}, t)$, that is, a positive perturbation about the background level, encounters a wave portion with locally reduced synaptic action, we expect partial cancellation of synaptic action in tissue masses containing large numbers of neurons. This interference effect may or may not be approximately linear depending partly on the magnitudes of the perturbations $\delta\Psi_e(\mathbf{r}, t)$.

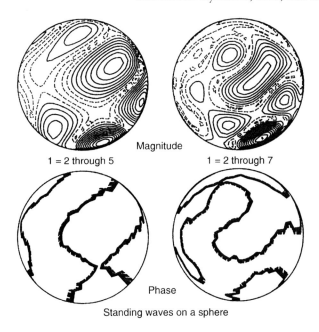

Magnitude

1 = 2 through 5   1 = 2 through 7

Phase

Standing waves on a sphere

Figure 11-8 Standing waves in a spherical shell similar to the *Schumann resonances* discussed in chapter 3. The surface waves were driven by 100 point sources, random in both location and time (for example, lightning strikes in the atmosphere). The resulting spatial patterns (analogous to fig. 11-7) are quite complicated and not shown here. Rather we Fourier transform these data and show magnitude (upper row) and cosine (phase) plots (lower row) for the broad frequency bands associated with the sum of several of the spherical harmonic functions. (*Left column*) ($n = 2$ through 5, labeled l in the plot). (*Right column*) ($n = 2$ through 7) showing more contributions from higher spatial frequencies. Reproduced with permission from Srinivasan (1995) and Nunez (1995).

Predicted global modes for *standing brain waves in a spherical shell* fig. 3-12) were obtained by Katznelson (1981) as a solution to the global wave equation (Nunez 1972, 1974, 1981). The model assumptions listed above are all unchanged except that the closed loop becomes a spherical shell of radius R (reviewed and updated in Nunez 1995). The nondimensional mode frequencies ($\omega_n R/v$) and damping ($\gamma_n R/v$) are plotted versus the spherical control parameter β_S in fig. 11-9 (mode $n = 1$), fig. 11-10 (mode $n = 2$), and fig. 11-11 (mode $n = 3$). With the choice of parameters $(L, R, \lambda, v) = (80\text{ cm},\ 12.7\text{ cm},\ 0.1\text{ cm}^{-1},\ 750\text{ cm/s})$, the fundamental mode f_1 is about 9 Hz when the nondimensional frequency $\omega_1 R/v$ equals one. With this choice of $\lambda R = 1.27$, the two-dimensional control parameter used here (β_S) is roughly equivalent to the one-dimensional version β (for details see pages 521−528 of Nunez 1995). Mode damping is independent of mode number in the simplest version of the one-dimensional linear theory; all modes become unstable for $\beta > 1$. By contrast, the spherical model exhibits a *mode scanning property* in following sense. As β_S increases from values less than one, lower modes become more weakly damped and oscillate at progressively lower frequencies.

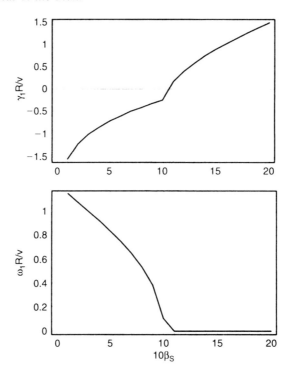

Figure 11-9 The fundamental mode ($n = 1$) in the spherical global model. (*Upper*) The nondimensional global mode damping ($\gamma_1 R/v$) is plotted versus the spherical cortical excitability parameter β_S, chosen here to match approximately the equivalent one-dimensional parameter β for the case $\lambda R = 1.27$. (*Lower*) The nondimensional global mode frequency ($\omega_1 R/v$) is plotted versus the spherical cortical excitability parameter β_S. See Katznelson (1981) and Nunez (1995) for more detail.

At still larger β_S these lower modes become unstable (in the strictly linear theory); their frequencies fall to zero and become nonoscillatory.

An example of this mode scanning feature (adopting the above parameters for ease of the description) is as follows. For very small β_S, the fundamental mode ($n = 1$) oscillates at about 9 Hz, but is strongly damped as shown in fig. 11-9. We might guess that this mode can be observed in EEG only if the global field is coupled to local oscillatory networks with similar resonance frequencies (perhaps generating the multiple alpha rhythms discussed in section 1). As β_S increases towards one, the fundamental mode frequency falls sharply while its damping decreases. The fundamental mode becomes nonoscillatory for $\beta_S > 1$ as shown in fig. 11-9. The second mode (first overtone, $n = 2$) is strongly damped for small β_S, but damping falls to zero for $\beta_S \approx 1.6$ as indicated in fig. 11-10. At this point the second mode oscillates with a frequency of about 13 Hz. Larger values of β_S then cause the frequency of the second mode to fall while instability increases (in the strictly linear theory). The second mode becomes nonoscillatory at $\beta_S \approx 3.2$. When β_S reaches about 1.7, the third mode becomes unstable and oscillates at about 23 Hz, as indicted by the solid curves in fig. 11-11. As β_S increases further, the

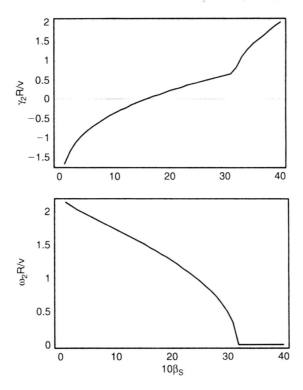

Figure 11-10   The first overtone ($n = 2$) in the spherical global model. (*Upper*) The nondimensional global mode damping ($\gamma_2 R/v$) is plotted versus the spherical cortical excitability parameter β_S. (*Lower*) The nondimensional global mode frequency ($\omega_2 R/v$) is plotted versus the spherical cortical excitability parameter β_S.

frequency of the third mode progressively decreases and becomes non-oscillatory at $\beta_S \approx 6.1$. This general behavior is repeated for higher modes with additional increases in β_S except that multiple branches of the dispersion relation appear as indicated in the fig. 11-11; the (dashed) branches shown are strongly damped. In summary, *at about the same time that lower modes disappear from the field oscillations, higher modes become progressively more weakly damped and oscillate with lower frequencies.* As in the one-dimensional version of the global theory, we conjecture enhanced negative feedback in healthy brains to prevent instability.

5   More Realistic Approximations to the Neocortical Dynamic Global Theory

Because of the extreme oversimplification inherent in the "toy brain" outlined in section 4, its predictive value is expected to be quite limited. Nevertheless, it may provide a genuine "entry point" to more comprehensive brain theory. One obvious place to start is to re-examine the assumed linear relation between action potential output $\Theta(x, t)$ and excitatory synaptic input given by (11.6). By backtracking one step in the

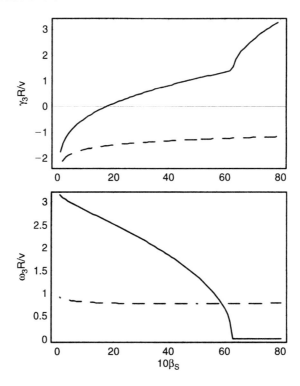

Figure 11-11   The second overtone ($n = 3$) in the spherical global model. (*Upper*) The nondimensional global mode damping ($\gamma_3 R/v$) is plotted versus the spherical cortical excitability parameter β_S. (*Lower*) The nondimensional global mode frequency ($\omega_3 R/v$) is plotted versus the spherical cortical excitability parameter β_S. The solid and dashed lines indicate two branches of the dispersion relation.

one-dimensional global theory (see appendix L) we obtain equation (A.10) of the appendix of Nunez (1995) or equation (46) of Jirsa and Haken (1997), both of which are of the form

$$\frac{\partial^2 \Psi}{\partial t^2} + 2v\lambda \frac{\partial \Psi}{\partial t} + v^2\lambda^2\Psi - v^2\frac{\partial^2 \Psi}{\partial x^2} = \rho(v^2\lambda^2 + v\lambda\frac{\partial}{\partial t})\delta\Theta + Z(x,t) \quad (11.12)$$

Here $\Psi(x,t) \equiv \delta\Psi_e(x,t)$ and $\delta\Theta(x,t)$ are the modulations of the excitatory synaptic action and action potential fields about their background levels, respectively, and $Z(x,t)$ includes additional cortical input, such as sensory input. In the simplest case of no local circuit effects, we may expect a sigmoid relation between excitatory input and action potential output (Freeman 1975). A straightforward mathematical approach to this general idea is to expand the sigmoid function in a Taylor series (Nunez 1995). By suitable linear transformation of $\Psi(x,t)$ and keeping the first nonzero nonlinear term, Jirsa and Haken (1997) obtain the simple relation

$$\rho\delta\Theta(x,t) = 2\beta\Psi(x,t) - \alpha\Psi(x,t)^3 \quad (11.13)$$

With the approximation (11.13), equation (46) of Jirsa and Haken (1997) is of the form

$$\frac{\partial^2 \Psi}{\partial t^2} - 2v\lambda(\beta - 1 - \frac{3\alpha}{2}\Psi^2)\frac{\partial \Psi}{\partial t} + v^2\lambda^2(1 - 2\beta + \alpha\Psi^2)\Psi = v^2\frac{\partial^2 \Psi}{\partial x^2} + Z(x,t)$$

(11.14)

In the linear limit ($\alpha \to 0$), the spatial-temporal Fourier transform of (11.14) recovers equation (A.10) of Nunez (1995) and the dispersion relation (11.4). The most important effect of the nonlinear terms is to prevent the instability that occurs in the one-dimensional linear theory when $\beta > 1$. Equation (11.14) may be solve numerically and/or one may seek approximate solutions of the form

$$\Psi(x, t) \cong \sum_{n=-N}^{N} \xi_n(t)\exp\left(\frac{j2nx}{L}\right)$$

(11.15)

Equation (11.15) is the one-dimensional version of (11.2) with the complex spatial function chosen to satisfy periodic boundary conditions; that is, forcing $\Psi(x, t)$ and its spatial derivatives to be continuous functions of x everywhere in the cortical loop $(-L/2, L/2)$. Note that only integer waves are allowed in the closed loop, in contrast to also allowing half integer waves in (say) a violin string fixed at each end.

While (11.14) is apparently an improvement over the linear theory, treatment of $Z(x,t)$ simply as a known forcing function neglects local circuit effects. Furthermore, our conjecture that natural selection may have provided multiple mechanisms for negative feedback to prevent instabilities in healthy brains suggests that the assumption of the sigmoidal input/output relation is probably inadequate. Thus, a more accurate dynamic theory might couple the equation for the excitatory modulation field $\Psi(x,t) \equiv \delta\Psi_e(x,t)$ given by (11.12) with separate equations for the inhibitory modulation field $\delta\Psi_i(x, t)$ and action potential field $\delta\Theta(x,t)$, for example

$$\delta\Theta = \delta\Theta[\delta\Psi_e(x, t), \delta\Psi_i(x, t)]$$

(11.16)

$$Z = Z[\delta\Psi_e(x, t), \delta\Psi_i(x, t), S(x, t)]$$

(11.17)

where $S(x,t)$ is due only to sensory input. Various models of large-scale neocortical dynamics have been published that mostly fit this general approach as outlined in section 9.

6 Experimental Connections to Global Theory

Any neocortical dynamic theory that attempts to include cortical or thalamocortical network effects must contain several (more likely many) physiological parameters that vary with brain state and are probably poorly known (if at all), as suggested by fig. 11-4. This provides motivation to start simply in our attempts to connect theory to EEG data. Thus, we consider several experimental implications of (11.4) that may enjoy some very approximate connections to brains in their more globally dominated states: apparently anesthesia, deep sleep, and the more globally dominant components of resting alpha rhythms. The reader should note that we only claim *connections* not comprehensive *explanations* to complex physiological processes!

(i) *The faster the propagation, the faster the global mode temporal frequencies.* If all parameters except the corticocortical propagation velocity v are fixed, brains with faster velocities will tend to produce higher global frequencies. Axon velocity depends on axon diameter and myelination. Myelination of axons increases propagation velocity by a factor of perhaps five or ten. Thus, corticocortical velocities are distributed according to these factors. Velocities tend to increase in the developing human brain because corticocortical axon myelination is not fully developed until roughly age 25 to 30 (Yakovlev and Lecours 1967; Courchesne 1990). What about brain size differences during maturation? A typical brain weight for a 5-year-old child is 93% of the adult weight (Blinkov and Glezer 1968), corresponding to 98% of the adult linear scale L. Thus, the approximation of constant L with maturation appears valid (Nunez 1995). What about EEG maturation? A posterior rhythm of about 4 Hz develops in babies in the first few months. It attenuates with eye closure and is believed to be the precursor of a corresponding adult alpha rhythm (Bickford 1973; Kellaway 1979; Niedermeyer and Lopes da Silva 1999). This dominant rhythm's frequency gradually increases until the adult-like 10 Hz rhythm is achieved at about age 10. In addition to this dominant rhythm, a more constant 8 Hz rhythm is usually evident by age 2 (Pilgreen 1995). *We are not claiming that axon myelination is the only contributor or even the major contributor to EEG frequency increases during maturation.* For example, even in the very limited context of (11.4), we expect frequency changes due to changes in the feedback gain parameter β. Rather, these data are consistent with the existence of multiple alpha rhythms with the more global rhythms partly dependent on characteristic axon speed v. More detailed discussion of this issue may be found in a critical commentary (Wright 2000) and the reply to this commentary (Nunez 2000b).

(ii) *The larger the cortex, the slower the global mode frequencies.* Suppose we were to compare a large number of brains in which the longest corticocortical fiber tracts scale with cortical size, that is, with $\lambda L \approx$ constant. Suppose further that axon diameters and myelination do not tend to increase with brain size (no change in axon velocity v). In this case, each global mode frequency ω_n would be inversely proportional to characteristic cortical size L. We are aware of only one human study in which this predicted size–frequency relationship was tested (Nunez et al. 1978; Nunez 1995). Participants were chosen through newspaper advertisements seeking volunteers with either very large or very small heads. Brain size is strongly correlated with skull volume (correlation coefficient $= 0.83$) (Blinkov and Glezer 1968). Head sizes and peak alpha frequencies were measured (blind) in 123 subjects with identifiable spectral peaks in the alpha band. Linear regression revealed a small ($r = -0.206$) but significant ($p = 0.02$) negative correlation between peak alpha frequency and head size. In addition, a "maximum frequency" was defined for each subject by the peak power histogram. That is, for each four-second epoch, the single frequency within the alpha band with the largest power was identified. A similar correlation between maximum frequency and head size was obtained (correlation coefficient $= -0.233$; $p = 0.01$). Strong correlations cannot be expected in such studies because brain sizes vary over only a small range, and many other parameters are expected to influence oscillation frequencies.

(iii) *Both standing and traveling waves with long spatial wavelengths should occur across neocortex and be measurable on the scalp.* As background, note that several studies have reported propagating activity when recording from animal cortex with small electrodes (Petsche et al. 1984, 1988; Lopes da Silva and Storm van Leeuwen 1978). These cortical spatial wavelengths are in the mm range and phase velocities are generally in the 1 mm/s range. Such waves apparently propagate by means of intracortical processes. These short-wavelength waves cannot be recorded from the scalp; volume conduction removes essentially all power at the mid and high ends of the spatial spectrum. That is, wave components with wavelengths shorter than a few centimeters cannot be recorded on the scalp. The data cited in chapter 10 show that (long-wavelength) traveling scalp waves can indeed be recorded in several experimental conditions.

(iv) *Phase velocities measured at the scalp should be in the general range of the characteristic corticocortical propagation speed v.* This is confirmed; supporting data are outlined in chapter 10.

(v) *Higher temporal frequencies should be associated with higher spatial frequencies above the fundamental mode. Group velocities should be in the general range of v.* Phase and group velocity are defined by

$$v_P \equiv \frac{\omega(k)}{k} \qquad v_G \equiv \frac{d\omega(k)}{dk} \qquad (11.18)$$

Application of (11.4) to the definitions (11.15) yields

$$v_P v_G = v^2 \qquad (11.19)$$

The data presented in chapter 10 are consistent with the (approximate) existence of dispersion relations for oscillations above the low end of the alpha band. Both phase and group velocities apparently occur in some (globally dominant) brain states and the velocities are in the general range of v. Our experimental estimates are not sufficiently refined to check (11.19) to see if group and phase velocities change in opposite directions. In any case, this test may be asking too much of such a crude theory.

(vi) *The ECoG should contain more high-frequency content above the low end of the alpha band than the corresponding EEG.* We know that volume conduction causes low-pass spatial filtering of potentials passing from cortex to scalp. We also know that the amplitudes and phases of scalp potentials generated by implanted dipole sources are unaltered by source frequency; tissue is purely resistive at large scales (Cooper et al. 1965). If our proposed global wave picture is correct, higher temporal frequencies should tend to occur with higher spatial frequencies in ECoG (above the low end of the alpha band). In this case, spatial filtering by the volume conductor implies temporal filtering of frequencies above the lower alpha band between cortex and scalp, as reported in a number of studies (Penfield and Jasper 1954; Delucchi et al. 1975; Pfurtscheller and Cooper 1975; Nunez 1981).

(vii) *Higher frequency oscillations should tend to have lower scalp amplitudes.* Scalp EEG amplitudes depend on two factors: the magnitude of the cortical mesosource function $\mathbf{P}(\mathbf{r}, t)$ and the phase synchrony of the oscillations. Source function magnitude is roughly proportional to the modulation depth of the excitatory synaptic field $\Psi(\mathbf{r}, t)$. Source synchrony over large distances (*long effective correlation lengths*) is closely associated with large power in the low end of the spatial frequency spectrum. Thus, if the magnitude of the cortical mesosource function is fixed and higher temporal frequencies are associated with higher spatial frequencies (only above the lower end of the alpha band), we expect high-end alpha, beta, and gamma oscillations to have progressively lower scalp amplitudes. This is roughly consistent with observations.

However, we cannot apply these arguments to delta and theta bands. First, we have no evidence of wave dispersion for frequencies lower than the lower end of the alpha band. More importantly, the large frequency difference between alpha and delta rhythms cannot be accounted for by changes in the spatial spectrum (by means of some putative dispersion relation). Nevertheless, increases in the cortical excitability parameter β is predicted to lower frequency in (11.4) and increase the amplitude of the synaptic action field modulation in (11.14). While the details of these changes depend on model specifics, several versions predict larger Ψ and lower mode frequencies with increasing β (Nunez 2000a).

(viii) *Globally dominated EEG generally consists of multiple modes (frequency components) that increase and decrease together as the cortical excitability parameter β changes.* The general effect of several modes going up and down together is demonstrated for one subject under varying concentrations of halothane anesthesia in fig. 11-2 and in fig. 11-12. These oscillations have large amplitudes over the entire scalp, generally in the range of

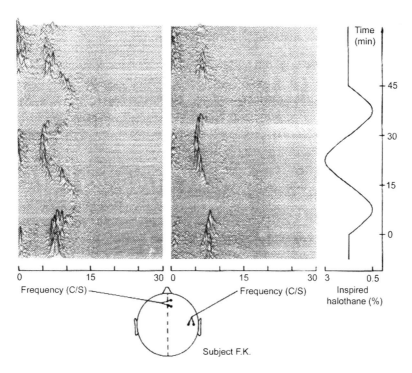

Figure 11-12 Anesthesia time-frequency plot. One subject is anesthetized to varying depths with halothane. Inspired concentration is shown as a function of time at right side. Increased halothane concentrations cause frequency reductions and amplitude increases in several modes. The oscillations generally have large amplitudes over the entire scalp, but different modes are emphasized by electrode pairs with different locations and orientations as shown. In the case of standing waves, placing both electrodes near a (cortical) nodal line of one mode is expected to reduce substantially the scalp amplitude of that particular mode, but not the amplitudes of other modes. Data recorded in connection with a separate cardiovascular study by Nunez et al. (1976). Reproduced with permission from Katznelson (1981).

approximately 50–100 μV at moderate inspired concentrations of halothane. However, different modes are emphasized by different electrode pairs as expected of standing waves and indicated in fig. 11-12 (Nunez 1995). Furthermore, the inverse relationship between amplitude and frequency expected of limit cycle modes was observed in all eight subjects (Nunez et al. 1976).

Equation (11.4) may be differentiated with respect to β to predict fractional changes in mode frequency as a function of excitability changes (due perhaps to halothane concentration changes), that is

$$f_n \Delta f_n \approx - \left(\frac{v\lambda}{2\pi} \right)^2 \beta \Delta \beta \tag{11.20}$$

To provide a numerical example, we choose the parameters (11.10) leading to $f_2 = 10.5$ Hz and suppose a brain state change causing a $\Delta\beta = 0.2$. In this case (11.14) predicts a frequency reduction of the nth mode $\Delta f_n \approx 3.5$ Hz, that is, from 10.5 Hz to 7.0 Hz. Of course, this is just a numerical example; we have very little idea of the magnitude of β and no idea of the size of Δβ associated with any state change. However, a more accurate quasi-linear approximation might predict the relationship between the amplitudes of (conjectured) limit cycle-like modes C_n and their frequencies (Nunez 2000b), that is

$$C_n = C_n(\beta) \tag{11.21}$$

For example, a combination of coordinate transformations and numerical solutions of (11.14) suggests the following approximation:

$$C_n \propto \sqrt{\beta - 1} \tag{11.22}$$

for β somewhat larger than one. In summary, brain state changes provide experimental amplitude and frequency changes $(\Delta C_n, \Delta f_n)$. In principle, equations like (11.21) and (11.4) provide partly independent equations to estimate β, Δβ, or both. A measure of the consistency of these estimates provides a rough quantitative test of theory. For example, by combining (11.20) with (11.22), we obtain an estimate for β based only on fraction changes in field amplitude and frequency:

$$\beta(\beta - 1) \approx - \left(\frac{2\pi f_n}{v\lambda} \right)^2 \left(\frac{C_n}{2\Delta C_n} \right) \left(\frac{\Delta f_n}{f_n} \right) \tag{11.23}$$

The first factor on the right-hand side of (11.23) is of the order of one if f_n is in the alpha band. In principal, the fractional changes of amplitude and frequency may be estimated in transitions involving hyperventilation or drugs that alter alpha frequency and amplitude (alcohol, for example) or anesthesia. A lot of assumptions are required to obtain (11.23) so this estimate should be viewed mainly as providing ideas for more sophisticated studies.

(ix) *Transitions between states due to increasing the parameter β can involve both decreases and increases in dominant frequencies.* Consider the following EEG behavior of a patient after introduction of cyclopropane anesthesia (Sadove et al. 1967); these general changes are common to the actions of many anesthetics (Stockard and Bickford 1975). (30 *seconds after anesthesia induction*: 20 μV resting alpha rhythm disappears and is replaced by low voltage "fast activity" ≈ 5 to 10 μV), (90 *seconds*: low voltage fast activity superimposed on 4 to 8 Hz dominant rhythm ≈ 30 μV), (100 *seconds*: low voltage fast activity superimposed on 3 to 4 Hz dominant rhythm ≈ 35 μV), (120 *seconds*: deep anesthesia, 3 Hz irregular rhythm ≈ 40 μV), (3 minutes: respiration depressed, 1 Hz irregular waveforms more–"nonlinear looking" ≈ 40 μV), (*Very deep anesthesia*: progressively longer intervals of near-isoelectric EEG with occasional bursts of fast activity in the 5 to 10 μV range).

The actions of anesthetics on neural tissue are quite complicated so that corresponding EEG changes are believed to reflect the actions of many different neurotransmitters on both cortical and subcortical tissue. Therefore, any attempt to "explain" EEG in anesthesia by the single parameter β (or $β_S$) is likely to be viewed as farfetched. Nevertheless, the simple global theory provides us with some general ideas of how the observed EEG behavior during progressively deeper anesthesia might occur. Consider the plots of mode frequency versus cortical excitability $β_S$ in figs. 11-9 through 11-11. The initial abrupt transition from alpha to low voltage fast activity is not well explained by the purely global theory; perhaps the inclusion local alpha networks that interact with the global field might accomplish this. However, imagine a progressive increase in $β_S$ associated with deepening anesthesia. For small $β_S$, the higher modes are strongly damped. As $β_S$ increases lower mode frequencies become progressively slower until they become unstable in the linear theory. Again, we conjecture that, in healthy brains, additional negative feedback is recruited to prevent instability as in the example of (11.14). *Brains that fail to accomplish this may suffer excessive net positive feedback, perhaps resulting in epilepsy.* At the same time the lower modes become nonoscillatory, higher modes become more weakly damped and begin to appear as high-frequency oscillations in the total signal. Thus, for each β (or $β_S$) we expect a characteristic mixture of slow and fast frequencies, roughly consistent with EEG observations in anesthesia.

7 Weakly Connected Resonant Oscillators and Binding by Resonance

Here we outline a general mathematical theory by Hoppensteadt and Izhikevich (1998) and Izhikevich (1999) to suggest how "soft-wired" brain networks might continually interact and disconnect on roughly 10 on 100 ms timescales. A very general class of weakly connected oscillators was considered. The main attraction of this approach is that very minimal restrictions need be placed on the oscillators—the results are largely independent of specific network model. An arbitrary number N *of semiautonomous oscillators* is assumed to be *pair-wise weakly connected* to themselves and to a central oscillator $\mathbf{X}_0$. By this we mean that the system is described in terms of vector dynamic variables $\mathbf{X}_n$ of the form

$$\frac{d\mathbf{X}_n}{dt} = \mathbf{F}_n(\mathbf{X}_n) + \varepsilon \sum_{j=1}^{N} \mathbf{G}_{nj}(\mathbf{X}_n, \mathbf{X}_j, \mathbf{X}_0, \varepsilon) \quad n = 1, N \quad \varepsilon \ll 1 \quad (11.24)$$

The vector functions $\mathbf{F}_n$ and $\mathbf{G}_{nj}$ are largely arbitrary. For example, simple mechanical or electrical oscillators, whether linear or nonlinear, might each be described by two scalar variables x_n and y_n (say position and velocity or current and voltage) so that $\mathbf{X}_n = (x_n, y_n)$. When disconnected from the larger system (the limit $\varepsilon \to 0$), each oscillator (n) is assumed to undergo quasi-periodic motion consisting of a set of discrete characteristic frequencies $f_{n1}, f_{n2}, f_{n3} \ldots$. For example, the coupled van der Pol oscillators in chapter 9 fit these criteria. Hoppensteadt and Izhikevich (1998) showed that the *individual oscillators cannot substantially interact (that is, interact on a time scale of the order of $1/\varepsilon$) unless certain resonant relations exist between the characteristic frequencies of the autonomous oscillators.*

To consider one example, suppose a central oscillator with dependent variables $\mathbf{X}_0$, perhaps representing tissue in thalamus, is assumed to have a single characteristic frequency f_{01}. The central oscillator is weakly connected to a pair of other oscillators $(\mathbf{X}_1, \mathbf{X}_2)$ also weakly connected to each other. This later pair of oscillators may represent two cortical networks of arbitrary size, as long as the conditions of semiautonomy and quasi-periodic oscillations are satisfied. Assume that each of the two cortical networks has a single characteristic frequency (f_{11} and f_{21}). In this example, the cortical networks *substantially interact* (that is, on a time-scale $1/\varepsilon$) only when the three frequencies (f_{01}, f_{11}, f_{21}) satisfy the resonant relation

$$m_0 f_{01} + m_1 f_{11} + m_2 f_{21} = 0 \quad (11.25)$$

where (m_1, m_2) are any combination of nonzero integers and m_0 is any integer including zero. Two simple cases are

$$f_{11} = f_{21} \quad \text{and} \quad f_{01} = f_{11} - f_{21} \tag{11.26}$$

The first case is the well-known resonant interaction between two oscillators with the same resonant frequency. The second case is illustrated by the following example. Suppose that two cortical networks composed of groupings of columns (at any scale) are formed as a result of *strong internal interconnections*. Let the two networks with characteristic gamma frequencies $f_{21} = 37$ Hz and $f_{11} = 42$ Hz be *weakly connected to each other and to the thalamus* (f_{01}). The two cortical networks may substantially interact, perhaps even forming a temporary single network in some sense, when the thalamic characteristic frequencies satisfy (11.26); several examples are $f_{01} = 2.5, 5, 15.67, 23.5$ Hz.

Suppose several networks $(\mathbf{X}_1, \mathbf{X}_2, \ldots \mathbf{X}_N)$ each have several characteristic frequencies, that is $(f_{11}, f_{12}, \ldots f_{1a}), (f_{21}, f_{22}, \ldots f_{2b}), \ldots (f_{n1}, f_{n2}, \ldots f_{nz})$, where the subscripts $a, b, \ldots z$ indicate the number of characteristic frequencies associated with each network. The central network $\mathbf{X}_0$ is then able to control interactions between the peripheral networks by changing its own characteristic frequencies $(f_{01}, f_{02}, \ldots f_{0a})$. Furthermore, the central network $\mathbf{X}_0$ may allow cortical network $\mathbf{X}_n$ to interact with several other networks $\mathbf{X}_j, \mathbf{X}_k, \ldots$ that do not interact among themselves, that is, by *multiplexing*. Following the analysis of Izhikevich (1999), we conjecture that cortical columns or larger networks may use rhythmic activity to communicate selectively. Such oscillating systems may not interact even when they are directly connected. Or, the systems may interact even with no direct connections, provided their characteristic frequencies satisfy the appropriate resonance criteria. Functional coupling between small elements or networks is then pictured as dynamic rather than hard-wired. Coupling strengths may easily change on short timescales.

8 Synaptic Action Fields and Global (Top–Down) Control of Local Networks

This section begins with yet another metaphor, but readers are reminded that *metaphor is not theory*. Our metaphor is used only to facilitate communication between the global theory of sections 1-4 through 1-6 and the oscillator theory of section 1-7 and to suggest new or modified physiologically based theory. A metaphor that roughly describes the putative local and global brain processes suggested by fig. 1-8 involves sound in an opera hall, analogous to the system composed of neocortex and corticocortical axons (Nunez 2000b). The synaptic and action potential fields $[\Psi_e(\mathbf{r}, t), \Psi_i(\mathbf{r}, t), \Theta(\mathbf{r}, t)]$ are analogous to physical fields in the opera hall like air pressure, density, temperature, molecular velocity, and so forth. Note that we comfortably use the label "field" for these physical variables even though they all originate with the dynamics of individual molecules (*active synapses*).

We replace the opera singers (*pacemakers*) by external sound sources (*subcortical input*). Global sound resonance occurs at multiple frequencies (*fundamental and overtones*) depending on sound speed (*corticocortical axon propagation speed*) and the opera hall size and shape. To avoid physiologically unrealistic reflective boundary conditions at the walls of a normal opera hall, let the opera hall take the shape of a torus or spherical shell with sound-absorbing walls. External sound sources (say from speakers on the wall) cause traveling waves in the air that interfere because of the *periodic boundary conditions* due to the hall's size and shape. Thus, certain spatial wavelengths (and corresponding temporal frequencies) dominate the sound (pressure) field. These frequencies and their corresponding spatial patterns (the *eigenfunctions*) are called the *normal modes* of the opera hall, the resonant frequencies of air pressure modulations around background pressure (analogous to *short time synaptic field modulations*).

Our imagined opera hall contains many water glasses of different sizes and shapes (*local and regional networks*) that vibrate when driven by global sound waves at glass resonant frequencies. Valves (*neurotransmitters*) control the amount of water in each glass, thereby controlling local resonant frequencies. Sensors on an outside wall of the hall (*scalp electrodes*) record only the long-wavelength part of the internal sound because of the opera wall's physical properties (*CSF, skull, scalp*) and physical separation of sensors from air molecules (*active synapses*). A purely global opera hall theory (*the purely global theory of section 4*) might attempt to predict resonant frequencies of air pressure modulations around background pressure (*synaptic field modulations*) by ignoring all influences of the internal glass structures as a first approximation. The normal modes of the opera hall can be controlled by heating the air (changing the molecular velocities), but here our metaphor breaks down since the neocortical global mode frequencies in section 4 are controlled by the background excitability parameter β.

In the next approximation, an oversimplified local/global theory of the opera hall might attempt to consider some of the effects of air–glass interactions. For example, we might generally expect *selective top-down interactions* between the sound (pressure field or *synaptic field*) and the water glasses. Each water glass should respond to sound waves at one of its particular resonant frequencies (interaction F-A in fig. 1-8). We also expect *bottom-up interactions*. That is, the resonating glasses will generally modify the air waves (interaction A-F in fig.1-8). In this manner, widely separated glasses with at least one resonant frequency in common can become parts of the same network if driven by a sound wave field containing substantial power in a "matching" (in the sense of section 7) frequency band. A particular glass having several resonant frequencies could easily participate simultaneously in multiple networks. Adding water to each glass (*long-timescale neuromodulation by chemical input to cortex*) changes its resonant frequencies so that it participates in a different collection of networks, perhaps contributing to a global phase change (*brain state change*).

To make the opera hall a more realistic metaphor for neocortex, hierarchical interactions that appear critical to neocortical dynamic behavior may be included (Freeman 1975; Ingber 1982, 1995). Replace the water glasses by complex networks of test tubes and beakers connected by glass rods that fill a substantial part of the space in the opera hall. Imagine rods inside tubes inside small beakers inside larger vessels with overlapping structures (*cortical columns at various scales*), the chemistry laboratory from hell! One can imagine progressively more complications of opera hall glass networks. However, if an important source of experimental data for this system is externally measured sound, the idea of macroscopic waves should be maintained, despite the enormous complexity of dynamics within the glass networks. One obvious reason is that the externally measured sound will be substantially biased towards low spatial frequencies (*scalp potentials*), and with nearly any wave phenomenon, low spatial frequencies imply low temporal frequencies. Thus, our external measurements (sound, *EEG*) will be biased towards more towards global fields than local networks.

These arguments suggest that we should retain synaptic field concepts as long as EEG is an important data source, even as discrete networks believed to underlie behavior and cognition become better understood. Separation of synaptic field and network concepts, even when they interact strongly and the separation is somewhat artificial, helps to simplify a very messy picture.

Given the general picture provided by the opera hall metaphor, we now consider how these general ideas might apply to the oscillator theory outlined in section 7. In that description, we imagined a central oscillator X_0, perhaps a small midbrain structure like thalamus or hippocampus. However, the mathematical analysis summarized in section 7 is more general; it does not restrict the size or location of this oscillator. Suppose now we identify X_0 as the synaptic action field in (11.1) which has multiple global resonant frequencies given (in this very crude approximation) by (11.4), that is

$$f_{01}(\beta), f_{02}(\beta), f_{03}(\beta), \ldots \qquad (11.27)$$

Suppose also that several brain networks $(X_1, X_2, \ldots X_N)$ are embedded within this global field, and each network has its own set of characteristic frequencies determined by local control parameters. In this imagined system, the global field X_0 is able to control interactions between the local networks by changing its own characteristic frequencies; that is, by changing β. Furthermore, the global field $\mathbf{X}_0$ may allow cortical network $\mathbf{X}_n$ to interact simultaneously with several other networks X_j, X_k, ... that do not interact among themselves. Given this general framework, it is not so implausible to conjecture that diffuse chemical input to the cortex may change global dynamic behavior, especially characteristic global frequencies, by changing β. Similarly, we imagine networks with local control parameters that modify local resonant frequencies (van Rotterdam et al. 1982; Nunez 1989, 1995). This global neocortical dynamics can perhaps act (top down) to influence functional coupling between specific networks embedded within the global neocortical/corticocortical system. In principle, these networks could be cortical, corticothalamic, or any other combination of brain structures, large or small.

9 Relationships to Other Theoretical Models and Criticisms of the Global Theory

Perhaps a dozen serious *large-scale neocortical dynamic theories* have been published over the past four decades that attempt to explain various aspects of EEG dynamic behavior. Many more excellent small-scales theories of interacting neurons have been developed, but our restriction to the adjective "large scale" is critical if our goal is to explain EEG dynamics recorded with large electrodes on the scalp and cortex. Some published theories are competitive with the global theory of section 4 while others are more complementary; many have both features. To the best of our knowledge, no general survey of these works has been published. It is not hard to see why. Any comprehensive survey would require quite a large effort and could easily fill an entire book—a book that would probably be read by only a few of today's scientists, some fraction of EEG scientists having appropriate mathematical and theoretical backgrounds. Future generations with strong training in both physical science and neuroscience will be required to fill the gap.

We do not attempt any survey of neocortical dynamic theories here; however, several general citations seem appropriate. One is Ingber's (1982, 1995) ambitious statistical mechanics of neocortical interactions, which derives large-scale dynamic variables from the smaller scales in the spirit of our alcohol metaphor of section 3. This work identifies multiple stable firing patterns that are candidates for storing short-term memory. A widely cited paper is Wilson and Cowan's (1973) quasi-linear treatment of *coarse-grained synaptic and action potential fields* predicting local limit cycle behavior in corticothalamic cell assemblies. Their coarse graining operation is also similar to our metaphor in section 3. Similar theories of note were published by Freeman (1975, 1992), van Rotterdam et al. (1982), and Zhadin (1984).

The theory of van Rotterdam et al. (1982) and Lopes da Silva (1991, 1995) is based on thalamocortical feedback with PSP delays. Nunez (1989,

1995, 2000a,b) showed that the original linear global theory (Nunez 1972, 1974) combines naturally with the linear local theory of van Rotterdam et al. (1982) so that observed oscillation frequencies may occur naturally as a result of both local synaptic and corticocortical axon delays. The idea is based on differential equations for local tissue networks of the form

$$D[\delta\Theta(x,t)] = f\left[\Psi(x,t)\right] \tag{11.28}$$

Here D is some local differential operator acting on the modulation of action potential density $\delta\Theta(x,t)$ with the synaptic action modulation function $f[\Psi(x,t)]$ appearing as a forcing function. Equation (11.28) may then replace (11.13) so that (11.12) and (11.28) provide a coupled set of differential equations, thereby allowing for both global and local contributions to oscillation frequencies. Linear approximations of (11.28) lead to multiple local-global branches of dispersion relations (see pages 494−498 and 694−698 of Nunez 1995). *Local networks and global fields interact in both directions (bottom up and top down) in contrast to the usual pacemaker idea (exclusively bottom up).*

In more complicated versions of this approach, inhomogeneous local properties may be modeled by varying the parameters in (11.28). For example, local resonant frequencies may vary because of neurotransmitter-based differences in local or regional feedback gains (Silberstein 1995b). Because of the many idealizations of genuine tissue, we expect most details to be wrong even if the general approach is correct. Nevertheless, this model provides a compelling argument that macroscopic fields of synaptic action and local or regional neural networks coexist naturally. *Different dominant frequencies are expected at different cortical locations, but local dynamic behaviors (including local oscillation frequencies) are due to combined local and global mechanisms. We further propose that local networks are bound to each other by the global field.*

Comprehensive theoretical work by Jirsa and Haken (1997) and Haken (1999) advanced this idea of complementary local and global processes by showing that the Wilson and Cowan local model and the Nunez global model are fully compatible. These scientists conclude that *the brain may act as a parallel computer at small scales by means of local or regional neural networks, while simultaneously producing global field patterns at macroscopic scales.*

Haken's (1999) work also showed that the global field equations have a general character, in the sense that the synaptic field dispersion relation for long-wavelength dynamics is relatively insensitive to corticocortical fiber distribution, thereby adding additional support to similar studies (Nunez 1995). The latter work also considered effects of distributed axon propagation velocities, which tends to eliminate higher modes by increasing their damping. Some effects of inhomogeneity of dynamic parameters on a linear cortex, say $\beta \rightarrow \beta(x)$ can be anticipated from studies of waves in physical media (Morse and Ingard 1968; Nunez 1995). For example, each mode frequency can be expected to oscillate with a range of spatial frequencies, thereby "smearing" simple dispersion relations. In an inhomogeneous closed loop

$$\omega_n = \omega_n(k_n) \quad \text{might be replaced by} \quad \omega_n = \omega_n(k_1, k_2, k_3 \ldots) \qquad (11.29)$$

where the wavenumbers (spatial frequencies) k_n are still required to satisfy the periodic boundary conditions. However, even with smeared version of the dispersion relation, we expect some correspondence between higher spatial and temporal frequencies, for example in the frequency–wavenumber spectra shown in chapter 10.

Jirsa and Haken's local-global theory was used to describe evoked magnetic field behavior (Jirsa and Haken 1997; Kelso et al. 1999; Fuchs et al. 1999; Jirsa et al. 1999, 2002). Subject performance on a motor task identified a brain state change or *phase transition* in the parlance of complex physical systems. The spatial-temporal MEG dynamics were described in terms of a competition between two spatial modes, with time-dependent amplitudes as *order parameters* as in (11.2). The first order parameter $\xi_1(t)$ (the first time-dependent spatial mode coefficient) dominated the pre-transition state and oscillated with the stimulus frequency. The second order parameter $\xi_2(t)$, having twice the stimulus frequency, dominated the posttransition state. A differential equation was derived with auditory and sensory cortices considered as local circuits embedded within the global field of (11.12). The theoretical model was able to reproduce essential features of MEG dynamics, including the phase transition. Thus, a triple correspondence was achieved relating behavior, MEG data and physiologically based theory. In later work from this group, spreading of wave fronts in folded cortex and scalp have been generated with a dynamic brain model coupled to a volume conductor model (Jirsa et al. 2002).

Robinson et al. (1997, 1998, 2002) have argued that the isolated cortex is relatively stable, leading to strongly damped waves and minimal influence of boundary conditions. When corticothalamic feedback is included, weakly damped waves become possible at low frequencies and near the alpha frequency; these are sensitive to boundary conditions and can display modal structure (Robinson et al. 2003). These authors have obtained a number of analytic results for their model in its linear regime. In the context of the local-global framework advocated in this chapter, these scientists are essentially saying that weakly damped waves require local network contributions. In another version of this work (Robinson et al. 2004), EEG data are used to "work backwards" to determine ranges of the model's physiological parameters that might plausibly account for experimental observations. More studies of this kind can be expected in the future by attempting to include progressively more of observed spatial temporal dynamics on the scalp and cortex, thereby narrowing the plausible range of theory parameters.

The work of Liley et al. (2002, 2003) and Bojak et al. (2003, 2004) is also a field theory that minimizes the effects of boundary conditions. Here EEG rhythms emerge as a consequence of reverberant activity within and between cortical excitatory and inhibitory neuronal populations, rather than through thalamocortical or corticocortical delays. This model predicts a variety of cortical oscillations by focusing on different magnitudes and time courses of postsynaptic excitation and inhibition; it is mostly a "local" theory in our chosen parlance. A range of EEG effects induced by sedatives and anesthetic agents is predicted by the model based on the experimentally determined influence of the agents on postsynaptic potentials. For example, insights into some of the effects of anesthesia outlined in section 5 and a basis for benzodiazepine-induced accelerations of resting EEG are suggested.

The works described above rely on a large number of physiological parameters. As in the case of all models, questions arise about the sensitivity of model predictions to parameter uncertainty. Nevertheless, we regard these studies as plausible approaches to (mainly) local theory and consistent with the idea of local networks immersed in a global environment, although the authors may argue (correctly) that such separation of the dynamics into two distinct parts is somewhat artificial (Liley 2000). The counter argument is that the purely global theory outlined above is able to make perhaps a dozen testable qualitative (and some semiquantitative) predictions that are a relatively robust to parameter uncertainty. Furthermore, many of the dynamic effects generated by local models are not directly observable at the scalp because of severe spatial filtering. Thus, we argue that *separation of the dynamic behavior into two parts provides convenient entry into more complex dynamic models and generally facilitates our primitive attempts at thinking about thinking.* Similar separations have proved quite convenient in the physical sciences. The separation of (global) longitudinal waves due to particle motion from (local) particle collisions in hot plasma theory comes to mind in this context.

A plausible criticism of the global theory outlined in section 4 is that genuine operating ranges of the physiological parameters cause propagating cortical waves to be spatially overdamped (Robinson et al. 1997; Liley et al. 1999; Wright 2000; Wright et al. 2001). If this criticism is correct, EEG may owe its origins more to local networks: cortical, thalamocortical, or both. In this view long-range corticocortical interactions are not required to explain EEG phenomena. It then follows that global boundary conditions may be neglected as in the local theories developed by these same scientists. Our answers to this criticism are as follows.

(i) We readily acknowledge the importance of local network effects on EEG and that cortical waves may be strongly damped in many brain states. However, our experimental focus for testing the global theory has been directed to brain states of minimal cognition where cortical waves may be weakly damped.

We contrasted EEG recorded in these resting states with recordings during mental calculations (see chapters 9 and 10). We also note that theories attempting contacts with intracranial recordings naturally focus more on local network effects that may dominate any possible global behavior in the recorded data.

(ii) Spatial damping is proportional to temporal damping through the group velocity of the wave packet. The two parameters involved with global damping are the fall-off rate λ^{-1} of the long corticocortical fiber system and the cortical excitability parameter β. Longer fibers and higher excitability reduce damping and produce instability in the purely linear theory or perhaps limit cycle-like modes in quasi-linear approximations; λ is fixed by the anatomy and is in the appropriate range for undamped cortical wave propagation provided that β is sufficiently large. A very crude estimate of β suggests it can be in the range to produce undamped or unstable waves (Nunez 1995, see pages 492–494 with $B \equiv 2\beta$). However, we are skeptical that accurate knowledge of the *effective* β *range* for cortical tissue will be available anytime soon, noting the vast complexity of local cortical networks.

(iii) The question of cortical wave damping is addressed experimentally by measurement of EEG propagation at the scalp. As shown in chapter 10, such propagation is observed in several brain states, and phase and group velocity estimates match corticocortical axon speeds. Of course, critics may point out that weak damping of cortical waves could require local network influences.

(iv) EEG recorded on the scalp is spatially filtered by the volume conductor. Thus, scalp EEG is strongly biased towards the low end of the spatial frequency spectrum. In the case of resting alpha rhythm, most scalp power occurs in the first few spherical harmonics as discussed in chapters 7 through 10. This has several implications. One question concerns the neglect of global boundary conditions when describing a phenomenon whose dominant wavelengths are comparable to brain dimensions. Local theories appear quite appropriate for local alpha rhythms, but only the parts of such fields with large-scale phase synchrony are observed at the scalp. The corticocortical fibers provide a compelling means to facilitate such synchrony as shown clearly in studies of EEG maturation (Thatcher et al. 1987; Srinivasan 1999; Thatcher 2004) and split brain subjects (Nunez 1981). It may be a bit implausible to recruit corticocortical fibers into a theory to obtain the required synchrony, and at the same time neglect the influence of their propagation delays (were this to be proposed by competing theories).

(v) The relative importance of corticocortical versus thalamocortical dynamics appears to be much higher in humans than lower mammals that provide much of the intracranial data (see fig. 1-2). That is, the number of thalamocortical axons entering (or leaving) a typical patch of the underside of human cortex is only a few percent of the number of corticocortical fibers (Braitenberg and Schuz 1991). Theoretical strategies that focus on the (minority) thalamocortical interactions but neglect the (majority) corticocortical interactions require compelling justification. This issue is discussed in more detail in the context of possibly stronger thalamocortical interactions (at least in primary sensory cortex) in Nunez (1995).

While we disagree with this criticism of the basic global theory for the reasons given above, such issues raised by critics are essential to genuine scientific progress and will likely be debated and (hopefully) tested experimentally in the future.

10 Summary

We have outlined the rationale for our conceptual framework in which cell assemblies are embedded within synaptic and action potential fields as summarized in fig. 1-8. The inclusion of the synaptic fields in our conceptual framework is motivated first by the close relationship of synaptic fields to scalp potentials, a connection more easily justified than putative (direct) relationships between neural networks and scalp potentials. Furthermore, this conceptual framework does not appear restrictive. It does not prejudge issues like the relative importance of local versus global delays to EEG dynamics or whether various behavioral and cognitive states are better associated with functional localization or integration. Such questions may be conveniently addressed experimentally in the context of the chosen framework.

Some of the most robust dynamic properties of scalp recorded EEG are summarized here. A global theory of large-scale neocortical dynamics is shown to have some limited predictive value for EEG despite its neglect of all network effects. This "toy brain" is presented first as a plausible entry point to more realistic theory in which cell assemblies (or networks) play a central role in cognition and behavior. Second, we conjecture that the synaptic action fields of the global theory may act (top-down) on local networks in a manner analogous to human cultural influences on social networks (Nunez 2000a). Such interactions across spatial scales are generally expected in a wide range of complex systems (for some simple examples, see Nunez 1995). The ubiquitous phenomenon of top-down/bottom-up interactions across scales in complex systems has been labeled *circular causality* by Haken (1983, 1987) and studied widely under the rubric *synergetics*. Systems in which circular causality forms an essential part of dynamic behavior include weather, magnetic materials, DNA dynamics, combat, societies, and financial markets (Ingber 1995). *The preeminent complexity of human brains suggests that circular causality should be treated as a central issue in both EEG and cognitive theory.*

Our conjecture that cell assembly interactions may be substantially facilitated by resonance effects is based on three known phenomena: (i) cognitive and behavioral events are associated with power changes in certain preferred EEG frequency bands; (ii) coherence and other measures of phase synchronization change during mental tasks, also in preferred frequency bands; and (iii) resonance interactions are critical in a wide range of physical and biological systems. Circuit resonance of analog filters, resonant interactions between the strings and wooden bodies of violins, and quantum wave function resonance associated with chemical bonds provide prominent examples.

Several local EEG theories are cited. We argue that much of this work complements the global theory because local networks must operate while immersed in a global field environment. There is no shortage of physiological mechanisms able to predict many of EEG's dynamic pro- perties; rather, the difficulty is picking the right ones. The large number of parameters that must be included in most serious brain theories presents a major obstacle to the cornerstone of genuine theory: *the opportunity for experimental falsification.* We emphasize the global theory here because of its ability to make several correct experimental predictions of general EEG properties, while acknowledging its vast oversimplification of genuine brain dynamics. Perhaps the greatest shortcoming of the global theory is that it is difficult to falsify. We could, for example, conjecture that any dynamic behavior not predicted by the global theory is due to embedded networks not included in the theory. Nevertheless, we adopt the strategy of searching for brain states and other experimental conditions that appear to minimize network effects; thereby providing opportunities to check the global theory in these limited circumstances. Our emphasis on (low spatial frequency) scalp-recorded data and resting alpha and anes- thesia states supports this goal. With this strategy in mind, "falsification" may be associated with failing to find brain states in which the simplified global theory has substantial predictive value.

Finally, we note that local characteristic timescales like rise and decay times of postsynaptic potentials and global timescales like the cortico- cortical transmission times across the entire brain appear to be in the same general range. Perhaps this is no coincidence. The dynamic properties of individual neurons and small neural assemblies appear to be quite variable and critically dependent on the details of the experimental envi- ronment. Thus, we offer one additional conjecture—*top-down, multiscale, neocortical dynamic plasticity*—in which individual neurons and networks adjust their time constants for (perhaps resonant) compatibility with other networks and the global environment. By "top-down plasticity" we imply that fixed global boundary conditions might constrain global mode frequencies, thereby forcing networks at multiple spatial scales to conform to the global field in healthy brains. Perhaps nonconforming networks become schizophrenic and these brains tend to be eliminated by natural selection. Who knows? *Maybe consciousness is a resonance phenomenon and only properly tuned brains can orchestrate beautiful music of sentience.*

References

Aminoff MJ, 1999, Electroencephalography: general principles and clinical applications. In: MJ Aminoff (Ed.), *Electrodiagnosis in Clinical Neurology*, 4th Edition, Amsterdam: Elsevier.

Andrew C and Pfurtscheller G, 1997, On the existence of different alpha band rhythms in the hand area of man. *Neuroscience Letters* 222: 103–106.

Barlow JS, 1993, *The Electroencephalogram. Its Patterns and Origins*, Cambridge, MA: MIT Press.

Bickford RG, 1950, Automatic electroencephalographic control of general anesthesia. *Electroencephalography and Clinical Neurophysiology* 2: 93–96.

Bickford RG, 1973, *Clinical Electroencephalography*, New York: Medcom.

Blinkov SM, Glezer II, 1968, *The Human Brain in Figures and Tables*, New York: Plenum Press.

Bojak I, Liley DTJ, Cadusch PJ, and Kan Cheng K, 2004, Electrorhythmogenesis and anaesthesia in a physiological mean field theory. *Neurocomputing* 58–60: 1197–1202.

Braitenberg V and Schuz A, 1991, *Anatomy of the Cortex. Statistics and Geometry*, New York: Springer-Verlag.

Bressler SL, 1995, Large scale cortical networks and cognition. *Brain Research Reviews* 20: 288–304.

Cooper R, Winter AL, Crow HJ, and Walter WG, 1965, Comparison of subcortical, cortical, and scalp activity using chronically indwelling electrodes in man. *Electroencephalography and Clinical Neurophysiology* 18: 217–228.

Courchesne E, 1990, Chronology of postnatal brain development: event-related potential, positron emission tomography, myelinogenesis, and synaptogenesis studies. In: JW Rohrbaugh, R Parasuraman, and R Johnson (Eds.), *Event-Related Potentials of the Brain*, New York: Oxford University Press, pp. 210–241.

Dale AM, Fischl B and Sereno MI, 1999, Cortical surface-based analysis: I. Segmentation and surface reconstruction, *NeuroImage* 9: 179–194.

Dale AM and Sereno MI, 1993, Improved location of cortical activity by combining EEG and MEG with MRI cortical surface reconstruction: a linear approach. *Journal of Cognitive Neuroscience* 5: 162–176.

Delucchi MR, Garoutte B, and Aird RB, 1975, The scalp as an electroencephalographic averager. *Electroencephalography and Clinical Neurophysiology* 38:191–196.

Edelman GM and Tononi G, 2000, *A Universe of Consciousness*, New York: Basic Books.

Fischl B, Sereno MI, and Dale AM, 1999, Cortical surface-based analysis: II. Inflation, flattening, a surface-based coordinate system. *NeuroImage* 9: 195–207.

Florian G, Andrew C, and Pfurtscheller G, 1998, Do changes in coherence always reflect changes in functional coupling? *Electroencephalography and Clinical Neurophysiology* 106: 87–91.

Freeman WJ, 1975, *Mass Action in the Nervous System*, New York: Academic Press.

Freeman WJ, 1992, Predictions on neocortical dynamics derived from studies in paleocortex. In: E Basar and TH Bullock (Eds.), *Induced Rhythms in the Brain*, Birhauser.

Fuchs A, Jirsa VK, and Kelso JAS, 1999, Transversing scales of brain and behavioral organization: II. Analysis and reconstruction. In: C Uhl (Ed.), *Analysis of Neurophysiological Brain Functioning*, Berlin: Springer-Verlag, pp. 90–106.

Gevins AS and Cutillo BA, 1995, Neuroelectric measures of mind. In: PL Nunez (Au.), *Neocortical Dynamics and Human EEG Rhythms*, New York: Oxford University Press, pp. 304–338.

Gevins AS, Smith ME, McEvoy L, and Yu D, 1997, High-resolution mapping of cortical activation related to working memory: effects of task difficulty, type of processing, and practice. *Cerebral Cortex* 7: 374–385.

Haken H, 1983, *Synergetics: An Introduction*, 3rd Edition, Berlin: Springer-Verlag.

Haken H, 1999, What can synergetics contribute to the understanding of brain functioning? In: C Uhl (Ed.), *Analysis of Neurophysiological Brain Functioning*, Berlin: Springer-Verlag, pp. 7–40.

Hoppensteadt FC and Izhikevich EM, 1998, Thalamo-cortical interactions modeled by weakly connected oscillators: could brain use FM radio principles? *Biosystems* 48: 85–92.

Ingber L, 1982, Statistical mechanics of neocortical interactions: I. Basic formulation. *Physica D* 5: 83–107.

Ingber L, 1995, Statistical mechanics of multiple scales of neocortical interactions. In: PL Nunez (Au.), *Neocortical Dynamics and Human EEG Rhythms*, New York: Oxford University Press, pp. 628–681.

Izhikevich EM, 1999, Weakly connected quasi-periodic oscillators, FM interactions, and multiplexing in the brain. *SIAM Journal of Applied Mathematics* 59: 2193–2223.

Jasper HD and Penfield W, 1949, Electrocorticograms in man. Effects of voluntary movement upon the electrical activity of the precentral gyrus. *Archiv. Fur Psychiatrie und Zeitschrift Neurologie* 183: 163–174.

Jirsa VK and Haken H, 1997, A derivation of a macroscopic field theory of the brain from the quasi-microscopic neural dynamics. *Physica D* 99: 503–526.

Jirsa VK, Jantzen KJ, Fuchs A, and Kelso JAS, 2002, Spatiotemporal forward solution of the EEG and MEG using network modeling. *IEEE Transactions on Medical Imaging* 21: 493–504.

Jirsa VK, Kelso JAS, and Fuchs A, 1999, Traversing scales of brain and behavioral organization: III. Theoretical modeling. In: C Uhl (Ed.), *Analysis of Neurophysiological Brain Functioning*, Berlin: Springer-Verlag, pp. 107–125.

Katznelson RD, 1981, Normal modes of the brain: neuroanatomical basis and a physiological theoretical model. In PL Nunez (Au.), *Electric Fields of the Brain: The Neurophysics of EEG*, 1st Edition, New York: Oxford University Press, pp. 401–442.

Kellaway P, 1979, An orderly approach to visual analysis: the parameters of the normal EEG in adults and children. In: DW Klass and DD Daly (Eds.), *Current Practice of Clinical Electroencephalography*, New York: Raven Press, pp. 69–147.

Kelso JAS, Fuchs A, and Jirsa VK, 1999, Traversing scales of brain and behavioral organization: I. Concepts and experiments. In: C Uhl (Ed.), *Analysis of Neurophysiological Brain Functioning*, Berlin: Springer-Verlag, pp. 73–89.

Klimesch W, 1999, EEG alpha and theta oscillations reflect cognitive and memory performance: a review and analysis. *Brain Research Reviews* 29: 169–195.

Lachaux JP, Rodriguez E, Martinerie J, and Varela FJ, 1999, Measuring phase synchrony in brain signals. *Human Brain Mapping* 8: 194–208.

Liley DTJ, 2000, Local and global dynamic control parameters are not so easily separated. *Behavioral and Brain Sciences* 23: 407–408.

Liley DTJ, Cadusch PJ, and Dafilis MP, 2002, A spatially continuous mean field theory of electrocortical activity network. *Computation in Neural Systems* 13: 67–113.

Liley DTJ, Cadusch PJ, Gray M, and Nathan PJ, 2003, Drug-induced modification of the system properties associated with spontaneous human electroncephalographic activity. *Physical Review E* 68: 051096.

Liley DTJ, Cadusch PJ, and Wright JJ, 1999, A continuum theory of electro-cortical activity. *Neurocomputing* 26–27: 795–800.

Lopes da Silva FH, 1991, Neural mechanisms underlying brain waves: from membranes to networks. *Electroencephalography and Clinical Neurophysiology* 79: 81–93.

Lopes da Silva FH, 1995, Dynamics of electrical activity of the brain, local networks, and modulating systems. In: PL Nunez (Au.), *Neocortical Dynamics and Human EEG Rhythms*, New York: Oxford University Press, pp. 249–271.

Lopes da Silva FH and Storm van Leeuwen W, 1978, The cortical alpha rhythm in dog: the depth and surface profile of phase. In: MAB Brazier and H Petsche (Eds.), *Architectonics of the Cerebral Cortex*, New York: Raven Press, pp. 319–333.

Morse PM and Ingard KU, 1968, *Theoretical Acoustics*, New York: McGraw-Hill.

Mountcastle VB, 1979, An organizing principle for cerebral function: the unit module and the distributed system. In: FO Schmitt and FG Worden (Eds.), *The Neurosciences 4th Study Program*, Cambridge, MA: MIT Press.

Niedermeyer E and Lopes da Silva FH (Eds.), 1999, *Electroencephalography. Basic Principals, Clinical Applications, and Related Fields*, 4th Edition, London: Williams and Wilkins.

Nunez PL, 1972, The brain wave equation: a model for the EEG, paper presented to the American EEG Society meeting, Houston, TX.

Nunez PL, 1974a, The brain wave equation: a model for the EEG. *Mathematical Biosciences* 21: 279–297.

Nunez PL, 1974b, Wave-like properties of the alpha rhythm. *IEEE Transactions on Biomedical Engineering* 21: 473–482.

Nunez PL, 1981, *Electric Fields of the Brain: The Neurophysics of EEG*, 1st Edition, New York: Oxford University Press.

Nunez PL, 1989, Generation of human EEG by a combination of long and short range neocortical interactions. *Brain Topography* 1: 199–215.

Nunez PL, 1995, *Neocortical Dynamics and Human EEG Rhythms*, New York: Oxford University Press.

Nunez PL, 2000a, Toward a large-scale quantitative description of neocortical dynamic function and EEG (Target article). *Behavioral and Brain Sciences* 23: 371–398.

Nunez PL, 2000b, Neocortical dynamic theory should be as simple as possible, but not simpler (Response to 18 commentaries on target article). *Behavioral and Brain Sciences* 23: 415–437.

Nunez PL, Reid L, and Bickford RG, 1977, The relationship of head size to alpha frequency with implications to a brain wave model. *Electroencephalography and Clinical Neurophysiology* 44: 344–352.

Nunez PL, Silberstein RB, Shi Z, Carpenter MR, Srinivasan R, Tucker DM, Doran SM, Cadusch PJ, and Wijesinghe RS, 1999, EEG coherence: II. Experimental measures of multiple EEG coherence measures. *Electroencephalography and Clinical Neurophysiology*, 110: 469–486.

Nunez PL, Srinivasan R, Westdorp AF, Wijesinghe RS, Tucker DM, Silberstein RB, and Cadusch PJ, 1997, EEG coherency: I. Statistics, reference electrode, volume conduction, Laplacians, cortical imaging, and interpretation at multiple scales. *Electroencephalography and Clinical Neurophysiology* 103: 516–527.

Nunez PL, Stockard JJ, and Smith NT, 1976, Data recorded at the VA Hospital, San Diego.

Nunez PL, Wingeier BM, and Silberstein RB, 2001, Spatial-temporal structures of human alpha rhythms: theory, micro-current sources, multiscale measurements, and global binding of local networks. *Human Brain Mapping* 13: 125–164.

Penfield W and Jasper HD, 1954, *Epilepsy and the Functional Anatomy of the Human Brain*, London: Little Brown.

Petsche H and Etlinger SC, 1998, *EEG and Thinking. Power and Coherence Analysis of Cognitive Processes*, Vienna: Austrian Academy of Sciences.

Petsche H, Kaplan S, von Stein A, and Filz O, 1997, The possible meaning of the upper and lower alpha frequency ranges for cognitive and creative tasks. *International Journal of Psychophysiology* 26: 77–97.

Petsche H, Pockberger H, and Rappelsberger P, 1984, On the search for sources of the electroencephalogram. *Neuroscience* 11: 1–27.

Pfurtscheller G and Cooper R, 1975, Frequency dependence of the transmission of the EEG from cortex to scalp. *Electroencephalography and Clinical Neurophysiology* 38: 93–96.

Pfurtscheller G and Lopes da Silva FH, 1999, Event related EEG/MEG synchronization and desynchronization: basic principles. *Electroencephalography and Clinical Neurophysiology* 110: 1842–1857.

Pfurtscheller G and Neuper C, 1992, Simultaneous EEG 10 Hz desynchronization and 40 Hz synchronization during finger movements. *Neurology Report* 3: 1057–1060.

Pilgreen KL, 1995, Physiologic, medical and cognitive correlates of electroencephalography. In: PL Nunez (Au.), *Neocortical Dynamics and Human EEG Rhythms*, New York: Oxford University Press, pp. 195–248.

Robinson PA, Rennie CJ, Rowe DL, and O'Conner SC, 2004, Estimation of multiscale neurophysiologic parameters by electroencephalographic means. *Human Brain Mapping* 23: 53–72.

Robinson PA, Rennie CJ, and Wright JJ, 1997, Propagation and stability of waves of electrical activity in the cerebral cortex. *Physical Review E* 55: 826–840.

Robinson PA, Whitehouse RW, and Rennie CJ, 2003, Nonuniform corticothalamic continuum model of electroencephalographic spectra with application to split alpha peaks. *Physical Review E* 68: 021922; 1–10.

Robinson PA, Wright JJ, and Rennie CJ, 1998, Synchronous oscillations in the cerebral cortex. *Physical Review E* 57: 4578–4580.

Sadove MS, Becka D, and Gibbs FA, 1967, *Electroencephalography for Anesthesiologists and Surgeons*, Philadelphia: JB Lippincott.

Sarnthein J, Petsche H, Rappelsberger P, Shaw GL, and von Stein A, 1998, Synchronization between prefrontal and posterior association cortex during human working memory. *Proceedings of the National Academy of Sciences USA* 95: 7092–7096.

Schack B, Vath N, Petsche H, Geissler HG, and Moller E, 2002, Phase-coupling of theta-gamma EEG rhythms during short-term memory processing. *International Journal of Psychophysiology* 44: 143–163.

Shaw GR, 1991, *Spherical Harmonic Analysis of the Electroencephalogram*. Ph.D. Dissertation. Alberta, Canada: The University of Alberta.

Silberstein RB, 1995a, Steady-state visually evoked potentials, brain resonances, and cognitive processes. In: PL Nunez (Au.), *Neocortical Dynamics and Human EEG Rhythms*, New York: Oxford University Press, pp. 272–303.

Silberstein RB, 1995b, Neuromodulation of neocortical dynamics. In: PL Nunez (Au.), *Neocortical Dynamics and Human EEG Rhythms*, New York: Oxford University Press, pp. 591–627.

Silberstein RB, Danieli F, and Nunez PL, 2003, Fronto-parietal evoked potential synchronization is increased during mental rotation. *NeuroReport* 14: 67–71.

Silberstein RB, Nunez PL, Pipingas A, Harris P, and Danieli F, 2001, Steady state visually evoked potential (SSVEP) topography in a graded working memory task. *International Journal of Psychophysiology* 42: 219–232.

Silberstein RB, Song J, Nunez PL, and Park W, 2004, Dynamic sculpting of brain functional connectivity is correlated with performance measures. *Brain Topography* 16: 249–254.

Singer W, 1993, Synchronization of cortical activity and its putative role in information processing and learning. *Annual Reviews of Physiology* 55: 349–374.

Srinivasan R, 1995, *A Theoretical and Experimental Study of Neocortical Dynamics*, Ph.D. Dissertation, New Orleans: Tulane University.

Srinivasan R, 1999, Spatial structure of the human alpha rhythm: global correlation in adults and local correlation in children. *Clinical Neurophysiology* 110:1351–1362.

Srinivasan R, Russell DP, Edelman GM, and Tononi G, 1999, Frequency tagging competing stimuli in binocular rivalry reveals increased synchronization of neuromagnetic responses during conscious perception. *Journal of Neuroscience* 19: 5435–5448.

Stockard JJ, 1976, *Epileptogenicity of General Anesthetics. Basic Mechanisms and Clinical Significance*, Ph.D. Dissertation, San Diego: University of California.

Stockard JJ and Bickford RG, 1975, The neurophysiology of anesthesia. In: E Gordon (Ed.), *A Basis and Practice of Neuroanesthesia II*, Amsterdam: Excerpta Medica, pp. 3–46.

Szentagothai J, 2004, Architectonics, modular of neural centers. In: G Adelman and BH Smith (Eds.), *Encyclopedia of Neuroscience*, 3rd Edition, New York: Elsevier.

Thatcher RW, 2004, Neuroimaging of cyclic cortical reorganization during human development. In: RW Thatcher, LG Reid, J Rumsey, and N Krasnegor (Eds.), *Developmental Neuroimaging: Mapping the Development of Brain and Behavior*, San Diego: Academic Press.

Thatcher RW, Walker WA, and Giudice S, 1987, Human cerebral hemispheres develop at different rates and ages. *Science* 236: 1110–1113.

Tononi G and Edelman GM. 1998, Consciousness and complexity. *Science* 282: 1846–1851.

Uhl C, 1999, *Analysis of Neurophysiological Brain Functioning*, Berlin: Springer-Verlag.

Van Rotterdam A, Lopes da Silva FH, van der Ende J, Viergever MA, and Hermans AJ, 1982, A model of the spatial-temporal characteristics of the alpha rhythm. *Bulletin of Mathematical Biology* 44: 283–305.

Wilson HR and Cowan JD, 1973, A mathematical theory of the functional dynamics of cortical and thalamic nervous tissue. *Kybernetik* 13: 55–80.

Wingeier BM, 2004, *A High resolution Study of Coherence and Spatial Spectra in Human EEG*, Ph.D. Dissertation, New Orleans: Tulane University.

Wingeier BM, Nunez PL, and Silberstein RB, 2001, Spherical harmonic decomposition applied to spatial-temporal analysis of human high-density EEG. *Physical Review E* 64: 051916-1, 9.

Wright JJ, 2000, Developing testable theories of brain dynamics: the global mode theory and experimental falsification. *Behavioral and Brain Sciences* 23: 414–415.

Wright JJ, Robinson PA, Rennie CJ, Gordon E, Bourke PD, Chapman CL, Hawthorn N, Lees GJ, and Alexander D, 2001, Toward an integrated continuum model of cerebral dynamics: the cerebral rhythms, synchronous oscillations and cortical stability. *Biosystems* 63: 71–88.

Yakovlev PI and Lecours AR, 1967, The myelogenetic cycles of regional maturation of the brain. In: A Minkowski (Ed.), *Regional Development of the Brain in Early Life*, Philadelphia: FA Davis, pp. 3–70.

Zhadin MN, 1984, Rhythmic processes in cerebral cortex. *Journal of Theoretical Biology* 108: 565–595.

APPENDIX A

Introduction to the Calculus
of Vector Fields

This appendix attempts to relieve symptoms of *vectorphobia* known to afflict engineering students when they encounter their first course in mechanics, electromagnetic theory, or fluid mechanics. There are at least two compelling reasons to adopt vector calculus. First, it often makes cumbersome calculations easy. Second, vector expressions are independent of coordinate systems. Genuine physical laws must be expressible in vector form because nature is not constrained by human choices of coordinate systems. Here we summarize the properties of vector fields in terms of the three component scalar fields. The treatment is brief since vector calculus is developed extensively in the literature. We stick mostly to rectangular coordinate systems, but the reader should not lose sight of the fact that physical laws do not depend on coordinate system.

Consider two vectors $\mathbf{A}$ and $\mathbf{B}$ and a scalar T. These are mathematical functions that need not represent physical quantities; however, the ideas are perhaps rendered less abstract by thinking in terms of the movement objects through a fluid, say a bird flock flying through an air stream. In this case, the vectors $\mathbf{A}$ and $\mathbf{B}$ might be identified as the individual velocities of birds and local air particles and T might be local bird density.

The dot product of the two vectors is defined as

$$\mathbf{A} \cdot \mathbf{B} = \text{scalar} = A_x B_x + A_y B_y + A_z B_z \tag{A.1}$$

The cross product is

$$\mathbf{A} \times \mathbf{B} = \text{vector}$$
$$= (A_y B_z - A_z B_y)\mathbf{i} + (A_z B_x - A_x B_z)\mathbf{j} + (A_x B_y - A_y B_x)\mathbf{k} \tag{A.2}$$

Here the vectors are defined in terms of their components along the x, y, and z axes and the corresponding unit vectors $\mathbf{i}$, $\mathbf{j}$, $\mathbf{k}$, which point in the directions of the three axes. Thus, (A.2) involves three distinct quantities and the unit vectors are just category labels.

The vector operator ∇ (*Del* or *Grad*) was introduced in the context of ion diffusion in a concentration gradient and in the definition of electrostatic potential. By the term "operator," we mean that ∇ does something to (operates on) whatever is written just to its right by following a fixed rule. The *Grad* operator is defined in terms of spatial derivatives such that

$$\nabla T = \text{vector} = \frac{\partial T}{\partial x}\mathbf{i} + \frac{\partial T}{\partial y}\mathbf{j} + \frac{\partial T}{\partial z}\mathbf{k} \tag{A.3}$$

Thus the *gradient of T* is defined as the spatial rate of change of the scalar field T, where T might represent temperature, altitude, ion concentration, potential, and so forth.

Although T is a scalar, ∇T is a vector. The x component of ∇T is a measure of how fast T changes in the x direction; the y and z components have similar interpretations. What is the direction of the vector ∇T? It is the direction in which T changes fastest. For example, if T were to represent altitude at horizontal location (x, y) of a mountain range, as on a geological survey map, ∇T points in the direction of the steepest local uphill slope. Of course, ∇T itself is a function of position; the direction of steepest slope generally changes as we follow a mountain trail. In another example, electric potential is defined in terms of the electric field by

$$\mathbf{E}(\mathbf{r}) = -\nabla\Phi(\mathbf{r}) = -\left(\frac{\partial\Phi}{\partial x}\mathbf{i} + \frac{\partial\Phi}{\partial y}\mathbf{j} + \frac{\partial\Phi}{\partial z}\mathbf{k}\right) \tag{3.4}$$

Thus, electric field is a vector that points "downhill" in the direction of the steepest local change in electric potential. In appendix B we indicate that electric potential can be defined by (3.4) only for relatively low frequency fields, a category that includes all of EEG.

Two common kinds of vector multiplication are defined, the dot product and the cross product. The operator *Del* may also operate on a vector, thus we define

$$\nabla \cdot \mathbf{A} = \frac{\partial A_x}{\partial x} + \frac{\partial A_y}{\partial y} + \frac{\partial A_z}{\partial z} \tag{A.4}$$

"*Del dot* $\mathbf{A}$" is also called the "*Divergence of* $\mathbf{A}$." Like the gradient, the divergence is a measure of spatial rate of change of a field; however, the divergence itself is a scalar. Of special interest in electrophysiology is the expression for divergence in spherical coordinates

$$\nabla \cdot \mathbf{A} = \frac{1}{r^2}\frac{\partial^2}{\partial r^2}\left(r^2 A_r\right) + \frac{1}{r\sin\theta}\frac{\partial}{\partial\theta}\left(A_\theta\sin\theta\right) + \frac{1}{r\sin\theta}\frac{\partial A_\phi}{\partial\phi} \tag{A.5}$$

For example, consider a spherically symmetric point source of current flux I from the origin $r = 0$. Since current is conserved, the current density at any radial location r is the current divided by the surface area of a sphere of radius r, that is

$$\mathbf{J} = \frac{I\mathbf{a}_r}{4\pi r^2} \tag{A.6}$$

where $\mathbf{a}_r$ is a unit vector in the radial direction. Application of (A.5) to (A.6) yields

$$\nabla \cdot \mathbf{J} = 0 \tag{A.7}$$

We emphasize that (A.4) and (A.5) have identical physical meanings: only the coordinate system is different. That is, if the divergence of $\mathbf{J}$ is zero in spherical coordinates, it is also zero in any other coordinate system, it may just be a little harder to show this.

The cross product of *Del* with a vector is

$$\nabla \times \mathbf{A} = \text{vector}$$
$$= \left(\frac{\partial A_z}{\partial y} - \frac{\partial A_y}{\partial z} \right) \mathbf{i} + \left(\frac{\partial A_x}{\partial z} - \frac{\partial A_z}{\partial x} \right) \mathbf{j} + \left(\frac{\partial A_y}{\partial x} - \frac{\partial A_x}{\partial y} \right) \mathbf{k} \tag{A.8}$$

"*Del cross* $\mathbf{A}$" is also called the "*Curl of* $\mathbf{A}$." Again it is a kind of spatial rate of change of a vector field. An important kind of electric field is one in which the net rotation or circulation of the field around any closed loop is zero. Most fields in nature have nonzero curl, the velocity field of water in a flushed toilet is one example. It can be shown that a field with zero circulation is also one in which the right side of (A.8) is zero. Only electric fields having this property can be expressed as the gradient of a scalar potential.

Finally, since ∇T is itself a vector, it can also be operated on by *Del*, that is

$$\nabla \cdot (\nabla T) = \text{scalar} = \frac{\partial^2 T}{\partial x^2} + \frac{\partial^2 T}{\partial y^2} + \frac{\partial^2 T}{\partial z^2} \tag{A.9}$$

We normally write $\nabla \cdot (\nabla T)$ as $\nabla^2 T$, which is called the *Laplacian* of T. The Laplacian of a scalar field is a measure of the spatial rate of change of the spatial rate of change of the field. It is the low-frequency approximation of electrophysiology (neglect of magnetic induction) that allows the EEG investigator to use the relatively simple scalar formulas of later chapters and to avoid most of vector field theory. However, magnetic field calculations require vectors even at low frequency. The Laplacian in spherical coordinates is given by

$$\nabla^2 T = \frac{1}{r^2} \frac{\partial}{\partial r} \left(r^2 \frac{\partial T}{\partial r} \right) + \frac{1}{r^2 \sin\theta} \frac{\partial}{\partial \theta} \left(\sin\theta \frac{\partial T}{\partial \theta} \right) + \frac{1}{r^2 \sin^2\theta} \frac{\partial^2 T}{\partial \phi^2} \tag{A.10}$$

Again, (A.9) and (A.10) have the same physical meaning, only the coordinate system has changed. The two terms on the far right-hand side of (A.10) involving the angles (θ, ϕ) form the surface Laplacian for a spherical surface. We make extensive use of the surface Laplacian of the scalp potential in chapters 8 through 10.

Two vector identities that are often useful are

$$\nabla \cdot (\nabla \times \mathbf{A}) \equiv 0 \qquad (A.11)$$

$$\nabla \times (\nabla T) \equiv 0 \qquad (A.12)$$

Relations (A.11) and (A.12) are not physical laws. They are mathematical identities that hold for any well-behaved functions $\mathbf{A}$ and T, that is, functions whose first and second derivatives exist. Naturally, these identities are valid in any coordinate system. An excellent physical description of vector and scalar fields is given in the first three chapters of Feynman's famous introduction to electromagnetic theory (Feynman 1963).

Reference

Feynman R, 1963, *Lectures on Physics*, Vol. 2, Palo Alto, CA: Addison-Wesley.

APPENDIX B

Quasi-Static Reduction of Maxwell's Equations

Maxwell's macroscopic equations for fields in material media (including living tissue) are

$$\nabla \cdot \mathbf{D} = \rho \tag{3.21}$$

$$\nabla \times \mathbf{E} = -\frac{\partial \mathbf{B}}{\partial t} \tag{3.22}$$

$$\nabla \cdot \mathbf{B} = 0 \tag{3.23}$$

$$\nabla \times \mathbf{H} = \mathbf{J} + \frac{\partial \mathbf{D}}{\partial t} \tag{3.24}$$

The constitutive relations are based on experimental evidence for media that are linear in the conductive, dielectric and magnetic senses, that is

$$\mathbf{J} = \sigma \mathbf{E} \tag{3.15}$$

$$\mathbf{D} = \varepsilon \mathbf{E} \tag{3.10}$$

$$\mathbf{B} = \mu \mathbf{H} \tag{3.26}$$

Equation (3.24) tells us that magnetic fields may be generated in two distinct ways, either by currents $\mathbf{J}$ of any frequency or by a time varying electric field (the displacement vector $\mathbf{D}$). Equation (3.22) tells us that any time-varying magnetic field will act back on the electric field, which then influences the magnetic field through (3.24) and so forth. Thus, when this coupling process is significant, *electric and magnetic fields* are properly labeled as *electromagnetic fields*.

1 Comparison of Conductive Effects with
   Capacitive Effects

Take the dot product of (3.24) and make use of the mathematical identity (A.11) to obtain

$$\nabla \cdot \left(\mathbf{J} + \frac{\partial \mathbf{D}}{\partial t} \right) = 0 \qquad (B.1.1)$$

Consider a component of the electric field oscillating with frequency f

$$\mathbf{E}(\mathbf{r}, t) = \mathbf{E}_1(\mathbf{r}) \exp [j2\pi ft] \qquad (B.1.2)$$

and express (B.1.1) in terms of the electric field using (3.15) and (3.10):

$$\nabla \cdot (\sigma \mathbf{E} + j2\pi f \varepsilon \mathbf{E}) = 0 \qquad (B.1.3)$$

The two terms inside the parentheses represent conductive and capacitive effects in a material medium, that is, the effects of free charge and stored (or bound) charge, respectively. In living tissue, the free charges of interest are positive and negative ions; additionally charges are stored locally by cell membranes. Thus we find that capacitive effects in macroscopic tissue masses may be neglected if

$$\text{Ratio} = \frac{2\pi f \varepsilon(f)}{\sigma(f)} \ll 1 \qquad (4.3)$$

As an example, consider the above ratio for muscle tissue at frequencies near $100\,\text{Hz}$. From fig. 4-5, the tissue resistivity is approximately

$$\eta \equiv \frac{1}{\sigma} \simeq 400\,\text{ohm cm} \quad \text{or} \quad \sigma = \frac{1}{400}\,\text{ohm}^{-1}\,\text{cm}^{-1} \times \frac{100\,\text{cm}}{\text{m}} = \frac{1}{4}\,\text{ohm}^{-1}\,\text{m}^{-1}$$

Also, from Fig. 4-5, the relative dielectric constant of muscle tissue is roughly

$$\kappa \equiv \frac{\varepsilon}{\varepsilon_0} \simeq 10^6 \text{ (unitless)}$$

The permittivity of free space is a fixed constant

$$\varepsilon_0 = 8.84 \times 10^{-12}\,\text{s ohm}^{-1}\,\text{m}^{-1}$$

Thus, the ratio of capacitive to resistive current (4.3) in this example is

$$\text{Ratio} = \frac{2\pi \times 100\,\text{s}^{-1} \times 8.84 \times 10^{-6}\,\text{s} \cdot \text{ohm}^{-1} \cdot \text{m}^{-1}}{0.25\,\text{ohm}^{-1} \cdot \text{m}^{-1}} \sim 0.02$$

As a second example, consider the ratio (4.3) for the passive membrane of the squid giant axon. In order to estimate the conductivity of the membrane, use

$$\sigma = \frac{\varepsilon}{\tau} \tag{4.18}$$

where τ is the membrane time constant, about 10^{-3} s. Thus, (4.3) and (4.18) yield

$$\text{Ratio} = 2\pi f \tau$$

It is also of interest to estimate passive membrane conductivity and dielectric constant from fundamental equations. Permitivity is related to capacity C by

$$\varepsilon = \frac{C \Delta r}{A} \tag{4.19}$$

Biological membranes are known to have a capacity per unit area of surface of

$$\frac{C}{A} \sim 1 \ \mu F/cm^2$$

and a thickness of

$$\Delta r \sim 10^{-6} \ cm$$

Thus

$$\varepsilon \sim \left(10^{-6} \ F/cm^2\right)\left(10^{-6} \ cm\right)(100 \ cm/m) \sim 10^{-10} \ F/m$$

or $10^{-10} \ s \cdot ohm^{-1} \cdot m^{-1}$

The relative dielectric constant of the membrane is then given by

$$\kappa \sim 12 \ (\text{unitless})$$

To first approximation the relative dielectric constant of the membrane is independent of biological material or field frequency. This is apparently also valid for the *active membrane*. Passive membrane conductivity may also be estimated from (4.18), that is, for the squid giant axon

$$\sigma \sim \frac{10^{-12} \ s \cdot ohm^{-1} \cdot cm^{-1}}{10^{-3} \ s} \sim 10^{-9} \ ohm^{-1} \cdot cm^{-1}$$

In contrast to dielectric constant, conductivity can be expected to vary considerably with biological material and to a much lesser degree with field frequency. The conductivity of the active squid membrane is roughly 40 times that of the passive membrane (Plonsey 1969).

2 Comparison of Conductive Effects with Magnetic Effects

The fundamental equations that describe electric field behavior in living tissue are summarized at the beginning of chapter 4. No magnetic field appears. Thus, all solutions of the equations for electric fields or potentials are independent of any magnetic field that might be present in the tissue. While this is only an approximation, we show here that it is an excellent approximation in EEG. Take the *Curl* of (3.22) to obtain

$$\nabla \times \nabla \times \mathbf{E} = -\nabla \times \left(\frac{\partial \mathbf{B}}{\partial t}\right) = -\frac{\partial}{\partial t}(\nabla \times \mathbf{B}) \qquad (B.2.1)$$

Combine (3.24), (3.15), (3.10), and (3.26) to obtain

$$\nabla \times \nabla \times \mathbf{E} = -\mu\frac{\partial}{\partial t}\left(\sigma\mathbf{E} + \varepsilon\frac{\partial \mathbf{E}}{\partial t}\right) \qquad (B.2.2)$$

Comparison of (B.2.2) with (3.22) reminds us that the right-hand side of (B.2.2) represents the "feedback effect" of a time-varying magnetic field acting back on the electric field, that is, *magnetic induction*. For example, inductors in electric circuits consist of coils of wire that produce magnetic fields, mainly directed along the axis of the coils, that act on the electric field in and around the wire, thereby producing a potential difference across the inductor proportional to the first time derivative of electric field (or potential), that is, proportional to field frequency. We may calculate the inductance of any wire coil geometry using (B.2.2), dropping the capacitive term on the far right, which is negligible in copper wires. From (3.22) we see that magnetic induction may be neglected when

$$\nabla \times \mathbf{E} \cong 0 \qquad (B.2.3)$$

However, we must have something to compare to this *Curl* in order to quantify the approximation. From (B.2.2) the condition is

$$\frac{\mu\left|\frac{\partial}{\partial t}\left(\sigma\mathbf{E} + \varepsilon\frac{\partial \mathbf{E}}{\partial t}\right)\right|}{|\nabla \times \nabla \times \mathbf{E}|} \ll 1 \qquad (B.2.4)$$

Like the condition for neglect of capacitive effects with respect to conductive effects (4.3), (B.2.4) *is a frequency-dependent condition; however, it is quite a different condition.* For example, the ratio (4.3) *decreases* with medium conductivity σ, so the approximation (4.3) becomes progressively better in better conductors. By contrast, the ratio (B.2.4) *increases* with conductivity, so the approximation (B.2.4) becomes progressively worse in better conductors. Furthermore, (B.2.4) involves spatial derivatives of the electric field as well as the time derivative leading to (4.3). To estimate the ratio (B.2.4) we note that smallest values in the denominator occur for relatively smooth spatial changes in electric field. Consider a Fourier component of the electric field component of the form

$$\mathbf{E}(\mathbf{r}, t) = \exp[j(2\pi ft + \mathbf{K} \cdot \mathbf{r})]\mathbf{i} \qquad (B.2.5)$$

where x indicates the "smoothest" direction for electric field changes. Here the wavenumber vector is defined by

$$\mathbf{K} = k_x\mathbf{i} + k_y\mathbf{j} + k_z\mathbf{k} \qquad (B.2.6)$$

The *Curl(Curl)* operation of (B.2.4) applied to (B.2.5) yields

$$\nabla \times \nabla \times \mathbf{E} = \left[\left(k_y^2 + k_z^2\right)\mathbf{i} - k_x k_y\mathbf{j} - k_x k_z\mathbf{k}\right] \exp[j(2\pi ft + \mathbf{K} \cdot \mathbf{r})] \qquad (B.2.7)$$

$$|\nabla \times \nabla \times \mathbf{E}| = \left[K\sqrt{\left(k_x^2 + k_z^2\right)}\right]E \sim K^2 E \qquad (B.2.8)$$

where K and E are the magnitudes of the associated vectors. Substitution into (B.2.4) yields the condition for neglect of magnetic induction in terms of field frequency f, smallest characteristic wavenumber K, and medium properties, that is

$$\left[\frac{2\pi f\mu(f)\sigma(f)}{K^2}\right]\sqrt{1 + \frac{4\pi^2 f^2\varepsilon^2(f)}{\sigma^2(f)}} \ll 1 \qquad (B.2.9)$$

A numerical estimate of (B.2.9) is as follows. The permeability μ of a nonmetallic material like tissue is essentially that of empty space

$$\mu \simeq \mu_0 \equiv \frac{1}{c^2\varepsilon_0}\,\text{ohm} \cdot \text{s} \cdot \text{m}^{-1}$$

where the velocity of light is $c = 3 \times 10^8$ m/s. A conservative (largest) value for the characteristic spatial wavelength on a human body is (say) 1 m or $K \sim 6$ m^{-1}. Take a conservative (large) estimate for the conductivity (see table 4-1) of $\sigma \sim 1$ ohm$^{-1} \cdot$ m^{-1} and dielectric constant $\kappa \sim 10^8$ (unitless). Then (B.2.9) yields

$$\frac{2\pi f\left(1.25 \times 10^{-6}\,\text{ohm} \cdot \text{s} \cdot \text{m}^{-1}\right)\left(1\,\text{ohm}^{-1} \cdot \text{m}^{-1}\right)}{36\,\text{m}^{-2}}$$

$$\times \sqrt{1 + \frac{4\pi^2 f^2\left(8.84 \times 10^{-4}\,\text{s} \cdot \text{ohm}^{-1} \cdot \text{m}^{-1}\right)^2}{\left(1\,\text{ohm}^{-1} \cdot \text{m}^{-1}\right)^2}} \ll 1$$

or

$$2 \times 10^{-7} f \sqrt{1 + 3 \times 10^{-5} f^2} \ll 1$$

Thus, the neglect of magnetic induction is an excellent approximation in the calculation of electric fields generated in the brain, apparently for frequencies up to roughly one mega Hz.

References

Plonsey R, 1969, *Bioelectric Phenomena*, New York: McGraw Hill.
Polk C and Postow E, 1986, CRC *Handbook of Biological Effects of Electromagnetic Fields*, Boca Raton, FL: CRC Press.

APPENDIX C

Surface Magnetic Field Due to a Dipole at an Arbitrary Location in a Volume Conductor

The radial and tangential magnetic fields at spherical coordinates (r, θ, ϕ) due to a tangential current dipole located at coordinates (r_1, θ_1, ϕ_1) in a volume conductor are derived here (see fig. C-1). The expression for the radial field component when the dipole is located on the z axis is readily available in the MEG literature. If only one dipole is present, the coordinate system may be rotated so the dipole is located on the z axis; however, with more than one dipole, this more general expression is required (Nunez 1986a). This derivation (Nunez 1986b) has undoubtedly been published earlier by others, but they are unknown to us.

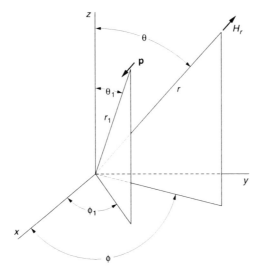

Figure C-1 Spherical coordinate system and radial component of the magnetic field H_r due to current dipole **p**. The angle between the radial vectors **r** and $\mathbf{r_1}$ is γ (not shown). The distance between the dipole and field point is $R = |\mathbf{r} - \mathbf{r_1}|$.

Maxwell's equation (3.24) shows that even when the displacement current is negligible (that is, magnetic induction may be neglected), any static or low-frequency current produces a magnetic field. The dipole source $\mathbf{p} = I\mathbf{d}$ consists of a current element flowing over a distance d as shown in fig. C-1. The Biot–Savart law is a special case of (3.24) when magnetic induction is negligible, that is

$$\mathbf{H} = \frac{\mathbf{p} \times \mathbf{R}}{4\pi R^3} \tag{C.1}$$

Here $\mathbf{R}$ is the vector from the dipole at $\mathbf{r}_1$ to the field (measurement) point $\mathbf{r}$. By inspection of fig. C-1, the unit vectors along $\mathbf{r}_1$ and $\mathbf{r}$ are given by

$$\begin{aligned}
\mathbf{a}_{r1} &= (\cos \phi_1 \mathbf{i} + \sin \phi_1 \mathbf{j}) \sin \theta_1 + \cos \theta_1 \mathbf{k} \\
\mathbf{a}_r &= (\cos \phi \mathbf{i} + \sin \phi \mathbf{j}) \sin \theta + \cos \theta \mathbf{k}
\end{aligned} \tag{C.2}$$

Here $\{\mathbf{i}, \mathbf{j}, \mathbf{k}\}$ are the usual unit vectors along the (x, y, z) axes. Using (C.2) the vector distance between dipole and field point may be expressed

$$\begin{aligned}
\mathbf{R} = \mathbf{r} - \mathbf{r}_1 &= (r \sin \theta \cos \phi - r_1 \sin \theta_1 \cos \phi_1)\mathbf{i} \\
&+ (r \sin \theta \sin \phi - r_1 \sin \theta_1 \sin \phi_1)\mathbf{j} + (r \cos \theta - r_1 \cos \theta_1)\mathbf{k}
\end{aligned} \tag{C.3}$$

If the dipole moment is directed along the positive x axis, $\mathbf{p} = p\mathbf{i}$, and the radial component of the magnetic field follows directly from (C.1), that is

$$H_r = \frac{\mathbf{p} \times \mathbf{R}}{4\pi R^3} \cdot \mathbf{a}_r \tag{C.4}$$

The relationship between the distance R and the angle γ between $\mathbf{r}$ and $\mathbf{r}_1$ is given by the following trigonometric relations (Jackson 1975):

$$\begin{aligned}
R^2 &= r^2 + r_1^2 - 2rr_1 \cos \gamma \\
\cos \gamma &= \cos \theta \cos \theta_1 + \sin \theta \sin \theta_1 \cos(\phi - \phi_1)
\end{aligned} \tag{C.4}$$

Substitution of (C.2), (C.3), and (C.5) into (C.4) yields the radial magnetic field due to an x-directed dipole:

$$H_r = \frac{pr_1(\cos \theta_1 \sin \theta \sin \phi - \cos \theta \sin \theta_1 \sin \phi_1)}{4\pi \{r^2 + r_1^2 - 2rr_1 [\cos \theta \cos \theta_1 + \sin \theta \sin \theta_1 \cos(\phi - \phi_1)]\}^{3/2}} \tag{C.6}$$

When the dipole is located on the z axis, (C.6) reduces to the familiar expression (Cuffin and Cohen 1977)

$$H_r = \frac{pr_1 \sin \theta \sin \phi}{4\pi (r^2 + r_1^2 - 2rr_1 \cos \theta)^{3/2}} \tag{C.7}$$

In this case, the surface radial magnetic field increases from zero (at $\theta = 0$) in directions perpendicular to the dipole axis ($\phi = \pm\pi/2$) to a maximum magnitude at the angle

$$\theta_{\text{MAX}} = \text{ArcCos}\left[\frac{\sqrt{r^4 + 14r^2 r_1^2 + r_1^4} - (r^2 + r_1^2)}{2rr_1}\right] \tag{C.8}$$

A numerical example is as follows. Let the dipole be located at $r_1 = 7.2$ cm (say, 0.8 cm below a 8.0 cm brain radius). Let the MEG sensor location be $r = 12$ cm (say 2.8 cm above a 9.2 cm scalp radius). In this example, the peak radial field occurs at $\theta_{\text{MAX}} = 20.5°$ or a surface distance of 4.3 cm on the 12 cm sphere defined by MEG sensor locations. The field then falls to half its maximum magnitude at $\theta_{1/2} = 54.0°$ or 11.3 cm along the same sensor sphere. When the dipole is y-directed $\mathbf{p} = p\mathbf{j}$, the derivation of the radial magnetic field is identical except for the evaluation of the cross product in (C.4).

The expression for the tangential magnetic fields due to a tangential dipole may also be derived in a similar manner. From fig. C-1, the two tangential unit vectors are

$$\begin{aligned}\mathbf{a}_\theta &= \cos\theta\cos\phi\,\mathbf{i} + \cos\theta\sin\phi\,\mathbf{j} - \sin\theta\,\mathbf{k} \\ \mathbf{a}_\phi &= -\sin\phi\,\mathbf{i} + \cos\phi\,\mathbf{j}\end{aligned} \tag{C.9}$$

The tangential fields due to an x-directed dipole are obtained from (C.1) and (C.9)

$$H_\theta = \frac{p[r_1\sin\theta\sin\theta_1\sin\phi_1 + \sin\phi(r_1\cos\theta\cos\theta_1 - r)]}{4\pi\{r^2 + r_1^2 - 2rr_1[\cos\theta\cos\theta_1 + \sin\theta\sin\theta_1\cos(\phi - \phi_1)]\}^{3/2}} \tag{C.10}$$

$$H_\phi = \frac{p\cos\phi[r_1\cos\theta_1 - r\cos\theta]}{4\pi\{r^2 + r_1^2 - 2rr_1[\cos\theta\cos\theta_1 + \sin\theta\sin\theta_1\cos(\phi - \phi_1)]\}^{3/2}} \tag{C.11}$$

The magnetic field expressions derived here provide only contributions from the primary (dipole) source current. In anisotropic and inhomogeneous media, the magnetic field may be expressed

$$\mathbf{H} = \mathbf{H}_{\text{primary}} + \mathbf{H}_{\text{secondary}} \tag{C.12}$$

The so-called secondary currents are actually mathematical constructs used to quantify the distortion of current patterns by inhomogeneity and anisotropy (Cuffin and Cohen 1977; Nunez 1986a;

Hamaleinen et al. 1993). These fictitious sources "turn off" when the primary sources turn off. If the volume conductor is a spherically symmetric layered medium, as in our standard volume conductor model used to calculate scalp electric potentials, the contribution of secondary sources to the radial magnetic field is zero and (C.6)–(C.8) may be used with impunity. However, the contribution of secondary sources to the tangential fields (C.10) and (C.11) is generally not zero, evidentally making them more difficult to interpret in terms of the underlying sources.

References

Cuffin BN and Cohen D, 1977, Magnetic fields of a dipole in special volume conductor shapes. *IEEE Transactions on Biomedical Engineering* 24: 372–381.

Hamaleinen M, Hari R, Ilmoniemi RJ, Knuutila J, and Lounasmaa OV, 1993, Magnetoencephalography theory, instrumentation, and application to noninvasive studies of the working human brain. *Reviews of Modern Physics* 65: 413–497.

Jackson JD, 1975, *Classical Electodynamics*, 2nd Edition, New York: Wiley.

Nunez PL, 1986a, The brain's magnetic field: some effects of multiple sources on localization methods. *Electroencephalography and Clinical Neurophysiology* 63: 75–82.

Nunez PL,1986b, Locating sources of the brain's electric and magnetic fields: some effects of inhomogeneity and multiple sources with implications for the future. Biophysics Lab, Navy Personnel Research and Development Center, San Diego, Technical Note 71-86-12.

APPENDIX D

Derivation of the Membrane Diffusion Equation

Here we obtain the differential equation describing the potential difference across the membrane of a cylindrical fiber due to an external current source $\mathbf{J}_S$, as shown in fig. 4-9. It is assumed that $\mathbf{J}_S$ is symmetrical about the z axis. Capacitive effects are assumed to be negligible except inside the membrane, as discussed in appendix B. From (3.27), (4.6), and (4.12) we obtain the fundamental equation for current conservation with an external source term

$$\nabla \cdot \left(\sigma \mathbf{E} + \varepsilon \frac{\partial \mathbf{E}}{\partial t} \right) = -\nabla \cdot \mathbf{J}_S(\mathbf{r}, t) \tag{D.1}$$

In order to integrate (D.1) over the cylindrical volume of intracellular fluid of radius $r_1 + \Delta r/2$ and height Δz as in fig. 4-9, we make use of the mathematical identity relating volume and surface integrals of any vector $\mathbf{B}$:

$$\int_V \nabla \cdot \mathbf{B} dV = \int_A \mathbf{B} \cdot d\mathbf{A} \tag{D.2}$$

to obtain

$$\int_{A_1} \left(\sigma \mathbf{E} + \varepsilon \frac{\partial \mathbf{E}}{\partial t} \right) \cdot d\mathbf{A}_1 = -\int_{A_1} \mathbf{J}_S \cdot d\mathbf{A}_1 = +I_S \tag{D.3}$$

where I_S is the source current injected into the axon, due either to electrode stimulation or synaptic input. If the conductivity of the membrane is much less than that of the intracellular fluid, and the axon length is much larger than its radius, the axial current flow $J_{1z} = \sigma_1 E_{1z}$ is approximately constant with radial location. Furthermore, current inside the membrane will be mostly in the radial direction. Using these approximations, (D.3) can be approximated by

$$\sigma_1 \left[E_{1z}|_{z+\Delta z} - E_{1z}|_z \right] \pi r_1^2 + 2\pi r_1 \Delta z \left[\sigma_2 E_{2r} + \varepsilon_2 \frac{\partial E_{2r}}{\partial t} \right]_{r=r_1+\Delta r/2} = +I_S \quad \text{(D.4)}$$

where the axial and radial components of the electric field are given by E_z and E_r, respectively, in regions given by the numbered subscript.

A second expression is obtained by integrating (D.1) over a volume of extracellular fluid located between the concentric cylindrical surfaces, $r_1 + \Delta r/2 \leq r \leq r_3$ and height Δz. It is assumed that adjacent axons contain both conductive and capacitive current flow inside the outer cylindrical wall $r = r_3$. Extracellular axial current flow is also assumed to be constant over the radial dimension. No current source contributes here since J_S is assumed to be supplied externally, for example by a stimulating electrode. In this case (D.1) can be approximated by

$$\sigma_3 \left[E_{3z}|_{z+\Delta z} - E_{3z}|_z \right] \left[\pi \left(r_3^2 - r_1^2 \right) \right] - (2\pi r_1 \Delta z) \left[\sigma_2 E_{2r} + \varepsilon_2 \frac{\partial E_{2r}}{\partial t} \right]_{r=r_1+\Delta r/2} = 0$$

$$\text{(D.5)}$$

Subtract (D.5) from (D.4) to obtain

$$\frac{1}{\Delta z} \left[(E_{1z} - E_{3z})|_{z+\Delta z} - (E_{1z} - E_{3z})|_z \right]$$

$$+ 2 \left[\frac{1}{r_1 \sigma_1} + \frac{r_1}{(r_3^2 - r_1^2)\sigma_3} \right] \cdot \left[\sigma_2 E_{2r} + \varepsilon_2 \frac{\partial E_{2r}}{\partial t} \right]_{r=r_1+\Delta r/2} = +\frac{I_S}{\pi r_1^2 \sigma_1 \Delta z}$$

$$\text{(D.6)}$$

We are interested in the potential difference across the membrane

$$V \equiv \Phi_1 - \Phi_3 \quad \text{(D.7)}$$

The electric field is related to the potential by derivatives such as

$$E_{1z} = -\frac{\partial \Phi_1}{\partial z} \quad \text{(D.8)}$$

Since the membrane is very thin, we can make use of the approximation

$$E_{2r}|_{r+\Delta r/2} \equiv -\frac{\partial \Phi_2}{\partial r}\bigg|_{r+\Delta r/2} \cong \frac{\Phi_1 - \Phi_3}{\Delta r} \equiv \frac{V}{\Delta r} \quad \text{(D.9)}$$

and allow $\Delta z \to 0$ to write (D.6) as

$$-\frac{\partial^2 V}{\partial z^2} + 2\left[\frac{1}{r_1\sigma_1} + \frac{r_1}{(r_3^2 - r_1^2)\sigma_3}\right] \cdot \left[\frac{\sigma_2}{\Delta r}V + \frac{\varepsilon_2}{\Delta r}\frac{\partial V}{\partial t}\right] = +\frac{I_S}{\pi r_1^2 \sigma_1 \Delta z} \quad \text{(D.10)}$$

which may be rearranged to yield

$$\lambda^2 \frac{\partial^2 V}{\partial z^2} - \tau\frac{\partial V}{\partial t} - V = \frac{-\lambda^2 I_S}{\pi r_1^2 \sigma_1 \Delta z} \quad \text{(D.11)}$$

Here the space constant of the axon and extracellular space is given by

$$\lambda^2 = \frac{r_1 \Delta r}{2}\frac{\left(\frac{r_3^2}{r_1^2} - 1\right)\frac{\sigma_1}{\sigma_2}}{\left(\frac{r_3^2}{r_1^2} - 1 + \frac{\sigma_1}{\sigma_3}\right)} \quad \text{(4.17)}$$

and the time constant of the membrane is

$$\tau = \frac{\varepsilon_2}{\sigma_2} \quad \text{(4.18)}$$

in accordance with the text. When the appropriate geometrical factors are inserted, (4.18) identical to the membrane time constant (4.20) derived from the usual core conductor network (Davis and Lorente de No 1947; Plonsey 1969).

The usual expression for the space constant of the core conductor model may be retrieved from (4.17) as follows. From (4.19), membrane conductivity σ_2 is related to the radial current resistance R_2 of a length Δz and thickness Δr of membrane by the relation

$$\sigma_2 = \frac{\Delta r}{2\pi r_1 \Delta z R_2} \quad \text{(D.12)}$$

The inner σ_1 and outer σ_3 conductivities of the same section of cylindrical fiber are related to axial current resistances R_1 and R_3 by the relations

$$\sigma_1 = \frac{\Delta z}{\pi r_1^2 R_1} \qquad \sigma_3 \cong \frac{\Delta z}{\pi(r_3^2 - r_1^2)R_3} \quad \text{(D.13)}$$

Substitute (D.12) and (D.13) into (4.17) to obtain the space constant in its more familiar form

$$\lambda^2 = \frac{R_2 \Delta z^2}{R_1 + R_3} \quad \text{(4.21)}$$

Some scientists may find (4.17) and (4.18) to be a bit more physical than the more familiar forms (4.20) and (4.21).

References

Davis L and Lorente de No R, 1947, Contribution to the mathematical theory of electronics. In: *A study of nerve physiology*, New York: Rockefeller Institute for Medical Research, Chapter 9.

Plonsey R, 1969, *Bioelectric Phenomena*, New York: McGraw-Hill.

APPENDIX E

Solutions to the Membrane Diffusion Equation

1 Transmembrane Potential Due to a Local Impulse Input to an Infinite, Cylindrical Fiber

The basic cable equation with point (delta function) input at $z = 0$ and $t = 0$ is

$$\frac{\partial^2 g}{\partial z^2} - \frac{\partial g}{\partial t} - g = -\delta(z)\,\delta(t) \tag{E.1.1}$$

Here $g(z, t)$ is nondimensional transmembrane potential and the independent variables are expressed in nondimensional form in terms of cable parameters, that is, $z \to \lambda z$ and $t \to t\tau$. Define the Fourier transform pair

$$G(k, \omega) = \int\limits_{-\infty}^{+\infty} e^{jkz} dz \int\limits_{-\infty}^{+\infty} g(z, t)\, e^{j\omega t} dt \tag{E.1.2}$$

$$g(z, t) = \frac{1}{4\pi^2} \int\limits_{-\infty}^{+\infty} e^{-jkz} dk \int\limits_{-\infty}^{+\infty} G(k, \omega)\, e^{-j\omega t} d\omega \tag{E.1.3}$$

Use (E.1.2) to take the (double) Fourier transform of (E.1.1) and substitute $G(k, \omega)$ into (E.1.3) to obtain

$$g(z, t) = \frac{j}{4\pi^2} \int\limits_{-\infty}^{+\infty} e^{-jkz} dk \int\limits_{-\infty}^{+\infty} \frac{e^{-j\omega t} d\omega}{\omega + j(k^2 + 1)} \tag{E.1.4}$$

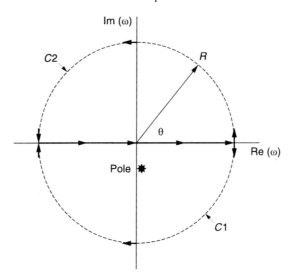

Figure E.1 The complex ω plane used to invert the Fourier transform.

The ω-integrand has a simple pole at $-j(k^2+1)$. Consider the closed contour in the ω plane shown in fig. E.1. The clockwise integral around the closed path C may be expressed as the sum of the integral along the real ω axis and the integral along the semicircular contour $C1$ in the lower half plane, that is

$$\oint_C \frac{e^{-jt\omega}d\omega}{\omega+j(k^2+1)} = \int_{-R}^{R} \frac{e^{-jt\omega}d\omega}{\omega+j(k^2+1)} + \oint_{C1} \frac{e^{-jt\omega}d\omega}{\omega+j(k^2+1)} \qquad (E.1.5)$$

To evaluate the integral over contour $C1$, let $\omega = R\,e^{j\theta}$, where R is constant on $C1$, obtaining

$$I_{C1} = \oint_{C1} \frac{e^{-jt\omega}d\omega}{\omega+j(k^2+1)} = jR\int_0^{-\pi} \frac{\exp[j(\theta - tR\cos\theta) + tR\sin\theta]d\theta}{Re^{j\theta}+j(k^2+1)} \qquad (E.1.6)$$

We now let the radius R of the semicircle approach infinity. Note that $\sin\theta$ is negative everywhere in the lower half plane, and the imaginary parts of exponential functions have magnitudes less than or equal to one. Thus

$$\lim_{R\to\infty} I_{C1} = 0 \quad t > 0 \qquad (E.1.7)$$

Using (E.1.7), evaluate the contour integral (E.1.5) to find the ω integral in (E.1.4) for $t > 0$ using Cauchy's integral formula for clockwise integration around the lower semicircle in fig. E-1 (Morse and Feshbach 1953), that is

$$I_\omega \equiv \int_{-\infty}^{+\infty} \frac{e^{-j\omega t}\,d\omega}{\omega + j(k^2+1)} = (-j2\pi)\left[(\text{Residue of pole at } \omega = -j(k^2+1)\right] (E.1.8)$$

$$I_\omega = -j2\pi e^{-t(k^2+1)} \quad t > 0 \qquad (E.1.9)$$

Substitute (E.1.9) into (E.1.4) and note that on the interval $\{-\infty, +\infty\}$ integrals of odd functions of k vanish and integrals of even functions are double their semi-infinite values, that is

$$g(z,t) = \frac{e^{-t}}{2\pi}\int_{-\infty}^{+\infty} e^{-tk^2 - jkz}\,dk = \frac{e^{-t}}{\pi}\int_{0}^{\infty} e^{-tk^2}\cos(kz)\,dk \quad z>0 \qquad (E.1.10)$$

$$g(z,t) = \frac{1}{2\sqrt{\pi t}}\exp\left[-\frac{z^2}{4t} - t\right] \qquad (E.1.11)$$

Or in terms of dimensional variables and cable parameters

$$g(z,t) = \frac{1}{2\sqrt{\pi}}\left(\frac{\tau}{t}\right)\exp\left[-\frac{(z/\lambda)^2}{4(t/\tau)} - t/\tau\right] \qquad (E.1.12)$$

2 Transmembrane Potential Due to Local Sinusoidal Input to an Infinite, Cylindrical Fiber

In this example, an oscillatory input with frequency Ω occurs at a point $(z=0)$ on the axis of the cylindrical fiber. The basic axon cable equation in nondimensional variables is

$$\frac{\partial^2 g}{\partial z^2} - \frac{\partial g}{\partial t} - g = -\delta(z)\cos(\Omega t) \qquad (E.2.1)$$

We seek a steady-state solution of the form

$$g(z,t) = \text{Re}[q(z)e^{j\Omega t}] \qquad (E.2.2)$$

Equation (E.2.1) then becomes

$$\frac{d^2 q}{dz^2} - (1 + j\Omega)q = -\delta(z) \qquad (E.2.3)$$

Take the Fourier transform of (E.2.3) and apply the inverse spatial transform in (E.1.3) to obtain

$$q(z) = \frac{1}{2\pi} \int\limits_{-\infty}^{+\infty} \frac{e^{-jzk}dk}{k^2 - k_0^2} \tag{E.2.4}$$

The integrand in (E.2.4) has simple poles at $k = \pm k_0$, where

$$k_0^2 = -(1 + j\Omega) \tag{E.2.5}$$

Let $k_0 = a - jb$ or $k_0^2 = a^2 - b^2 - j2ab$. Thus, $b = \Omega/2a$ and $a^2 - b^2 = -1$. Combine these last two expressions to obtain

$$a^4 + a^2 - \frac{\Omega^2}{4} = 0 \tag{E.2.6}$$

$$a^2 = -\frac{1}{2} \pm \frac{1}{2}\sqrt{1 + \Omega} \tag{E.2.7}$$

$$a = \pm\sqrt{\frac{1}{2}\left(\sqrt{1 + \Omega^2} - 1\right)} \tag{E.2.8}$$

$$b = \pm\sqrt{\frac{1}{2}\left(\sqrt{1 + \Omega^2} + 1\right)} \tag{E.2.9}$$

Since $b = \omega/2a$, a and b have the same sign for $\omega > 0$. Thus, taking only positive roots for a and b is consistent with poles at

$$k_0 = \pm(a - jb) \tag{E.2.10}$$

Consider the closed contour in the k plane similar to the equivalent contour in the ω plane shown in fig. E-1. The integral around the closed path C may be expressed as the sum of the integral along the real k axis and the integral along the semicircular contour $C2$ in the upper half plane. The same arguments are applied as in (E.1.5) and (E.1.6). That is, to evaluate the integral over contour $C2$, let $k = R\,e^{j\theta}$, where R is constant on $C2$, obtaining

$$I_{C2} = \oint\limits_{C2} \frac{e^{-jzk}dk}{k^2 - k_0^2} = jR \int\limits_{0}^{\pi} \frac{\exp[j(\theta - zR\cos\theta) + zR\sin\theta]d\theta}{R^2 e^{j2\theta} - k_0^2} \tag{E.2.11}$$

We now let the radius of the semicircle R approach infinity. Note that $\sin\theta$ is positive everywhere in the upper half plane. Also, imaginary parts of exponential functions are limited to maximum magnitudes equal to one. Thus

$$\lim_{R\to\infty} I_{C2} \to \infty \quad z > 0$$
$$\lim_{R\to\infty} I_{C2} \to 0 \quad z < 0$$

(E.2.12)

Using (E.2.11) and (E.2.12), we evaluate the contour integral (E.2.4) to find the function $q(z)$ for $z < 0$, again using Cauchy's integral formula based on counterclockwise integration

$$q(z) = \frac{1}{2\pi} \oint_C \frac{e^{-jzk}dk}{k^2 - k_0^2} = \frac{1}{2\pi}(j2\pi)[\text{Res pole at } k = -k_0] \quad z < 0$$

(E.2.13)

$$q(z) = j\left(\frac{e^{-jkz}}{k - k_0}\right)_{k=-k_0} = \frac{(b - ja)e^{bz+jaz}}{2(a^2 + b^2)} \quad z < 0 \qquad (E.2.14)$$

To evaluate the contour integral (E.2.4) for $z > 0$, we follow a similar procedure except we close the contour in the lower half plane. In this case, the integral over the semicircle C1 has limits $\theta = 0$ to $-\pi$ (clockwise). Noting that Cauchy's integral formula treats closed integrals in the counterclockwise direction as positive, we obtain

$$q(z) = \frac{1}{2\pi} \int_{-\infty}^{+\infty} \frac{e^{-jzk}dk}{k^2 - k_0^2} = \frac{1}{2\pi}(-j2\pi)[\text{Res pole at } k = +k_0] \quad z > 0$$

(E.2.15)

$$q(z) = -j\left(\frac{e^{-jkz}}{k + k_0}\right)_{k=+k_0} = \frac{(b - ja)e^{-bz-jaz}}{2(a^2 + b^2)} \quad z > 0 \qquad (E.2.16)$$

Comparison of (E.2.14) and (E.2.16) shows that the solution for $q(z)$ may be written more concisely as

$$q(z) = \frac{(b - ja)e^{-b|z|-ja|z|}}{2(a^2 + b^2)} \quad -\infty < z < +\infty \qquad (E.2.17)$$

Substitute (E.2.17) into (E.2.2) to obtain

$$g(z, t) = \frac{1}{2(a^2 + b^2)} \text{Re}\{(b - ja) \exp[-b|z| + j(\Omega t - a|z|)]\}$$

$$= \frac{e^{-b|z|}}{2(a^2 + b^2)}[b\cos(\Omega t - a|z|) + a\sin(\Omega t - a|z|)]$$

(E.2.18)

The solution may be expressed more usefully by making use of the identity

$$\cos(C - D) \equiv \cos C \cos D + \sin C \sin D \qquad (\text{E.2.19})$$

$$D = \Omega t - a|z| \qquad (\text{E.2.20})$$

$$\cos C = \frac{b}{\sqrt{a^2 + b^2}} \qquad \sin C = \frac{a}{\sqrt{a^2 + b^2}} \qquad (\text{E.2.21})$$

$$g(z, t) = \frac{e^{-b|z|}}{2\sqrt{a^2 + b^2}} \cos\left[\Omega t - a|z| - \mathrm{ArcTan}\left(\frac{a}{b}\right)\right] \qquad (\text{E.2.22})$$

Express a and b in terms of $\Omega\tau$ and the membrane potential in terms of dimensional variables and cable parameters to obtain

$$g(z, t) = \left\{ \frac{\exp\left[-\sqrt{0.5\left(\sqrt{1 + \Omega^2\tau^2} + 1\right)}\left(\frac{|z|}{\lambda}\right)\right]}{2\sqrt[4]{1 + \Omega^2\tau^2}} \right\}$$

$$\times \cos\left\{ \Omega t - \sqrt{0.5\left(\sqrt{1 + \Omega^2\tau^2} + 1\right)}\left(\frac{|z|}{\lambda}\right) - \mathrm{ArcTan}\left(\frac{\sqrt{0.5\left(\sqrt{1 + \Omega^2\tau^2} - 1\right)}}{\sqrt{0.5\left(\sqrt{1 + \Omega^2\tau^2} + 1\right)}}\right) \right\}$$

$$(\text{E.2.23})$$

APPENDIX F

Point Source in a Five-Layered Plane Medium

Here we consider a point source located at $(z=0, r=0)$ in the five-layered plane medium. Dipole and other source distributions may be constructed from the monopole solution by linear superposition. The general problem of a source located in layered media was solved before the Great Depression by Stefanesco and Schlumberger (1930) and applied more recently to neocortical potentials by Zhadin (1969). The approach is to solve Poisson's equation (4.12) for $\Phi(r,z)$, where r and z refer to cylindrical coordinates. The potential in each of the five regions is given by Φ_1 through Φ_5 (top to bottom). The interface boundary conditions are given by (4.7) and (4.8), which require the *normal component* of current density and the tangential component of electric field to be continuous at the four interfaces ($z = h_i, i = 1, 4$), that is

$$\sigma_i \frac{\partial \Phi_i}{\partial z} = \sigma_{i+1} \frac{\partial \Phi_{i+1}}{\partial z} \quad i = 1, 4 \tag{F.1}$$

$$\frac{\partial \Phi_i}{\partial r} = \frac{\partial \Phi_{i+1}}{\partial r} \quad i = 1, 4 \tag{F.2}$$

Here h_4 is the vertical distance between the monopolar source and 4–5 interface (lowest interface), h_3 is measured to the 3–4 interface, and so forth. We require *symmetry* about the z axis such that

$$\left. \frac{\partial \Phi_i}{\partial r} \right|_{r=0} = 0 \quad i = 1, 5 \tag{F.3}$$

We also require *finite* solutions in the appropriate limits, that is

$$\Phi_i(r,z) \quad \text{finite for} \quad r=0 \quad \text{and} \quad r \to \infty \quad i=1,5 \tag{F.4}$$

$$\Phi_1(r,z) \quad \text{finite for } z \to +\infty$$
$$\Phi_5(r,z) \quad \text{finite for } z \to -\infty \tag{F.5}$$

The conditions (F.5) are required since the upper and lower media are semi-infinite. We further require that the potential in the lower layer approach the potential due to a point source in a homogenous medium, that is

$$\Phi_5\big|_{\substack{r \to 0 \\ z \to 0}} \to \frac{I}{4\pi\sigma_5\sqrt{r^2+z^2}} \tag{F.6}$$

Within each of the five layers, σ_i is constant so we seek solutions of Laplace's equation

$$\nabla^2\Phi_i = 0 \quad i=1,5 \tag{F.7}$$

The usual separated solution to (F.7) yields

$$\Phi(r,z) = (ae^{+kz} + be^{-kz})[cJ_0(kr) + dN_0(kr)] \tag{F.8}$$

Here, (a,b,c,d) are arbitrary constants, $J_0(kr)$ and $N_0(kr)$ are zero-order Bessel functions of the first and second kinds, respectively, and k is the separation constant. The Bessel functions of the second kind are infinite at $r=0$, thus boundary condition (F.4) forces us to choose $d=0$. This choice occurs in all similar problems in cylindrical coordinates when the cylinder axis ($r=0$) occurs inside the medium. However, when problems involving the Laplacian operator are solved in the cylindrical shell $r_1 < r < r_2$, both Bessel functions are retained and boundary conditions must be specified at the inner surface $r = r_1$. The calculation of external fields due to cylindrical fibers provides one biological example. A physical example is that of heat transfer in a heated toilet paper holder in an Alaskan outhouse, a problem chosen more to bedevil engineering students than to prevent frostbite.

Due to the linearity of Laplace's equation, we may add up (or integrate) solutions associated with different arbitrary constants. Thus, using (F.4) and (F.8) solutions in each layer are expressed in the form

$$\Phi_1 = \int_0^\infty A_1(k)J_0(kr)e^{-kz}dk \tag{F.9}$$

$$\Phi_2 = \int_0^\infty A_2(k)J_0(kr)e^{-kz}dk + \int_0^\infty B_2(k)J_0(kr)e^{+kz}dk \qquad (F.10)$$

$$\Phi_3 = \int_0^\infty A_3(k)J_0(kr)e^{-kz}dk + \int_0^\infty B_3(k)J_0(kr)e^{+kz}dk \qquad (F.11)$$

$$\Phi_4 = \int_0^\infty A_4(k)J_0(kr)e^{-kz}dk + \int_0^\infty B_4(k)J_0(kr)e^{+kz}dk \qquad (F.12)$$

$$\Phi_5 = \frac{1}{4\pi\sigma_5}\int_0^\infty J_0(kr)e^{-kz}dk + \int_0^\infty B_5(k)J_0(kr)e^{+kz}dk \qquad (F.13)$$

The integral at the near right side of (F.13) was chosen to satisfy (F.6), that is, use was made of the identity

$$\frac{1}{\sqrt{r^2+z^2}} \equiv \int_0^\infty J_0(kr)e^{-k|z|}dk \qquad (F.14)$$

The above formal solutions are expressed in terms of eight unknown parameters, $A_1(k)$ through $A_4(k)$ and $B_2(k)$ through $B_5(k)$. We make use of the derivative of the zero order Bessel function

$$\frac{\partial J_0(kr)}{\partial r} = -kJ_1(kr) \qquad (F.15)$$

There are eight interface boundary conditions (F.1) and (F.2) so that we may obtain the eight parameters in terms of the various conductivities σ_i, interface separations h_i and current source I. The solution is outlined here for the special case when the uppermost medium is a perfect insulator ($\sigma_1 = 0$), which is of most interest in EEG. By applying boundary conditions at the $(1,2)$ interface, we obtain

$$\left(\frac{\partial\Phi_1}{\partial r}\right)_{z=h_1} = \left(\frac{\partial\Phi_2}{\partial r}\right)_{z=h_1} \quad \text{or} \quad -A_1(k) = -A_2(k) - B_2(k)e^{2kh_1} \qquad (F.16)$$

$$\left(\frac{\partial\Phi_2}{\partial z}\right)_{z=h_1} = 0 \quad \text{or} \quad -A_2(k) + B_2(k)e^{2kh_1} = 0 \qquad (F.17)$$

Applying boundary conditions at the $(2,3)$ and $(3,4)$ interfaces yields (for $i=2$ and 3)

$$\left(\frac{\partial\Phi_i}{\partial r}\right)_{z=h_i} = \left(\frac{\partial\Phi_{i+1}}{\partial r}\right)_{z=h_i} \quad \text{or}$$

$$-A_i(k) - B_i(k)e^{2kh_i} = -A_{i+1}(k) - B_{i+1}(k)e^{2kh_i} \qquad (F.18)$$

$$\sigma_i \left(\frac{\partial \Phi_i}{\partial z} \right)_{z=h_i} = \sigma_{i+1} \left(\frac{\partial \Phi_{i+1}}{\partial z} \right)_{z=h_i} \quad \text{or}$$

$$\sigma_i \left[-A_i(k) + B_i(k)e^{2kh_i} \right] = \sigma_{i+1} \left[-A_{i+1}(k) + B_{i+1}(k)e^{2kh_i} \right] \tag{F.19}$$

The boundary conditions at the lowest $(4, 5)$ interface are

$$\left(\frac{\partial \Phi_4}{\partial r} \right)_{z=h_4} = \left(\frac{\partial \Phi_5}{\partial r} \right)_{z=h_4} \quad \text{or}$$

$$-A_4(k) - B_4(k)e^{2kh_4} = -\frac{I}{4\pi\sigma_5} - B_5(k)e^{2kh_4} \tag{F.20}$$

$$\sigma_4 \left(\frac{\partial \Phi_4}{\partial z} \right)_{z=h_4} = \sigma_5 \left(\frac{\partial \Phi_5}{\partial z} \right)_{z=h_4} \quad \text{or}$$

$$\sigma_4 \left[-A_4(k) + B_4(k)e^{2kh_4} \right] = \sigma_5 \left[-\frac{I}{4\pi\sigma_5} + B_5(k)e^{2kh_4} \right] \tag{F.21}$$

(F.16) through (F.21) include eight linearly independent equations for the eight unknown coefficients $A_1(k)$ through $A_4(k)$ and $B_2(k)$ through $B_5(k)$. These equations were solved manually by brute force and a solution provided in the first edition of this book. With modern software, especially Mathematica (Wolfram Research, Inc.), finding the algebraic solution is trivial, but requires several pages to print out. Since any application of this solution is likely to be carried out within Mathematica, we omit the printed version here.

Given the algebraic solutions, it is then a simple matter to calculate the eight parameters for a range of k if k_{max} is large enough such that the integrals $\int_0^\infty \dots dk$ may be approximated by integrals $\int_0^{k_{max}} \dots dk$. The solution outlined here reduces to the following proper limiting cases.

- *Two-layered medium*
  (i) $h_1 = h_2 = h_3 = h_4 =$ distance of source below single interface, or
  (ii) $\sigma_2 = \sigma_3 = \sigma_4 = \sigma_5 =$ conductivity of lower medium

- *Three-layered medium* (Zhadin 1969)
  (iii) $h_1 = h_2 = h_3$
  (iv) $h_2 = h_3 = h_4$
  (v) $\sigma_2 = \sigma_3 = \sigma_4$
  (vi) $\sigma_3 = \sigma_4 = \sigma_5$

Due to the linearity of Poisson's equation, the potential due to any combination of sources and sinks located in layer five (including a dipole) may be obtained by adding up the contributions from each monopolar source, given by the analysis above.

References

Stefanesco S and Schlumberger CM, 1930, *J. de Physique* 1: 132.

Zhadin MN, 1969, Mechanisms of origin of synchronization of the biopotentials of the cerebral cortex: I. model of independent sources. *Biophysics* (Russian) 14: 734–743.

APPENDIX G

Radial Dipole and Dipole Layer Inside the 4-Sphere Model

Here we outline the method of calculating the potentials inside head models composed an inner sphere surrounded by concentric spherical shells with each having a different conductivity (see fig. 6.5). The source is either a single dipole that is oriented radial to the surfaces or a dipole layer composed of many radial dipoles located at equal radii in the innermost sphere.

These s-sphere models are used throughout the book, usually with four spherical regions (an inner sphere and three spherical shells) representing brain, cerebrospinal fluid (CSF), skull, and scalp or with three spherical regions by excluding the CSF layer. We refer to these models as the *n-sphere model*, *4-sphere model*, and *3-sphere model* in the text. Although the 4-sphere model is far from perfect, it provides an excellent means to estimate the consequences of many experimental designs, including reference electrode effects and distortion of coherence estimates by volume conduction. Such applications are discussed throughout this book.

1 Methods for a Single Radial Dipole in s Spheres

We consider solutions for radially oriented dipoles, which simplifies the mathematics due to azimuthal (ϕ) symmetry. In this case, the solutions to Laplace's equation

$$\nabla^2 \Phi = 0 \qquad (G.1.1)$$

for the potential Φ depend only on the two spherical coordinates r and θ and the formal solution can be expressed in each sphere as (Jackson 1976)

$$\Phi_L(r,\theta) = \sum_{n=0}^{\infty} [A_n r^n + B_n r^{-(n+1)}] P_n(\cos\theta) \qquad (G.1.2)$$

The functions $P_n(\cos\theta)$ are the Legendre polynomials of order n, which are described in appendix I. The coefficients A_n and B_n depend on the sources and boundary conditions of continuous tangential electric field (or continuous potential) and radial current flow at the interface between spheres. In addition, we require the solution to be finite at $r=0$ and as $r \to \infty$. The former condition requires that $B_n = 0$ in the innermost sphere and the latter condition requires that $A_n = 0$ in the infinite medium surrounding the outer surface (air).

The innermost sphere, with conductivity σ_1, contains a dipole source at radius r_z on the polar axis ($\theta = 0$) with current I and pole separation d_z. The potential at any location in this sphere is a solution to Poisson's equation:

$$\nabla^2\Phi = \frac{I}{4\pi\sigma_1} \delta(\cos\theta - 1)\left[\delta\left(r - r_z - \frac{d_z}{2}\right) - \delta\left(r - r_z + \frac{d_z}{2}\right)\right] \qquad (G.1.3)$$

The product of delta functions on the right-hand side locates the two poles of the dipole with radial orientation. A solution to (G.1.1) for Φ in an inhomogeneous medium is the sum of the solution to (G.1.3) for a dipole in a homogeneous medium Φ_H and the formal solution to Laplace's equation Φ_L as given in (G.1.2).

In order to compute the homogeneous potential due to the dipole source, we begin by noting that the potential due to a monopolar source in a homogeneous medium of conductivity σ_1 is

$$\Phi = \frac{I}{4\pi\sigma_1 R} \qquad (G.1.4)$$

where R is the distance from the source to the field point. The distance R can be expanded as a series of Legendre polynomials

$$\frac{1}{R} \equiv \sum_{n=0}^{\infty} \frac{r_z^n}{r^{n+1}} P_n(\cos\theta) \quad r > r_z \qquad (G.1.5)$$

where r_z and r are the radial coordinates of the source and field point, respectively, and θ is the angular separation between the two locations. The potential due to a dipole of pole separation d_z at radius r_z in a homogeneous medium can then be expressed as sum of the potential due to two monopolar sources:

$$\Phi_H = \frac{I}{4\pi\sigma_1} \sum_{n=0}^{\infty} \left[\frac{(r_z + d_z/2)^n}{r^{n+1}} - \frac{(r_z - d_z/2)^n}{r^{n+1}}\right] P_n(\cos\theta) \qquad (G.1.6)$$

Note that

$$\left(r_z + \frac{d}{2}\right)^n = r_z^n\left(1 + \frac{d}{2r_z}\right)^n \cong r_z^n\left(1 + \frac{nd}{2r_z} + \cdots\right) \qquad \text{(G.1.7)}$$

Since $d \ll r_z$ higher order terms in the expansion can be dropped. Substituting this approximation into (G.1.6) yields

$$\Phi_H \cong \frac{Id_z}{4\pi\sigma_1 r_z^2} \sum_{n=1}^{\infty} \left(\frac{r_z}{r}\right)^{n+1} nP_n(\cos\theta) \qquad r > r_z \qquad \text{(G.1.8)}$$

Note that terms corresponding to $n = 0$ cancel consistent with current conservation in the case of a dipole source.

The potential in the innermost sphere Φ^1 can then be written as

$$\Phi^1(r) = \Phi_H + \Phi_L = \frac{Id_z}{4\pi\sigma_1 r_z^2} \sum_{n=1}^{\infty} \left[A_n^1\left(\frac{r}{r_1}\right)^n + \left(\frac{r_z}{r}\right)^{n+1}\right] nP_n(\cos\theta) \qquad r_z < r \le r_1$$

$$\text{(G.1.9)}$$

Here r_1 is the radius of the innermost sphere. In each of the other spherical shells, $s = 2, 3 \ldots n$, the potential Φ^s follows from the formal solution to Laplace's equation given in (G.1.2)

$$\Phi^s = \frac{Id}{4\pi\sigma_1 r_z^2} \sum_{n=1}^{\infty} \left[A_n^s\left(\frac{r}{r_s}\right)^n + B_n^s\left(\frac{r_s}{r}\right)^{n+1}\right] nP_n(\cos\theta) \qquad r_{s-1} \le r \le r_s$$

$$\text{(G.1.10)}$$

The unknown coefficients in each spherical shell are determined from boundary conditions of continuous potentials

$$\Phi^{s-1}\big|_{r=r_s} = \Phi^s\big|_{r=r_s} \qquad \text{(G.1.11)}$$

and continuous radial current density

$$\sigma_{s-1}\frac{\partial\Phi^{s-1}}{\partial r}\bigg|_{r=r_s} = \sigma_s\frac{\partial\Phi^s}{\partial r}\bigg|_{r=r_s} \qquad \text{(G.1.12)}$$

at the $s - 1$ interfaces between s spheres. At the outermost shell $s = n$ of an n-sphere model, the surrounding medium (air) has a conductivity of zero, so that radial current density at the outer surface must be zero:

$$\sigma_n\frac{\partial\Phi^n}{\partial r}\bigg|_{r=r_n} = 0 \qquad \text{(G.1.13)}$$

Equations (G.1.11), (G.1.12), and (G.1.13) yield $2s - 1$ equations that are solved for an equal number of unknown coefficients.

2 Solution for the 4-Sphere Model (Srinivasan et al. 1998)

The 4-sphere model consists of brain ($s = 1$), CSF ($s = 2$), skull ($s = 3$), and scalp ($s = 4$). For convenience we introduce the notation $r_{ij} = r_i/r_j$ and $\sigma_{ij} = \sigma_i/\sigma_j$ to indicate radii and conductivity ratios. In addition, we define the quantities

$$V_n = \frac{\sigma_{34}\dfrac{n+1}{n} - \dfrac{r_{34}^n - r_{43}^{n+1}}{\dfrac{n+1}{n}r_{34}^n + r_{43}^{n+1}}}{\sigma_{34} + \dfrac{r_{34}^n - r_{43}^{n+1}}{\dfrac{n+1}{n}r_{34}^n + r_{43}^{n+1}}} \tag{G.2.1}$$

$$Y_n = \frac{\sigma_{23}\dfrac{n}{n+1} - r_{23}^n\dfrac{\dfrac{n}{n+1} - V_n r_{32}^{n+1}}{r_{23}^n + V_n r_{32}^{n+1}}}{\sigma_{23} + \dfrac{r_{23}^n\dfrac{n}{n+1} - V_n r_{32}^{n+1}}{r_{23}^n + V_n r_{32}^{n+1}}} \tag{G.2.2}$$

$$Z_n = \frac{r_{12}^n - \dfrac{n+1}{n}Y_n r_{21}^{n+1}}{r_{12}^n + Y_n r_{21}^{n+1}} \tag{G.2.3}$$

The model coefficients are

$$A_n^1 = \frac{r_{z1}^{n+1}\left[Z_n + \sigma_{12}\left(\dfrac{n+1}{n}\right)\right]}{(\sigma_{12} - Z_n)} \tag{G.2.4}$$

$$A_n^2 = \frac{A_n^1 + r_{z1}^{n+1}}{Y_n r_{21}^{n+1} + r_{12}^n} \tag{G.2.5}$$

$$B_n^2 = A_n^2 Y_n \tag{G.2.6}$$

$$A_n^3 = \frac{A_n^2 + B_n^2}{r_{23}^n + V_n r_{32}^{n+1}} \tag{G.2.7}$$

$$B_n^3 = A_n^3 V_n \tag{G.2.8}$$

$$A_n^4 = \frac{A_n^3 + B_n^3}{\frac{n+1}{n} r_{34}^n + r_{43}^{n+1}} \tag{G.2.9}$$

$$B_n^4 = A_n^4 \frac{n}{n+1} \tag{G.2.10}$$

The potential on the scalp surface due to a radial dipole on the polar axis of the coordinate system $(\theta = 0)$ is

$$\Phi^4(r_4, \theta) = \frac{Id}{4\pi\sigma_1 r_z^2} \sum_{n=1}^{\infty} (A_n^4 + B_n^4) n P_n(\cos\theta) = \frac{Id}{4\pi\sigma_1 r_z^2} \sum_{n=1}^{\infty} H_n P_n(\cos\theta)$$

$$\tag{G.2.11}$$

The coefficients H_n depend on the model parameters and the radial position of the source r_z. The potential on the surface of the brain sphere is given by (G.1.9) evaluated at $r = r_1$.

3 Dipole Layers

Equation (6.2.11) can be used for radial dipoles at arbitrary locations by computing the angular separation θ between source and scalp locations. As discussed throughout this book, a dipole layer of synchronous aligned dipole sources is a more realistic source geometry for EEG than a single dipole. In any case, the single dipole is merely a special case of the dipole layer when its size is much smaller than distance to the scalp surface. Here we provide the formula for the potential due to a dipole layer located at radius r_z in the form a spherical cap of width θ_z centered on the z axis.

The potential due to a dipole located at (r', θ', ϕ') can also be expressed by using the addition theorem for spherical harmonics to expand (6.2.11):

$$\Phi^4(\theta, \phi) = \frac{Id}{4\pi\sigma_1(r')^2} \sum_{n=1}^{\infty} \frac{4\pi}{2n+1} H_n(r') \sum_{m=-n}^{n} Y_{nm}(\theta, \phi) \cdot Y_{nm}^*(\theta', \phi') \tag{G.3.1}$$

The spherical harmonics $Y_{nm}(\theta, \phi)$ are discussed in appendix I. Equation (G.3.1) can be expressed in terms of the potential V_0 across a dipole layer of size A to obtain the normalized potential due to a small element of active surface area $\Delta A'$ at location (r', θ', ϕ'):

$$\frac{\Phi^4}{V_0} = \sum_{n=1}^{\infty} \frac{H_n(r')}{2n+1} \sum_{m=-n}^{n} Y_{nm}(\theta, \phi) Y_{nm}^*(\theta', \phi') \Delta A' \tag{G.3.2}$$

For a spherical cap, centered on the z axis and of extent θ_z, integration of (G.3.2) over the area of the cap yields the following expression for the normalized potential:

$$\frac{\Phi^4}{V_0} = \frac{1}{2} \sum_{n=1}^{\infty} \frac{H_n(r')}{2n+1} [P_{n-1}(\cos\theta_z) - P_{n+1}(\cos\theta_z)] P_n(\cos\theta) \qquad \text{(G.3.3)}$$

4 Approximation to the 4-Sphere Model

The surface potential generated by a single radial dipole in the 4-sphere model is expressed as an infinite sum over Legendre polynomials (G.2.11). Surface potential distributions due to multiple sources may be obtained by simply adding the effects of individual sources. In order to make such simulations more widely available (especially in laboratories with minimal physics expertise), we present simple analytic expressions that closely match three solutions for surface potentials in the 4-sphere model. These solutions all assume a spherical head with 9.0 cm radius, brain conductivity equal to scalp conductivity ($\sigma_1 = \sigma_4$), and CSF conductivity equal to five times brain conductivity ($\sigma_2 = 5\sigma_1$). The radial locations of the dipole, brain surface, top of CSF, outer skull surface and scalp are fixed as $\{r_z, r_1, r_2, r_3, r_4\} = \{7.8, 7.9, 8.0, 8.5, 9.0\}$. The black dots in fig. G.1 represent the potential on the scalp surface as a function of the angle θ (degrees) measured from the dipole axis as calculated from (G.2.11). Each degree corresponds to a scalp surface distance of 0.157 cm; the horizontal axis spans $50°$ or 7.86 cm on the outer surface. The solid lines are simple fits to these solutions, given below for brain-to-skull conductivity ratios $\sigma_1/\sigma_3 = 20, 40, 80$.

The equations used to fit the genuine solutions on $0° < \theta < 50°$ are

$$\frac{\Phi_{20}}{\Phi_0} = 34.1 \exp[-0.15\theta] + 1.29 - 0.123\theta + 0.00164\theta^2 \qquad \text{(G.4.1)}$$

$$\frac{\Phi_{40}}{\Phi_0} = 27.4 \exp[-0.10\theta] - 5.49 + 0.203\theta - 0.00234\theta^2 \qquad \text{(G.4.2)}$$

$$\frac{\Phi_{80}}{\Phi_0} = 13.4 \exp[-0.10\theta] - 0.155 - 0.0135\theta \qquad \text{(G.4.3)}$$

We emphasize that these functional forms are largely arbitrary; many other combinations might be used and even more accurate fits obtained. The fits on the dipole axis ($\theta = 0$) are rather poor, but this inaccuracy has minimal practical consequences. A scalp electrode and conductive gel covers an angular range of $2°$ or $3°$, such electrode records the potential averaged over this region. *One warning is appropriate for any reader that might*

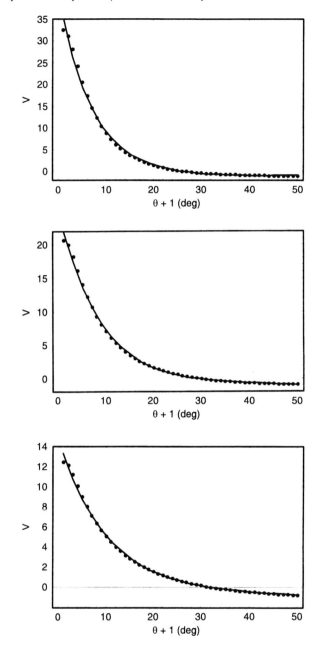

Figure G-1 Comparison of 4-sphere solutions (G.2.11) (dots) to approximate fits given by (G.4.1)–(G.4.3) (solid lines) for outer surface potential due to a radial dipole (parameters given in text). Normalized potential is plotted versus surface angle from dipole axis (degrees). Brain-to-skull conductivity ratios = 20, 40, and 80, plots top to bottom.

attempt to be too creative: do not attempt to estimate surface Laplacians by taking derivatives of these curve fit functions! Rather, one may use these simple functions to simulate scalp potentials due to an arbitrary number of dipoles at fixed depth ($r_z = 7.8$ cm), either as single time slices or as time series.

The potentials (G.4.1)–(G.4.3) are normalized with respect to the potential that would be generated in an infinite medium of conductivity σ by a dipole at distance $R = r_4$ (radius of scalp surface), that is

$$\Phi_0 = \frac{Id}{4\pi\sigma R^2} \tag{G.4.4}$$

As an example, consider a current of 1 μA passing between poles separated by $d = 1$ mm in a cortical-like medium of resistivity $\eta = 1/\sigma = 300$ Ω cm. If such dipole were placed at the location of the center of the spheres (but in an infinite, homogeneous and isotropic medium), the potential at the location of the outer surface would be

$$\Phi_0 = 0.0295 \ \mu V \tag{G.4.5}$$

The potentials directly above dipoles close to the scalp are larger by factors of 12 to 35 in the examples of fig. G.1, yielding scalp surface potentials in roughly the 0.1 to 0.4 μV range. Multiple synchronous dipoles that form a dipole layer will, of course, produce much large potentials due to linear superposition.

APPENDIX H

Tangential Dipole Inside
Concentric Spherical Shells

1 Tangential Dipole in Homogeneous Sphere

In order to calculate potentials generated by a tangential dipole in head models consisting of concentric spherical shells, we first require the solution for the case of a single homogeneous sphere in terms of a spherical harmonic expansion. The following derivation is rather cumbersome, but has the advantage of illustrating several subtle issues in mathematical physics. The potential $\Phi(r, \theta, \phi)$ in a homogeneous, isotropic conducting sphere of conductivity σ due to (point) monopolar current sources of strength $+I$ located at (r_1, θ_1, ϕ_2) and $-I$ located at (r_1, θ_1, ϕ_1) is a solution of Poisson's equation (4.12):

$$\nabla^2\Phi = \frac{-I}{\sigma r^2}\delta(r - r_1)\delta(\cos\theta - \cos\theta_1)[\delta(\phi - \phi_2) - \delta(\phi - \phi_1)] \quad \text{(H.1.1)}$$

Figure C-1 (appendix C) shows the appropriate spherical coordinates. When the monopoles are close together, they form a dipole. In contrast to the (mathematically) equivalent electrostatics problem involving charges in a dielectric, we require a balance of sources and sinks because of the physical requirement of current conservation. To find the solution to (H.1.1), note the expression for the Laplacian of $\Phi(r, \theta, \phi)$ in spherical coordinates

$$\nabla^2\Phi = \frac{1}{r^2}\frac{\partial}{\partial r}\left(r^2\frac{\partial\Phi}{\partial r}\right) + \nabla_S^2\Phi \quad \text{(H.1.2)}$$

where the surface Laplacian is given by

$$\nabla_S^2 \Phi = \frac{1}{r^2} \left[\frac{1}{\sin\theta} \frac{\partial}{\partial\theta} \left(\sin\theta \frac{\partial\Phi}{\partial\theta} \right) + \frac{1}{\sin^2\theta} \frac{\partial^2\Phi}{\partial\phi^2} \right] \tag{H.1.3}$$

The spherical harmonic functions $Y_{nm}(\theta, \phi)$ have the property (Jackson 1975)

$$\nabla_S^2 Y_{nm}(\theta, \phi) = -\frac{n(n+1)Y_{nm}(\theta, \phi)}{r^2} \tag{H.1.4}$$

Any well-behaved function $h(\theta, \phi)$ may be expanded in the generalized Fourier series (spherical harmonic expansion):

$$h(\theta, \phi) = \sum_{n=0}^{\infty} \sum_{m=-n}^{n} A_{nm} Y_{nm}(\theta, \phi) \tag{H.1.5}$$

The expansion coefficients follow directly from the orthogonal property of the spherical harmonic functions and are given by the surface integral

$$A_{nm} = \iint_S h(\theta, \phi) Y_{nm}^*(\theta, \phi) d\Omega \tag{H.1.6}$$

Thus, we expand the angular function on the right-hand side of (H.1.1), that is

$$\delta(\cos\theta - \cos\theta_1)[\delta(\phi - \phi_2) - \delta(\phi - \phi_1)] = \sum_{n=0}^{\infty} \sum_{m=-n}^{n} A_{nm} Y_{nm}(\theta, \phi) \tag{H.1.7}$$

$$A_{nm} = Y_{nm}^*(\theta_1, \phi_2) - Y_{nm}^*(\theta_1, \phi_1) \tag{H.1.8}$$

Note that the spherical harmonics are defined in terms of the associated Legendre functions by (Jackson 1975)

$$Y_{nm}(\theta, \phi) \equiv \sqrt{\frac{(2n+1)(n-m)!}{4\pi(n+m)!}} P_n^m(\cos\theta) e^{jm\phi} \tag{H.1.9}$$

The associated Legendre functions are defined in terms of the Legendre polynomials

$$P_n^m(x) = (-1)^m (1-x^2)^{m/2} \frac{d^m}{dx^m} P_n(x) \tag{H.1.10}$$

Suppose we place the two monopoles close together in the y-z plane such that θ_1 is small and $(\phi_1, \phi_2) = (-\pi/2, +\pi/2)$. These sources create a dipole with axis directed in the positive y-direction (see fig. C-1). Note that the

$P_n(x)$ are polynomials with powers ranging from x^0 to x^n. With $x \to \cos\theta_1$, the term in front of the derivative is $(\sin\theta_1)^m$. Thus, if we expand the coefficients $A_{nm}(\theta_1)$ in (H.1.8) in a Taylor series about $\theta_1 = 0$, the only first-order contributions in θ_1 occur for $m = \pm 1$. (This step is easier using Mathematica). For the case $(\phi_1, \phi_2) = (-\pi/2, +\pi/2)$, we expand the coefficients A_{n1} about $\theta_1 = 0$ to obtain

$$A_{n1} = \frac{j}{2\sqrt{\pi}}\sqrt{n(n+1)(2n+1)}\theta_1 + \vartheta(\theta_1^3)$$

$$A_{n,-1} = A_{n1}$$

$$A_{nm} = \vartheta(\theta_1^3) \quad m = \pm 3, 5, 7 \dots$$

$$A_{nm} = 0 \quad m = \pm 0, 2, 4, \dots \tag{H.1.11}$$

The last result in (H.1.11) occurs because A_{nm} is proportional to $\sin(m\pi/2)$. The double sum in (H.1.7) may be reduced to a single sum using (H.1.10), (H.1.11), and the following relation:

$$Y_{n,-m}(\theta, \phi) = (-1)^m Y_{nm}^*(\theta, \phi) \tag{H.1.12}$$

thereby reducing the double sum in (H.1.7) to

$$\sum_{n=0}^{\infty}\sum_{m=-n}^{n} A_{nm}Y_{nm}(\theta, \phi) \cong \sum_{n=1}^{\infty}[A_{n1}Y_{n1}(\theta, \phi) + A_{n,-1}Y_{n,-1}(\theta, \phi)]$$

$$= \frac{j2\sin\phi}{\sqrt{4\pi}}\sum_{n=1}^{\infty}A_{n1}\sqrt{\frac{(2n+1)(n-1)!}{(n+1)!}}P_n^1(\cos\theta)$$

$$= \frac{-\theta_1\sin\phi}{2\pi}\sum_{n=1}^{\infty}(2n+1)P_n^1(\cos 0) \tag{H.1.13}$$

We seek a solution to Poisson's equation of the form

$$\Phi(r, \theta, \phi) = \sum_{n=0}^{\infty}\sum_{m=-n}^{n} g_{nm}(r)Y_{nm}(\theta, \phi) \tag{H.1.14}$$

Substitute (H.1.14) into (H.1.1), make use of (H.1.4) and (H.1.12), and equate terms with $m = \pm 1$, that is

$$\sum_{n=0}^{\infty}\left[\frac{d}{dr}\left(r^2\frac{dg_{n1}}{dr}\right) - n(n+1)g_{n1}\right]P_n^1(\cos\theta)$$

$$= \frac{I\theta_1}{2\pi\sigma}\delta(r - r_1)\sum_{n=1}^{\infty}(2n+1)P_n^1(\cos\theta) \tag{H.1.15}$$

From (H.1.15) obtain an ordinary differential equation for the radial functions $g_{n1}(r)$:

$$\frac{d}{dr}\left(r^2 \frac{dg_{n1}}{dr}\right) - n(n+1)g_{n1} = \frac{I\theta_1(2n+1)}{2\pi\sigma}\delta(r - r_1) \qquad (\text{H.1.16})$$

Because of the equation discontinuity at $r = r_1$, we seek separate solutions to the homogeneous version of (H.1.16) in two regions, that is

$$g_{n1}^a(r) = a_n r^n + b_n r^{-(n+1)} \qquad r < r_1 \qquad (\text{H.1.17})$$

$$g_{n1}^d(r) = c_n r^n + d_n r^{-(n+1)} \qquad r > r_1 \qquad (\text{H.1.18})$$

In order to find relations between the coefficients in (H.1.17) and (H.1.18), we apply boundary conditions at the surface $r = r_1$; however, the presence of the delta function makes this procedure a little tricky in this case. Application of continuous tangential electric field (4.8) to (H.1.16) and (H.1.17) is identical to forcing a continuous potential across the boundary. However, the presence of the dipole source on the boundary means that the normal derivative of potential is discontinuous even though conductivity is constant, thus (4.7) does not apply at $r = r_1$. With this in mind, boundary conditions are applied as follows:

(i) $g_{n+1}^a(0)$ is finite, thus $b_n = 0$
(ii) Solution continuous $g_{n1}^a(r_1) = g_{n1}^d(r_1)$, thus $a_n r_1^n = c_n r_1^n + d_n r_1^{-(n+1)}$
(iii) Derivative discontinuous at $r = r1$ as shown by (H.1.19)

$$\int_{r_1-\varepsilon}^{r_1+\varepsilon} \left[\frac{d}{dr}\left(r^2 \frac{dg_{n1}}{dr}\right) - n(n+1)g_{n1}\right] dr = K_n \int_{r_1-\varepsilon}^{r_1+\varepsilon} \delta(r - r_1) dr \qquad (\text{H.1.19})$$

For a dipole with pole separation d, located at radial location r_1, the angular separation of the poles is $\theta_1 = d/2r_1$. The terms K_n are defined by (H.1.15), that is

$$K_n = \frac{Id(2n+1)}{4\pi\sigma r_1} \qquad (\text{H.1.20})$$

Relation (H.1.19) then yields

$$n r_1^{2n+1}(c_n - a_n) - (n+1)d_n = K_n r_1^n \qquad (\text{H.1.21})$$

Combine (H.1.21) with (ii) to obtain

$$d_n = \frac{-K_n r_1^n}{2n+1} = \frac{-Id r_1^{n-1}}{4\pi\sigma} \qquad (\text{H.1.22})$$

From (H.11.14), (H.11.15), and (H.11.18):

$$\Phi(r, \theta, \phi) = \sin\phi \sum_{n=0}^{\infty} \left(c_n r^n + \frac{d_n}{r^{n+1}} \right) P_n^1(\cos\theta) \tag{H.1.23}$$

where the d_n are given by (H.1.22) and the c_n are determined by the boundary condition on the surface of the outer sphere $r = R$. Consider first the case of a dipole located at the origin ($r_1 \to 0$). A finite solution then requires that $d_0 = 0$. The constant term involving c_0 may be subtracted from (H.1.23) without loss of generality since only potential gradients have physical meaning. We can generally drop the $n = 0$ terms in (H.1.14) for all problems in which current is conserved inside the volume conductor (in contrast to the mathematically equivalent electrostatics problem involving charges). Apply boundary condition (4.9) at the surface $r = R$ indicating that all current is confined inside to obtain

$$c_n = \frac{n+1}{nR^{2n+1}} d_n \tag{H.1.24}$$

Thus, the potential due to a y-directed tangential dipole in a homogeneous sphere is

$$\Phi(r, \theta, \phi) = \frac{-Id \sin\phi}{4\pi\sigma r^2}$$
$$\times \sum_{n=1}^{\infty} \left[\frac{n+1}{n} \left(\frac{r}{R} \right)^{n+2} + \left(\frac{R}{r} \right)^{n-1} \right] \left(\frac{r_1}{R} \right)^{n-1} P_n^1(\cos\theta) \tag{H.1.25}$$

We can check (H.1.25) against the expression for a radial dipole in the center of the sphere by letting $r_1 \to 0$. In this limit only the $n = 1$ term in the sum is nonzero. The associated Legendre function follows from (H.1.10), $P_1^1(\cos\theta) = -\sin(\theta)$, so the potential due to a central dipole with axis along the y axis is given by

$$\Phi(r, \theta, \phi) = \frac{Id \sin\theta \sin\phi}{4\pi\sigma r^2} \left[1 + 2\left(\frac{r}{R} \right)^3 \right] \tag{H.1.26}$$

Compare (H.1.26) to the expression (6.18), noting that the dipole axis is aligned with the z axis. Replace θ in (6.18) by the angle γ between the y axis and the vector $\mathbf{r}$:

$$\Phi(r, \theta, \phi) = \frac{Id \cos\gamma}{4\pi\sigma r^2} \left[1 + 2\left(\frac{r}{R} \right)^3 \right] \tag{H.1.27}$$

Use (C.5) and fig. C-1 to find that $\cos\gamma = \sin\theta \, \sin\phi$ so that (H.1.26) and (H.1.27) agree. In the case of an infinite homogeneous medium ($R \rightarrow \infty$), both equations reduce to the basic dipole formula (1.7).

2 Tangential Dipole in Concentric Spheres Model

Equation (H.1.23) may be used as the basis for constructing solutions for head models consisting of concentric spherical shells. Formal solutions are constructed for each shell and interface boundary conditions used to find the unknown coefficients in the expansions as described in appendix G. Rewrite (H.1.23) using (H.1.22) and the notation of appendix G:

$$\Phi(r, \theta, \phi) = - \sin\phi \sum_{n=1}^{\infty} \left[C_n^1 r^n + \frac{Id}{4\pi\sigma_1 r_4^2} \left(\frac{r_4}{r_z}\right)^2 \left(\frac{r_z}{r}\right)^{n+1} \right] P_n^1(\cos\theta) \quad \text{(H.2.1)}$$

Here we have changed the label for the radial location of the dipole r_1 to r_z to be consistent with appendix G. In order to simplify the following expressions, we normalize potentials with respect to

$$\Phi_0 = \frac{Id}{4\pi\sigma_1 r_4^2} \quad \text{(G.4.4)}$$

and normalize sphere radii with respect to outer sphere radius by setting $r_4 = 1$. CSF and skull conductivities (σ_2, σ_3) are normalized with respect to brain (or scalp) conductivity by setting $\sigma_1 = \sigma_4 = 1$. Thus, (H.2.1) expressed in nondimensional form is

$$\frac{\Phi(r, \theta, \phi)}{\Phi_0} = - \sin\phi \sum_{n=1}^{\infty} \left[C_n^1 r^n + r_z^{-2} \left(\frac{r_z}{r}\right)^{n+1} \right] P_n^1(\cos\theta) \quad \text{(H.2.2)}$$

where all radii are interpreted as fractions of r_4 in the following expressions. Solutions are expressed formally in each of the four shells as in appendix G. For example, the potential in the outer (scalp) shell is given by

$$\frac{\Phi(r, \theta, \phi)}{\Phi_0} = - \sin\phi \sum_{n=1}^{\infty} \left[C_n^4 r^n + D_n^4 r^{-(n+1)} \right] P_n^1(\cos\theta) \quad \text{(H.2.3)}$$

Applying the usual boundary condition of zero current flux normal to the scalp at the scalp surface ($r = 1$) allows the coefficients D_n^4 to be expressed in terms of the C_n^4 so that (H.2.3) simplifies to

$$\frac{\Phi(1, \theta, \phi)}{\Phi_0} = - \sin\phi \sum_{n=1}^{\infty} C_n^4 \left(\frac{2n + 1}{n + 1}\right) P_n^1(\cos\theta) \quad \text{(H.2.4)}$$

Here the coefficients are given in terms of ratios of radii and conductivities by

$$C_n^4 = \frac{-(n+1)(2n+1)^3 \sigma_2 \sigma_3 r_z^{n-1}(r_2 r_3)^{n+1}}{GF + J[H + n^2(K_1 + K_2 + K_3) + n(P_1 + P_2)]} \tag{H.2.5}$$

where individual terms in the denominator are defined as follows:

$$G = n(2n+1)r_2^{n+1}r_3^{-n}\left(n + r_3^{2n+1} + nr_3^{2n+1}\right) \tag{H.2.6}$$

$$\begin{aligned} F = \sigma_3 \Big[&(\sigma_2 - 1)(\sigma_2 + n\sigma_2 + n\sigma_3)r_1^{2n+1} \\ &+ (\sigma_3 - \sigma_2)(n + \sigma_2 + n\sigma_2)r_2^{2n+1} \Big] \end{aligned} \tag{H.2.7}$$

$$J = -n(r_2 r_3)^{-n}\left[1 + (\sigma_3 - 1)r_3^{2n+1} + n\left(1 + \sigma_3 + (\sigma_3 - 1)r_3^{2n+1}\right)\right] \tag{H.2.8}$$

$$H = \sigma_2 \sigma_3 (r_2 r_3)^{2n+1} \tag{H.2.9}$$

$$K_1 = (\sigma_2 - 1)(\sigma_3 - \sigma_2)(r_1 r_3)^{2n} \tag{H.2.10}$$

$$K_2 = (\sigma_2 + 1)(\sigma_3 - \sigma_2)r_2^{4n+2} \tag{H.2.11}$$

$$K_3 = r_2(\sigma_2 + \sigma_3)\left[(\sigma_2 - 1)r_1(r_1 r_2)^{2n} + (\sigma_2 + 1)r_3(r_2 r_3)^{2n}\right] \tag{H.2.12}$$

$$P_1 = r_1(\sigma_2 - 1)\left[\sigma_2 r_2(r_1 r_2)^{2n} + (\sigma_3 - \sigma_2)r_3(r_1 r_3)^{2n}\right] \tag{H.2.13}$$

$$P_2 = r_2\left[\sigma_2(\sigma_3 - \sigma_2)r_2^{4n+1} + (\sigma_2^2 + \sigma_3 + 2\sigma_2\sigma_3)r_3(r_2 r_3)^{2n}\right] \tag{H.2.14}$$

3 Checking the Solution

Four-shell solutions in appendices G and H may be checked by considering several limiting cases, for example

(i) Applying either of the limits $\{\sigma_2 \to 1, \sigma_3 \to 1\}$ or $\{r_1 \to 1, r_2 \to 1, r_3 \to 1\}$ to (H.2.5) yields the solution for a dipole in a homogeneous sphere

$$C_n^4 = \frac{n+1}{n}r_z^{n-1} \tag{H.3.1}$$

Substitution of (H.3.1) into (H.2.4) yields

$$\frac{\Phi(1,\theta,\phi)}{\Phi_0} = -\sin\phi \sum_{n=1}^{\infty} \left(\frac{2n+1}{n}\right) r_z^{n-1} P_n^1(\cos\theta) \qquad \text{(H.3.2)}$$

Equation (H.3.2) agrees with (H.1.25) for the case of potentials on the sphere's surface $r = R = 1$.

(ii) Other checks involve comparing different ways to obtain three-shell solutions

$$\left|C_n^4\right|_{\sigma_2=1} = \left|C_n^4\right|_{r_1=r_2} = \left|C_n^4\right|_{\sigma_3=\sigma_2} = \left|C_n^4\right|_{r_2=r_3} \qquad \text{(H.3.3)}$$

(iii) The tangential dipole solution may be checked against the radial dipole solution in appendix G when the dipole is located at the center of the shells. For example, the tangential coefficient for a two-shell model may be obtained from (H.2.5) in the limit $\{r_2 \to 1, r_3 \to 1, n \to 1\}$ yielding

$$C_1^4 = \frac{-6}{1 + 2\sigma_2 - 2(\sigma_2 - 1)r_1^3} \qquad \text{(H.3.4)}$$

Equation (H.3.4) agrees with the two-shell radial dipole solution when angles are interpreted to account for rotation of the dipole axis by $90°$ as in the example of the one-sphere case (H.1.27).

APPENDIX I

Spherical Harmonics

The spherical harmonics $Y_{nm}(\theta, \phi)$ are a set of orthogonal basis functions on a spherical surface. Any physical quantity measured on a spherical surface can be expressed as a sum of spherical harmonics, in the same general manner that a time series can be expressed as a sum of its Fourier components. For instance, the potential $\Phi(\theta, \phi)$ on a spherical surface can be expanded as an infinite series of spherical harmonics as

$$\Phi(\theta, \phi) = \sum_{n=0}^{\infty} \sum_{m=-n}^{n} F_{nm} Y_{nm}(\theta, \phi) \tag{I.1}$$

The double sum is over the spherical harmonic *degree* n and *order* m, and F_{nm} are the spherical harmonic expansion coefficients. The terms are ordered such that larger n and m indicate higher spatial frequencies.

The derivation of the spherical harmonics can be found in almost any mathematical physics book as the solution to the eigenvalue problem for Laplace's equation in spherical coordinates, including the classic text by Morse and Feshbach (1953). The spherical harmonics are written as

$$Y_{nm}(\theta, \phi) = \sqrt{\frac{2n+1}{4\pi} \frac{(n-|m|)!}{(n+|m|)!}} e^{jm\phi} P_n^{|m|}(\cos \theta) \tag{I.2}$$

where the $P_n^{|m|}(\cos \theta)$ are the associate Legendre functions. If $m = 0$, the associated Legendre functions reduce to the Legendre polynomials $P_n(\cos \theta)$. The Legendre polynomials are the basis functions for solutions to concentric spheres models of the head when the solution is independent of the angle ϕ as in the case of the radial dipole treated in appendix G.

The spherical harmonics have a number of applications in this book. We have used spherical harmonics to estimate the transfer function between cortical source distribution and scalp potential or surface Laplacian in chapters 6 and 8. In chapter 9 we make use of spherical harmonic expansions to define a spatial white noise source distribution to estimate the effects of volume conduction on coherence between potentials recorded at different locations on the sphere. In chapter 10 we have calculated spherical harmonic expansions of EEG data to plot their spatial spectra. The global dynamic theory outlined in chapter 11 may be applied to any geometry; when applied to a spherical shell, the solutions are expressed in spherical harmonic expansions.

To improve readers' intuition about these basis functions, we have made plots of spherical harmonics using the real-valued formulation of the spherical harmonics:

$$Y_{nm}(\theta, \phi) = \sqrt{\frac{2n+1}{4\pi} \frac{(n-|m|)!}{(n+|m|)!}} \cos m\phi P_n^{|m|}(\cos \theta) \quad m \geq 0 \qquad (\text{I.3})$$

$$Y_{nm}(\theta, \phi) = \sqrt{\frac{2n+1}{4\pi} \frac{(n-|m|)!}{(n+|m|)!}} \sin m\phi P_n^{|m|}(\cos \theta) \quad m < 0 \qquad (\text{I.4})$$

Figure I-1a shows the spherical harmonics of degree $n = 1$ and orders $m = -1, 0$, and 1. In each case, one hemisphere is positive and the other half is negative. Figure I-2b shows the spherical harmonics for $n = 2$ and $m = -2, 1, -1, 0, 1, 2$. Note that the only difference between spherical harmonics with positive and negative m (of the same degree n) is a rotation

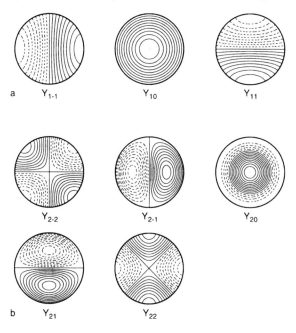

Figure I-1 (a) Spherical harmonics of degree $n = 1$ and order $m = -1, 0, +1$. (b) Spherical harmonics of degree $n = 1$ and order $m = -2, -1, 0, +1, +2$.

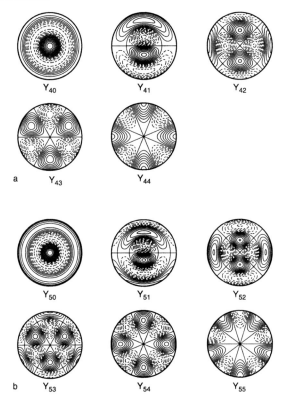

Figure I-2 (a) Spherical harmonics of degree $n = 4$ and order $m = 0$, 1, 2, 3, 4. (b) Spherical harmonics of degree $n = 5$ and order $m = 0$, 1, 2, 3, 4, 5.

of 90°, consistent with a change of basis from $\sin \phi$ to $\cos \phi$. Also, the spherical harmonics of order 0 (the Legendre polynomials) are always spherically symmetric. Figure I-2 shows the spherical harmonics of degree $n = 4$ and $n = 5$ and nonnegative m. As the degree n increases the spatial frequency increases in the same way as frequency increases in a Fourier series expansion. Latitudinal wavenumber or spatial frequency k on a spherical surface is approximately related to the (n, m) indices and sphere radius R by

$$k \approx \frac{n}{(2\pi)R} \tag{I.5}$$

Here spatial frequency is expressed in cycles/cm if the factor (2π) is included in the denominator or cm^{-1} if not included. This approximation is valid only if the index m is small. The index n is a measure of the "overall spatial frequency" of each spherical harmonic Y_{nm} involving a sort of "average" over the m indices.

Reference

Morse PM and Feshbach H, 1953, *Methods of Theoretical Physics, Parts I and II*, New York: McGraw-Hill.

APPENDIX J

The Spline Laplacian

The surface Laplacian algorithm is the principal high-resolution EEG method described in this book. Our discussion applies specifically to the New Orleans spline Laplacian algorithm developed by the Brain Physics Group at Tulane University. Various versions were created and tested during the period 1988–1995. The first version relied on planar interpolation based on the seminal work of the French group (Perrin et al. 1987). The discussion here refers to our latest version which involves interpolation of potential in three-dimensional space. While other spline Laplacian algorithms (often based on interpolation on a sphere) are expected to behave similarly, we only have experience with the New Orleans algorithm. However, the Melbourne dura imaging algorithm (Cadusch et al. 1992), which is based on a 3-sphere model, uses interpolation on a sphere. As shown in chapters 8 and 10, the New Orleans spline Laplacian and Melbourne dura imaging algorithms yield nearly identical spatial patterns when applied to either EEG or simulated data obtained with the 4-sphere head model, provided dense sampling is used (say more than 100 electrodes or simulated surface samples). With 131 electrodes, the electrode-by-electrode correlation coefficients comparing the two methods are typically in the 0.95 range. With 64 electrodes, the correlation coefficients fall to roughly the 0.80 to 0.85 range.

Chapter 8 presents the theoretical background to the surface Laplacian, while chapters 9 and 10 consider the use and interpretation of the surface Laplacian with experimental EEG data. The surface Laplacian is the second spatial derivative of the scalp potential estimated along a geometric model of the scalp surface that passes through the electrode positions. To estimate the surface Laplacian, a continuous potential distribution $\Phi(x, y, z)$ is estimated on the model scalp surface from the discrete potentials $V_i(t)$ measured at $i = 1, 2, \ldots n$ electrode sites distributed (mostly) over the upper surface of the head.

Splines are apparently the best choice for the interpolation of EEG data. The surface Laplacian is estimated by applying the surface Laplacian operator to the interpolating function. This spline Laplacian estimate is then evaluated at each electrode position and any other location on the model scalp. Spherical splines (Perrin et al. 1989; Wahba 1981) have come into widespread use to interpolate potentials for topographic maps, by approximating the electrode positions on a sphere. In section 1 of this appendix we provide the formulation of a three-dimensional spline interpolation that can be used to interpolate potentials on any surface that approximates head shape and passes through each electrode. The details of calculation of the surface Laplacian on a spherical surface are given in section 3. Better approximations to the scalp surface, perhaps derived from MRI can be used with this algorithm potentially to improve Laplacian estimates. For instance, the New Orleans spline Laplacian algorithm has been applied to prolate spheroidal and ellipsoidal surfaces (Law et al. 1993). MATLAB (Natick, MA) programs to implement the interpolation on arbitrary surfaces and the surface Laplacian on a spherical surface are provided here and may be downloaded from www.electricfieldsofthebrain.com.

1 Three-Dimensional Spline Interpolation

A three-dimensional interpolation of the potential distribution Φ at one instant in time can be obtained from n electrode sites using a third-order thin-plate spline, defined as

$$\Phi(x, y, z) = \sum_{i=1}^{n} p_i K(x - x_i, y - y_i, z - z_i) + Q(x, y, z) \tag{J.1.1}$$

where (x_i, y_i, z_i) are the Cartesian coordinates of the electrode sites and (x, y, z) are the interpolated coordinates. Table J-1 provides a set of coordinates for 111 electrodes on a spherical surface. In principle, these coordinates can be on an arbitrary surface that passes through the electrode positions. While we have tested this spline on prolate spheroidal and ellipsoidal surfaces, our experience with spherical surfaces is much more extensive. That is, we have run several thousand simulations over 12 years using different noise levels, sampling densities, and head models (for forward solutions) with the spline algorithm based on a spherical surface. This version appears to be quite robust.

The basis function $P(x, y, z)$ is the sum in (J.1.1) whose terms are

$$K(x, y, z, x_i, y_i, z_i, w) = K(x - x_i, y - y_i, z - z_i, w)$$
$$= (d^2 + w^2)^2 \log(d^2 + w^2) \tag{J.1.2}$$

Table J-1 The positions of 111 electrodes on a sphere of radius 9.2 cm are listed

Electrode	X (cm)	Y (cm)	Z (cm)
1	−5.014	6.901	−3.447
2	−6.691	6.240	−0.962
3	−7.511	5.066	1.598
4	−7.864	2.556	4.033
5	−6.687	1.422	6.156
6	−4.875	0.000	7.802
7	−2.052	−1.490	8.843
8	−6.901	5.014	−3.447
9	−8.224	4.011	−0.962
10	−8.664	2.649	1.598
11	−8.269	0.000	4.033
12	−6.687	−1.422	6.156
13	−3.944	−2.865	7.802
14	−8.112	2.636	−3.447
15	−9.037	1.431	−0.962
16	−9.060	0.000	1.598
17	−9.037	−1.431	−0.962
18	−8.617	−2.800	1.598
19	−7.864	−2.556	4.033
20	−5.531	−4.018	6.156
21	−8.112	−2.636	−3.447
22	−8.224	−4.011	−0.962
23	−7.330	−5.326	1.598
24	−6.689	−4.861	4.033
25	−6.901	−5.014	−3.447
26	−6.691	−6.240	−0.962
27	−5.578	−7.139	1.598
28	−4.861	−6.689	4.033
29	−3.418	−5.921	6.156
30	−1.507	−.637	7.802
31	0.784	−2.411	8.843
32	−5.014	−6.901	−3.447
33	−4.574	−7.924	−0.962
34	−3.247	−8.459	1.598
35	−2.556	−7.864	4.033
36	−0.715	−6.800	6.156
37	1.507	−4.637	7.802
38	−2.636	−8.112	−3.447
39	−2.059	−8.915	−0.962
40	−0.632	−9.038	1.598
41	0.000	−8.269	4.033
42	2.113	−6.502	6.156
43	0.000	−8.530	−3.447
44	0.638	−9.127	−0.962
45	2.038	−8.828	1.598
46	2.556	−7.864	4.033
47	3.279	−8.542	−0.962
48	4.530	−7.847	1.598

Continued

Electrode	X (cm)	Y (cm)	Z (cm)
49	4.861	−6.689	4.033
50	4.574	−5.080	6.156
51	3.944	−2.865	7.802
52	2.536	0.000	8.843
53	3.317	−7.859	−3.447
54	5.633	−7.210	−0.962
55	6.626	−6.179	1.598
56	6.689	−4.861	4.033
57	6.246	−2.780	6.156
58	4.875	0.000	7.802
59	5.565	−6.465	−3.447
60	7.495	−5.248	−0.962
61	8.143	−3.971	1.598
62	7.864	−2.556	4.033
63	6.837	0.000	6.156
64	7.234	−4.520	−3.447
65	8.702	−2.827	−0.962
66	8.949	−1.418	1.598
67	8.269	0.000	4.033
68	8.401	−1.481	−3.447
69	9.150	0.000	−0.962
70	8.949	1.418	1.598
71	7.864	2.556	4.033
72	6.246	2.780	6.156
73	3.944	2.865	7.802
74	0.784	2.411	8.843
75	8.401	1.481	−3.447
76	8.702	2.827	−0.962
77	8.143	3.971	1.598
78	6.689	4.861	4.033
79	4.574	5.080	6.156
80	1.507	4.637	7.802
81	7.312	4.394	−3.447
82	7.495	5.248	−0.962
83	6.626	6.179	1.598
84	4.861	6.689	4.033
85	2.113	6.502	6.156
86	5.597	6.438	−3.447
87	5.633	7.210	−0.962
88	4.530	7.847	1.598
89	2.556	7.864	4.033
90	3.333	7.852	−3.447
91	3.279	8.542	−0.962
92	2.038	8.828	1.598
93	0.000	8.269	4.033
94	−0.715	6.800	6.156
95	−1.507	4.637	7.802
96	−2.052	1.490	8.843
97	0.638	9.127	−0.962

Continued

Table J-1 Continued

Electrode	X (cm)	Y (cm)	Z (cm)
98	−0.632	9.038	1.598
99	−2.556	7.864	4.033
100	−3.418	5.921	6.156
101	−3.944	2.865	7.802
102	0.000	8.530	−3.447
103	−2.059	8.915	−0.962
104	−3.247	8.459	1.598
105	−4.861	6.689	4.033
106	−5.531	4.018	6.156
107	−2.636	8.112	−3.447
108	−4.574	7.924	−0.962
109	−5.578	7.139	1.598
110	−6.689	4.861	4.033
111	0.000	0.000	9.200

where

$$d^2 = (x - x_i)^2 + (y - y_i)^2 + (z - z_i)^2 \qquad (J.1.3)$$

is the square of the distance between the interpolation point (x, y, z) and the electrode position (x_i, y_i, z_i). The osculating function

$$Q(x, y, z) = q_1 + q_2 x + q_3 y + q_4 x^2 + q_5 xy + q_6 y^2 + q_7 z + q_8 zx + q_9 zy + q_{10} z^2 \qquad (J.1.4)$$

serves to smooth the resulting distribution. The interpolation has been tested on spherical and ellipsoidal surfaces (Srinivasan et al. 1996; Law et al. 1993). The p and q coefficients depend on the potential as given in section 2 of this appendix.

The parameter w serves to distribute the loading of the interpolation function over a finite-sized region of width w rather than a point. In EEG applications it makes sense to select $w = 0.5 - 1.0$ cm, which is the typical effective electrode size (with gel or other conductive contact material). The simulations shown here and examples in chapters 8−10 were calculated with $w = 1.0$ cm. The effect of loading the spline over a finite size region is to spatially low-pass filter the potential distribution reducing the contribution of very high spatial frequencies, thereby tending to minimize spatial aliasing (Srinivasan et al. 1996).

2 Method of Solution for the Three-Dimensional Spline

Law et al. (1993) published a general method of solution for the three dimensional spline of different orders. We present here the solution for the third-order spline, which is implemented as MATLAB code.

Let $\mathbf{Q} = [q_1, q_2 \ldots, q_{10}]^T$, $\mathbf{P} = [p_1, p_2, \ldots, p_n]^T$ represent the spline coefficients in (J.1.1) and (J.1.4) and $\mathbf{V} = [V_1, V_2, \ldots, V_n]^T$ are the scalp potentials (with any reference strategy) at n electrode positions. $\mathbf{Q}$ and $\mathbf{P}$ are solutions to the following matrix equations (Law et al. 1993):

$$\mathbf{KP} + \mathbf{EQ} = \mathbf{V} \tag{J.2.1}$$

$$\mathbf{E}^T\mathbf{P} = \mathbf{0} \tag{J.2.2}$$

where $\mathbf{K}$ is a square matrix whose elements are

$$K_{ij} = K(x_i, y_i, z_i, x_j, y_j, z_j) \quad i, j = 1, 2 \ldots n \tag{J.2.3}$$

and $\mathbf{E}$ is an n by 10 matrix whose n rows are given by

$$E_i = \begin{bmatrix} 1 & x_i & y_i & x_i^2 & x_i y_i & y_i^2 & z_i & z_i x_i & z_i y_i & z_i^2 \end{bmatrix} \tag{J.2.4}$$

The solutions to (J.2.1) and (J.2.2) for the coefficient vectors $\mathbf{P}$ and $\mathbf{Q}$ are

$$\mathbf{Q} = [\mathbf{E}^T\mathbf{K}^{-1}\mathbf{E}]^{-1} \mathbf{E}^T\mathbf{K}^{-1}\mathbf{V} \tag{J.2.5}$$

$$\mathbf{P} = \mathbf{K}^{-1}\mathbf{V} - \mathbf{K}^{-1}\mathbf{EQ} \tag{J.2.6}$$

The solution is presented in two MATLAB functions in figs. J-1 and J-2. The algorithm is separated into two separate functions for computational speed. The first function calculates quantities that only depend on the electrode positions. The second function solves the matrix equations (J.2.5) and (J.2.6). The use of these two functions to interpolate potentials at another set of coordinates (x_s, y_s, z_s) is given as a function in fig. J-3.

3 Solution for the Surface Laplacian on a Spherical Surface

The surface Laplacian operator is defined as

$$\nabla_S^2 \Phi = \frac{1}{h_1 h_2 h_3} \left[\frac{\partial}{\partial u_2} \left(\frac{h_3 h_1}{h_2} \frac{\partial}{\partial u_2} \Phi \right) + \frac{\partial}{\partial u_3} \left(\frac{h_2 h_1}{h_3} \frac{\partial}{\partial u_3} \Phi \right) \right] \tag{J.3.1}$$

where u_2 and u_3 are two spatial coordinates on the surface, and the coordinate u_1 is normal to the surface. Spheres, prolate spheroids, and ellipsoids can all be described in their own coordinate systems using two surface coordinates with the other coordinate held fixed. The parameters h_1, h_2, and h_3 are scale factors that depend on the coordinate system (Morse and Feshbach 1953). Law et al. (1993) provide the details for

```
function [k,kinv,a,ainv,e] = k_and_e(w,x,y,z)
%This function calculates the matrix K, its inverse, the matrix E, and intermediate matrix A
%and its inverse in the three-dimensional spline fit. All of these matrices only depend on the
%electrode positions an parameter w. The outputs are passed to mateqs to solve for P and Q
%INPUTS
%x,y,z   : electrode positions
%w       : smoothing parameter
%
%OUTPUTS
%k,kinv : The matrix K (I.2.3)
%e       : The matrix E (I.2.4)
%a,ainv : intermediate quantities used by mateqs

n = size(x,2);     % number of electrodes
for i=1:n           % Add noise to electrode coordinates that are exactly zero.
        if x(i) == 0
                x(i) = 0.001;
        end;
        if y(i) == 0
                y(i) = 0.001;
        end;
        if z(i) == 0
                z(i) = 0.001;
        end;
end;
for i=1:n           % Calculate matrix K
        for j=1:n
                s = x(i) − x(j);
                t = y(i) − y(j);
                r = z(i) − z(j);
                str = s.^2 + t.^2 + r.^2;
                k(i,j) = ((str + w.^2). ^2)*log(str + w.^2);
        end;
end;
kinv = inv(k);     % Invert K
for i=1:n           % Calculate matrix E
e(i,1) = 1;
e(i,2) = x(i);
e(i,3) = y(i);
e(i,4) = x(i).^2;
e(i,5) = x(i)*y(i);
e(i,6) = y(i).^2;
e(i,7) = z(i);
e(i,8) = z(i)*x(i);
e(i,9) = z(i)*y(i);
e(i,10) = z(i).^2;
end;
ke = kinv*e;       % Intermediate matrix A and its inverse
et = e';
a = et*ke;
ainv = inv(a);
```

Figure J-1 MATLAB program to calculate matrices **K**, **E**, **A**, **K**$^{-1}$, and **A**$^{-1}$.

```
function [p,q,error_check] = mateqs(v,k,kinv,a,ainv,e)
%Implements solution for P and Q. Requires variables calculated by k_and_e.m
%
%INPUTS
%v        : row vector of potential distribution at 1 time sample
%k,kinv,a,ainv,e        : all outputs from k_and_e.m
n = size(x,2); %number of electrodes
%SOLUTION FOR Q (I.2.4)
et = e';
kv = kinv*v';
ev = et*kv;
q = ainv*ev;
%SOLUTION FOR P (I.2.5)
eq = e*q;
keq = kinv*eq;
p = kv - keq;
%ERROR CHECK - SHOULD BE ZERO
kp = k*p;
verror = v' - (kp + eq);
etp = et*p;
error_check(1) = sum(verror);
error_check(2) = sum(etp);
```

Figure J-2 MATLAB program to calculate matrices **P** and **Q**.

```
function image_3d = interp_3d(w,xelec,yelec,zelec,xs,ys,zs,p,q)
%Interpolates the potentials at locations (xs,ys,zs) from the coefficients P and Q obtained
%from mateqs.
%INPUTS
%w        : smoothing parameter
%xelec,yelec,xelec        : row vectors of electrode position coordinates
%xs,ys,zs                : matrices of interpolation position coordinates
%p,q      : the coefficient vectors obtained from mateqs
%OUTPUT
%image_3d = interpolated values
n = size(xelec,2); % number of electrodes
ms = size(xs,1);
ns = size(xs,2);
image_3d = zeros(ms,ns);
qm = zeros(ms,ns);
qm = q(1) + q(2)*xs + q(3)*ys + q(4)*xs.^2 + q(5)*xs.*ys + q(6)*ys.^2 + q(7)*zs
+ q(8)*zs.*xs + q(9)*zs.*ys + q(10)*zs.^2;
sum = zeros(ms,ns);
s = zeros(ms,ns);
t = zeros(ms,ns);
r = zeros(ms,ns);
str = zeros(ms,ns);
for i=1:n
        s = xs - xelec(i)*ones(ms,ns);
        t = ys - yelec(i)*ones(ms,ns);
        r = zs - zelec(i)*ones(ms,ns);
        str = s.^2 + t.^2 + r.^2;
        sum = sum + p(i)*((str + w*ones(ms,ns).^2).^2).*log(str + w*ones(ms,ns).^2);
end;
image_3d = sum + qm; %output interpolated values
```

Figure J-3 MATLAB program to interpolate potentials on any surface using the 3-dimensional spline.

586

calculating surface Laplacians on prolate spheroidal and ellipsoidal surfaces. In spherical coordinates (θ, ϕ), the surface Laplacian is written as

$$\nabla_S^2 \Phi = \frac{1}{r^2 \sin \theta} \frac{\partial}{\partial \theta} \left(\sin \theta \frac{\partial}{\partial \theta} \Phi \right) + \frac{1}{r^2 \sin^2 \theta} \frac{\partial^2 \Phi}{\partial \phi^2} \qquad (\text{J.3.2})$$

Alternatively, the surface Laplacian can be calculated by first calculating the three-dimensional Laplacian:

$$\nabla^2 \Phi = \left[\frac{\partial^2}{\partial x^2} + \frac{\partial^2}{\partial y^2} + \frac{\partial^2}{\partial z^2} \right] \Phi \qquad (\text{J.3.3})$$

and then subtracting the radial Laplacian:

$$\nabla_S^2 \Phi = \nabla^2 \Phi - \frac{1}{r^2} \frac{\partial}{\partial r} \left(r^2 \frac{\partial}{\partial r} \Phi \right) \qquad (\text{J.3.4})$$

The surface Laplacian operator is applied to the interpolating function (J.1.1) to obtain the spline interpolation for the surface Laplacian. For computational speed and numerical stability, we have made use of the definition (J.3.2) to calculate the surface Laplacian of the osculating function $Q(x, y, z)$ and the definition (J.3.4) to calculate the surface Laplacian of the basis function $P(x, y, z)$. To calculate the surface Laplacian for a set of potential measurements $\mathbf{V}$ at locations (x, y, z), the spline interpolation coefficients $\mathbf{P}$ and $\mathbf{Q}$ are calculated using the functions given in figs. J-1 and J-2. Figure J-4 provides a function that uses these spline coefficients to evaluate the surface Laplacian at a set of positions on the sphere (x_s, y_s, z_s). Since the accuracy of the interpolation is best at the electrode locations, we normally evaluate the surface Laplacian at electrode locations.

Table J-2 provides two examples using potentials due to a single radial dipole source in a four concentric spheres model of the head. The 4-sphere model of the head is described in appendix G. The potentials were calculated at 111 simulated electrode sites whose (x, y, z) coordinates are given in table J-1. Head model parameters are spherical shell radii $(r_1, r_2, r_3, r_4) = (8, 8.1, 8.6, 9.2)$ cm and conductivity ratios are $(\sigma_{12}, \sigma_{13}, \sigma_{14}) = (0.2, 40, 1)$. The dipoles were placed directly under the vertex electrode (111). In example 1, the dipole is 4.2 cm below the scalp surface, while in example 2 the dipole is 2.2 cm below the scalp surface. Scalp potentials and analytic surface Laplacians were calculated at the 111 simulated electrode sites using the 4-sphere model. The spline Laplacian was calculated from the potentials at these sites using the functions in figs. J-1, J-2, and J-4. The spline Laplacian is very strongly correlated to the analytic surface Laplacian in both examples. Note that in EEG applications we are only interested in relative values of the spline Laplacian over the surface.

```
function v_lap = spherical_lap(w,x,y,z,xs,ys,zs,p,q)
%calculates Laplacian on spherical surface
%INPUTS
%w        : smoothing parameters
%x,y,z    : electrode position coordinates
%xs,ys,zs      : Laplacian position coordinates
%p,q           : Spline coefficients calculated using mateqs
%OUTPUT
%v_lap         : surface Laplacian at positions given by xs,ys,zs
w = w.^2;
n = size(x,2);
ns = size(xs,2);
[azs,els,rs] = cart2sph(xs,ys,zs);
els = (pi/2)*ones(size(els,1),size(els,2)) − els;
[az,el,r] = cart2sph(x,y,z);
el = (pi/2)*ones(size(el,1),size(el,2)) − el;
%calculate trig functions to keep things easier
st = sin(els);
ct = cos(els);
sp = sin(azs);
cp = cos (azs);
s2t = sin(2*els);
c2t = cos(2*els);
s2p = sin(2*azs);
c2p = cos(2*azs);
%surface Laplacian of osculating function Q(x,y,z)
uuxyz = 2*q(4) + 2*q(6) + 2*q(10) − (2*st.*(q(2)*cp + q(3)*sp)./rs + 2*q(7)*ct./rs ... %line contd
+ 6*(st.^2).*(q(4)*(cp.^2) + q(6)*(sp.^2) + q(5)*sp.*cp) + 6*st.*ct.*(q(8)*cp + q(9)*sp) + 6*q(10)*ct.^2);
smpp = zeros(size(st,1),size(st,2));
smtt = zeros(size(st,1),size(st,2));
smp = zeros(size(st,1),size(st,2));
smt = zeros(size(st,1),size(st,2));
ttcomp = zeros(size(st,1),size(st,2));
rrcomp = zeros(size(st,1),size(st,2));
%surface Laplacian of spline fiction P(x,y,z). The three dimensional Laplacian is
%calculated and then the second derivative in the radial direction is subtracted.
for j = 1:n
        a = r(j)*(st.*cp − sin(el(j))*cos(az(j))*ones(size(st,1),size(st,2)));
        b = r(j)*(st.*sp − sin(el(j))*sin(az(j))*ones(size(st,1),size(st,2)));
        c = r(j)*(ct − cos(el(j))*ones(size(st,1),size(st,2)));
        str = a.^2 + b.^2 + c.^2;
        strw = str + w*ones(size(st,1),size(st,2));
        comterm = 4*str./strw − ((str./strw).^2) + 2*log(strw);
        comterm2 = 2*(2*str.*log(strw) + (str.^2)./strw);
        tcomp = 3*compterm2 + 4*str.*comterm;
        dr = 2*(a.*st.*cp + b.*st.*sp + c.*ct);
        d2r2 = 2;
        rcomp = dr.*comterm2 + d2r2*r(j)*comterm2/2 + r(j)*(dr.^2).*comterm;
        ttcomp = ttcomp + p(j)*tcomp;
        rrcomp = rrcomp + p(j)*rcomp/r(j);
end;
v_lap = − (ttcomp + uuxyz − rrcomp)
```

Figure J-4 MATLAB program to calculate surface Laplacian on a sphere at electrode positions.

Table J-2 Examples of the spline Laplacian. Two examples due to a radial dipole source in a four concentric spheres model are presented

Electrode	Example 1			Example 2		
	Potential	Analytic Laplacian	Spline Laplacian	Potential	Analytic Laplacian	Spline Laplacian
1	−0.838	−0.017	−0.020	−0.819	−0.012	−0.023
2	−0.574	−0.020	−0.019	−0.639	−0.017	−0.018
3	−0.185	−0.023	−0.028	−0.349	−0.024	−0.060
4	0.384	−0.023	−0.019	0.125	−0.035	−0.005
5	1.193	−0.007	−0.009	0.922	−0.046	−0.071
6	2.273	0.059	0.055	2.302	−0.033	−0.015
7	3.446	0.239	0.237	4.694	0.298	0.189
8	−0.838	−0.017	−0.020	−0.819	−0.012	−0.026
9	−0.574	−0.020	−0.019	−0.639	−0.017	−0.018
10	−0.185	−0.023	−0.024	−0.349	−0.024	−0.029
11	0.384	−0.023	−0.021	0.125	−0.035	−0.018
12	1.193	−0.007	−0.009	0.922	−0.046	−0.072
13	2.273	0.059	0.061	2.302	−0.033	0.036
14	−0.838	−0.017	−0.020	−0.819	−0.012	−0.016
15	−0.574	−0.020	−0.020	−0.639	−0.017	−0.021
16	−0.185	−0.023	−0.025	−0.349	−0.024	−0.034
17	−0.574	−0.020	−0.019	−0.639	−0.017	−0.014
18	−0.185	−0.023	−0.024	−0.349	−0.024	−0.034
19	0.384	−0.023	−0.020	0.125	−0.035	−0.012
20	1.193	−0.007	−0.011	0.922	−0.046	−0.093
21	−0.838	−0.017	−0.019	−0.819	−0.012	0.008
22	−0.574	−0.020	−0.021	−0.639	−0.017	−0.025
23	−0.185	−0.023	−0.022	−0.349	−0.024	−0.019
24	0.384	−0.023	−0.022	0.125	−0.035	−0.028
25	−0.838	−0.017	−0.019	−0.819	−0.012	−0.003
26	−0.574	−0.020	−0.019	−0.639	−0.017	−0.007
27	−0.185	−0.023	−0.023	−0.349	−0.024	−0.020
28	0.384	−0.023	−0.023	0.125	−0.035	−0.031
29	1.193	−0.007	−0.008	0.922	−0.046	−0.069
30	2.273	0.059	0.056	2.302	−0.033	−0.014
31	3.446	0.239	0.240	4.694	0.298	0.212
32	−0.838	−0.017	−0.019	−0.819	−0.012	−0.001
33	−0.574	−0.020	−0.021	−0.639	−0.017	−0.019
34	−0.185	−0.023	−0.026	−0.349	−0.024	−0.044
35	0.384	−0.023	−0.020	0.125	−0.035	−0.014
36	1.193	−0.007	−0.010	0.922	−0.046	−0.084
37	2.273	0.059	0.055	2.302	−0.033	−0.004
38	−0.838	−0.017	−0.018	−0.819	−0.012	0.005
39	−0.574	−0.020	−0.016	−0.639	−0.017	0.017
40	−0.185	−0.023	−0.025	−0.349	−0.024	−0.035
41	0.384	−0.023	−0.020	0.125	−0.035	−0.013
42	1.193	−0.007	−0.010	0.922	−0.046	−0.087
43	−0.838	−0.017	−0.018	−0.819	−0.012	0.007
44	−0.574	−0.020	−0.020	−0.639	−0.017	−0.014
45	−0.185	−0.023	−0.026	−0.349	−0.024	−0.044
46	0.384	−0.023	−0.020	0.125	−0.035	−0.014

Continued

Table J-2 Continued

Electrode	Example 1			Example 2		
	Potential	Analytic Laplacian	Spline Laplacian	Potential	Analytic Laplacian	Spline Laplacian
47	−0.574	−0.020	−0.018	−0.639	−0.017	0.001
48	−0.185	−0.023	−0.020	−0.349	−0.024	0.000
49	0.384	−0.023	−0.025	0.125	0.035	−0.048
50	1.193	−0.007	−0.004	0.922	−0.046	−0.044
51	2.273	0.059	0.060	2.302	−0.033	0.013
52	3.446	0.239	0.233	4.694	0.298	0.160
53	−0.838	−0.017	−0.019	−0.819	−0.012	0.002
54	−0.574	−0.020	−0.023	−0.639	−0.017	−0.035
55	−0.185	−0.023	−0.022	−0.349	−0.024	−0.014
56	0.384	−0.023	−0.024	0.125	−0.035	−0.040
57	1.193	−0.007	−0.009	0.922	−0.046	−0.076
58	2.273	0.059	0.054	2.302	−0.033	−0.008
59	−0.838	−0.017	−0.018	−0.819	−0.012	0.006
60	0.574	−0.020	−0.016	−0.639	−0.017	0.015
61	−0.185	−0.023	−0.025	−0.349	−0.024	−0.034
62	0.384	−0.023	−0.019	0.125	−0.035	−0.003
63	1.193	−0.007	−0.007	0.922	−0.046	−0.060
64	−0.838	−0.017	−0.021	−0.819	−0.012	−0.016
65	−0.574	−0.020	−0.020	−0.639	−0.017	0.016
66	−0.185	−0.023	−0.024	−0.349	−0.024	−0.032
67	0.384	−0.023	−0.025	0.125	−0.035	−0.041
68	−0.838	−0.017	−0.018	−0.819	−0.012	−0.002
69	−0.574	−0.020	−0.020	−0.639	−0.017	−0.020
70	−0.185	−0.023	−0.024	−0.349	−0.024	−0.033
71	0.384	−0.023	−0.019	0.125	−0.035	−0.002
72	1.193	−0.007	−0.009	0.922	−0.046	−0.071
73	2.273	0.059	0.060	2.302	−0.033	0.020
74	3.446	0.239	0.241	4.694	0.298	0.219
75	−0.838	−0.017	0.020	−0.819	−0.012	−0.021
76	−0.574	−0.020	−0.020	−0.639	−0.017	−0.025
77	−0.185	−0.023	−0.025	−0.349	−0.024	−0.036
78	0.384	−0.023	−0.024	0.125	−0.035	−0.038
79	1.193	−0.007	−0.004	0.922	−0.046	−0.031
80	2.273	0.059	0.055	2.302	−0.033	0.006
81	−0.838	−0.017	−0.020	−0.819	−0.012	−0.022
82	−0.574	−0.020	−0.018	−0.639	−0.017	−0.007
83	−0.185	−0.023	−0.022	−0.349	−0.024	−0.017
84	0.384	−0.023	−0.025	0.125	−0.035	−0.044
85	1.193	−0.007	−0.011	0.922	−0.046	−0.082
86	−0.838	−0.017	−0.020	−0.819	−0.012	−0.027
87	−0.574	−0.020	−0.025	−0.639	−0.017	−0.056
88	−0.185	−0.023	−0.020	−0.349	−0.024	−0.005
89	0.384	−0.023	−0.019	0.125	−0.035	−0.003
90	−0.838	−0.017	−0.021	−0.819	−0.012	−0.033
91	−0.574	−0.020	−0.019	−0.639	−0.017	−0.019
92	−0.185	−0.023	−0.028	−0.349	−0.024	−0.056
93	0.384	−0.023	−0.022	0.125	−0.035	−0.021

Continued

Table J-2 Continued

Electrode	Example 1			Example 2		
	Potential	Analytic Laplacian	Spline Laplacian	Potential	Analytic Laplacian	Spline Laplacian
94	1.193	−0.007	−0.005	0.922	−0.046	−0.042
95	2.273	0.059	0.055	2.302	−0.033	−0.009
96	3.446	0.239	0.237	4.694	0.298	0.193
97	−0.574	−0.020	−0.022	−0.639	−0.017	−0.042
98	−0.185	−0.023	−0.021	−0.349	−0.024	−0.013
99	0.384	−0.023	−0.020	0.125	−0.035	−0.012
100	1.193	−0.007	−0.008	0.922	−0.046	−0.062
101	2.273	0.059	0.062	2.302	−0.033	0.048
102	−0.838	−0.017	−0.020	−0.819	−0.012	−0.031
103	−0.574	−0.020	−0.017	−0.639	−0.017	−0.006
104	−0.185	−0.023	−0.028	−0.349	−0.024	−0.056
105	0.384	−0.023	−0.022	0.125	−0.035	−0.023
106	1.193	−0.007	−0.011	0.922	−0.046	−0.086
107	−0.838	−0.017	−0.020	−0.819	−0.012	−0.030
108	−0.574	−0.020	−0.022	−0.639	−0.017	−0.036
109	−0.185	−0.023	−0.020	−0.349	−0.024	−0.007
110	0.384	−0.023	−0.020	0.125	−0.035	−0.007
111	4.033	0.403	0.425	7.050	2.381	2.390

The 4-sphere model parameters are radii $(r_1, r_2, r_3, r_4) = (8, 8.1, 8.6, 9.2)$ cm and conductivity ratios $(\sigma_{12}, \sigma_{13}, \sigma_{14}) = (0.2, 40, 1)$ of the spheres. The sources are a radial dipole under the vertex electrode (111), either 4.2 cm (example 1) or 2.2 cm (example 2) below the outer sphere (scalp). The first column is the electrode number, with locations on the sphere specified in table J-1.

References

Cadusch PJ, Breckon W, and Silberstein RB, 1992, Spherical splines and the interpolation, deblurring and transformation of topographic EEG data. *Brain Topography* 5: 59.

Law SK, Nunez PL, and Wijesinghe RS, 1993, High-resolution EEG using spline-generated surface Laplacians on spherical and ellipsoidal surfaces. *IEEE Transactions on Biomedical Engineering* 40: 145–152.

Morse PM and Feshbach H, 1953, *Methods of Theoretical Physics*, Parts I and II, New York: McGraw-Hill.

Perrin F, Bertrand O, and Pernier J, 1987, Scalp current density mapping: value and estimation from potential data. *IEEE Transactions on Biomedical Engineering*. 34: 283–388.

Perrin F, Pernier J, Bertrand O, and Echalier JF, 1989, Spherical splines for scalp potential and current density mapping. *Electroencephalography and Clinical Neurophysiology* 72: 184–187.

Srinivasan R, Nunez PL, Tucker DM, Silberstein RB, and Cadusch PJ, 1996, Spatial sampling and filtering of EEG with spline Laplacians to estimate cortical potentials. *Brain Topography* 8: 355–366.

Wahba G, 1981, Spline interpolation and smoothing on the sphere. *SIAM Journal on Scientific and Statistical Computing* 2: 5–16.

APPENDIX K

Impressed Currents and Cross-Scale Relations in Volume Conductors

1 Simple Interpretation of the "Impressed Current" in a Volume Conductor

Low-frequency current in a volume conductor satisfies

$$\nabla \cdot \mathbf{J} = 0 \tag{4.10}$$

In electrophysiology, it is useful to introduce a fictitious macroscopic current density $\mathbf{J}_S$ called the "impressed current" such that Ohm's law (3.15) is modified to read (Geselowitz 1967; Malmivuo and Plonsey 1995)

$$\mathbf{J} = \sigma \mathbf{E} + \mathbf{J}_S \tag{4.11}$$

Substitute (4.10) into (4.9) and make use of the definition of electric potential (3.4) to obtain

$$\nabla \cdot [\sigma(\mathbf{r})\nabla\Phi] = -s(\mathbf{r}, t) \tag{4.12}$$

where the volume source current is defined by

$$s(\mathbf{r}, t) \equiv -\nabla \cdot \mathbf{J}_S(\mathbf{r}, t) \tag{4.13}$$

A simple interpretation of the impressed current and source function makes use of fig. K-1. Imagine a spherical region of radius a that uniformly produces current in the radial direction with volume current

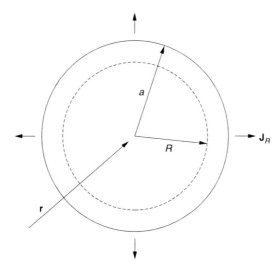

Figure K-1 Current source region with sources uniformly distributed over a sphere of radius a. Boundary surface is chosen at radius R.

density s_0 (say in units of $\mu A/mm^3$). The total current produced inside any inner sphere of radius $R < a$ (dashed line) is

$$I_R = \frac{4}{3}\pi R^3 s_0 \quad R < a \tag{K.1.1}$$

The surface current density J_R at the dashed surface R is then obtained by dividing by its surface area, that is

$$J_R = \frac{R s_0}{3} \quad R < a \tag{K.1.2}$$

Since the current is assumed to be exclusively radial, the general expression for divergence of a vector in spherical coordinates (A.5) yields

$$\nabla \cdot \mathbf{J}_R = \frac{1}{R^2}\frac{\partial}{\partial R}\left(R^2 J_R\right) = s_0 \quad R < a \tag{K.1.3}$$

Comparison of (K.1.3) with (4.13) above suggests that the function $s(\mathbf{r}, t)$ may be identified as a volume current source density for current generated at macroscopic location $\mathbf{r}$ provided that $\mathbf{J}_S$ is interpreted as $-\mathbf{J}_R$. The negative sign is due to the fact that the outward normal coordinates from the inner regions of fig. 4-7 point in the opposite direction to outward normal coordinates of the outer regions. This sign discrepancy could have been avoided by changing the original definition of impressed current (4.11) to $\mathbf{J} = \sigma\mathbf{E} - \mathbf{J}_S$; however, we retained the form (4.11) to be consistent with the historical definition of J_S. At locations outside the source region, current conservation yields

$$J_R = \frac{I_a \mathbf{a}_R}{4\pi R^2} = \frac{a^3 s_0 \mathbf{a}_R}{3R^2} \quad R > a \tag{K.1.4}$$

Here I_a is the total current produced inside the sphere of radius a and $\mathbf{a}_R$ is the unit vector in the radial direction. The general expression for the divergence of a vector in spherical coordinates (A.5) shows that

$$\nabla \cdot \mathbf{J}_R = 0 \quad R > a \tag{K.1.5}$$

Comparison of (K.1.2) with (K.1.4) shows that the current source density is continuous across the interface $R = a$, whereas comparison of (K.1.3) with (K.1.5) shows that the divergence is discontinuous at $R = a$. Thus, if we place the boundaries of our general volume conductor in fig. 4-7 just inside the source region boundaries, we may reasonably identify J_S as the negative source current density crossing these boundaries. However, if the boundary surface is chosen outside the source region ($R > a$), the connection between the fictitious J_S and the genuine J_R is lost. In this case we interpret J_S only as a construct to specify boundary conditions on the inner surfaces of fig. 4-7.

2 Interpretation of the Impressed Current Using Green's Theorem

With the help of Green's theorem, a convenient general form for the solution to Poisson's equation (4.12) inside a volume conductor of constant conductivity σ is given by (equation (1.42) of Jackson 1975) with the identification $\rho \to s/4\pi\sigma$

$$\Phi(\mathbf{r}) = \frac{1}{4\pi\sigma} \iiint_{\text{Volume}} s(\mathbf{r}_1) G(\mathbf{r}, \mathbf{r}_1) d^3 r_1 + \frac{1}{4\pi} \iint_{\text{Surface}} \left[G(\mathbf{r}, \mathbf{r}_1) \frac{\partial \Phi}{\partial u_1} - \Phi(\mathbf{r}_1) \frac{\partial G}{\partial u_1} \right] d^2 r_1$$

$$\tag{K.2.1}$$

Here $G(\mathbf{r}, \mathbf{r}_1)$ is the (scalar) Green's function for the volume conductor and the coordinate u_1 is the local outward normal coordinate of the closed surface of the volume conductor. A unique solution to Poisson's equation may be obtained if we specify either the potential (*Dirichlet boundary condition*) or its normal derivative (*Neumann boundary condition*) everywhere on the outer surface. Alternatively, we may specify potential on parts and normal derivative on other parts (*mixed boundary condition*). Consider the case where all current is confined to the volume in question.

In this case, the normal derivative of potential in (K.2.1) is zero on the outer surface. Furthermore, we may choose the Green's function such that (Jackson 1975, equation (1.45))

$$\frac{\partial G_N}{\partial u_1}(\mathbf{r}, \mathbf{r}_1) = -\frac{4\pi}{S_1} \quad \text{for } r_1 \text{ on } S_1 \tag{K.2.2}$$

where S_1 is the total surface area. In this case, the solution (K.2.1) reduces to

$$\Phi(\mathbf{r}) = \langle \Phi \rangle_{S1} + \frac{1}{4\pi\sigma} \iiint\limits_{\text{Volume}} s(\mathbf{r}_1) G_N(\mathbf{r}, \mathbf{r}_1) d^3 r_1 \tag{K.2.3}$$

The first term on the right-hand side is the potential averaged over the entire surface. If all currents are confined inside the volume, this average potential is zero. In cases where current can cross part of the chosen boundary of the volume (say the lower head or neck region), an integral involving the normal derivative of surface potential must be added to (K.2.3), as in Jackson (1975), equation (1.46).

3 Mesosource as Dipole Moment per Unit Volume in Electrophysiology

The mathematical formalism required for the transition from "microscopic" (synaptic scale) to mesoscopic (columnar scale) source functions in electrophysiology is based largely on the mathematical equivalence of two versions of Poisson's equation: the electric potential due to a charge distribution in a dielectric

$$\nabla \cdot [\varepsilon(\mathbf{r})\nabla\Phi(\mathbf{r}, t)] = -\rho(\mathbf{r}, t) \tag{4.14}$$

and the electric potential generated by multiple small-scale (synaptic or other) current sources in a conductive medium (the brain, heart, muscle, and so forth) given by (4.12), above. In either case, the solution for potential is expressed as a volume integral over the source region by (K.2.3). Generally, in neurophysiology, this "source region" may be any mass of neural tissue. In EEG applications, the entire neocortex may contribute to scalp potentials.

How can we make practical use of (K.2.3)? The surface density of synapses in neocortex is roughly $10^{14}/\text{mm}^2$ and the scalp electrode records potentials averaged over perhaps 10 cm^2, a space average over something like 10^{17} synaptic sources at cell membranes plus the return currents required for current conservation. Our answer is to make full use of a century of advances in classical physics by dozens of physicists, many who devoted entire careers to establishing connections between micro-scopic and macroscopic fields in dielectric media. A brief (mostly qualitative) outline of similar cross-scale connections applied in electro-physiology follows.

The first step is to express the volume integral in (K.2.3) in terms of subvolumes W at location $\mathbf{r}$ that are sufficiently large such that local current is conserved within the volumes (see fig. 4-12):

$$\iiint_{W} s(\mathbf{r}, \mathbf{w}, t)dW(\mathbf{w}) \cong 0 \qquad (4.27)$$

Here the coordinate $\mathbf{w}$ locates current sources within the volume W, for example, inside a millimeter-scale cortical column. Within such small volume W, the Green's function is essentially that of an infinite homo-geneous medium $|\mathbf{r} - \mathbf{r}_1|^{-1}$. Define the (vector) current dipole moment per unit volume at the mesoscale W, that is

$$\mathbf{P}(\mathbf{r}, t) = \frac{1}{W} \iiint_{W} \mathbf{w}s(\mathbf{r}, \mathbf{w}, t)dW(\mathbf{w}) \qquad (4.26)$$

If the mesoscopic volume W is taken at the millimeter scale (or smaller), scalp potentials at macroscopic (centimeter) scales receive negligible contributions from quadrupole and higher order terms resulting from the multipole expansion of the microscopic Green's function in (K.2.3). If, in addition, the monopole contribution is zero because of (4.27), scalp potential may be expressed in terms of an integral over the cortical mesosource function, that is, over contributions from all brain tissue

$$\langle \Phi(\mathbf{r}, t) \rangle = \iiint_{\text{Brain}} \mathbf{G}(\mathbf{r}, \mathbf{r}') \cdot \mathbf{P}(\mathbf{r}', t)dV(\mathbf{r}') \qquad (2.2)$$

Here the volume Green's function $\mathbf{G}(\mathbf{r}, \mathbf{r}')$ contains all macroscopic information about the volume conductor. The brackets around the poten-tial emphasize that this is a macroscopic potential to be recorded with centimeter-scale scalp electrodes. Most scalp EEG is believed to be gen-erated by cortical sources. In this case (2.2) may be conveniently replaced by a surface integral over the cortical mesosource function (essentially over cortical columns) involving the surface Green's function, that is

$$\langle \Phi(\mathbf{r}, t) \rangle = \iint_{S} \mathbf{G}_S(\mathbf{r}, \mathbf{r}') \cdot \mathbf{P}(\mathbf{r}', t)dS(\mathbf{r}') \qquad (4.39)$$

References

Geselowitz DB, 1967, On bioelectric potentials in an inhomogeneous volume conductor, *Biophysical Journal* 7: 1–11.

Jackson JD, 1975, *Classical Electrodynamics*, 2nd Edition, New York: Wiley.

Malmuvino J and Plonsey R, 1995, *Bioelectromagetism*, New York: Oxford University Press.

APPENDIX L

Outline of Neocortical Dynamic Global Theory

---

1 Brief Description

The label *global theory* is used here to indicate mathematical models in which action potential delays in the corticocortical fibers forming most of the white matter in humans provide the underlying timescale for the large-scale EEG dynamics. Periodic boundary conditions are generally essential to global theories because the cortical–white matter system of each hemisphere is topologically close to a spherical shell.

As used in this book, the label *local theory* indicates mathematical models of cortical or thalamocortical interactions for which corticocortical propagation delays are neglected. The underlying timescales in these theories are typically PSP (postsynaptic potential) rise and decay times due to membrane capacitive-resistive properties. Thalamocortical networks are also "local" from the viewpoint of a surface electrode, which cannot distinguish purely cortical from thalamocortical networks. These theories are also "local" in the sense of being independent of global boundary conditions.

A brief outline of the simplest version of the global theory follows in sections 2 and 3 of this appendix. More detail may be found in chapters 11 and 12 and the appendix of Nunez (1995) and in Nunez (2000a, b). These references also discuss methods to combine local and global theories. The global theory proposes equations for the three field variables:

$\Psi_e(\mathbf{r}, t)$ excitatory synaptic action density, or

$\delta\Psi_e(\mathbf{r}, t) \equiv \Psi(\mathbf{r}, t)$ modulation of excitatory synaptic action density

$\Psi_i(\mathbf{r}, t)$ inhibitory synaptic action density

$\Theta(\mathbf{r}, t)$ action potential density

The excitatory synaptic action density is the number of active excitatory synapses per unit area of cortical surface in the two-dimensional version of theory or number per unit length of a strip of cortex in the one-dimensional version. The modulation of cortical synaptic output $\delta\Psi_e(\mathbf{r}, t)$ due to modulation of action potential input $\delta\Theta(\mathbf{r}, t)$ about background is considered first. In the linear version of the theory, a dynamic transfer function (or its inverse, the dispersion function) is obtained. The dispersion relation is determined by the poles of the transfer function in the usual manner of linear systems analysis. A linear differential equation in the variable $\delta\Psi_e(\mathbf{r}, t) \equiv \Psi(\mathbf{r}, t)$ follows directly from the dispersion relation. Nonlinear versions of this equation are suggested based on plausible physiological conjectures, especially the postulate that instability is prevented in healthy brains by recruitment of additional inhibitory mechanisms (negative feedback) from thalamus, contiguous cortex (lateral inhibition), or both.

2 Derivation of a Nonlinear One-Dimensional Differential Equation for Excitatory Modulation of Synaptic Action

The excitatory synaptic action at cortical location $\mathbf{r}$ may be expressed in terms of an inner integral over the cortical surface and outer integral over distributed axon propagation speeds as

$$\delta\Psi_e(\mathbf{r}, t) = \delta\Psi_0(\mathbf{r}, t) + \int_0^\infty dv_1 \iint_{\text{Cortex}} \Re(\mathbf{r}, \mathbf{r}_1, v_1)\delta\Theta\left(\mathbf{r}_1, t - \frac{|\mathbf{r} - \mathbf{r}_1|}{v_1}\right)d^2r_1$$

(L.2.1)

The corticocortical and thalamocortical fibers are believed to be exclusively excitatory (or nearly so). Thus, (L.2.1) is based on the simple, noncontroversial idea that excitatory synaptic action at cortical location $\mathbf{r}$ is due to excitatory subcortical input $\delta\Psi_0(\mathbf{r}, t)$ plus excitatory action potential density $\delta\Theta(\mathbf{r}, t)$ integrated over the entire neocortex. The inner integrals in (L.2.1) are over cortical surface coordinates, but action potentials at location $\mathbf{r}_1$ produce synaptic activity at location $\mathbf{r}$ only after a delay that is assumed to be proportional to cortical separation distance and inversely proportional to axon speed v_1. Distances are defined on an equivalent smooth cortex as indicated in fig. 11-3. All the complications of white matter (corticocortical) fiber tracts (after smoothing) are included in the distribution function $\Re(\mathbf{r}, \mathbf{r}_1, v_1)$. The outer integral is over the generally distributed corticocortical propagation velocities v_1.

In the simplest one-dimensional version of the global theory (Nunez 1972, 1974), axons are assumed to run only in the anterior–posterior direction of each hemisphere (perhaps not such a bad assumption based on known anatomy). The corticocortical axons are parceled into M fiber systems with connection densities that fall off exponentially with separation $|x - x_1|$, that is

$$\Re(x, x_1, v_1) = \frac{1}{2} \sum_{m=1}^{M} \rho_m \lambda_m f_m(v_1) \exp[-\lambda_m |x - x_1|] \qquad (L.2.2)$$

where ρ_m is the number of excitatory synapses per m-system axon. Substitution of (L.2.2) into (L.2.1) and obtaining its spatial-temporal Fourier transform (based on an infinite medium) yields

$$\delta\Psi_e(k, \omega) = \delta\Psi_0(k, \omega) + \delta\Theta(k, \omega) \sum_{m=1}^{M} \rho_m \int_0^\infty \frac{\lambda_m^2 v_1^2 + j\omega\lambda_m v_1}{(\lambda_m v_1 + j\omega)^2 + k^2 v_1^2} f_m(v_1) dv_1$$

$$(L.2.3)$$

We can convert (L.2.3) to a plausible differential equation and apply boundary conditions afterwards, a procedure with some precedent in physical theories. For a model cortex with a single fiber system containing axons with equal propagation velocity v, the velocity distribution function is $f_m(v_1) = \delta(v_1 - v)$ and (L.2.3) reduces to

$$\delta\Psi_e(k, \omega) = \delta\Psi_0(k, \omega) + \rho \left[\frac{\lambda^2 v^2 + j\omega\lambda v}{(\lambda v + j\omega)^2 + k^2 v^2} \right] \delta\Theta(k, \omega) \qquad (L.2.4)$$

Here we have dropped the fiber system subscripts on ρ and λ since the following analyses are limited to a single fiber system. The differential equation equivalent to (L.2.4) is

$$\frac{\partial^2 \Psi}{\partial t^2} + 2v\lambda \frac{\partial \Psi}{\partial t} + v^2\lambda^2 \Psi - v^2 \frac{\partial^2 \Psi}{\partial x^2} = \rho \left(v^2\lambda^2 + v\lambda \frac{\partial}{\partial t} \right) \delta\Theta + Z(x, t) \quad (11.12)$$

Here the notation has been simplified with the definition $\delta\Psi_e(\mathbf{r}, t) \equiv \Psi(\mathbf{r}, t)$, and the subcortical driving terms involving $\delta\Psi_0(x, t)$ are lumped into the variable $Z(x, t)$. By expanding an assumed sigmoid relationship between action potential density and synaptic action, one may obtain the relation (Jirsa and Haken 1997)

$$\rho\delta\Theta(x, t) = 2\beta\Psi(x, t) - \alpha\Psi(x, t)^3 \qquad (11.13)$$

Substitute (11.13) into (11.12) to find a relatively simple nonlinear equation for the modulation of synaptic action density:

$$\frac{\partial^2 \Psi}{\partial t^2} - 2v\lambda\left(\beta - 1 - \frac{3\alpha}{2}\Psi^2\right)\frac{\partial \Psi}{\partial t} + v^2\lambda^2(1 - 2\beta + \alpha\Psi^2)\Psi = v^2\frac{\partial^2 \Psi}{\partial x^2} + Z(x, t)$$

$$(11.14)$$

3 Dispersion Relation Obtained with Linear Theory

We can shed a little light on the origin of the parameter β in (11.13) and the expected behavior of (11.14) as follows. The relation between inhibitory synaptic action field $\Psi_i(x, t)$ and action potential density provides an additional equation relating inhibitory action to action potential density; however, this relation is much simpler than (L.2.1) since inhibitory synapses occur only on (local) intracortical axons so zero inhibitory delays are assumed. That is, for the scalp waves of moderate to long wavelength $k \ll \lambda_i$, the equivalent of (L.2.4) is simply (Nunez 1995)

$$\delta\Psi_i(k, \omega) \approx \rho_i\delta\Theta(k, \omega) \tag{L.3.1}$$

The third equation relating the three field variables is the basic linear approximation (Nunez 1972, 1974, 1995)

$$\delta\Theta = \frac{\partial \Theta}{\partial \Psi_e}\delta\Psi_e + \frac{\partial \Theta}{\partial \Psi_i}\delta\Psi_i \equiv Q_e\delta\Psi_e - Q_i\delta\Psi_i \tag{L.3.2}$$

The Qs in (L.3.2) are defined as the partial derivatives indicating the incremental changes in action potential output from a neural mass due to excitatory or inhibitory input. The incremental increase in action potentials $\delta\Theta$ produced in a cortical tissue mass is assumed proportional to the weighted difference between incremental increases in excitatory synaptic input and inhibitory synaptic input. Essentially, we expand about a fixed background "state" of the brain where the above partial derivatives are assumed to be constant over the short timescales of interest. An infinite cortex is assumed to allow for easy Fourier transform and the above three equations combined so that the basic input–output relation for cortex may be expressed in terms of Fourier transform variables as

$$\delta\Psi_e(k, \omega) = \frac{\delta\Psi_0(k, \omega)}{D_G(k, \omega)} \tag{L.3.3}$$

Here the global cortical dispersion function is defined as the inverse global cortical dynamic transfer function

$$D_G(k, \omega) = T_G^{-1}(k, \omega) \tag{L.3.4}$$

Consider the idealized case where all but one ($m = M$) corticocortical axon systems have essentially infinite propagation speeds (zero global delays). The dispersion relation then takes on the form

$$1 - B(k) \int_0^\infty \frac{\lambda_M^2 v_1^2 + j\omega\lambda_M v_1}{(\lambda_M v_1 + j\omega)^2 + k^2 v_1^2} f_M(v_1)dv_1 = 0 \qquad (L.3.5)$$

where the excitatory control function is defined by

$$B(k) \equiv \frac{\dfrac{\rho_M Q_e}{\rho_i Q_i}}{\left[1 - \dfrac{Q_e}{Q_i}\sum_{m \neq M}\dfrac{\rho_m}{\rho_i}\left(1 + \dfrac{k^2}{\lambda_m^2}\right)^{-1}\right]} \qquad (L.3.6)$$

Here the sum in the denominator of (L.3.6) is over all excitatory systems with negligible global delays. With this idealization, we have separated the corticocortical and intracortical fiber systems into two categories—a single long fiber system M with substantial global delays and multiple systems ($m \neq M$) that provide the background excitability of neocortex as measured by $B(k)$ in (L.3.6). If we restrict the analysis to moderate to long wavelengths such that

$$\left(\frac{k}{\lambda_m}\right)^2 \ll 1 \quad \text{for all } m \neq M \qquad (L.3.8)$$

the control function becomes the excitability parameter $B(k) \to 2\beta$. To a first approximation, we assume only a single propagation speed for the Mth fiber system, that is

$$f_M(v_1) = \delta(v_1 - v) \qquad (L.3.9)$$

The complex frequency is given in terms of real and imaginary parts by

$$\omega(k) = \omega_R(k) - j\gamma(k) \qquad (L.3.10)$$

This yields the dispersion relation in terms of real and imaginary frequencies

$$\omega_R = v_M k \sqrt{1 - \left(\frac{\beta\lambda_M}{k}\right)^2} \qquad (L.3.11)$$

$$\gamma = v_M\lambda_M(\beta - 1)$$

For dynamics in a closed cortical loop of length L, periodic boundary conditions require

$$k = \frac{2n\pi}{L} \quad n = 1, 2, 3, \ldots \qquad (L.3.12)$$

In this case the real mode frequencies in (L.3.11) are restricted to

$$f_n = \frac{v_M}{L} \sqrt{n^2 - \left(\frac{\beta \lambda_M L}{2\pi}\right)^2} \quad n = 1, 2, 3, \ldots \quad \text{(L.3.13)}$$

Equation (L.3.13) is identical to (11.4) if we drop the M subscripts to simplify notation. Equation (L.3.11) indicates that all modes are unstable for $\beta > 1$ in this crude linear theory. The equivalent differential equation is

$$\frac{\partial^2 \Psi}{\partial t^2} + 2v\lambda(1 - \beta)\frac{\partial \Psi}{\partial t} + (1 - 2\beta)v^2\lambda^2\Psi = v^2\frac{\partial^2 \Psi}{\partial x^2} + Z(x, t) \quad \text{(L.3.14)}$$

which is identical to (11.14) when the nonlinear parameter $\alpha \to 0$. Because of the different physiological assumptions leading to (11.13) and (L.3.2), the excitability parameter β has a somewhat different interpretation in the nonlinear version (11.14) than in the linear version (L.3.14). The nonlinear version appears more physiologically realistic, whereas the linear version has the advantage of allowing an analytic solution.

4 More Elaborate Global Theory

Various assumptions characterize the basic global theory. These may be evaluated in the context of more detailed focus on specific issues, including:

(i) Linear solution in a spherical shell (Katznelson 1981, Nunez 1995).
(ii) Interface with neocortical statistical mechanics (Ingber 1995).
(iii) Inclusion of local feedback processes (Nunez 1989, 1995, 2000a, b; Jirsa and Haken 1997; Jirsa et al. 1999; Haken 1999).
(iv) Effects of multiple fibers systems and alternative corticocortical distribution functions on the linear version of the theory (Nunez 1995; Haken 1999).
(v) Distributed corticocortical velocities (Nunez 1974, 1995).
(vi) More realistic brain geometry (Jirsa et al. 2002).
(vii) Heterogeneous fiber systems (Jirsa and Kelso 2000; Jirsa 2004).

References

Haken H, 1999, What can synergetics contribute to the understanding of brain functioning? In: C Uhl (Ed.), *Analysis of Neurophysiological Brain Functioning*, Berlin: Springer-Verlag, pp. 7–40.
Ingber L, 1995, Statistical mechanics of multiple scales of neocortical interactions. In: PL Nunez (Au.), *Neocortical Dynamics and Human EEG Rhythms*. New York: Oxford University Press, pp. 628–681.

Jirsa VK, 2004, Information processing in brain and behavior displayed in large-scale topographies such as EEG and MEG. *International Journal of Bifurcation and Chaos* 14: 679–692.

Jirsa VK and Haken H, 1997, A derivation of a macroscopic field theory of the brain from the quasi-microscopic neural dynamics. *Physica D* 99: 503–526.

Jirsa VK, Jantzen KJ, Fuchs A, and Kelso JAS, 2002, Spatiotemporal forward solution of the EEG and MEG using network modeling. *IEEE Transactions on Medical Imaging* 21: 493–504.

Jirsa VK and Kelso JAS, 2000, Spatiotemporal pattern formation in continuous systems with heterogeneous connection topologies. *Physical Review E* 62: 8462–8465.

Jirsa VK, Kelso JAS, and Fuchs A, 1999, Traversing scales of brain and behavioral organization: III. Theoretical modeling. In: C Uhl (Ed.), *Analysis of Neurophysiological Brain Functioning*, Berlin: Springer-Verlag, pp. 107–125.

Katznelson RD, 1981, Normal modes of the brain: neuroanatomical basis and a physiological theoretical model. In PL Nunez (Au.), *Electric Fields of the Brain: The Neurophysics of EEG*, 1st Edition, New York: Oxford University Press, pp. 401–442.

Nunez PL, 1972, The brain wave equation: a model for the EEG, paper presented to the American EEG Society meeting, Houston, TX.

Nunez PL, 1974, The brain wave equation: a model for the EEG, *Mathematical Biosciences* 21: 279–297.

Nunez PL, 1981, *Electric Fields of the Brain: The Neurophysics of EEG*, 1st Edition, New York: Oxford University Press.

Nunez PL, 1989, Generation of human EEG by a combination of long and short range neocortical interactions. *Brain Topography* 1: 199–215.

Nunez PL, 1995, *Neocortical Dynamics and Human EEG Rhythms*, New York: Oxford University Press.

Nunez PL, 2000a, Toward a large-scale quantitative description of neocortical dynamic function and EEG (Target article). *Behavioral and Brain Sciences* 23: 371–398.

Nunez PL, 2000b, Neocortical dynamic theory should be as simple as possible, but not simpler (Response to 18 commentaries on target article). *Behavioral and Brain Sciences* 23: 415–437.

Index